Thomson Delmar Learning's
Pharmacy Practice for Technicians

Third Edition

SR. JANE DURGIN, CIJ, RPh, EdD
ZACHARY I. HANAN, RPh, MS, FASHP

THOMSON

DELMAR LEARNING   Australia Canada Mexico Singapore Spain United Kingdom United States

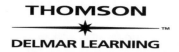

THOMSON
DELMAR LEARNING

Thomson Delmar Learning's Pharmacy Practice for Technicians, Third Edition
by Sr. Jane Durgin and Zachary Hanan

Vice President, Health Care Business Unit:
William Brottmiller

Editorial Director:
Cathy L. Esperti

Acquisitions Editor:
Maureen Rosener

Developmental Editor:
Darcy M. Scelsi

Marketing Director:
Jennifer McAvey

Marketing Channel Manager:
Tamara Caruso

Marketing Coordinator:
Chris Manion

Editorial Assistant:
Elizabeth Howe

Project Editor:
David Buddle

Production Coordinator:
Bridget Lulay

Art/Design Specialist:
Connie Lundberg-Watkins

Library of Congress Cataloging-in-Publication Data
Thomson Delmar Learning's pharmacy practice for technicians / [edited by] Sr. Jane M. Durgin, Zachary I. Hanan.—3rd ed. p. ; cm.
Rev. ed. of: Pharmacy practice for technicians / [edited by] Sr. Jane M. Durgin, Zachary I. Hanan, Janet Mastanduono.
Includes bibliographical references and index.
ISBN-10: 1-4018-4857-5
ISBN-13: 978-1-4018-4857-6
1. Pharmacy technicians—Handbooks, manuals, etc. 2. Pharmacy—Handbooks, manuals, etc.
[DNLM: 1. Pharmacy. 2. Pharmaceutical Preparations. 3. Pharmacists' Aides. QV 735 D359 2005] I. Title: Pharmacy practice for technicians. II. Durgin, Jane M. III. Hanan, Zachary I. IV. Pharmacy practice for technicians.
RS122.95.P43 2005
615'.1—dc22   2004048036

Notice to the Reader

Contents

Preface   xvi
Reviewers   xvii
Acknowledgments   xviii
Contributors   xix
Introduction   xxiii

PART I   OVERVIEW OF HEALTH CARE

Chapter 1   Historical Developments in Pharmacy and Health Care   **3**

Greek Influence   4
  Hippocrates, circa 400 B.C.   4
  Hippocratic Corpus   4
  Theophrastus   5
  Pedanios Dioscorides (A.D. 100)   5
Roman Influence   6
  Claudius Galen (A.D. 130–200)   6
Jewish Influence   6
  Biblical Records (1200 B.C.)   6
  Ancient Hebrews (1200 B.C.)   6
  Moses ben Maimon (Maimonides) (1135–1204)   7
Christian Influence   7
  Cosmas and Damian (d. A.D. 303)   7
  Monastic Manuscripts (A.D. 500–1200)   7
  Christian Renaissance Period   8
Eastern Influence   8
  Clay Tablets of Mesopotamia (3000–2500 B.C.)   8
  Pen T'sao (3000 B.C.)   8
  China (500 B.C.)   8
  Mithradates VI (d. 63 B.C.)   8
  Arabia and Persia (A.D. 700–800)   9
  India (1000 B.C.)   9
  Egyptian Influence   9
Military Influence   9
Western Influences   10
  Western Europe   10
International Influence   13
  Canadian Contribution   13
  World Health Organization   13

iii

Developments in the United States Related to Health Care
  and Drug Therapy   13
Nonmilitary Hospitals   13
Psychiatric Care   13
Surgical Care   14
Contemporary Medical Practices   14
Polio Vaccine   14
Steptomycin   14
Surgical Procedures   15
Governmental Interventions in Medical Practice   15
Review of Therapeutic Advances Discovered in the Nineteenth
  and Twentieth Centuries   15
Drug Standards Set by Pharmacopoeias   15
Biologicals   16
Hormones   16
Anti-Infectives   16
Synthetics   16
Immunomodulators   16
Drug Development   16
Hospital Development   16

Chapter 2   **Organizational Structure and Function
                  of the Hospital**   **21**

Hospital Functions   21
Hospital Organization   23

Chapter 3   **Home Health Care**   **29**

Home Health Care Services   31
Home Health Services   31
Personal Care and Support Services   32
Home Equipment Management Services   32
Home Pharmacy Services   33
Role of Pharmacy in Home Health Care   33
Home Infusion Therapy   33
Pharmacy Services   33
Home Nursing Services   34
Equipment Management Services   34
Types of Home Infusion Providers   35
Retail or Community Pharmacies   36
Institutional or Long-Term Pharmacies   36
Hospital Pharmacies   36
Home Health Agencies   37
HME-Based Providers   37
Infusion Therapy Specialty Providers   37
Ambulatory Infusion Centers   37
Types of Care and Therapies Provided   38
Antibiotic Therapy   38
Antiviral Therapy   39
Total Parenteral Nutrition   39
Enteral Nutrition   40
Pain Management   41

Cancer Chemotherapy 42
Hydration 42
Miscellaneous Drugs 42
Ancillary Drugs 43
Preparing and Dispensing Medications for Home Care 43
Infusion Devices 44
Factors in the Selection of an Infusion Device or Pump 49
Equipment Management 49
Complications of Home Infusion Therapy 50
Phlebitis 50
Infiltration 50
Sepsis 50
Embolism 51
Allergic Reactions 51
Free Flow 51
Role of Technicians in Home Infusion Therapy 51
Driver or Delivery Representative 52
Warehouse Supervisor/Technician 52
Patient Service Representative 52
Purchasing Manager 52
Billing Clerk/Case Manager 52

Chapter 4   Long-Term Care   57
Types of Long-Term Care Facilities 57
Regulation of Long-Term Care Facilities 58
Income Sources 58
Medicare and Medicaid 58
Private Pay 58
Third-Party Payers 58
Population 59
Pharmaceutical Personnel in Long-Term Care 60
Consultant Pharmacist 60
Emerging Challenges for the Pharmaceutical Professional 60
The Future of Pharmacy in Long-Term Care 61

Chapter 5   Community Pharmacy Practice   65
Prescription Processing 66
Types of Community Pharmacies 67
Surgical Supply 68
Long-Term Care 68
Home Infusion 68
Specialty Compounding Services 68
Clinical Services 69

PART II   THE PROFESSION OF PHARMACY

Chapter 6   Regulatory Standards in Pharmacy Practice   75
Federal and State Statutes 76
Rules and Regulations 76
Quasi-Legal Standards 76

Regulatory Agencies and Quasi-Legal Standards   76
Federal Versus State Drug-Control Laws   76
State Regulatory Agencies   77
State Board of Pharmacy   77
Long-Term Care Facilities   77
Federal Regulatory Agencies   78
   Tax-Free Alcohol   78
   Taxable Alcohol   78
Federal Food, Drug, and Cosmetic Act   79
   Durham-Humphrey Amendments   79
   An FDA Regulation   80
Adverse Drug Reactions   80
Drug Recalls   80
   Classes of Recalls   80
   Repackaging of Drugs   81
Investigational Drugs   82
   Preclinical Studies   82
   Clinical Studies   82
Use of Marketed Products for Unapproved Uses   83
Institutional Review Board   84
Orphan Drugs   84
The Controlled Substances Act   84
   Schedules of Controlled Drugs   84
   Symbols   85
   Records and Reports   85
   Order Forms   86
   Registration   86
   Lost or Stolen Order Forms   87
   Inventory Requirements   87
   Destruction of Controlled Substances   87
Federal Hazardous Substances Act   87
   Poison Prevention Packaging Act   87
Occupational and Safety Act   88
   Hazardous Drugs and Chemicals   88
   Air Contaminants   89
   Flammable and Combustible Liquids   89
   General Concerns about Hazardous Materials   89
Omnibus Budget Reconciliation Act   90
Health Insurance Portability and Accountability Act of 1996   91
   Overview of Administrative Simplification   92
   Results of Implementation of the HIPAA Regulations   92
   Definitions   92
   Some Preexisting Pharmacy Privacy Requirements   93
Quasi-Legal Standards   93
   Practice Standards, Guidelines, and Statements   93
Joint Commission on Accreditation of Healthcare Organizations   94
   JCAHO Accreditation   94
   JCAHO Standards   95
   The JCAHO Survey Process   96
   JCAHO Survey Results   99
Patient's Bill of Rights   100
   Patients' Rights   100

Chapter 7   **Drug Use Control: The Foundation**
of Pharmaceutical Care   **105**
    The Drug Use Process   106
        Drug Distribution   106
        The Drugs   106
        Distribution of Drugs from Pharmaceutical Manufacturers   108
        Distribution of Drugs from Drug Wholesalers   108
    Self-Care and the Role of Over-the-Counter Medication   109
        Self-Care   109
        Over-the-Counter (OTC) Medication   109
    Prescribing Drugs   110
        The Prescription   110
        Writing the Prescription   112
        Drug Samples   112
    Dispensing   113
        Types of Retail Pharmacies   113
        The Dispensing Process   114
    Drug Distribution in Organized Health Care Settings   115
        Floor Stock   115
        Unit-Dose   115
        IV Admixtures   116
    Medication Use in the United States   117
    Medication Administration   117
        Compliance with Taking the Medication as Prescribed   118
    Pharmaceutical Care   119
        The Elements of Pharmaceutical Care   120
    Quality Drug Therapy   121
    Medication Safety and Drug Misadventures   122
        Side Effects   122
        Adverse Drug Reactions   122
        Allergic Drug Reactions   122
        Drug-Drug Interactions   122
        Medication Errors   122
    Control of the Drug Use Process   123
    Current Issues in the Drug Use Process   123
        The Rising Number of Prescriptions and Limited Numbers
          of Pharmacists   123
        Pharmacy Automation   123

Chapter 8   **Ethical Considerations for the Pharmacy Technician**   **127**
    The Changing Health Care Environment   127
    Pharmaceutical Care   128
        The Role of the Pharmacy Technician   128
    Codes of Professional Behavior   129
        The Code of Ethics for Pharmacy Technicians   130
        The Pharmacist's Code of Ethics   130
        Ethical Decision-Making   130
        Ethical Principles   132
        The Decision-Making Process   132
        Practical Applications   133
        Risk/Benefit Response   134

Chapter 9   **Organizations in Pharmacy**   **139**
Historical Development   139
National Associations of Pharmacists and Pharmacy Technicians   141
   Other Associations   143
Association Publications   145

PART III   **PROFESSIONAL ASPECTS OF PHARMACY TECHNOLOGY**

Chapter 10   **The Prescription, Terminology, and Medical Abbreviations**   **147**
Common Word Elements   149
Common Medical Terms   150
Common Medical/Pharmacy Abbreviations and Terminology   154
Commonly Used Apothecary Symbols   157
Brand/Trade Names and Generic Names   157
Common Look-Alike and Sound-Alike Drug Names   161
The Prescription   161

Chapter 11   **Pharmaceutical Dosage Forms**   **165**
Classification   166
   Liquid Dosage Forms   166
   Solid Dosage Forms   170
   Miscellaneous Dosage Forms   173
Gastrointestinal System   176
Ocular System   176
Transdermal System   177

Chapter 12   **Pharmaceutical Calculations**   **181**
Interpreting the Drug Order   181
Ratio and Proportion   185
   Ratio   185
   Proportion   185
Practice Problems   187
Conversion Between Systems of Measurements   187
   Review of the Metric System   187
Practice Problems   189
   Apothecary System of Weights   190
   Apothecary System of Volume (Liquid) Measure   190
   Apothecary System Notation   190
   Converting from the Apothecary System to the Metric System 190
Practice Problems   192
Calculation of Fractional Doses   192
Practice Problems   194
Calculation of Dosages Based on Weight   194
Practice Problems   196
Pediatric Dosage Calculations   196
Practice Problems   197
Calculations Involving Intravenous Administration   197
   Calculating the Rate of IV Administration   198

Practice Problems   199
   Calculations Involving Piggyback IV Infusion   200
Practice Problems   201
Calculations Related to Solutions   202
   Percentage Solutions   202
Prevention of Medication Errors   203
Suggested Activities   203
Answers to Practice Problems   204

Chapter 13   Extemporaneous Compounding   207
Equipment   208
   Traditional Equipment   208
Weighing Techniques   210
   Modern Equipment   212
Compounding Principles   214
   Liquids   214
   Solids   214
   Suspensions   214
   Ointments and Creams   215
   Transdermal Gels   215
   Troches, Lollipops, and Gummy Bears   216
   Flavoring   216
   Suppositories   217
   Capsules   217
   Lotions   218
   Enteral Preparations   218
   Sterile Compounding, On-Site Sterility, and Pyrogen Testing   219
   Sterilization   219
   Labeling of Finished Products and Record-Keeping   220
   Cleaning Equipment   221

Chapter 14   Parenteral Compounding   225
Background   225
Routes of Administration   226
Characteristics of Parenteral Products   226
   Intravenous Products   227
   Types of IV Solutions   228
Preparation of Parenteral Products   230
   Laminar Airflow Hoods   230
   Ampules and Vials   234
   Working With Needles and Syringes   234
Safety Considerations   235
   Opening Glass Ampules   235
   Local and Systemic Effects of Medication   235
   Needle Sticks   236
Role of the Technician   237

Chapter 15   Administration of Medications   241
Medication Orders   242
   Information Needed on Drug Orders   242
The Medication Administrator or Medication Technician   243

Administration of the Drug	244
Patient Rights	244
Oral Drug Administration	246
Topical Drug Administration	247
Eyedrop and Eye Ointment Application	247
Administration of Ear and Nose Preparation	248
Application of Transdermal Drugs	248
Insertion of Suppositories	248
Injectable Drug Administration	249
Discontinuence of Drug Administration	249
Unit-Dose Administration	250
Crushing Medications	250
Internal and External Medications	250
Medication Teaching	251
Readiness to Learn	251
Age and Education Level	251
Learning Method	252
Teaching Plan	252
Teaching Process	252
Reinforcement	253
Evaluation of Learning	253
Professional Responsibility for Drug Administration	253
Legal Responsibilities in Drug Administration	254
Trends in Drug Administration	255
Chapter 16 **Drug Information Centers**	**259**
Drug Information Specialists	260
Drug Information Centers	260
Definition of Drug Information	261
The Systematic Approach to Answering a Drug Information Question	261
Requestor Demographics	261
Background Information	261
Determination and Categorization of the Ultimate Question	264
Search Strategy and Information Collection	264
Evaluation, Analysis, and Synthesis of Information	265
Formulate and Provide Response	265
Follow-up and Documentation	265
Drug Information Resources	265
Tertiary Resources	266
Secondary Resources	266
Primary Resources	266
The Internet	270
Necessary Skills for the Pharmacy Technician	270
Other Pharmacy Technician Responsibilities	272
Chapter 17 **Drug Distribution Systems**	**275**
Drug Distribution Systems	276
Floor Stock System	276
Individual Prescription System	276
Combined Floor Stock and Patient Prescription System	277
Unit-Dose Drug Distribution System	277

Centralized Dispensing 278
Decentralized Dispensing 278
Physician's Original Order 278
Basic Requirement of a Compete Medication Order 279
Transmittal of Orders to Pharmacy 279
Electromechanical Systems 279
Computerization 280
Bar Code Applications 281
Physician's Order Entry Process 281
Receiving the Medication Order 282
The Pharmacist's Role 282
The Technician's Role 283
Medication Delivery Systems 285
Transportation Courier 285
Equipment 285
Unit-Dose Picking Area 286
Medication Dispensing Units 287
Drug Distribution of the Future 287
Robotics 288
Pyxis, Omnicell, and HBOC/McKesson 288
ATC Profile 288
ROBOT-Rx 289
The Future 289
A Caveat 289

Chapter 18 Infection Control and Prevention in the Pharmacy 293
Contamination of Pharmaceuticals 294
Infection Control Fundamentals 296
The Goals of Infection Control and Prevention Programs 296
The Principles of Aseptic Techniques 296
Preventing Infections in Health Care Workers 296
Health Care Worker Infection Control Education 297
Infections 298
Sources of Infectious Agents 298
Host 299
Transmission 299
Control of Infections 300
Universal-Standard Precautions 300
Personal Protective Equipment (PPE) 300
Prevention of Needle-Stick and other Sharps Injuries 301
Handwashing 301
Cleaning and Decontamination of Surfaces and Spills 302
Engineering and Work Place Controls 302
Hepatitis B Vaccination 303
Hospital Isolation Precautions 303
Transmission-Based Precautions 304
Occupational Exposures 305
Bloodborne Pathogen Exposures 305
What to Do If Exposed 305
Post-Bloodborne Pathogen Exposure Evaluation and Follow-up 306
Tuberculosis 306
Health Care Worker Work Restrictions 307

PART IV — CLINICAL ASPECTS OF PHARMACY TECHNOLOGY

Chapter 19   Introduction to Biopharmaceutics   315
Routes of Administration   315
Factors Affecting Drug Absorption   316
  Drug Release from the Dosage Form   316
  Dissolution   316
  Diffusion   317
  Anatomic and Physiologic Considerations   317
First-Pass Metabolism in the Liver   318
Bioavailability   319
Drug Distribution, Metabolism, and Elimination   319
Methods to Assess Bioavailability   320
Bioavailability Studies   321

Chapter 20   The Actions and Uses of Drugs   325
Factors That Affect Drug Response   325
  Route of Administration   325
  Patient Variability   328
Classification of Drugs   330
  Bone and Joint Disorders   331
  Cardiovascular Disorders   332
  Endocrine Disorders   335
  Gastrointestinal Disorders   338
  Gynecologic and Obstetric Disorders   338
  Infectious Diseases   340
  Neurologic Disorders   340
  Respiratory Disorders   343

Chapter 21   Nonprescription Medications   349
Dosage Forms   350
Pain   350
Cold and Allergy   352
Gastrointestinal Problems   353
  Constipation   353
  Diarrhea   355
  Acid/Peptic Disorders   356

Chapter 22   Natural Products   361
How Are Drugs and Herbals Regulated in the USA?   362
  Drug Regulation in the United States   362
  Regulation of Herbals, Botanicals, and Dietary Supplements   364
The Chemical Structure of Herbals: Secondary Plant Metabolites   365
Preparation and Routes of Administration of Herbals   368
The Safety of Herbals   368
Hypersensitivity (Allergic) Reactions   369
Content and Concentration of the Herbal Product   369
Potential Contamination of the Herbal Product   369
Potential Herbal-Drug Interactions   370

Where to Get More Information on Herbals 370
Some Traditional Uses of Herbals 372

PART V   ADMINISTRATIVE ASPECTS OF PHARMACY TECHNOLOGY

Chapter 23   The Policy and Procedure Manual   379
Need for Policies and Procedures 379
Composing a Policy and Procedure Manual 382
  Format 382
The Approval Process 385
Contents of a Policy and Procedure Manual 386
  Distribution 388
  Problems 389

Chapter 24   Materials Management of Pharmaceuticals   393
Procurement 395
  Drug Selection 395
  Source Selection 395
  Cost Analysis 396
  Group Purchasing and Prime-Vendor Relationships 396
  Purchasing Procedures 396
  Impact of Drug Shortages 397
  Record-Keeping 398
  Receiving Control 399
Drug Storage and Inventory Control 399
  Storage 399
  Security Requirements 400
Repackaging and Labeling Considerations 402
  Benefits Associated with Bar Coding 404
Distribution Systems 405
Recapture and Disposal 406
  Returned Medications 406
  Expiration Dates 406
  Environmental Considerations 406

Chapter 25   The Pharmacy Formulary System   411
The Formulary System 412

Chapter 26   Computer Applications in Drug-Use Control   419
Computer Terminology 420
Components of Computer Applications 420
  Computer Hardware 420
  Application Software 424
  System Network 424
  Information Server 425
System Management 425

Hospital Information System Application Relationships   427
  Patient Flow Cycle   427
  Ancillary Systems   427
  Business Systems   428
The Hospital Pharmacy Application   429
  Inventory Management   429
  Purchasing/Receiving   429
  Clinical Support   430
The Future of Pharmacy Information Systems   431

Chapter 27   Preventing and Managing Medication Errors:
              The Technician's Role   435
Background   436
Ordering Medications   436
  Illegible Handwriting   436
  Look-Alike Drug Names   437
  Sound-Alike Drug Names   439
  Ambiguous Orders   439
  Abbreviations to Avoid   441
Preparing and Dispensing Medications   444
  Steps in Prescription-Filling   444
  Selecting Medications   445
  Selecting Auxiliary Labels   448
Sterile Admixture Preparation   449
Effective Medication Error Prevention and Monitoring Systems 450

Chapter 28   Reimbursement for Pharmacy Services   453
Ambulatory Care (Community Pharmacy) Reimbursement   453
Reimbursement for Ambulatory Care Parenteral Therapy   454
Reimbursement for Long-Term Care   455
Reimbursement for Acute Care   456
Reimbursement for Cognitive Services   457
The Role of Pharmacy Technicians in Increased Reimbursement 458

Chapter 29   Accreditation of Technician Training Programs 461
The Need for a Differentiated Workforce   461
ASHP Initiatives   462
  Accreditation Program   463

Chapter 30   Pharmacy Technician Certification Board   465
Background   466
Structure   466
Current Examination Practices   466
Technology   467
Get Involved with PTCB   467
  Item Writers   467
  Stakeholder Policy Council   467
Communication Vehicles   468
Regulation of Pharmacy Technicians   468
Future for Pharmacy Technicians   468

APPENDIXES

Appendix A   **Long-Term Care**   **471**
A-1   Examples of Guidelines for Automatic Stop-Order Policy in a Skilled Nursing Facility (Unless Otherwise Specified by Physician)   471
A-2   Medication Order Entry Flow Chart   472

Appendix B   **The Hospital Formulary System**   **473**
B-1   The Pharmacy and Therapeutics Committee   473
B-2   Definitions and Categories of Drugs to Be Stocked in the Pharmacy   474
B-3   Additions to the Formulary   475
B-4   Deletions from the Formulary   475

Appendix C   **Body Surface Area Nomogram**   **476**

Appendix D   **Common Sound-Alike Drug Names**   **477**

Glossary   481
Index   497

Preface

Pharmacy technicians are becoming ever more important in the pharmacy profession. In this age of clinical and scientific advancements and pharmacy technology, the role of the pharmacy technician is becoming even more critical. Helping pharmacists to fulfill their potential as providers of pharmaceutical care as pharmacy practice is expanding at an unprecedented rate due to the pharmacist workforce shortage, the increased volume of prescriptions, the demand for pharmaceutical care services, and the need to provide safe medication use. The increased use of technicians is one obvious way of reducing workload pressures, reducing medication errors, and freeing pharmacists to spend more time with patients for the provision of a safe medication system. Pharmacy technicians are significant members of the health care team.

Pharmacy technicians may receive their training and be prepared for practice in a number of different ways, such as informal on-the-job training, formal training offered by some health care institutions, chain drugstores, the military, and academic training programs offering associate degrees and certificates. A national pharmacy certification exam is also offered and is a meaningful component of a technician's professional development. Certification recognizes the knowledge and competency demonstrated by the technician who successfully passes this national examination. This recognition furthers the technician's pharmacy career options.

To meet the needs of technicians and their respective training programs, it is the goal and focus of the editors to provide technicians with an understanding of the background and history of the profession of pharmacy and to bring current professional, clinical, and administrative information and practice trends to the student to increase his or her understanding, knowledge, and competencies of the pharmacy profession.

Each chapter in the third edition has been revised to reflect current practice, while additional chapters have been added in drug information, community pharmacy practice, OTCs, natural products, reimbursement for pharmacy services, and pharmacy technician certification, all in an effort to reinforce and emphasize the important technological component of pharmacy practice. Nationally recognized authors have contributed to this publication in their respective areas of expertise.

The vision and goal of the editors of this textbook is to provide the background necessary for the technician to achieve his or her respective goals by fostering the knowledge, values, attitudes and skills to assist the technician to meet his or her desired objectives in the practice of pharmacy.

Reviewers

Renee Ahrens, PharmD, MBA
Shenandoah University
Winchester, Virginia

Glenn D. Appelt, PhD, RPh
Columbia Southern University
Orange Beach, Alabama

Cheri Boggs, BA, CPhT
El Paso Community College
La Mesa, New Mexico

Carol Miller, EdD, RRT
Miami-Dade Community College
Miami, Florida

Jim Mizner, RPh, MBA
Applied Career Training
Rosslyn, Virginia

Reviewers of Second Edition
Patricia K. Anthony, BSPhS, BS Biology, MS, PhD
Pima Medical Institute
Tucson, Arizona

Carolyn Bunker, RPh
Salt Lake Community College
Salt Lake City, Utah

Jane Doucette, RPh
Salt Lake Community College
Salt Lake City, Utah

Emery C. Fellows, Jr., CPhT
Pima Medical Institute
Denver, Colorado

Tova R. Wiegand-Green
Ivy Tech State College
Fort Wayne, Indiana

Percy M. Johnson
Bidwell Training
Pittsburgh, Pennsylvania

Elizabeth Johnson
Houston Community College System
Southeast College
Houston, Texas

Kathy Moscou, BS Pharmacy
North Seattle Community College
Seattle, Washington

Larry Nesmith, BS Ed
Academy of Health Sciences, AMEDD Center &
    School
Pharmacy Branch, Fort Sam Houston, U.S. Army
San Antonio, Texas

Glen E. Rolfson, RPh
Salt Lake Community College
Salt Lake City, Utah

Peter E. Vonderau, RPh
Cuyahoga Community College
Highland Falls Village, Ohio

Sharon Burton-Young, RN
POLYtech Adult Education
Woodside, Delaware

Acknowledgments

Sincere thanks to our professional colleagues, personal friends, peers, and associates whose time, effort, clinical expertise, and contributions to the book made this publication possible. Each contributor has enhanced this text with his or her knowledge, experience, and dedication in support of the education and training of pharmacy technicians.

We especially thank Darcy Scelsi, our Developmental Editor; Connie Lundberg-Watkins, our Art and Design Coordinator; David Buddle, our Project Editor; and Bridget Lulay, our Production Coordinator for their untiring efforts in the coordination of the numerous details during the production of this textbook. We also thank Laura Horowitz for her management of the coordination of the final draft revisions.

Contributors

Sister Jane Marie Durgin, CIJ, RN, RPh, EdD
Former Professor of Pharmacy
St. John's University
Jamaica, New York
Chapter 1: Historical Developments in Pharmacy
and Health Care

Kevin M. Spiegel, Sr.
Chief Operating Officer
Trumbull Memorial Hospital
Warren, Ohio
Chapter 2: Organizational Structure and Function
of the Hospital

Vito Cassata, RPh, MBA
Vice President, General Services and Facilities
Planning
New York Hospital Queens
Flushing, New York
Chapter 2: Organizational Structure and Function
of the Hospital

Darryl S. Rich, PharmD, MBA, FASHP
Associate Director, Surveyor Development and
Management
Joint Commission on Accreditation of Healthcare
Organizations
Oakbrook Terrace, Illinois
Chapter 3: Home Health Care

Barbara Limburg Mancini, PharmD, BCNSP
President, Home Care Consulting Services
Indian Head Park, Illinois
Chapter 3: Home Health Care

Janet Ungar, MPA
Administrator
Chapin Home for the Aging
Jamaica, New York
Chapter 4: Long-Term Care

Maria Marzella Sulli, PharmD, CGP
Assistant Clinical Professor
Department of Clinical Pharmacy Practice
St. John's University
College of Pharmacy and Allied Health Professions
Jamaica, New York
Chapter 5: Community Pharmacy Practice

Zachary I. Hanan, RPh, MS, FASHP
Former Director of Pharmaceutical Services
Mercy Medical Center
Rockville Centre, New York
President
ZIH Pharmacy Associates, Inc.
Chapter 6: Regulatory Standards in Pharmacy
Practice

William N. Kelly, PharmD
Professor and Chairman, Department of
Pharmacy Practice
School of Pharmacy
Mercer University
Atlanta, Georgia
Chapter 7: Drug Use Control: The Foundation of
Pharmaceutical Care

Martha L. Mackey, JD
Assistant Professor of Pharmacy Administration
St. John's University
College of Pharmacy and Allied Health Professions
Jamaica, New York
Chapter 8: Ethical Considerations for the
Pharmacy Technician

Kenneth W. Miller, PhD
Vice President for Graduate Education, Research,
and Education
American Association of Colleges of Pharmacy
Alexandria, Virginia
Chapter 9: Organizations in Pharmacy

Christine Martin, RPh, MS
Clinical Pharmacist
Department of Pharmacy
Good Samaritan Hospital
West Islip, New York
Chapter 10: The Prescription, Terminology, and
    Medical Abbreviations

P.L. Madan, PhD
Professor of Pharmacy and Administrative
    Sciences
St. John's University
College of Pharmacy and Allied Health
    Professions
Jamaica, New York
Chapter 11: Pharmaceutical Dosage Forms

Barry S. Reiss, BS, MS, PhD, RPh
Professor Emeritus, Albany College of
    Pharmacy
Albany, New York
Chapter 12: Pharmaceutical Calculations

Ronald L. McLean, RPh, MS
Past Interim President and Dean
Albany College of Pharmacy
Albany, New York
Chapter 12: Pharmaceutical Calculations

Joseph A. Duprey, RPh, MS
Education Coordinator
Department of Pharmacy
Lancaster General Hospital
Lancaster, Pennsylvania
Chapter 13: Extemporaneous Compounding

Steve Laddy, RPh, President
Master Compounding Pharmacy
Richmond Hill, New York
Chapter 13: Extemporaneous Compounding

Thomas Mastanduono, RPh
Master Compounding Pharmacy
Richmond Hill, New York
Chapter 13: Extemporaneous Compounding

Michael J. Ficurilli, RPh, MS
Information Systems Coordinator
Department of Pharmacy
Good Samaritan Hospital
West Islip, New York
Chapter 14: Parenteral Compounding

Julie Brunnell, RN, BS
Service Director, Specialty Services
Champlain Valley Physician's Hospital Medical
    Center
Plattsburgh, New York
Chapter 15: Administration of Medications

Laura Gianni Augusto, PharmD
Director, Drug Information Service
North Shore-Long Island Jewish Health
    System
Assistant Clinical Professor
St. John's University
College of Pharmacy and Allied Health
    Professions
Jamaica, New York
Chapter 16: Drug Information Centers

Sheldon Lefkowitz, RPh, MS
Director of Pharmacy Services
St. Mary's Medical Center
901 45th Street
West Palm Beach, Florida
Chapter 17: Drug Distribution Systems

Jeffrey Spicer, MBA
Operations Supervisor
Department of Pharmacy
Martin Memorial Medical Center
300 Hospital Way
Stewart, Florida
Chapter 17: Drug Distribution Systems

Vita J. Padrone, RN, MPA, CIC
Infection Control Practitioner
North Shore, Manhasset
Manhasset, New York
Chapter 18: Infection Control and Prevention in
    the Pharmacy

Robert S. Kidd, MS, PharmD
Associate Professor and Vice Chair
Department of Biopharmaceutical Sciences
Bernard J. Dunn School of Pharmacy
Shenandoah University
Winchester, Virginia
Chapter 19: Introduction to Biopharmaceutics
Chapter 20: The Actions and Uses of Drugs

Robert A. Mangione, RPh, EdD
Dean and Clinical Professor of Pharmacy
St. John's University
College of Pharmacy and Allied Health Professions
Jamaica, New York
Chapter 8: Ethical Considerations for the
   Pharmacy Technician

L. Michael Marcum, PharmD
Department of Biopharmaceutical Sciences
Bernard J. Dunn School of Pharmacy
Shenandoah University
Winchester, Virginia
Chapter 20: The Actions and Uses of Drugs

Nicole M. Maisch, PharmD
Assistant Clinical Professor
Department of Clinical Pharmacy Practice
St. John's University
College of Pharmacy and Allied Health Professions
Jamaica, New York
Chapter 21: Nonprescription Medications

Dudley G. Moon, PhD
Professor
Basic and Pharmaceutical Sciences
Albany College of Pharmacy
Albany, New York
Chapter 22: Natural Products

Martha Hass, PhD
Associate Professor
Basic and Pharmaceutical Sciences
Albany College of Pharmacy
Albany, New York
Chapter 22: Natural Products

Dennis Hoffman, PharmD
Oncology Medical Liaison
Roche Laboratories
Middle Island, New York
Chapter 23: The Policy and Procedure Manual

Steven J. Ciullo, RPh, MS, MPS
Region Director
Health Systems—New England
Pharmaceutical Distribution
Cardinal Health
Peabody, Massachusetts
Chapter 24: Materials Management of
   Pharmaceuticals

Joseph N. Gallina, PharmD
Vice President, Clinical Support Services
Western Maryland Health System
Cumberland, Maryland
Chapter 25: The Pharmacy Formulary System

Edmund Hayes, RPh, MS, PharmD
Senior Clinical Pharmacist–Parenteral
   Nutrition
University Medical Center, Stony Brook
Health Sciences Center, State University of New
   York
Stony Brook, New York
Chapter 26: Computer Applications
   in Drug-Use Control

Matthew Grissinger, RPh
Medication Safety Analyst
Institute for Safe Medication Practices
Huntington Valley, Pennsylvania
Chapter 27: Preventing and Managing Medication
   Errors: The Technician's Role

Susan Proulx, PharmD
Vice President, Operations
Institute for Safe Medication Practices
Huntington Valley, Pennsylvania
Chapter 27: Preventing and Managing Medication
   Errors: The Technician's Role

Kenneth R. Cohen, PhD, RPh, PCD
Chief of Clinical Pharmacology and
   Therapeutics
Brookhaven Memorial Hospital Medical
   Center
Patchogue, New York
Chapter 28: Reimbursement for Pharmacy
   Services

Lisa S. Lifshin, RPh
Manager, Program Services
Coordinator, Technician Training Programs
Accreditation Services Division
American Society of Health-System
   Pharmacists
Bethesda, Maryland
Chapter 29: Accreditation of Technician
   Programs

Donald E. Letendre, PharmD
Dean of Pharmacy
College of Pharmacy
University of Rhode Island
Kingston, Rhode Island
Chapter 29: Accreditation of Technician Programs

Melissa M. Murer, RPh
Executive Director/Chief Executive Officer
Pharmacy Technician Certification Board
Washington, DC
Chapter 30: Pharmacy Technician Certification
    Board

Phara G. Rodigue, MA
Administrative Manager
Pharmacy Technician Certification Board
Washington, DC
Chapter 30: Pharmacy Technician Certification
    Board

Introduction

Five Years of Progress in the Training of Pharmacy Technicians

It's difficult to believe that five years have gone by since the publication of the second edition of *Pharmacy Practice for Pharmacy Technicians*. We are now well into the first decade of the twenty-first century. This is a perfect time to reflect on the positive progression of the role of the pharmacy technician, further warranting the importance of cultivating a highly-trained workforce. The pharmacist shortage, an increased number of prescriptions for our aging population, and a public awareness for the absolute need for a safe process for medication use have played an integral role in placing the pharmacy technician in a brighter light to be an active member of the health care team.

Pharmacy organizations have increased advocacy activities to substantiate the need for technicians to participate in tasks which will allow the pharmacist to have a greater role in the care of patients. This promotes a better environment for the public health of our nation. The second Scope of Pharmacy Practice was conducted early in 2000 by the Pharmacy Technician Certification Board (PTCB) to review specific tasks performed by pharmacy technicians and how they have evolved since the last review in the mid-1990s. Upon completion of the task analysis, the second edition of the Model Curriculum for Pharmacy Technician Training was compiled to serve as an outline of the many areas that a pharmacy technician could receive training to become active participants in assisting the pharmacist in participating in direct patient care activities. The revision included the original collaborators (AAPT, APhA, ASHP, PTEC), and an additional organization—the National Association of Chain Drug Stores (NACDS)—joined the ranks of support of the document.

In 2001, the PTCB expanded its corporate membership to include the National Association of Boards of Pharmacy (NABP). Prior to 2001, PTCB's corporate partners included ASHP, APhA, Illinois Society of Health-System Pharmacists (ICHP), and Michigan Society of Health-System Pharmacists. Over 150,000 pharmacy technicians are now PTCB certified, as compared to 18,000 in 1999!

The "Sesquicentennial Stepping Stone Summit Two, Pharmacy Technicians" convened representatives from the Council of Credentialing in Pharmacy (representatives from the Academy of Managed Care Pharmacy, AACP, the American College of Apothecaries, the American College of Clinical Pharmacy, the American Council of Pharmaceutical Education, the American Society of Consultant Pharmacists, the Commission for Certification in Geriatric Pharmacy, PTCB, and PTEC), NACDS, and the National Community Pharmacy Association (NCPA) in Baltimore, Maryland, in 2002. Much of the time spent during the two-day period was spent discussing the importance of education and training for pharmacy technicians. A summit attended by such a great number of pharmacy organizations convened to discuss the educational needs of pharmacy technicians was not conducted prior to this event since 1988. The "White Paper on Pharmacy Technicians 2002: Needed Changes Can No Longer Wait" was written as a response to the Summit to address the need for the profession of pharmacy to develop a shared vision for pharmacy technicians and other supportive personnel.

There are now over 90 pharmacy technician training programs that have undertaken the peer review process to be accredited by ASHP. Some states are even investigating requiring standardized education for technicians to be recognized by their individual states.

So, as we look back over the past five years, much has evolved for the pharmacy technician. There are new career options that were not available before. Clinical pharmacy technicians, pharmacy database operators, investigational drug customer service agents, point-of-use drug distribution operation representatives, and pharmacy managers in hospitals are just a few of the new areas that pharmacy technicians can make their careers.

What is in the future? It is difficult to predict. In order to make sure pharmacy technicians are able to undertake future challenges and opportunities, it is important for each of them to utilize tools available to make them the best educated to be prepared for these new endeavors. The third edition of this text represents a major contribution to education and training that will provide a foundation for those who wish to excel as pharmacy technicians. Students using this reference will gain valuable information to advance them in their practices and be integral in the advancement of the role of the pharmacy technician into the next decade.

Lisa S. Lifshin, R.Ph
American Society of Health-System Pharmacists
Bethesda, Maryland

PART

I

Overview of Health Care

Chapter 1:   Historical Developments in Pharmacy
             and Health Care
Chapter 2:   Organizational Structure and Function
             of the Hospital
Chapter 3:   Home Health Care
Chapter 4:   Long-Term Care
Chapter 5:   Community Pharmacy Practice

CHAPTER

1

Historical Developments in Pharmacy and Health Care

COMPETENCIES

Upon completion of this chapter, the reader should be able to

1. Cite examples from history of the care of the sick in different cultural settings.

2. Describe the Greek and/or Roman influence on present-day health care.

3. List the contributions of Hippocrates, Maimonides, Basil, Camillus, and the Crusaders.

4. Name the father of medicine, father of botany, father of toxicology, and father of pharmacology.

5. Briefly describe six dosage forms found in the Hippocratic Corpus.

6. Briefly describe the role of the town of Gheel in Belgium in the care of the mentally ill.

7. List a contribution of each of the following to health or treatment care: Dioscorides, Galen, Shen-Nung, Sirach, Theophrastus, Benjamin Franklin, Abraham Lincoln, King George III, Louisa May Alcott, Crawford Long, Benjamin Rush

8. Trace the treatment of tuberculosis from the beginning of the 20th century to the beginning of the 21st century.

9. Describe the cause and effects of deinstitutionalization of persons with mental health problems.

10. State the name of the person who discovered, isolated, or synthesized each of the following: codeine, insulin, smallpox vaccine, penicillin, arsphenamine, streptomycin, digitalis, prontosil, quinine, diphtheria antitoxin

Introduction

This chapter provides the student with the knowledge and an appreciation of the values, the evolution, and the development of the healing arts and health care.

Literature records remarkable developments in health care facilities and methods of treatment over many centuries. Hospitality and care for the sick have been and continue to be cultural concerns wherever communities of persons gather. The facilities designed to carry out these functions have gone through architectural, administrative, and clinical changes. They have been modified by environmental factors and diagnostic treatment needs brought about by wars, **epidemics**, and scientific discoveries.

From the beginning of time, individuals have searched for remedies to heal the various maladies that affect the mind and the body. The history of the search is fascinating. Healing often requires the help and intervention of others. Originally provided almost exclusively in the family or within the clan or tribe, eventually places were established dedicated to the care of the sick (e.g., monastic infirmaries, almshouses, and later, hospitals). Remedies for nearly 2,000 years were found in plants and minerals. The last part of this century has achieved healing remedies so remarkable that they are called "miracle drugs."

This chapter briefly describes the evolution of health care facilities at home and abroad. The historical development and present-day trends in drug therapy are also highlighted to give a mosaic of health care from a historical perspective.

The approach is based on the contribution of the various cultures from early Greece through modern-day America.

Greek Influence

The Greek temple dedicated to Aesculapius, the mythical god of medicine, and the temple on the Greek Island of Cos where **Hippocrates**, the renowned father of medicine, practiced medicine and pharmacy (400–300 B.C.) are early examples of healing centers where gods were implored, physicians practiced medicine, and apprentices learned the art of healing. Patients who came to these temples were diagnosed, treated, and cared for until they were able to return home. Treatments included herbal remedies, mineral baths, exercise, fresh sea air, and sunshine. Archaeologists have found admission records and other medical records inscribed in the columns of these temples.

Hippocrates, circa 400 B.C.

For thousands of years, the writings of Hippocrates, the famous philosopher, physician, and pharmacist, occupied a place in medicine corresponding to that of the Bible in the literature and ethics of Western people. Through the use of rational concepts based on objective knowledge, he liberated medicine from the mystic and the demonic. The concept of **homeostasis**—the attainment and retainment of equilibrium in the body through appropriate drugs and diet—was the traditional benchmark of his numerous practices and writings. Hippocrates is considered to be the "father of medicine."

Hippocratic Corpus

Through the writings and practice of Hippocrates and his colleagues, medicine moved from the magical to the rational. The theory of humoral **pathology** considers disease as a disturbance of a body fluid (e.g., blood, **phlegm**, and yellow and black **bile**). Disease is treated by restoring equilibrium. Health is preserved by caring for the internal environment (e.g., diet, sleep, exercise) and properly reacting to the external environment (e.g., rain, excess sun, climate changes) to enhance the physical harmony of the body. Restoration of the physical harmony of the body or the restoration of bodily equilibrium is a basic health concept developed by Hippocrates and is medically known as homeostasis. Over 200 herbal remedies and a dozen minerals are recommended in the Hippocratic writings. These drugs were available as **pills**, **troches**, **gargles**, eye washes, **ointments**, and inhalants. In the Corpus, the word for *drug*—pharmakon—was defined as a purifying remedy; later it was described as a healing remedy.

Allopathy, the common medical practice in the Western world, treats symptoms and diseases with drugs that restore health by causing the opposite effect, e.g., antacids, antibiotics, antidiarrheals etc. This is in contrast to an infrequently used therapy known as **homeopathy**, which treats health problems with very dilute substances that cause the same effect as the symptom, e.g., a person with a fever is treated with minute doses of a fever–producing agent to reinforce the body's defense system.

To purify the body of excess fluids, drugs were frequently used as **expectorants**, **emetics**, **cathartics**, **diuretics**, and **sudorifics**. The common cold, seen as cold and damp, was treated with mustard, which is hot and dry. This example conveys the concept of allopathy employed by the Greeks. The juice of the poppy, which today we recognize as opium, was among the 200 drugs mentioned in the Hippocratic writings.

Theophrastus

Theophrastus was a Greek philosopher and botanist who lived circa 300 B.C. Botany, the study of plants, is closely related to **pharmacognosy**, the science that deals with the medicinal ingredients in living plants. Theophrastus classified plants by their leaves, roots, seeds, and stems. His accurate pharmaceutical and pharmacologic observations related to the classification and action of medicinal plants won for him the title of "father of botany."

Pedanios Dioscorides (A.D. 100)

The noted botanist and pharmacologist Dioscorides was the major authority on drugs for sixteen centuries. He added to the work of Hippocrates the knowledge he gained while accompanying the Roman armies on their conquests. A major focus of his studies and writings was the use and biological effects of early remedies. For this reason, perhaps he should be called the "father of pharmacology."

Dioscorides's herbal

The information in Dioscorides's herbal, known in Latin as *De Materia Medica,* was the major authority on drugs for sixteen centuries. More than 600 plants and ninety minerals were included. Knowledge was collected by Dioscorides from his extensive travels in Africa, Gaul, Persia, Armenia, and Egypt. The remedies of these countries were incorporated into the herbal, which gave plant/mineral descriptions, instructions for growing and preservation, dosage, medicinal uses, and side effects. Considered the most important pharmaceutical guide of antiquity, 35 translations and commentaries had been issued by 1540.

Roman Influence

In early Rome (A.D. 200–500), hospitals were often endowed by wealthy citizens who frequently cared for the sick as volunteers. Fabiola, a wealthy Roman woman, donated her palace for the care of the sick and injured and personally cared for their needs. With the fall of the Roman Empire, major changes occurred. The care of the sick became a civil responsibility and prostitutes and prisoners were assigned health care tasks.

Claudius Galen (A.D. 130–200)

Until 1950, pharmacy students took a course entitled "Galenical Pharmacy." Galen practiced and taught both pharmacy and medicine in Rome. His principles, derived from Hippocrates' theory for the preparation and compounding of medicines, were followed in the Western world for 1,500 years. This Greek-born physician who practiced in Rome organized the **pharmacotherapy** of humoral pathology into a scientific system.

On the art of healing (A.D. 1500)

Galen compiled and added to drug information available in Rome in the most famous of his writings, *On the Art of Healing*. The properties and mixtures of simple remedies and compounded drugs are described. Pharmacotherapy of humoral pathology was systematically classified according to the theories of Hippocrates. The treatments described such **galenicals** as **tinctures**, **fluidextracts**, **syrups**, and ointments. Galenicals have recently lost popularity due to the present use of synthetic chemicals, antibiotics, and **biologicals**.

Jewish Influence

Biblical Records (1200 B.C.)

The Old Testament book of Sirach (38:4–8) states, "The Lord created medicines from the earth and a sensible man will not despise them. Was not water made sweet with a tree in order that His power might be known? And he gave skill to men that He might be glorified in His marvelous works. By them He heals and takes away pain; the pharmacist makes of them a compound. His works will never be finished; and from Him health is upon the face of the earth." Genesis, the first book of the Bible, mentions myrrh, a remedy used throughout history as an appetite stimulant, **carminative**, and skin protectant with healing properties. Olibanum (frankincense) is gum resin mentioned in the books of Exodus, Ezra, Jeremiah, Ezekiel, and the Song of Solomon. The pharmacist's role, professional norms, and many drug examples are included in the Old Testament of the Bible.

Ancient Hebrews (1200 B.C.)

"God hath created medicines out of the earth and let not a discerning man reject them" (Sirach 38:4). Several drugs mentioned in the Old Testament are still in use today. Garlic (Numbers 11:5), with a history of thousands of years, is currently being investigated as a means to reduce blood pressure, lower cholesterol, and possibly inhibit growth of cancer cells. Aloe, mentioned in the New Testament (John 19:39) but available much earlier, is an official ingredient in compound benzoin tincture. Acacia (Exodus 26:15), used earlier for building purposes, is now commonly used as an emulsifying agent. Other items still in use include coriander, myrrh, almond, and anise. Presently, they are mainly used as foods or flavors.

The Jewish influence on health care is demonstrated by the teachings and works of the famous rabbi and physician, **Moses Maimonides**. The Prayer of Maimonides for many years continued the pledge of service made by pharmacists as they completed school and began professional practice.

Moses ben Maimon (Maimonides) (1135–1204)

For many decades, pharmacy students were presented with a scroll at graduation containing the Prayer of Maimonides, a Spanish rabbi and scientist. Included are the phrases, "May I be filled with love for my art. Preserve my strength that I may be able to preserve the strength of (others) may there never rise in me the notion that I know enough." Although Maimonides is best known for this document, he also published a glossary of drug terms and a manual of poisons.

Christian Influence

The spread of Christianity brought the teachings of Jesus to the care of the sick and infirm. At the Council of Nicaea in the fourth century A.D., bishops were required to provide a shelter for the care of the sick in each diocese. The Basilius, built by St. Basil the Great in the fourth century, has influenced hospital design to this day. Bishop Landry founded the Hotel Dieu in Paris in A.D. 660. This hospital still cares for the sick from its location on the Seine River in Paris.

Cosmas and Damian (d. A.D. 303)

While the early Greeks had their mythical gods and goddesses of healing (e.g., Aesculapius, Hygeia, and Panacea), the early Christians venerated those saints who significantly contributed to healings. Cosmas was a physician; Damian, his twin brother, practiced pharmacy. They were among many who were martyred for their Christian beliefs during Diocletian's persecutions (303–313). Over the years, they have been honored as the patron saints of medicine and pharmacy.

The early Christian **monasteries** included an infirmary in their structural design. These infirmaries served the sick monks and persons in the neighborhood who required special care. During periodic plagues, the monks cared for persons with deadly and frightening diseases. Monasteries also contributed to health service by growing, preserving, and preparing herbal medicines and retaining and printing drug information available at the time. These early manuscripts were the medical textbooks of the day.

Monastic Manuscripts (A.D. 500–1200)

The impact of political, intellectual, religious, social, and cultural upheavals of the Middle Ages gave rise to medieval monasteries as centers of learning and science, including medical/pharmacy knowledge. Manuscripts from throughout the world were translated or copied in the famous monastic scriptoria (libraries). Among the most famous treaties are *De Viribus Herbarum* ("herbs used by people") composed in a French abbey by Abbott Odo and *Causae et Curae* written by the Abbess Hildegard in a monastery in Bingen, Germany. Both manuscripts were completed during the eleventh to twelfth centuries. In addition to compiling existing knowledge, the monks added to the knowledge through studying the effects of the numerous plants grown in the monastery gardens.

Christian Renaissance Period

At the beginning of the Renaissance, several encouraging events occurred. In 1586, St. Camillus de Lellis founded a religious order, Clerics Regular Servants of the Sick, at the Hospital of St. James in Rome. Through his efforts the deplorable, filthy conditions in hospitals and miserable treatment by civil servants were scrutinized. St. Camillus took his new community of men and centered their activities in the Hospital of the Holy Spirit, which had been founded in 717 and was one of the largest hospitals in Europe. The brothers provided personal care for the patients with special attention to diet. Holy Spirit Hospital soon became a major site for the education of lay physicians with nearly 100 physicians in attendance. The hospital still contains an impressive library of medical literature. Thus, hospitals were beginning to emerge from the Dark Ages.

After St. Camillus founded his religious order, Pope Sixtus V authorized the red cross as a special insignia designating the special service provided by the order in the care of patients, many with diseases. To this day, a fourth vow of service which originated at the time of pestilence is made by members of this order who wear the red cross on the breast of their habit. The red cross was soon seen on battlefields and ultimately became the insignia of the famous relief organization, the International Red Cross (recently renamed the International Movement of the Red Cross and Red Crescent).

Eastern Influence

Clay Tablets of Mesopotamia (3000–2500 B.C.)

Among thousands of clay tablets unearthed in the present Persian Gulf region, over 800 tablets contained materia medica information. These first pharmaceutical texts contained over 500 remedies from plant, mineral, and other sources. The Code of Hammurabi was also discovered containing a section on ethical standards for health practitioners.

Pen T'sao (3000 B.C.)

The Chinese document *Pen T'sao,* freely translated as "the botanical basis of pharmacy," describes over 1,000 plants and 11,000 prescriptions handed down by oral tradition from Shen-Nung, considered the father of Chinese pharmaceutics. The early Chinese texts were inscribed on bamboo slats. They indicated the name of the drug, the **dosage**, and the symptoms it was used to treat.

About 500 B.C., Lao-tsu, a Taoist philosopher, composed a herbal compendium called "Tao te Ching" (The Way).

China (500 B.C.)

Drugs used in early China include ephedra, cassia, rhubarb, camphor, and ginseng. Yin drugs were cold and wet, and yang drugs were warm and dry. Red drugs treated heart conditions, and yellow drugs were used to treat liver problems.

Mithradates VI (d. 63 B.C.)

Early in history, the adverse or poisonous effects of drugs were a matter of concern. Mithradates might be called the "father of toxicology" for his investigation and writings related to the prevention and counteraction of the poisonous effects of drugs through the use of appropriate **antidotes**.

Arabia and Persia (A.D. 700–800)

In Arab countries, attitudes were humane and compassionate. Asylums for **psychiatric** patients were built that provided gardens, fountains, pleasant music, and a healthy setting where drugs, baths, and good nutrition were given to the patients.

New **dosage forms** were introduced as syrups and jams that contained active ingredients such as aloes, senna, nutmeg, clover, camphor, and musk. The *Minhaj* (*Handbook for the Apothecary Shop*) stated that a pharmacist "ought to have deep religious convictions, consideration for others, especially the poor and needy, a sense of responsibility and be careful and God-fearing."

Avicenna (Ibn Sina) (A.D. 980–1037)

Avicenna, also known as Ibn Sina, is called the "Persian Galen." His Arabic writings unified pharmaceutical and medical knowledge known at the time. His teachings were accepted in the West until the seventeenth century and to this day remain influential in the East.

India (1000 B.C.)

More than 2,000 drugs are mentioned in Charaka's writings, including cinnamon, cardamom, ginger, pepper, aconite, and licorice. These condiments and spices are in use today. Mercury was used in numerous preparations and is used today as an external antiseptic in Mercurochrome and Merthiolate.

Egyptian Influence

The great Al-Mansur Hospital in Cairo, Egypt is an example of the Arabs' interest and dedication to health care. The hospital had special wards for particular diseases, outpatient clinics, convalescent areas, diet kitchens, and a large medical library. Both men and women were trained to provide care for the sick.

Ebers papyrus (1500 B.C.)

The parchment (papyrus) scroll found in Egypt by George Ebers (1837–1898) is one of eleven medical scrolls that preserve the knowledge of early Egyptian medicine. Over 700 drugs are mentioned, with formulas for more than 800 remedies. According to these scrolls, the pharmacist selected the drugs, prepared them in a magically correct way, and then said prescribed benediction over them. The use of mortars and pestles, hand mills, sieves, and weighing scales is mentioned in the papyrus.

Military Influence

Wars accelerate the need for health care. Military medicine throughout history has provided the stimulus for improvement in infection control, surgical interventions, and trauma management. The Crusaders brought personal and financial support to the hospitals in the areas of conquest between A.D. 1096 and 1291. The Crusaders built hospitals in the Holy Lands. During this period, the Hospitalers of the Order of St. John of God were established to staff the hospitals and care for the wounded on the battlefield. This order continues to maintain health facilities throughout the world.

Hospitals began to take shape in what is now the United States in approximately the same way. It is known that military hospitals functioned during the

Revolutionary War in New York (Manhattan), Pennsylvania (Lititz), Massachusetts, and other areas of battle. For the most part, these were temporary field hospitals.

A historic example of a hospital formulary was compiled in Pennsylvania during the Revolutionary War. Known as the "Lititz Pharmacopoeia," it was used in preparing medications for the military hospital located in that town.

During the Civil War in the United States, Louisa May Alcott served as a volunteer and observed the wanton conditions of poor sanitation, depressing environment, and patient and staff misery at the Union Hospital in Georgetown, Virginia. She describes these conditions in detail in her published book, *Hospital Sketches*. This book influenced President Abraham Lincoln to establish the U.S. Sanitary Commission, which has as its goal a single desire and resolute determination to secure for the men who have enlisted in this war and that care which it is the duty of the nation to give them. Lincoln also requested the Sisters of Charity to care for the wounded on the battlefields in the Civil War.

During the ensuing decades, rapid changes took place. The wars of the twentieth century have seen significant changes in hospitals and health care delivery systems. World War I brought about the need to care for patients suffering from major trauma, burns, poison gas, and infections of all kinds. Hospital design reflected these needs in dealing with the masses of the injured, maimed, and sick. Ships designed as floating hospitals (begun during the Civil War) were in great demand to handle large numbers of casualties away from the immediate battlefield. They were also used to transport the sick under treatment to land-based institutions. World War II saw major advances in trauma surgery, the introduction of systemic sulfonamides, penicillin, and the wide use of blood and plasma for transfusion. The volume of injured increased and very large hospitals were built to provide the services needed. The Cadet Nurse Corps was developed in the early 1940s to answer the need for large numbers of professionally trained people to nurse the sick. Because of the kinds of injuries, new forms of treatment of war injuries were developed. The professions of occupational therapist and physical therapist came into being. Emotional problems resulting from the war gave new impetus for hospital facilities to deal with war-related psychiatric problems. One vivid reminder of the Korean conflict was the television series *M*A*S*H*. The weekly series brought us the experience of war through the eyes and emotions of a mobile army surgical hospital staff. It was the close proximity of these mobile operating rooms and support resources that resulted in saving the lives of hundreds, if not thousands, of victims.

Western Influences

Western Europe (A.D. 500–1200)

Medieval physicians prescribed approximately 1,000 natural substances, most of plant origin. **Herbs** were the main source of medication. Materia medica was derived from the Greeks, Romans, and Arabs. The monasteries in England, Germany, and France preserved this information and added to it the medicinal herbs grown in the monastery gardens. Early explorers of American shores brought back to Europe native remedies such as quinine found in the bark of South American trees.

During the Middle Ages, medical advancement came close to a standstill. A church edict in 1163 forbade clerics from performing any surgery that caused a loss of blood. At this time, monks were the primary health care practitioners, so surgical procedures were eliminated. Between 1347 and 1350, the **Black Plague** killed almost one-third of the inhabitants of Europe. Although most people were cared for and/or died in their own homes, many either died on the street or were brought to overcrowded hospitals. Hotel Dieu, one of the finest hospitals in Europe at the time, was reported to dismiss up to 500 bodies a day to be buried during the height of the plague.

Throughout the centuries, persons afflicted with mental health problems were often secluded from society in confined custodial care. The poor conditions of care are reflected in the story of Bethlehem Hospital in London, called Bedlam. (The word continues in the English language to convey the idea of confusion and disorder.) Modern health care requires concern for those afflicted with mental disorders.

In Italy, mental hospitals were built in Metz, Uppsala, Bergamo, and Florence in which patients were treated in a humane way. Outstanding in the care of psychiatric patients was the town of Gheel in Belgium, where the focus of town employment and activities was on the care of psychiatric patients who were given residence in the homes of the townspeople. It was in this town that St. Dymphna, the patron saint for mental disorders, was murdered by her deranged father who was king of Ireland and who pursued his daughter in rage after she had fled his abuse. To this very day, the town of Gheel is given over to the care of the mentally ill with support from the Belgian government.

Swiss influence

Paracelsus (1493–1541) was born Philippus Aureolus Theophrastus Bombast von Hohenheim. This Swiss alchemist changed his name to indicate his superiority over the great herbalist, Celsus. A product of the Renaissance, Paracelsus revolutionized pharmacy from a botanical science to the beginnings of a chemical orientation in the profession. He replaced the four body fluids identified by Hippocrates (blood, phlegm, yellow bile, and black bile) with three chemical constituents of the body. Paracelsus was the prime mover in bringing pharmacy from a botanical to a chemical science. Sulfur, mercury, and salt were the materials of the body, and drugs were used to overcome excess acid or alkalinity in the body. Alcohols, spirits, acids, and oils were used and mercurials and other minerals.

German influence

The Magna Carta of pharmacy

For the first time in the history of Western Europe, pharmacy was declared an independent profession separate from medicine through the official Edict of 1231. Emperor Frederick II of Germany was the author of this edict, known as the Magna Carta of pharmacy. By it, pharmacies were subject to government inspections; the pharmacist was obliged, under oath, to prepare drugs as prescribed in a reliable and uniform method. This edict influenced the practice of pharmacy across all of western Europe.

Pharmacopoeias

Books that contain official drug standards have been known through the ages as recipe books, formularies, **dispensatories**, and pharmacopoeias. The distinction of having the first legal pharmacopoeia goes to the city of Nuremberg, Germany, where the municipal authorities in 1546 made it the official book of drug standards for that city. This book, known as *Dispensatorium Pharmacopolarum,* also became official in Augsburg, Cologne, Florence, and Rome.

Frederick Serturner (1783–1841), a pharmacist, won international recognition when he prepared salts of morphine (1804), a drug of universal acclaim in the control of intractable (not easily managed) pain.

Johannes Buchner (1783–1852), a pharmacist and professor of pharmacy in Munich, discovered salicin in willow bark and nicotine in tobacco. These discoveries paved the groundwork for aspirin (acetylsalicylic acid) and nicotinic acid. The latter was synthesized from nicotine in 1867 and is used today as niacin, a member of the vitamin B complex.

Rudolph Brandes isolated hyoscyamine (1819) and, with fellow pharmacist Philipp Geiger (1785–1836), collaborated in research to discover atropine (1835). Atropine, used to this day, is a prototype for antispasmodic drugs.

Although Emil von Behring (1854–1917) was a physician and not a pharmacist, his contribution to pharmacy was a landmark. His work with antitoxins to combat the effects of diphtheria, and later tetanus, initiated serum therapy. Diphtheria antitoxin (1892) created a whole new category of pharmaceuticals.

The concept of chemotherapy was introduced by Paul Ehrlich (1854–1915), who researched 606 chemical combinations until he found an arsenical that would be effective in combating the contemporary **pandemic**: syphilis. Arsphenamine was patented in 1907 and achieved fame as the "magic bullet" against syphilis. Ehrlich was a German physician and a pioneer in cellular pathology. Specific remedies, many of a chemical nature, were targeted at specific microbial and specific human cells. An intensive warfare against infection had begun.

Gerhard Domagk (1895–1964), a German scientist, discovered a sulfa drug, prontosil, to be effective against hemolytic streptococci. The use of this drug became widespread as its effectiveness against a wide range of microorganisms became evident.

Swedish influence

Karl Scheele (1742–1786) was a Swedish pharmacist who made numerous chemical discoveries in the laboratory of his pharmacy shop. Among his discoveries were arsenic (1771), chlorine (1774), glycerin (1783), and numerous organic acids.

English influence

During the eighteenth century, many hospitals were built in England to provide diagnosis and treatment of the poor. The Bristol Royal Hospital claims to be the first voluntary hospital in the provinces. One of the most famous hospitals, Guy's Hospital in London, was built in 1740 and provided free care through a ticket admission system.

William Withering (1741–1799), a clinician and a botanist in England, investigated the active ingredient in a folk remedy used to cure dropsy (an accumulation of fluids due to heart impairment). He called attention to digitalis (1741) as the active **alkaloid** in the foxglove plant. Digoxin, a form of digitalis, is widely used today as a cardiotonic drug.

Edward Jenner (1749–1823), an English physician, vaccinated against smallpox with the cowpox vaccine (1789). This discovery in turn led to the eradication of smallpox in the twentieth century.

Ten years later, a new class of anti-infective drugs became available in limited quantities. Penicillin (1942), the first antibiotic to be used in therapy, was available to treat 100 patients. It was first observed as an inhibitor of microbial growth by Alexander Fleming at St. Mary's Hospital in London in 1928. Later, Howard Florey (1898–1968) and his coworkers succeeded in first isolating and then making available this lifesaving antibiotic to treat gram-positive infections.

French influence

Bernard Courtois (1777–1838) discovered iodine (1811) in marine algae. In 1826, the year he graduated from pharmacy school in Montpellier, Antoine Balard discovered bromine in sea water. He later became a faculty member of the same school.

Joseph Caventou (1795–1877), a pharmacist, collaborated with Pierre Pelletier (1788–1842) in the discovery of quinine (1820), which has become a worldwide treatment for **malaria**. He made other discoveries as well, including the identification of caffeine (1821).

Pierre Robiquet (1788–1840), a pharmacist who was also a phytochemist, made a number of significant discoveries, including codeine (1832). Codeine, an analgesic weaker than but similar to morphine, is a drug widely used to control pain.

Henri Moissan (1852–1907) obtained free fluorine (1886) by electrolytic methods, thus completing the elements in the halogen family of drugs.

International Influence

Canadian Contribution

Another dramatic and lifesaving discovery was made by Frederick Banting (1891–1941) and Charles Best (1899–1978) when they collaborated to discover insulin (1922). The lives of millions of diabetic patients have been saved and enhanced by this major therapeutic breakthrough.

World Health Organization

The World Health Organization (WHO) published the first *International Pharmacopoeia* in Geneva, Switzerland in 1951. This book was published in English, French, and Spanish and later in German and Japanese. Although not a legal document, it assists in setting internationally acceptable drug standards. Drugs that are included in any pharmacopoeia are those of proven pharmaceutic and therapeutic value.

Developments in the United States Related to Health Care and Drug Therapy

Hospitals have emerged over the years from **almshouses** for the sick poor, **asylums** for the care and confinement of orphans and the mentally ill, **sanatoriums** for long-term care of tuberculosis patients and the victims of other chronic diseases, **hospices** for the terminally ill, and infirmaries for short-term acute care.

Nonmilitary Hospitals

Nonmilitary hospitals came into existence in New Amsterdam, New York; Salem, Massachusetts; and Philadelphia, Pennsylvania. Philadelphia General Hospital was started in 1713 by the Quakers as an almshouse to give relief to the sick, the incurable, the poor, orphans, and abandoned infants.

Benjamin Franklin obtained a grant in 1751 to found the first American hospital, known as the Pennsylvania Hospital. Jonathan Roberts was recruited as the pharmacist and enjoys the reputation of being the first American hospital pharmacist. This institution has had a reputation for excellence from its earliest beginnings. The New York Cornell Medical Center was initially supported by King George III in a charter granted in 1771. The apothecary-in-chief was one of the four administrative officers named in the original charter.

Psychiatric Care

In the United States, Benjamin Rush, who was a physician, introduced new methods of treatment for psychiatric patients based on moral principles. His concerns and methods were outlined in a treatise on the topic that he published in 1812. Dr. Rush was a friend of Benjamin Franklin and cared for the mentally ill at Pennsylvania Hospital. The hospital was a forerunner in the care of the mentally disturbed in a general hospital, although at that time, psychiatric patients were housed in the lower level of the hospital and separated from the medical treatment areas.

Custodial care

The nineteenth century continued the manner of dealing with mental patients by separating them from family and society. At the same time, the term *hospital* was substituted for the term *asylum*. The growth in the number and size of mental hospitals after the turn of the century was tremendous. Custodial care in gigantic facilities became the norm, with half the hospital beds in the United States occupied by mental patients. During the middle of the twentieth century, the trend reversed.

Deinstitutionalization

Appropriate use of psychiatric drugs and various psychiatric treatment methods allowed many psychiatric patients to leave custodial care and assume the activities of daily living in society. Under this concept of **deinstitutionalization**, large numbers of persons were discharged to communities and, in some cases, to fend for themselves in the streets. The movement received strong support from civil liberty groups. State governments were only too willing to unburden themselves of the financial responsibilities involved in institutional care. What seemed to be a humane approach only increased the number of homeless in society. Now efforts are being made by professionals to develop small housing facilities for their care. Some now recognize that continued structural support and care are still required.

Surgical Care

Massachusetts General Hospital in Boston was the first hospital to use general anesthesia in surgery. The first operation was performed in 1842 with anesthesia provided by Dr. Crawford Long. Soon chloroform and ether became standard anesthetic agents, which allowed for more frequent, less painful surgery.

Contemporary Medical Practices

"Miracle drugs" are a major part of the medical fabric of the twentieth century. Numerous researchers in universities, in pharmaceutical firms, and under government sponsorship have made and continue to make drug discoveries that stave off death and improve the quality of life.

Polio Vaccine

Poliomyelitis was a disease that crippled American President Franklin Roosevelt and killed and crippled many children. Eventually, two vaccines were developed: an injectable vaccine (by Jonas Salk, 1955) and an oral vaccine (by Albert Sabin, 1961). These vaccines have practically eliminated the disease commonly known as infantile paralysis.

Streptomycin

Selman Waksman (1888–1973) and his colleagues at Rutgers University in New Jersey began an intensive search to find another antibiotic to treat tuberculosis, known as the Great White Plague, which was claiming numerous lives. Streptomycin, discovered in 1944, was the first antibiotic to be effective against tubercle bacillus, the infective agent in tuberculosis.

Whole hospital buildings were changed or eliminated as a result of new treatments. Tuberculosis sanatoriums and poliomyelitis facilities are examples of treatment centers outmoded by new therapy. The famed Willard Parker Hospital of New York was declared obsolete after drug and antibiotic treatments reduced contagion and the need for isolation in hospital buildings. More recently, ambulatory (outpatient) treatment of childhood disease has caused a dramatic reduction in the need for pediatric hospital beds.

Surgical Procedures

Technology continues at an accelerated pace, making real what only a few years ago appeared to be science fiction. New technology has resulted in shorter hospitalization and has given rise to home health care. For example, **cataract** surgery in the 1930s and 1940s was followed by a long postoperative recovery. The patient was housed in a darkened room and the head immobilized between sandbags. Now surgery is performed on an ambulatory basis with the patient going home the same day, once surgery is completed. Increasingly, diagnostic procedures and treatments are conducted in outpatient facilities.

Governmental Interventions in Medical Practice

Government pressures and controls have had their impact on the health care delivery system. Part of the impetus for ambulatory surgery has resulted from pressures by government, insurance companies, and the public at large to perform procedures quickly, eliminate hospital stay, and provide patients with the opportunity for recovery in their own home environment. Second opinions have helped to reassure patients that surgery is, in fact, necessary and justified. In many instances, insurance companies or employers require that prior approval be given for hospitalization if the company or employer is expected to be responsible for payment. Fewer needed beds have forced hospitals to close or merge. Hospital mergers reduce costs and provide greater economic efficiency.

Review of Therapeutic Advances Discovered in the Nineteenth and Twentieth Centuries

Drug Standards Set by Pharmacopoeias

The first U.S. Pharmacopoeia (U.S.P.) was published in Philadelphia in 1820 by the U.S. Pharmacopoeia Convention. This convention, founded on the American principle of representation, had **physician** representatives from all the existing states. The goal of the convention was to select the "official" drugs and to set up standards for their identity, purity, and assay methods. By 1850, pharmacists and physicians were members of the convention. The pharmacopoeia is revised every 10 years. The first pharmacist to be chairman of the convention was Charles Rice, superintendent of the General Drug Department at Bellevue Hospital in New York. He laid the foundation for the sixth edition of the U.S.P., published in 1882.

Biologicals

Serum therapy was initiated with the discovery of the germ theory by Robert Koch, the discovery of **vaccination** to provide **immunity** by Edward Jenner, and the discovery of antitoxins to neutralize microbial toxins by Emil von Behring. The vaccines, toxoids, and antitoxins, which utilize the clear fluid of the blood, were the first biologicals used in serum therapy. Smallpox vaccine was introduced in the early 1900s, followed by vaccines for typhus, whooping cough, measles, mumps, rubella, diphtheria, tetanus, influenza, and polio. In 1987, a genetically engineered hepatitis B vaccine was marketed.

Hormones

Isolation of human hormones began in 1897 with adrenaline followed by thyroxine (1916), insulin (1922), cortisone, adrenocorticotropin (ACTH), estrone (1929), and testosterone (1935). These substances are important for replacement therapy and other therapeutic needs. Human insulin (humulin), a product of genetic engineering, was introduced in 1982.

Anti-Infectives

Anti-infective therapy began with salvarsan (1907) and then prontosil (1935). A major breakthrough occurred with the discovery of penicillin (1928–1940). Other antibiotics soon followed: streptomycin (1944) and chloramphenicol (1947), known as the first broad-spectrum antibiotic.

Synthetics

Synthetic chemicals were rapidly developed, including phenobarbital (1912), Raudixin (1953), Thorazine (1954), lithium (1960), and Valium (1963).

Antihypertensives, **antiarrhythmics**, **antianginals**, **vasodilators**, and **beta blockers** all improved cardiac and circulatory problems. Drugs were developed to meet problems in the major biologic systems.

Immunomodulators

The most recent category of drugs to be developed is the **immunomodulators**. Based on the theory of preserving the integrity of the immune system, immunostimulators are used when there is a deficiency, and immunosuppressants are used to prevent organ transplant rejection and to treat autoimmune diseases. These modulators preserve equilibrium in the second most complicated biologic system, the immune system. (The most complex is the nervous system.)

Drug Development

The use of medicinal substances is a part of every culture. Plants, minerals, and animal parts were the drug components until the early nineteenth century. The twentieth century has advanced drug therapy to a greater extent than the contributions of all ages past.

Hospital Development

Hospital care has moved within the evolution of the human race. The multifaceted health institutions of today, with all the advances of biomedical science, have retained the primary mission of hospitals. This mission is the humane, compassionate, contemporary goal to fight disease, control pain, and provide optimum quality of life through prevention, restoration, cure, or health maintenance. Human care remains a noble endeavor in which we, as health professionals, take our turns as consumer and provider.

Summary

Health maintenance organizations (HMOs), emergicenters, and other facilities have been developed to meet the public's desire for quick, early, and relatively inexpensive care. Much of the concern over the safety of performing surgery on an ambulatory basis has disappeared. Results of other health care delivery systems are being evaluated. Hospitals have been forced to find alternative means to bring in revenue to bolster flagging institutional finances. Some of the ideas have alarmed health care professionals. Advertising, television spots, candlelight dinners, exercise clubs, and day care centers are but a few of the trendy ideas being used to bring the name of the local hospital to the attention of the public.

At the close of the twentieth century, the demand for service, the method of reimbursement for health care services, and the practice of medicine greatly influenced hospitals. Most assuredly, the awesome specter of AIDS has had a great impact on research efforts related to the immune system. Hospitals will continue to change and grow or diminish as medicine, **biotechnology**, science, politics, and public concerns assert their influence. As a result of these factors, hospitals will continue to develop their own special character.

Pharmacy practice at the end of the twentieth century in the United States has, through many internal and external factors, reoriented from a product focus to a concern for the ways drugs are used by people. The incorporation of clinical studies in the pharmacy school curriculum, clinical drug research activities supported by the government, industry, and universities, and extensive drug information services are moving pharmacy into an esteemed health profession role in the twenty-first century.

Recently, there has been enthusiasm for tracing "roots." Knowledge of historical development provides a framework to clarify values, foster appreciation, and establish future focus. This chapter reviews the cultural, medical, pharmaceutical, and ethical dimensions of better care as documented in the history of the healing sciences. To fully appreciate this heritage as a member of a noble profession, it is important to relate to the major contributions that have been bequeathed to contemporaries in the service of the sick at various times in history.

TEST YOUR KNOWLEDGE

Multiple Choice Questions

1. Which of the following aspects of pharmacy are mentioned in the Old Testament?
   a. the role of the pharmacist
   b. professional norms of practice
   c. examples of healing herbs
   d. all of the above
   e. none of the above

2. The Edict of 1231, the Magna Carta of pharmacy, stated that
    a. pharmacists depend upon physicians to specify how prescriptions should be compounded
    b. no one has the right to inspect a pharmacy for standards
    c. drugs should be prepared in a reliable and uniform method
    d. all of the above
    e. none of the above

3. Pharmacopoeias contain
    a. herbal collections
    b. chemical drugs
    c. synthetic drugs
    d. official drug standards
    e. antidotes for herbal poisons

4. A famous rabbi-physician was
    a. Hippocrates
    b. Landry
    c. Mansur
    d. Maimonides
    e. Ezekiel

5. The town of Gheel is dedicated to the care of
    a. war veterans
    b. drug addicts
    c. the homeless
    d. psychiatric patients
    e. unwed mothers

6. Fabiola was a
    a. female physician
    b. Greek apothecary
    c. hospital benefactor
    d. mythical goddess of nursing
    e. Roman storyteller

7. The well-known military hospital in the town of Lititz was located in
    a. Pennsylvania
    b. New York
    c. Massachusetts
    d. Virginia
    e. New Amsterdam

8. The Pennsylvania Hospital was founded by
    a. George Washington
    b. Benjamin Franklin
    c. Abraham Lincoln
    d. Benjamin Rush
    e. William Penn

9. Deinstitutionalization has resulted in
    a. increased number of homeless
    b. bizarre street behaviors
    c. improved care for persons with emotional disorders
    d. empty institutions
    e. a, b, and d

10. The present health care system is being modified and refocused by
    a. economic pressures
    b. political influence
    c. scientific discoveries
    d. biotechnology
    e. all of the above

Matching Questions

11. _____ quinine

12. _____ arsphenamine

13. _____ streptomycin

a. heart problems

b. malaria

c. syphilis

14. _____ digitalis   d. tuberculosis

15. _____ vaccination   e. smallpox

True/False Questions

16. _____ Pharmacy has always been based on scientific findings.

17. _____ Galen and Paracelsus influenced the practice of medicine and pharmacy for hundreds of years.

18. _____ Garlic has been used since antiquity as a remedy for numerous health problems.

19. _____ Serum therapy uses only those herbs of therapeutic value.

20. _____ The early explorers who first came to American shores took some of the native American herbs back to Europe.

References

Cowen, D. L., & Helfand, W. H. (1990). *Pharmacy, an illustrated history.* New York: Harry N. Abrams, Inc.

Cowie, L. (1986). *Plague and fire.* London: Wayland Publishing.

Donahue, P. (1996). *Nursing, the finest art* (2nd ed.). St. Louis: C.V. Mosby.

Dorland's illustrated medical dictionary (30th ed.). (2003). Philadelphia: W.B. Saunders Company.

Dubos, R. (1988). *Mirage of health.* New York: Harper and Row.

Garrison, F. H. (1960). *History of medicine* (4th ed.). Philadelphia: Saunders.

Ziegler, P. (1984). *The black death.* New York: Penguin Books.

2 Organizational Structure and Function of the Hospital

COMPETENCIES

Upon completion of this chapter, the reader should be able to

1. Explain the primary function of a hospital.
2. List five functions related to patient "processing" activities.
3. Name four treatment modalities available in a hospital for patient care.
4. Explain the hospital's role in wellness programs.
5. Describe the roles of the hospital's governing board.
6. List the functions of the director of a medical department.
7. Mention the major diagnostic units in the hospital.

Introduction

Hospitals today are complex networks of health care services. These services focus on **diagnosis**, treatment, prevention, and health maintenance of the community which it serves. This chapter will explore the organizational structure and the functions of a hospital that enable it to maximize optimum therapeutic outcomes for the patients served.

When asked to explain what running a hospital was like, an experienced administrator once described it as running the largest hotel in town, the largest restaurant, the largest laundry, the largest laboratory, the largest employment office, the largest cleaning service, and so forth, all wrapped up into one. This scenario, although somewhat amusing, can be particularly helpful in understanding how patient care is delivered and how a hospital functions on a day-to-day basis. In this chapter we shall explore two concepts: (1) the functions of today's modern hospital and (2) how the hospital is organized to achieve those functions.

Hospital Functions

The primary functions of any hospital are to provide resources for and assist the physicians in diagnosing and treating their patients. In carrying out these primary

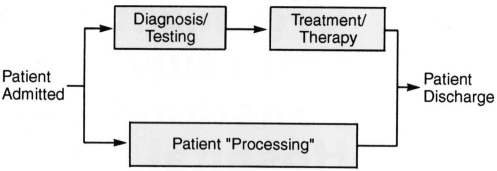

FIGURE 2-1 Simplified diagram of hospital functions

functions, a variety of secondary functions must also be performed (e.g., record keeping, billing, making plans for posthospital care). This simple breakdown of functions is shown in **Figure 2-1.**

The "processing" of patients refers to all the functions and paperwork associated with a patient's stay in the hospital. These include the admission process, the medical records function, utilization review, billing, and **discharge planning**, to name a few.

The physician orders tests to confirm or identify the patient's diagnosis or medical condition. These tests are carried out in the various departments (e.g., radiology, medical laboratory, cardiopulmonary). Once the diagnosis has been determined, treatment or therapy may be necessary and may include surgery, physical therapy, respiratory therapy, or drug therapy. Each is carried out by the appropriate clinical service. Some essential departments, such as nursing (patient care services), play an ongoing role in both the diagnosis and treatment functions.

The diagnosis and treatment of a patient is rarely a simple, straightforward process. Complications and unexpected ancillary test results can blur the distinction between diagnosis and treatment. It is not uncommon, for example, for one diagnosis to be treated only to have another health problem manifest (show) itself. In today's aging society, older patients frequently present themselves at the hospital with multiple diagnoses and conditions, all interrelated to varying degrees, making the diagnosis/treatment functions quite complex. For purposes of understanding the hospital's overall functions, however, it is of importance to recognize the sequence of diagnosis and treatment and the corresponding patient "processing" as being of primary significance to the structure and function of the hospital.

Another major function of hospitals that has gradually been developed over the past 10 to 15 years has been health education and wellness promotion. Hospitals have taken on responsibility for not only helping patients recover good health, but also for helping them stay healthy. To this end, hospitals have sponsored smoking cessation programs, stress reduction classes, weight loss programs, and instruction in how to identify potential health problems, such as self-examination for breast cancer. Community screening efforts for blood pressure, mammography, cholesterol, and glucose levels are representative of similar efforts to uncover those people at risk of becoming ill before their health actually begins to deteriorate (early detection). In addition, hospitals have developed support groups for patients and families with such health problems as diabetes and cancer. Finally, hospitals have begun to play a coordinating role in helping whole groups of patients assess their health care needs and gain access to the appropriate health care providers. One group of patients for whom this function is prevalent is senior citizens.

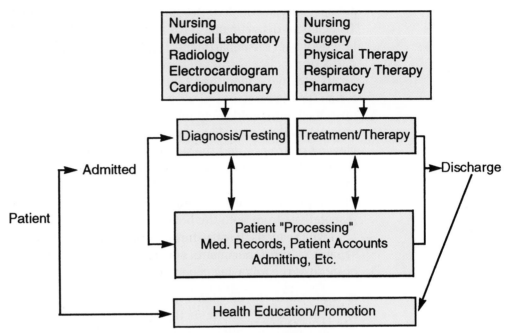

FIGURE 2-2 Expanded diagram of hospital functions

If we are to superimpose these additional functions on Figure 2-1, it will now appear as shown in **Figure 2-2**.

Anyone who has ever been in a hospital recognizes that there are a great many other things that go on that have not yet been addressed. Dietary service counsels patients and prepares and serves patient and employee meals. Housekeeping keeps the hospital clean and plays an integral role in infection control. Plant engineering maintains the facility and provides the necessary heating or air-conditioning and other utilities. Coordination of all of these activities, and others, are essential to the successful operation of a hospital.

Hospital Organization

Hospital organization and governance have traditionally been characterized as a three-legged stool: the governing body, the medical staff, and the hospital staff as led by the hospital's administration. It is a useful analogy since all three elements must be effectively integrated for a hospital to successfully support itself.

The governing body is usually called a **board of trustees** or **board of directors**. (In a governmental hospital these are sometimes known as a board of supervisors.) The board is charged with the ultimate responsibility of governing the hospital in the community's best interest. To this end, they are ethically, financially, and legally responsible for everything that goes on in the hospital. The board organizes itself into a variety of committees to perform the detailed activities required to govern the hospital. These committees encompass financial activities, community relations, planning, quality assurance, and personnel, as well as a variety of other areas of responsibility.

The medical staff consists of physicians, psychologists, podiatrists, dentists, and so forth, credentialled in their specialty or subspecialty to practice at the hospital. They are organized into departments such as medicine, surgery, family practice, ob/gyn, and pediatrics. The medical staff is sometimes further subdivided into subspecialty sections or groups such as cardiology, orthopedics, and neurology. The clinical departments have a department director or chair who oversees the functioning of the department. Typically, these functions include establishing standards of practice for the department's specialty, providing continuing education for its members, monitoring individual physicians' performance, and providing a forum for the exchange of ideas and new techniques. The medical staff also organizes itself into multidisciplinary committees to perform specific activities that the medical staff as a whole is responsible for. These committee activities include reviewing pharmacy and therapeutics, **credentialling**, tissue review, quality assurance, and utilization review. Both the medical staff and the board of trustees also have executive committees that coordinate the work of all the other committees. They typically share sponsorship of a joint conference committee made up of representatives from both the board and the medical staff.

Like the medical staff, the hospital staff is organized around common functions separated into departments or services. Each department or service performs one or more of the following general categories of functions:

- assist with the diagnosis via testing
- help treat the patient via therapy
- "process" the patient's paperwork or monitor the patient's treatment
- maintain the physical environment or support the patient's stay in the hospital
- support the functioning and management of the individual departments or hospital as a whole

Diagnostic testing is typically carried out in departments such as the laboratory, radiology, nuclear medicine, and EKG. Therapy is provided in the departments of pharmacy, physical therapy, speech therapy, and radiation therapy. Some departments, such as nursing, psychiatry, and respiratory therapy, spend significant amounts of time both determining diagnoses and providing treatments.

Other departments perform "processing" functions that assist the patient throughout the stay without directly affecting diagnosis or treatment. Examples of these departments include **medical records**, admitting, patient accounts (billing), **utilization review**, and social services.

Another group of departments support the patient's stay either by contributing to the physical environment or by supporting the coordination of services to the patient. Included in this group would be communications, housekeeping, volunteers, laundry, plant engineering and maintenance, safety and security, and pastoral care. The dietary department, while providing support to the patient through ongoing nutrition, can also play a **therapeutic** role and a health teaching role.

Finally, a variety of departments and services are vital to the overall success of a hospital, but patients may never hear of them while around the hospital. These departments support the ongoing operation of the hospital and the individual services and include the departments of materials management, human resources, **community relations and fund development,** planning, risk management, and accounting and finance. In addition, there are personnel who clerically support the activities of the medical staff.

Each hospital department/service is generally run by an administrative director or a section supervisor. These middle managers, in turn, report to representative members of the administration. These vice presidents report to either the executive vice president or directly to the president. Historically, the departments were grouped according to common operating characteristics into four categories: nursing services, clinical services (testing and treatment departments), support services (support and facilities departments), and financial services (accounting, patient accounts). The organizational chart in **Figure 2-3** reflects this historical division of responsibility.

However, hospital organizational structure has changed dramatically over the years and is now tailored specifically to each hospital's activities and the capabilities of its department heads and administrative staff. Although some elements are common to all organizational charts, there is no longer one dominant organizational structure.

Matrix management and **product line management** are only two examples of organizational theory applied to the rapid technological and service delivery evolution that has taken place in health care. Matrix management structurally emphasizes the overlapping areas of responsibility among departments and the common areas of decision-making. Product line management organizes the hospital not along the lines of comparable operating principles, but by the end product or category of service being delivered.

It is not essential to fully understand organizational theory to appreciate how a hospital functions. What is important is to appreciate the great variety in the ways hospitals organize themselves and that, in each case, communication and collaboration among departments is vital.

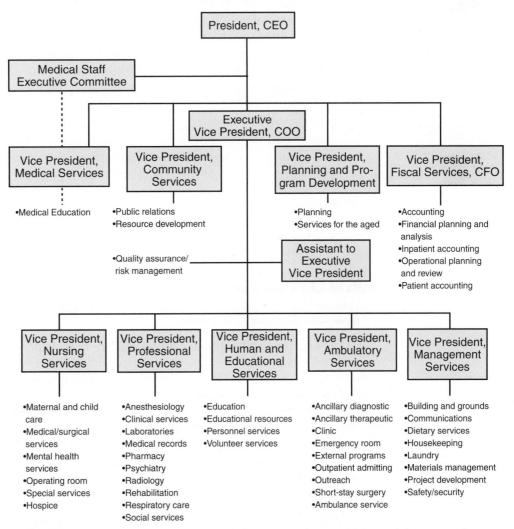

FIGURE 2-3 Hospital organizational chart according to traditional divisions of responsibility

As a way of enhancing communications the hospital staff, such as the board of trustees and the medical staff, forms committees. Some committees are ongoing ones, such as safety and quality assurance committees. Many, however, are ad hoc working groups brought together to address a specific problem or concern. Once the desired resolution is achieved, these groups disband or form new committees to address different problems and issues. These ad hoc committees bring various departments together in a problem-solving situation without dramatically altering the organizational structure of the hospital or interfering with the reporting relationships carefully developed over time. As such, they represent a flexible, informal organizational structure that allows the hospital to get its work done.

Summary

If there is one conclusion about hospital organizational structure and function that can be reached, it is that it will continuously change. New technologies are only now becoming available that will change whole departments or create new ones. New roles are continuously being proposed for the nation's hospitals and new organizational structures developed to meet the challenges that lie ahead. In short, it is far from clear what hospitals will look like in the future or precisely how they will function. In light of the financial crisis hospitals are facing today, compounded by the technological revolution we are experiencing, we can be sure that hospitals will remain complex organizations that patients depend upon to adequately provide the quality care that is required. We can also be sure that proper and appropriate health care will continue to depend on accurate and precise communication of information and, most importantly, on the skill and dedication of those who staff our hospitals.

TEST YOUR KNOWLEDGE

Multiple Choice Questions

1. The primary functions of a hospital are to provide for which of the following
   a. diagnosis
   b. treatment
   c. volunteer workers
   d. a and b
   e. a, b, and c

2. Patient "processing" activities include
   a. the admission process
   b. medical records function
   c. utilization reviews
   d. discharge planning
   e. all of the above

3. Most hospitals provide the following treatment modalities:
   a. surgery
   b. hypnosis
   c. acupuncture
   d. drug therapy
   e. a and d

4. Wellness programs in hospitals typically include
   a. smoking cessation programs
   b. handicap olympics
   c. strength training
   d. aerobics
   e. none of the above

5. The role of the hospital governing board includes responsibility for all the following except:
   a. ethical concerns
   b. hiring of supervisory personnel
   c. legal and financial matters
   d. monthly on-site inspections of facility
   e. b and d

Matching Questions

6. _____ maintains physical environment   a. board of trustees

7. _____ establishes medical standards of practice   b. medical staff

8. _____ overall hospital governance   c. hospital staff

9. _____ social services

10. _____ monitors physicians' performance

True/False Questions

11. _____ All hospitals conform to the same organizational structure.

12. _____ All hospitals function to provide required diagnostic and treatment services.

13. _____ Hospitals generally follow the patient into the community through discharge planning functions.

14. _____ Joint conference committees are made up of representatives from the board of directors and the medical staff.

15. _____ Clinical services include the testing and treatment departments.

Home Health Care

COMPETENCIES

Upon completion of this chapter, the reader should be able to

1. Describe the evolution and future of the home health care industry, particularly related to home infusion therapy and home care pharmacy practice.
2. Explain the scope of services available to a patient requiring home health care.
3. Describe the five most common drug categories of, medical indications for, and complications of home infusion therapy.
4. Describe the different types of infusion control devices used in home infusion therapy.
5. Describe the various roles for a pharmacy technician in a home infusion company.

Introduction

Home health care in the United States is a diverse and rapidly growing segment of the health care industry. It is rapidly becoming the predominant form of health care provision, replacing in-hospital care. Home health care, also called home care, can be defined as the provision of health care services to patients in their place of residence. The U.S. Census Bureau estimated that there were 19,670 home health care service establishments in 1997. The National Association for Home Care (NAHC) believes this number to currently be over 20,000. Home health care is as old as mankind; however, the first home health care agencies were established during the 1880s. On the basis of historical information obtained by NAHC, their numbers grew to 1100 by 1963 (2001). Pharmaceutical services were not a component of these early agencies, which consisted primarily of nurses, therapists, and home health aides. Retail pharmacies provided medications (primarily oral drugs) to patients in their home through home deliveries by the pharmacy or the home health care nurse who picked up the medications for the patient. Pharmacy's role in home health care was then minor and indistinguishable from retail pharmacy practice. Indeed, home health care patients may have received less pharmaceutical care (i.e., clinical care) than their outpatient counterparts because they rarely interacted with the pharmacist.

The first major boom in the number of home health care agencies occurred in 1965 with the enactment of Medicare. Medicare made home health care services available to the elderly and, beginning in 1973, to certain disabled younger Americans. Between 1967 and 1985, the number of home health agencies grew by more than threefold, from 1,753 to 5,983. However, pharmacy's role in home health care had increased very little because drugs were not a Medicare benefit. In 1983, Medicare initiated a prospective payment method of reimbursement for inpatient hospital care based on diagnosis-related groups (or DRGs) in an effort to reduce health care costs. This method of reimbursement provided economic incentives for hospitals to discharge patients as early as possible, reducing the length of a patient's stay in the hospital. This dramatically shifted patients from in-hospital care to receiving the provision of care in the home setting. Thus in over 34 years, the number of home health care agencies grew from 1,100 to over 20,000. The number of patients receiving home health care services by 1996 grew to 7.2 million individuals, roughly 2.7% of the U.S. population.

The role of pharmacy in the growth of home health care can be retraced to the birth of home infusion therapy during the early 1970s. Several university-based medical centers demonstrated the feasibility of providing nutritional support via the intravenous route, called total parenteral nutrition (TPN), in the home setting. This direct result of technological advances in infusion pumps allowed for smaller, yet more sophisticated, pumps and technological improvements in intravenous catheter materials and catheter placement techniques. These technological advances, with the implementation of the DRG-based method of hospital reimbursement and Medicare's willingness to pay for home TPN at one-third the inpatient rate, resulted in the birth of the home infusion therapy business. Once home TPN was established, other home infusion services were provided, including home antibiotic therapy and pain management. Prior to this, TPN and drug infusion therapy were primarily hospital inpatient procedures. Now there is almost no drug which cannot be administered safely in the home setting. Pharmacy's role in this field became prominent and, to this day, home infusion therapy remains pharmacy's predominant arena in home health care. In addition to hospitals as providers of home infusion therapy, the 1980s and 1990s saw entrepreneurial companies develop whose primary service was provision of home infusion therapy. During this time, both the number of providers and the number of patients served grew. From 1982 through 1987, the compounded annual growth rate of the home infusion therapy industry was 58%. In 1987, it was estimated by the U.S. Office of Technology Assessment that 250,000 patients were receiving home infusion therapy.

Today the organizations and employers who pay for health care (including the U.S. government) are increasingly looking for ways to manage the cost of it. One predominant way of doing this is by managing the provision of care itself. This concept is called "managed care." Sometimes insurance companies, health maintenance organizations (HMOs), or employers directly provide this management of care. Other times, they hire separate entities to manage the care for them. Under managed care, it has been increasingly realized that directing patients to the most appropriate and most cost-efficient health care setting at different cycles in their health care can reduce the cost of care without reducing (and sometimes increasing) the quality of care provided. Managed care is more prevalent in the employer-based health insurance market, where 3 out of 4 workers with health insurance receive it through a managed care plan. Managed care organizations typically finance health care services through a negotiated prepaid rate to health care providers. Often a home care provider will compete for a managed care contract to provide home care to all participants of a health care plan who may need those services within a geographical area. This requires home care providers to manage their expenses carefully and be very good at predicting the home care needs of the participants. Another feature of managed care is the desire for one bill for all home care services (i.e., one-stop shopping). This often requires home care providers to contract with other home care providers for services that they do not directly provide. The increasingly competitive home care market has created incentives for many home care providers to enter managed care provider networks.

Despite the tremendous growth of home health care in terms of number of patients and providers, the total cost of home health care is low. Based on CMS (Centers for Medicare and Medicaid Services) data, annual expenditures for home health care in 1998 amounted to an estimated $34–$35 billion, which represents only 3% of the $1,149 trillion spent for personal health care in the United States in the same year. Compared to 38% for hospital care, and 9% for nursing home care, home health care looks like a bargain. The cost of home health care is expected to be even lower, as CMS implemented a Prospective Payment System (PPS) for Medicare in October 2000. Under PPS, the organization is paid a flat fee for a 60-day episode of care, rather than payment for each visit. The incentive is to minimize the number of visits and provide care with the least expenses possible. Medicare payment for hospital care is also under a Prospective Payment System.

The number of healthcare workers employed by private, freestanding home care organizations steadily grew from 510,000 in 1993 to 707,000 in 1997. However, the advent of managed care has reduced those numbers to 659,000 in 1999. PPS is expected to reduce them further; however there is still a healthy number of employees in home care, and the numbers will grow as the population ages. In addition, on the basis of satisfaction surveys, patients prefer home health care to hospital care, and one can see that the growth of home health care has not yet peaked. Even home infusion therapy, which has seen virtually no breakthroughs in technology and new therapies administered in the home in the past few years, is still experiencing a 13% annual compounded growth rate. The growth of pharmacy in home health care will continue into the next century. Many predict it will become the predominant health care setting for the provision of drug therapies and pharmacy practice.

Home Health Care Services

Home Health Services

The most frequently provided home care services are **home health services**, defined as the provision of health care services by a health care professional in the patient's place of residence, usually on a per-visit basis. Home health services consist of a wide diversity of health care services. The predominant form of home health services is nursing. Other services include those of a dietitian, medical social worker, physical therapist, occupational therapist, and speech therapist. Some people also include respiratory therapists, dentists, and physicians in this group. Respiratory therapists are usually associated with the home medical equipment industry rather than with home health agencies. The provision of dental services in the home is relatively new and extremely rare at present. Most people prefer to differentiate physician services in the home, referring to them as *home medical services.* Providers of home health services are called *home health agencies.* Home health agencies can be classified as public (governmental) agencies, nonprofit agencies, proprietary agencies, and hospital-based agencies. Most states require home health agencies to be licensed. Approximately 55% of home health agencies are Medicare certified. To be Medicare certified, the organization must meet the Medicare Conditions of Participation and have a Medicare provider number. As part of the Conditions of Participation, the home health agency must provide nursing and one other home health service directly. Other services can be provided through a contracted provider. Nursing services can be high tech (e.g., infusion therapy) or low tech (e.g., diabetic teaching and monitoring) on an intermittent visit schedule or as 4- to 12-hour shifts.

Personal Care and Support Services

The second most common form of home care services is **personal care and support services**, defined as the provision of nonprofessional services for patients in their place of residence. These services include homemaking, food preparation, personal care, and bathing. The individuals who provide these services are usually called home health aides, homemakers, or personal care attendants. Most personal care and support services are provided by home health agencies, although some companies (non-Medicare certified) specialize in this form of care exclusively. One of the growing areas for personal care and support services is private duty services. Private duty involves the provision of personal care services round-the-clock or for 8–18 hours per day, sometimes by a live-in attendant. These services are generally not reimbursed by Medicare or Medicaid and rarely by insurance, so the predominant form of payment is personal out-of-pocket costs to the patients and/or their families. Home health or nursing services can also be provided on a private duty basis and it, too, is a growing area. It is estimated that 20.7% of all home care services are paid for out-of-pocket.

Home Equipment Management Services

The third most prevalent form of home care services is **home equipment management services**, also referred to as **home medical equipment (HME)** services or **durable medical equipment (DME)** services. Home equipment management services can be defined as the selection, delivery, setup, and maintenance of equipment and the education of the patient in the use of the equipment—all performed in the patient's place of residence. Medical equipment includes wheelchairs, canes, walkers, beds, and commodes. It also includes higher technology items such as oxygen tanks, oxygen concentrators, ventilators, apnea monitors, phototherapy lights, infusion pumps, enteral pumps, and uterine monitors. Many providers include the sale of medical equipment and supplies (such as ostomy supplies) in this home care definition. However, the federal government and the Joint Commission on Accreditation of Healthcare Organizations (JCAHO), which accredits such providers, do not include the provision of products without services in their definition of home care. So such sales, without the corresponding services, would not be considered home care.

Home medical equipment providers are not required to be licensed in most states, although the U.S. Food and Drug Administration (FDA) and the Department of Transportation (DOT) require registration for distribution and transportation of oxygen. A large number of pharmacies are involved in the provision of home medical equipment services and sales, which may be included in the definition of home care. Many HME organizations also provide clinical respiratory services, which include the professional services of a registered respiratory therapist for performing in-home assessments, monitoring of vital signs, oximetry testing, and/or administrating therapeutic treatments. Pharmacies are often involved in providing the respiratory drugs for these patients, either directly for the patient, or under contract with the HME provider.

Home Pharmacy Services

The last major form of home care service is the provision of home pharmacy services. Home pharmacy services do not have a clear and concise definition since there is considerable overlap with retail or community pharmacy practice. However, home care pharmacy generally has the following characteristics:

■ All medications are delivered, mailed, or shipped to the patients' home. The patient has never been present in the pharmacy or communicated face-to-face with a pharmacist (except perhaps in their home).

■ The patient is usually receiving home health (nursing) services and sometimes medical care in his or her home and may be homebound.

■ The pharmacy is usually responsible for monitoring the patient's medication therapy and clinical status on an ongoing basis while the patient is in his or her home. If not the pharmacy, then someone else is (e.g., home health nurse, hospice team, or another pharmacist).

Role of Pharmacy in Home Health Care

The predominant form of home pharmacy services is home infusion therapy (90% or more). However, pharmacies that specialize in providing services to hospice patients or hospice pharmacies are also categorized as providing home pharmacy services, as are a growing number of specialized mail-order pharmacies. The predominant specialty areas for such mail-order pharmacies include transplant/immunocompromised patients, cystic fibrosis patients, children with growth problems, and hemophilia patients, who often deal with biotech and injectable products.

Home Infusion Therapy

According to the U.S. Office of Technology Assessment, home infusion therapy is described as a medical therapy that involves the prolonged (and usually repeated) injection of pharmaceutical products, most often delivered intravenously, but sometimes delivered via other routes (e.g., subcutaneously or epidurally) into patients in their home environment. Home infusion therapy is generally thought of as consisting of three services: pharmacy, nursing (home health), and equipment management services.

Pharmacy Services

Pharmacy services generally involve both compounding and dispensing the intravenous solutions into a ready-to-administer form. In many ways, this process is similar to the IV room of a hospital pharmacy. Preparation of sterile admixtures for home administration may require special techniques and more stringent environmental controls than a hospital IV admixture room. Unlike in a hospital where a medication is usually prepared within 24 to 48 hours of administration, home care may involve up to one month between preparation and administration, thus allowing a greater potential for microbial growth. More extensive quality control and end-product testing are also performed on the prepared products for the same reasons.

Another significant difference between home care and hospital pharmacy practice involves labeling of the admixture. Home care pharmacists have usually researched the stability of IV medications over longer periods of time; when research results indicate, they provide expiration dating much longer than manufacturers' recommendations. Prescription labels must conform to the requirements for the state pharmacy laws for retail pharmacies. The pharmacy is also responsible for the packaging and delivery of the prepared products to the patient's home. Delivery techniques vary from the use of one's own delivery vehicles and drivers, to the use of external contracted delivery services—both local and national (e.g., Federal Express), to having the nurse pick up and deliver the medications. Regardless of the delivery method, the pharmacy must always ensure that the product is packed to control the factors that affect the stability of the product (temperature, light, humidity, etc.) during delivery to the patient's residence.

The pharmacist working in home infusion is also responsible for the pharmaceutical care and clinical monitoring of the patient. The pharmacy monitors the drug therapy through evaluation of information received from the patient's nurse, the patient or family member or caregiver, the delivery driver, and the pharmacist's review of laboratory test results, which are often sent directly to the pharmacy. There is extensive communication regarding the care of patients with their physician and nurse, as well as other health care professionals involved and sometimes the patients themselves. The pharmacy maintains not only the normal prescription and dispensing records, but also a clinical record of the patients called a chart or home care record. The home infusion pharmacy generally operates under outpatient or retail pharmacy laws, although many state boards of pharmacy have either additional or different regulations for home care pharmacies. The pharmacy is often involved in providing the nursing supplies, catheter care supplies, and the access device for the infusion therapy to patients. These infusion-related supplies and devices are sent with the medications to the patient, for use by the patient or nurse, in the patient's home.

Home Nursing Services

At least initially, most patients receiving home infusion therapy will also be receiving home nursing services. Nurses usually have considerable experience in handling IVs in an acute care setting before they care for home infusion patients. Major responsibilities of the home care nurse include educating the patient and/or family caregiver regarding administration of the infusion and care of the infusion site, performing dressing and infusion site changes, making in-home physical assessments, and monitoring the patient's health status. Nurses will also administer the medications initially, but the eventual goal is to train the patient or a caregiver to perform this task. Periodic visits are then made to monitor the patient's status and response to therapy. The nurse may also insert some types of IV access devices or catheters into the patient in the home. The choice of venous access device depends on the patient's condition, the length and type of infusion therapy, and the preferences of the patient, physician, and nurse. The selection of the access device can significantly affect the need for, quantity of, and type of supplies, the nursing time and visits, and thus the overall cost. Certain devices also require more skill for insertion or placement than others. For instance, peripherally inserted central catheters (PICC), which are commonly used for two- to eight-week home infusion therapy, are the most complicated venous access devices that can be inserted in the home. Insertion requires nurses who have undergone special training and are certified to perform this procedure. Sometimes nurses will also provide more traditional nursing home care to infusion patients (e.g., wound care), thus meeting all the patient's nursing care needs.

Equipment Management Services

Equipment management services primarily include the selection, delivery, and set up of an infusion control device (i.e., an infusion pump). These services are often performed by the pharmacy, but may also be performed by the home health agency or a separate HME provider. They also include the separation of clean (patient-ready) and dirty (returned) equipment, cleaning and disinfecting of equipment between patient use, and routine and preventative maintenance of the equipment including inspection, testing, and performing maintenance on the equipment. Equipment sent to patients also needs to be tracked and logged in compliance with the Safe Medical Devices Act (SMDA) of 1990. Backup equipment and/or services are needed for equipment malfunctions. As in a hospital or clinic setting, not all home infusion patients need an infusion pump. Gravity administration of the drug using the rate controller or clamp on the administration set or tubing can be safely used at home for some drugs and administration rates. Special infusion pumps and devices have been developed especially for the special needs of home infusion patients. Disposable administration devices and small lightweight pumps that do not require an IV pole are commonly used for home infusion therapy. When drug dilution is not required and the administration time is short, some patients may receive their medication as an IV push (a term used when the active ingredient goes directly into the vein). Home care pharmacists must be able to decide whether an infusion device is required and what device or pump is appropriate for the patient, drug, and administration rate.

A home infusion provider may provide all three services (pharmacy, nursing, and equipment) to a patient together, separately, or in any combination. Some pharmacies are involved in the provision of home pharmacy services only, although the vast majority also provide infusion and enteral pumps. These pharmacies rely on the home health agency nurse to communicate patient assessment data in a timely manner and to coordinate care with the patient. Some insurers may want to pay only one provider. In this case, the pharmacy may contract with a home health agency, collect payment from the insurer, and pay the agency for the nursing services. This scenario may decrease the pharmacist's time required to obtain the assessment data from and coordinate care with the nurse because the pharmacy controls the patient care and nursing service payment. The reverse scenario also occurs, however, in which the home health agency contracts with the pharmacy and the pharmacy receives payment from the home health agency. In this case, it is often difficult for the pharmacy to obtain the data needed in a timely manner. Decisions regarding the selection of a provider for a patient's home infusion therapy may be made by the insurers, patients, and physicians. Thus some patients may receive pharmacy services only, whereas others will receive both nursing and pharmacy services from the organization. The trend toward "one-stop shopping" by managed care providers and the increasing trend toward diversification by home care organizations will result in many home infusion providers being part of a large organization that provides a vast array of home care services. Many home infusion therapy providers have also expanded into the long-term care market (as many providers of long-term care services are expanding into home care) to capture what is called the *post-acute* or *alternate site market.*

Types of Home Infusion Providers

Home pharmacy services, as part of home infusion therapy, can usually only be provided by a licensed pharmacy either alone or as part of a broader health care organization. The exception is physician practices, which can provide these services without a pharmacist or pharmacy out of their office under the auspices of their physician's license. This type is most commonly seen in oncology and infectious disease practices. Usually, physicians run an ambulatory infusion center as part of their office. Patients receive cancer chemotherapy, antibiotics, or any type of infusion while they are in the physician's office. Between physician visits, patients may return to the infusion center to receive their IV medications or have them provided through home care. Even in cases when the patient predominately uses the infusion center, at times a nurse needs to visit the patient in the home (e.g., catheter problems in the middle of a weekend). Home care is usually provided by the nurses from the physicians' offices and is usually considered a sideline to their office-based practice. In these physician-based practices, nurses—not pharmacy technicians or pharmacists—are usually responsible for compounding and admixing the IV medications. Sometimes a local pharmacy is contracted to compound and deliver the medications to the physician's office, and occasionally a pharmacist is hired by the physician. Technicians are rarely used in this environment unless a pharmacist is present.

Other types of settings where home care pharmacy is practiced include retail or community pharmacies, institutional or long-term care pharmacies, hospital pharmacies, home health agencies, HME-based providers, infusion therapy specialty providers, and ambulatory infusion centers.

Retail or Community Pharmacies

Independent retail or community pharmacies are most likely to provide a variety of services including HME, ostomy care products, and diabetic care. Infusion therapy is usually a low volume component. Pharmacists, and sometimes technicians, usually provide home infusion therapy services in addition to retail and other pharmacy duties. Most are "pharmacy-only" providers; however, a few pharmacies hire nurses to help coordinate home infusion therapy services and perhaps provide a limited amount of home health services. Delivery services are provided by nurses or the same delivery mechanism as the retail pharmacy/HME business. Some are part of a franchise in home infusion or participate in a home infusion network. Many are one-owner operations.

Institutional or Long-Term Care Pharmacies

Institutional or long-term care (LTC) pharmacies primarily provide drug distribution services to a large number of nursing homes, prisons, and other institutional facilities, servicing an average 4,000 patients daily. Although the primary business is oral therapies, many also provide IV therapies to long-term care facilities with subacute units. Expanding the provision of IV services from the nursing home to the home care environment is very easy. Thus many LTC pharmacy providers have entered the home care market. However, home infusion therapy is usually a very low volume component of their services. These organizations have extensive internal delivery systems (e.g., their own fleet of vans) and provide at least enteral and infusion pumps, though some may also supply other HME. Although these pharmacies may employ a nurse to assist with care coordination and education of the long-term care facility staff, home health services are rarely provided directly by these organizations, which tend to be pharmacy-only operations.

Hospital Pharmacies

Home infusion therapy is often provided by the hospital department of pharmacy in the inpatient IV admixture room or the outpatient pharmacy utilizing the existing staff. A pharmacist is assigned clinical responsibilities in home care and for interacting with the home health care team. The hospital usually provides a broad array of home health services, although these are operationally in a different department and may not even be on the hospital premises. Infusion pumps are either handled by the biomedical engineering department, the home health services department, materials management or the pharmacy department, or a combination of these. Delivery services are usually provided by the home care nurses who pick up the medications from the pharmacy. Some hospitals have created a separate home infusion pharmacy independent of the inpatient pharmacy, especially when the volume remains high, which may be located on the campus of the hospital. Some hospitals have created a home infusion division (home health plus pharmacy) that resides off-campus, sometimes as a separate corporate entity, that looks and acts like an infusion therapy specialty provider.

Home Health Agencies

Home health agencies have purchased or implemented a pharmacy to supplement their home health services provision. These are usually large home health agencies that provide a wide array of home health services and may have multiple home health offices. The pharmacy may service multiple home health branches and usually looks and operates similar to an infusion therapy specialty provider.

HME-Based Providers

HME providers may also provide home infusion pharmacy services. Usually the primary role of pharmacies is to supply respiratory therapy medications which are needed for the home medical equipment and clinical respiratory needs of their patients. The home infusion pharmacy may operate similarly to a retail pharmacy-based infusion program or an infusion therapy specialty provider.

Infusion Therapy Specialty Providers

The infusion therapy speciality provider specializes only in the provision of home infusion therapy. Generally, this organization provides home health services, although the nurses specialize in home infusion therapy only. Pharmacy occupies a prominent role in this type of organization. Infusion and enteral pumps are usually the only type of medical equipment provided by this company. Maintenance of the infusion and enteral pumps is usually performed by the company's employees. The infusion therapy specialty providers tend to have their own delivery staff and vans, depending on the size of the organization. This type of provider may service up to 1,000 infusion patients per day. Smaller volume providers in this category also exist, however, and usually reside in suburban industrial office parks.

Ambulatory Infusion Centers

Ambulatory infusion centers consist of an office, usually in a doctor's office building. Patients are referred here to receive their infusions in a comfortable setting. The office consists of a series of rooms, each with a relaxing chair, infusion pump, and TV. Nurses manage and run the office and administer the drugs. The offices are generally licensed as pharmacies and have a pharmacy and pharmacist present to prepare the IV admixtures for the nurses to administer. The nursing staff may provide limited home care services to patients treated by the center. As discussed, a nurse will need to visit the patient in the home and provide almost all deliveries. Many ambulatory infusion centers are owned by infusion therapy specialty providers and operate in a similar manner. Others are owned by physicians.

　　In all of the preceding cases, the provider can be independent or part of a regional or national chain. Some pharmacies serve patients seen by multiple home health agencies or home medical equipment providers, and service patients in multiple states whose geography is limited only by the areas serviced by overnight delivery services (such as Federal Express). Others are single-site providers that only serve their local community.

Types of Care and Therapies Provided

Although virtually any infusion can now be given safely to patients in their homes, some forms of therapy have predominated, including antibiotic therapy, antiviral therapy, total parenteral nutrition, enteral nutrition, pain management, cancer chemotherapy, hydration, miscellaneous drugs, ancillary drugs, and preparing and dispensing medications for home care.

Antibiotic Therapy

Antibiotic therapy is by far the most common of the home infusion therapies provided. Presently, ceftriaxone (Rocephin), cefazolin, and vancomycin are the most frequently dispensed antibiotics in home care. All three drugs have long half-lives which allow for longer dosing intervals (less frequent doses) which increases patient acceptance and compliance in the home. All three drugs are effective for many of the common bacteria or disease states which may require administration of parenteral rather than oral antibiotics. Other antimicrobials which are used less frequently include the antifungals (amphotericin B and fluconazole [Diflucan]), the aminoglycosides (amikacin, gentamicin, and tobramycin), the cephalosporins (cefepime, ceftazidime, cefotetan, cefuroxime, and cefotaxime), penicillin G, ampicillin and ampicillin-sulbactam (Unasyn), nafcillin, clindamycin, and imipenem-cilastatin (Primaxin). Even drugs with short stabilities, such as ampicillin, are dispensed as vials for the patient to mix in the home.

Common diseases treated by home antibiotics are osteomyelitis (bone infection), Lyme disease (a tick-borne infection that makes people weak and tired), cellulitis (an infection of the skin and surrounding tissues), pneumonia and bronchitis (common respiratory diseases), pelvic inflammatory disease, urinary tract infections, endocarditis (infection of the heart), and cystic fibrosis (a childhood respiratory disorder that causes thick mucous secretions in the lung, making the child susceptible to respiratory infections), wound infections including surgical sites, foot ulcers (common in diabetic patients), sepsis (infection in the blood stream), and septic arthritis (infected joints). Many patients are being discharged home to finish their course of antibiotics started in the hospital. For example, a patient may need to receive six weeks of intravenous antibiotics for osteomyelitis. This patient may receive a few days to a week in the hospital and complete the course of treatment at home.

Some patients, including chemotherapy and home total parenteral nutrition (TPN) patients, may need treatment with home IV antibiotics for infections of their intravenous catheter, catheter exit site, or implanted venous access device (e.g., Port-a-Cath). Some immune compromised patients may receive home IV antibiotics for prevention of infections.

Acquired immune deficiency syndrome (AIDS) is a viral infection acquired *only* by transmission of bodily fluids. The virus involved is known as human immunodeficiency virus (HIV). Patients may acquire HIV, but not manifest AIDS for many years later. This disease, for which there is currently no cure, results in a breakdown of the patient's immune system, making the person susceptible to unusual infections (primarily unusual forms of pneumonia, tuberculosis, etc.), which ultimately leads to death. The most common causes of transmission of the virus are shared needles (in IV drug abuse situations) and sex. Health care staff who treat HIV-positive patients (patients with HIV infection) can only acquire the disease if stuck with a needle or object that has the patient's blood on it. Staff are usually trained in the appropriate precautions for handling products contaminated with patients' blood. Staff *cannot* acquire the disease through casual contact with the patient. In most cases, staff are more likely to give the patient an infection, or acquire other infections such as tuberculosis (TB) from the patient, hence the need for the strict use of infection control procedures in this population. These procedures commonly include hand washing, use of specially labeled containers for hazardous wastes, use of gloves, use of sharps containers for used needles and supplies, routine TB testing, and use of specially fitted TB masks. The procedures also require special training on the part of technicians and other staff in home care. Although some experimental treatments are being used to treat HIV infection, most antibiotic therapy is directed at prevention or treating the other infections the patient acquires. The course of AIDS is often prolonged, with the patient getting sicker and needing more medications over time. Because of this length of treatment needed and patients' desire for a decent lifestyle in their remaining days, home is the preferred site for care.

Antiviral Therapy

The predominant group of patients receiving antivirals are AIDS patients, although other immunosuppressed patients (e.g., cancer and transplant patients) may also receive this type of therapy. The predominant viral infections are cytomegalovirus, which affects the eyes and gastrointestinal tract, and herpes, which affects the skin and other tissues. The principal drugs in this group include acyclovir, ganciclovir, and foscarnet; however, new agents are constantly being introduced by the FDA or being used on an experimental basis. Ganciclovir is the only agent in this group considered **cytotoxic** and requiring special handling, such as a cancer chemotherapy agent.

Total Parenteral Nutrition

Total parenteral nutrition (TPN) was the first type of home infusion therapy, but the number of patients receiving home TPN has decreased over the years. This therapy involves providing nutrient solutions containing amino acids (the building blocks of proteins), glucose, or sugar and fats, with electrolytes or salts, vitamins, and essential elements or minerals directly into the right atrium of the heart. The purpose of TPN is to allow patients to receive all the nutrition/food they require to maintain normal body functions and survival. TPN should only be provided when patients cannot eat sufficient food or receive enteral solutions.

The primary reason for home TPN is that patients cannot absorb sufficient nutrients from their intestinal tract. The most common reason they receive home TPN is cancer. Cancer patients may have tumors which prevent nutrients from reaching their intestines and therefore cannot be absorbed or they may be too weak or emaciated (which is also seen with AIDS patients) to eat enough to survive. Other reasons for home TPN include Crohn's disease (an inflammatory disease of the gastrointestinal tract), surgical removal of the intestines, severe diarrhea from various causes, and hyperemesis gravidarum (severe vomiting during pregnancy). Some persons will require TPN for their entire life and some will receive home TPN only until whatever condition or disease has caused their inability to eat has been cured.

Peripheral parenteral nutrition (PPN) has a lower dextrose concentration than TPN because TPN solutions are too concentrated to be infused into peripheral veins without causing severe pain and irritation and possible tissue damage. Because PPN is a short-term therapy which provides most but not all nutrients to sustain life, it is rarely used in home care. TPN products are prescription items that require a large amount of preparation time by the pharmacy technician. Because the solution is infused directly into the patient's heart, perfect aseptic technique is essential. TPN admixtures often require five to ten components and supplemental additives. To improve the accuracy of the compounding of TPN solutions and to decrease the potential of contamination which may lead to an infection in the patient, various compounding devices called *TPN compounders* have been developed. The Accusource Monitoring System is a typical automated TPN compounder with a total nutrient admixture **(Figure 3-1)**. These TPN compounders generally involve a multichannel pump for the amino acids, dextrose, fats, and other additives that is connected to a personal computer. The personal computer helps with TPN admixture calculations and drives the pump. Microcompounding pumps have been developed for the electrolytes and other additives. Microcompounders are not commonly found in home infusion providers, although most of those providers who specialize in the provision of home TPN usually have a TPN compounder. Both of these compounding devices need to be calibrated and cleaned daily.

Enteral Nutrition

Enteral nutrition (EN) solutions are liquid nutrient solutions that are administered by mouth or through a feeding tube directly into the stomach or intestines. Enteral formulas contain all the essential nutrients that a person needs for survival. **Home enteral nutrition (HEN)** is safer than TPN because persons on HEN have fewer and less severe infections and complications than with home TPN. Care of the HEN patient is easier to learn for patients and their families and is less costly in the formulas and supplies and in the time required for the care. Enteral formulas are available in ready-to-use liquids or in powders that need to be reconstituted (usually in a blender). Powders are rarely compounded for the home care setting by the pharmacy because they are usually stable only 24 to 48 hours. Hence the patient is

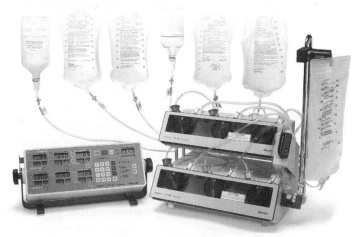

FIGURE 3-1 The Accusource Monitoring System *(Courtesy of Baxter Healthcare Corporation).*

usually responsible for reconstitution. Changes in the types of enteral formulas a person receives are relatively infrequent so the pharmacy will deliver these solutions up to a month in advance. A few enteral nutrition products are prescription items, but most are nonprescription and can be acquired in community pharmacies and discount and grocery stores. The main role of the pharmacy for the HEN patient is the provision of an enteral pump, which is a special pump used to instill the enteral nutrition into the stomach or gut of the patient at a controlled rate. An enteral pump, although similar to the infusion pumps used for intravenous solutions, is usually less costly, easier to operate, and requires fewer supplies **(Figure 3-2)**. The pharmacist may be responsible for monitoring the nutritional care of the patient, but sometimes the pharmacy is only a vendor for the products. Also, many patients on short-term TPN are transitioned from TPN to HEN before being allowed to return to a regular diet.

Pain Management

Many patients with cancer and AIDS have severe pain. Other patients may receive long-term pain therapy for nerve and muscle disorders or short-term pain therapy following surgery. Although most patients are initially prescribed oral pain control, many do not respond because of the level of pain involved. After trying intramuscular or subcutaneous injections or transdermal (skin) patches, patients may receive continuous infusions of pain medications to achieve pain relief. Sometimes the infusions are continuous subcutaneous infusions or continuous intravenous infusions. In severe cases, the pain medications are infused directly into the spinal cord fluid (epidural) or fluid surrounding the brain (intrathecal). In such cases, sterility and products without preservatives are important. Infusions of pain medications usually involve narcotic solutions. Most frequently, the narcotic infusion is administered by an infusion pump, known as a **patient-controlled analgesia (PCA) pump**, that provides a continuous flow of medication and also allows the patient to provide occasional boluses (large doses) of pain medication when the

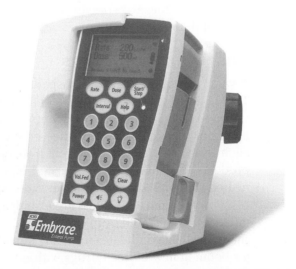

FIGURE 3-2   Enteral pump *(Courtesy of the Ross Products Division of Abbott Laboratories).*

continuous infusion does not provide sufficient relief. The pump controls the medication and bolus dose, the number of boluses, and the frequency that boluses may be given.

Cancer Chemotherapy

Almost any form of cancer chemotherapy can be given to patients at home, although predominantly they receive these products in the doctor's office or ambulatory infusion center. Almost all of these products are cytotoxic and require special labeling and precautions in handling. It is believed that prolonged and repeated exposure to these products may cause genetic defects and cancer. Special preparation techniques are used, including special garments and accessories. Preparation occurs in a class II biological containment hood, also called a **vertical hood**. This hood not only provides a sterile environment, but unlike other hoods, also protects the person working in the hood by containing any airborne product within the confines of the hood. These precautions prevent or minimize exposure to the cytotoxic agents by the technician or pharmacist who prepares them. Special spill kits are used to handle spills of these agents—again to minimize exposure. All staff and patients should be taught the special precautions for these agents. Please note that ganciclovir (an antiviral agent) shares these cytotoxic properties with cancer chemotherapy agents and requires the same special precautions for handling. Even when cancer chemotherapy is not administered in the home, the ancillary treatment of cancer symptoms and the treatment of the side effects of chemotherapy is administered there. Besides receiving home pain medications, TPN, and antibiotics, as previously discussed, these patients may also receive a number of other antinausea drugs, called antiemetic drugs (e.g., metoclopramide), blood products (e.g., erythropoietin, iron dextran, colony stimulating factor), and blood transfusions.

Hydration

Basic intravenous solutions such as normal saline, dextrose in water, Ringer's solution (a sterile solution of sodium chloride, potassium chloride, and calcium chloride used to replenish electrolytes) are given as primary hydration therapy. Hydration therapy is used for such problems as dehydration and hyperemesis (severe prolonged and repeated vomiting in some pregnant women). Regardless of whether it is used as the primary therapy or ancillary therapy, it is important to remember that these are prescription drugs. They must be dispensed and labeled as prescription drugs.

Miscellaneous Drugs

A variety of other drugs are dispensed to patients in the home care setting (see **Table 3-1**). Many of these products are newly developed through biotechnology—they are exact duplicates of products available in the body that are produced in the laboratory by genetically engineered biological organisms, for instance, bacteria such as *E. coli.* These are different from many drugs, which are chemically derived products, because they look or act like products in the body. Genetically engineered drugs tend to have fewer side effects than their chemical counterparts. Also, because most products are exactly like their human body counterparts, they must be administered by injection and cannot be given orally. This attribute makes them excellent candidates for home infusion therapy. There is expected to be a major boom in new biotech drugs within the next few years because a large number of companies are currently in the process of developing new biotech products.

TABLE 3-1

Other Drugs Used in Home Infusion Therapy

Drug	Indication
Methylprednisolone (Solu-Medrol)	Immunosuppressed patients
OKT-3 (Orthoclone)	Transplant patients
Deferoxamine	Hemophilia
Factors VIII, IX	Hemophilia
IV gammaglobulin	Immunosuppressed patients
Alpha-1-antitrypsin	Emphysema
Growth hormone	Growth deficiency in pediatrics
Beta-interferon	Multiple sclerosis
Erythropoietin	Red blood cell deficiency
Iron dextran	Iron deficiency
Colony stimulating factors (G-CSF, Gm-CSF)	White blood cell deficiency
Heparin	Thrombosis
Low molecular weight heparin	Thrombosis
Dobutamine	Severe congestive heart failure
Tocolytic therapy	Prolong or delay birth

Ancillary Drugs

The home infusion therapy nurse will provide a number of drugs to patients to assist in their main therapy. Most common are the line maintenance drugs—low dose heparin and saline—both of which are used to keep catheters from clogging due to blood clots. Low dose urokinase is also used for this purpose, but less frequently because of its higher costs. The pharmacy will also provide external products to clean catheter areas and prevent infections. Alcohol-based wipes and povidone-iodine products (e.g., gel, soap) are used in this capacity. Many nurses are given anaphylaxis kits to have available in case a patient experiences an anaphylactic or severe allergic reaction to the drugs given. These kits will include epinephrine, diphenhydramine, methylprednisolone or another steroid, and other drugs to be given in an emergency based on a standard physician's order or protocol.

Preparing and Dispensing Medications for Home Care

The preparation and dispensing of medications in home infusion therapy requires specialized knowledge and skills. Both pharmacists and technicians from hospital pharmacy practice often take a year before they are comfortable with the nuances and differences of home care practice.

The pharmacist and technician must first be aware of the differences of outpatient versus hospital pharmacy law. In most states, home infusion therapy (even if dispensed by the hospital pharmacy) must adhere to outpatient pharmacy laws and/or special home care regulations, which are different from those of inpatient hospital pharmacy practice. For instance, inpatient pharmacists can often accept verbal orders relayed from a nurse on a floor. In outpatient pharmacy regulations, most states prohibit the pharmacist from accepting the verbal prescription from anyone but the physician directly (or the physician's employee agent), often resulting in the need to call the physician back to verify orders transmitted to the home care nurse. Outpatient prescription records and labeling requirements are different from those of the inpatient ones. Second, the pharmacist and technician must be aware of expanded stability and expiration dates of the products they prepare, beyond those used in hospital pharmacy, including special packaging requirements for delivery. Products must often be packed in coolers or Styrofoam-lined boxes for delivery in extremely hot or cold weather. Third, pharmacists and technicians need to be aware of special preparation techniques based on the infusion pump the patient will be using. For instance, the use of a fluid dispensing pump may be needed in preparing drugs in elastomeric devices because of the tremendous pressure needed to fill them. Knowing that some pumps, such as the CADD pump, require that the drug be filled in a special cassette is an example of such expanded knowledge that is needed. Fourth, these patients (particularly those with HIV infections) have heightened needs for confidentiality, of which home infusion staff must be aware and thus show extra sensitivity. For example, staff should not leave supplies with a neighbor. Lastly, special preparation sterility techniques are required. The American Society of Health System Pharmacists (ASHP) has developed guidelines for the preparation of sterile drug products (ASHP Technical Assistance Bulletin, 1993). Most hospitals prepare drugs at risk level I—the lowest risk level for potential transmission of infections by the prepared drug product; however, home care is at risk level II or III. Hence, special techniques and added precautions must be exercised. In addition to ASHP, the U.S. Pharmacopeia (USP) also has guidelines for the preparation and dispensing of sterile drugs used in the home (Sterile Preparations, Pharmacy Practices, 2000). In some states, adherence to these is required by law and regulation. Many state pharmacy laws also have special requirements for IVs prepared for home use.

Most of these guidelines center around the use of a **class 100 environment** (hood or room) for the preparation of sterile products, which indicates that the environment has less than 100 particles of dust and particulates per cubic meter of air. Sometimes **clean rooms** (specially filtered rooms to create a sterile environment) are required. In all cases, the sterile preparation area must be functionally separate from areas where nonsterile drugs are prepared. Traffic flow in and around the sterile preparation area should be minimized. The area should be free of clutter and particulate-generating materials (e.g., paper, boxes). Work surfaces and equipment should be cleaned daily with an appropriate antiseptic agent, and the floors (and the walls and ceiling if the paint and ceiling tiles are appropriately coated) should be cleaned monthly using a dilute bleach solution. The inside of the hoods should be free of papers and labels. Appropriate aseptic techniques must be used, final products should be visually inspected for particles or signs of deterioration, and more quantitative quality control techniques must be used, such as end-product testing.

Most importantly, the timing of preparation and dispensing is critical in ensuring that the delivery of the product is coordinated with the needs of the patient and nurse who may be administering the product. This is considerably more complex and difficult than meeting the delivery needs of inpatients.

Infusion Devices

Medications can be given by injection into the blood system by three different methods, each of which is determined by the volume to be injected and the time required for administration.

1. **Bolus or IV push** is the administration of a drug by directly pushing the barrel of a syringe to inject its contents directly into the vein. This approach is used for the rapid injection of a drug into the vein and is reserved for situations when speed of response is key and when rate of administration or concentration of the drug will not negatively affect the patient. In home infusion therapy, antibiotics such as cefazolin and ceftriaxone are often administered by the IV push route. Advantages to this route in home care include less time for patient education in self-administration, fewer costly disposable supplies such as IV tubing, and increased patient satisfaction and compliance.

2. **Intermittent injection** is the administration of the drug over 15 minutes to 4 hours (usually 0.5 to 1 hour), after which there is a period of no drug administration followed by cycles of administration/no administration at intervals of 4, 6, 8, 12, 24, or more hours, hence the term "intermittent." Drugs administered by this technique are less concentrated than by IV push with a greater volume of fluid involved (usually 50–250 ml). Intermittent injection results in peak and valley effects in the level of drug in the blood. IV minibags are most commonly used for intermittent infusion, although infusion pumps and elastomeric devices (discussed in the next section) can also be used.

3. **Continuous infusion** is the administration of the drug at a constant rate and allows larger volumes of drug to be instilled over a longer period of time. Drugs administered by this technique are less concentrated than by intermittent infusion with a greater volume of fluid involved (usually 500–3000 ml). Continuous infusion results in a steady and continuous level of drug in the blood.

The preceding definitions assume that the drug is being administered into the blood. Alternate administration methods could be used, such as administering the drug **subcutaneously** (just under the skin), **intramuscularly** (into the muscle), **intrathecally** (into the brain's fluid), **intrasynovially** (into a joint's fluid), **epidurally** (into the spinal fluid), or into any body fluid or cavity. The volume, content, and concentration of the drug, however, may need to be varied. In addition, there are a variety of methods for accomplishing each approach. For instance, the IV push method can be administered manually (by hand), with the use of a syringe pump, or with the use of a bolus button on a PCA infusion pump. The intermittent and continuous infusions can be administered by a slow gravity drip method, by elevating the bag/bottle of drug above the access site (usually on an IV pole), or by using an infusion control device or pump when the accuracy of the infusion rate is important.

The function of an infusion control device, or infusion pump, is to regulate the rate of administration of a drug infusion. Following are several types of infusion control devices.

1. *Nonmechanical rate controller.* This type of device, sometimes called a "dial-calibrated gravity flow regulator," has no mechanical parts. It is not a pump because the main force of the infusion remains gravity. However, the device accurately controls the infusion rate by controlling the size of the device's orifice, through which the drug travels. Examples of this type of device are the Dial-a-Flow and the Rate Regulator.

2. *Nonmechanical external pump.* This type of device also has no mechanical parts. The device exerts a positive infusion force and thus does not rely on gravity to work.
   a. The most common type of nonmechanical external pump is the *disposable elastomeric pump.* The drug is put inside a balloon reservoir (made of an elastomeric material), which expands within a hard plastic container.

Because the pressure to expand the balloon is considerable, a special hand or mechanical pump must be used to fill the contents of this reservoir. The balloon provides the positive pressure. The diameter and length of a segment of tubing controls the rate of infusion. These devices are available in various sizes and flow rates. A specific device is selected based on the medication, amount of fluid, and rate at which the drug should be administered. These devices are small, extremely lightweight, and conveniently fit in the patient's pocket or in a small pouch. The convenience of a throwaway device and the freedom of movement during infusion makes these pumps preferred by most patients. Due to the disposable feature, the cost is often high and many payers will not reimburse for a device that is more costly than other infusion devices. Examples of this type of device **(Figure 3-3)** include the Intermate, ReadyMED, MedFlo II, Eclipse, and Homepump.

    b. Another less common version of this pump is the *spring-controlled pump*. A plastic disc-shaped bag containing the drug is placed between two halves of the pump. A strong spring exerts pressure on a plate next to the bag to create the positive pressure. As in the elastomeric pump, the diameter and length of a segment of tubing controls the rate of infusion. In this version, however, only the plastic bag containing the drug is disposable; the other components are reusable. An example of this type of pump is the Sidekick.

3. *Mechanical peristaltic pump.* This type of pump is a mechanical device that delivers the drug at a controlled rate by means of a system of rocking rollers or alternating motors. Many different manufacturers market these devices, which are useful for delivery of both large and small volumes of drugs as either continuous or intermittent infusions or both continuous and intermittent administration. Mechanical peristaltic pumps are available as pole-mounted pumps (common in many hospitals) or as portable or ambulatory pumps (commonly used in home care). Most of the pole-mounted pumps require electricity to operate, but have battery backup systems. The ambulatory pumps generally

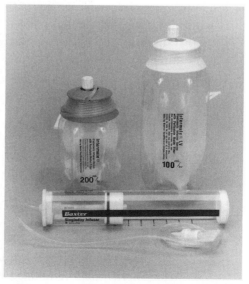

FIGURE 3-3   Elastomeric device *(Courtesy of Baxter Healthcare Corporation).*

use 9-volt batteries, although some have special batteries and electrical charging units. Examples of these ambulatory pumps include the Verifuse, CADD-PCA, and Aim Plus. Some of the more portable versions (e.g., CADD-PCA and WalkMed 350) require the drug be placed in a special plastic reservoir or cassette designed for the pump **(Figure 3-4)**. These devices usually are electronically controlled through visual displays and buttons. Multiple alarm systems prevent complications or alert the patient to pump failure problems. Most are programmed by the pharmacist or nurse before delivery to the patient, although others (e.g., Verifuse) may be programmed remotely via computer commands given over the telephone line using a modem. Also, some versions have multiple channels acting as multiple pumps in one unit and allowing up to four different drugs to be controlled by one pump. Examples of this type of pump include the Provider 6000. Some models are specifically designed for PCA pain management since they allow continuous flow plus bolus dosing, special programming, and lockout features.

Another version of the mechanical peristaltic pump worth noting is the microinfusion pump. This pump allows extremely small volumes of drug to be continuously infused over long periods of time. Although the way the pump works is the same, the regular peristaltic pump would not be able to deliver this small a volume as slowly as a microinfusion pump. This pump is important when highly concentrated solutions need to be administered very slowly to patients. Examples of this type of pump include the WalkMed 440 PIC.

4. *Mechanical piston pump*. This pump is similar to the peristaltic pump except the basis of the pump is a double-acting piston that is electromagnetically operated by means of a battery. As the first system is activated, a magnetic field is created moving the piston and forcing the drug from the piston cylinder. Simultaneously, the second cylinder is recharged and the drug is infused during the next piston cycle. The advantage of this system is miniaturization,

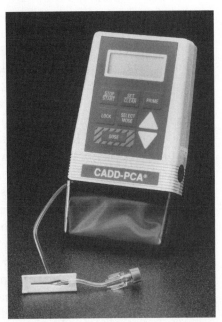

FIGURE 3-4 PCA pump *(Courtesy of Deltec, Inc., St. Paul, Minnesota)*.

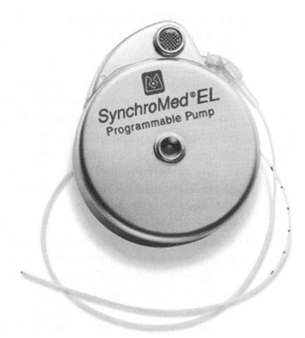

FIGURE 3-5 Implantable pump *(Courtesy of Medtronic, Inc.).*

although several large, nonportable pumps are in this category. An example of this type of pump is the multichannel Lifecare Omniflow 4000.

5. *Mechanical syringe pump.* This pump has been less popular in recent years, although it is extremely cost-effective. It uses regular syringes for the disposable reservoir and operates by several different mechanisms. One type uses an electromotor to drive the plunger at a slow rate. A screw assembly mechanism advances the plunger slowly, usually in pulses created by a motor drive variable. Examples of mechanical syringe pumps are the BARD Mini-infuser and the MS-16.

6. *Implantable pumps.* These pumps are surgically implanted just under the skin of the patient with a catheter entering a vein or other cavity **(Figure 3-5).** Implantable pumps usually work by a mechanical piston system or by means of gas pressure. In this latter type of system, pressure is created by a fluorocarbon vapor liquid mixture that forces against a collapsible diaphragm, discharging the drug through a flow-regulating tube. These pumps contain long-lasting batteries and systems that keep the pump operating continuously for up to 10 years. Implantable pumps have either a fixed flow rate that is set by the manufacturer or the rate is externally programmed using an external electromagnetic wand. The advantage of implantable pumps is they are able to provide extremely small volumes of drug. Because many are implanted intrathecally, the risk of infection is less than other pumps since most require filling only once every 30 to 60 days. The home care nurse fills the pump by injection into the pump chamber through the patient's skin. The disadvantages of these pumps are that they are extremely costly, they must be surgically implanted, and they cannot be shut off, so the internal reservoir must be continually filled with fluid or else serious complications can result. Implanted pumps include the Syncromed and the Infusaid.

Factors in the Selection of an Infusion Device or Pump

The selection of an appropriate infusion device or pump is complex. The pharmacy staff in cooperation with the home health nurse or agency, patient, payor, and others must consider what pump or device is appropriate for each patient. This decision includes factors related to the pump specifications such as flow range and volume; flow accuracy under optimal conditions; flow accuracy with temperature variations, low battery voltage, extended operation, back pressure and negative pressure; flow consistency; occlusion/flow restriction alarm and bolus volume after occlusion (blockage); and audible alarms and visual indicators. Other factors requiring consideration are equally important, such as quality of construction, design, ease of use, manufacturer support, operator's manual, and potential for **free flow** (a dangerous condition in which all of the infusion is accidentally administered in a short period of time). Practical considerations include the amount of time to train the patient, existing staff knowledge of pump operations, time of the infusion, patient's ability to ambulate, and the patient's home environment (e.g., stairs, carpeting).

A variety of devices are available for providing home infusion therapy. It was the advances in pump technology that led to the birth and growth of the home infusion therapy industry. Continuing advances to increase the features and reduce the size and expense of pumps will fuel the home infusion industry during the twenty-first century.

Equipment Management

A major role of the home infusion therapy company is the management of the infusion pumps and equipment provided to patients. This equipment may include IV poles, refrigerators, modems, and special telemonitoring devices (e.g., intrauterine monitors). If the organization is also a provider of home medical equipment, the range will expand even more. Home infusion companies have several responsibilities in this area. First, they are responsible for tracking each piece of equipment, whether it is with a particular patient, in the warehouse, or off-site for maintenance. In the event of a recall, the exact pump can be found. The FDA requires that home care companies accurately track the equipment they provide. Second, they are also responsible for ongoing routine and preventative maintenance of the equipment. Routine cleaning and maintenance should be performed between each patient use and at regular intervals (e.g., annually). Routine maintenance for infusion pumps should include, at a minimum,

1. A visual inspection of the structural integrity of the infusion pump casing and exposed operating parts (e.g., checking for cracks and broken external parts).
2. A check of the functionality of all buttons, switches, displays, and safety alarms. Alarms should be tested by simulating a malfunction to ensure that each alarm works.
3. A check of the battery charge and recharging or replacing it.
4. Determination of the accuracy of the rate at which the pump delivers fluid to ensure that it is within manufacturers' specifications.
5. Any other requirements or recommended procedures specified by the manufacturer in the operating manual for the pump.

A rate accuracy check (sometimes called a volumetric check) is important because it tests the basic function of the pump, which is to infuse solution at a controlled rate. Because reimbursement policies limit the use of infusion pumps to drugs that require a controlled rate of infusion, the accuracy of that rate of infusion becomes more important. All maintenance should be documented. There should also be a mechanism for tracking equipment that requires ongoing routine and preventative maintenance (e.g., annually).

When equipment is received from patients, it should be identified and placed in an area designated for recovered equipment to be cleaned. It should never be mixed with clean, patient-ready equipment. Also, obsolete equipment or equipment that needs maintenance or repair should be identified and separated from patient-ready and dirty equipment, including items not only in the warehouse but also in delivery vehicles. There should be appropriate systems for the delivery and set up of equipment in the patient's home. Finally, there should be a backup system for patients. Usually extra batteries are left with the patient or an extra pump. Extra backup pumps should be available. A 24-hour-a-day "on-call" system or the ability to replace the pump within a few hours, at any time, is also necessary.

Complications of Home Infusion Therapy

The complications of home infusion therapy are no different than hospital-based infusion therapy. Some believe the risk of infection by a serious, or resistant, organism is much less. Pharmacists and nurses often work together to monitor and prevent the complications of infusion therapy in home care. Complications that the provider may encounter include phlebitis, infiltration, sepsis, embolism, allergic reactions, and free flow.

Phlebitis

Phlebitis, the most frequently encountered complication of any infusion therapy, is inflammation at the site of the catheter insertion. If there is a blood clot involved, it is called **thrombophlebitis**. Depending on the situation, this complication has been estimated to occur in 3.5 to 7% of all patients receiving IV medications. Phlebitis can be caused by the drug, irritation by the catheter itself, or by an infection at the catheter site.

Infiltration

Infiltration occurs relatively frequently in patients with peripheral IVs, although it can occur with other types of venous access. The catheter is improperly placed or is dislodged from the vein and the drug is infused into the surrounding tissue rather than into the vein. This complication can be extremely painful, depending on the drug, and extremely serious in cases of infiltration by some cancer chemotherapeutic agents.

Sepsis

Sepsis is an infection in the blood which is a serious complication of infectious phlebitis left untreated. Sepsis is an overwhelming infection of the entire body and can be fatal. Each year it is estimated that 20,000 to 30,000 patients die from catheter-related sepsis.

Embolism

Embolism occurs when particulate matter, most commonly a blood clot, is introduced into the vein. This clot, or **embolus**, will travel through the bloodstream until it enters a blood vessel that is too small for it to flow through and then becomes lodged and eventually stops circulation. Because the tissue downstream of the embolism has its blood supply cut off, it will become oxygen starved and die, usually in the lung. The amount of damage varies but can include death. With the appropriate use of heparin or saline in catheter care, embolism from blood clots can be reduced. Air can also cause embolism. The delivery of air by the infusion pump is an issue that can be prevented.

Allergic Reactions

Allergic reactions may be the second most common cause of complication. The reaction may be mild, represented by a redness or rash, or it may be severe, represented by anaphylactic shock. The latter occludes the airway and results in death if not treated immediately. Patients are most commonly allergic to the drugs given (occurring in about 2% of patients), but more rarely are allergic to the plastic materials in the catheter or containers. Noting allergies in the medication history can often prevent disaster.

Free Flow

Free flow is a complication that results from a malfunction of the pump causing the entire infusion to be delivered into the catheter in an extremely short period of time. Free flow can create a variety of problems depending on the drug and IV solution. For instance, if the product is TPN, the high glucose can cause a diabetic reaction, called hyperglycemia, and insulin may need to be given to the patient. Newer pumps are designed to prevent free flow.

Role of Technicians in Home Infusion Therapy

The role of the technician is more varied and more progressive in home infusion therapy than almost any type of pharmacy. The traditional and key role of the technician in home infusion therapy is in the preparation of sterile products in the IV room, under the supervision of a pharmacist. It is important to note that most states have more stringent requirements for technician supervision by a pharmacist in outpatient and home care settings (e.g., a pharmacist must be physically present within eyesight of the technician at all times). As previously discussed, this requires added knowledge and skills related to home care practice. In pharmacy environments that are more expanded, such as combined with a retail pharmacy, institutional pharmacy, or hospital pharmacy, the technician's role may be more varied and include duties and responsibilities in these other areas as well. Other roles for pharmacy technicians in home infusion therapy include

- driver or delivery representative or coordinator
- warehouse supervisor
- equipment management technician
- patient service representative
- purchasing agent or manager
- billing clerk
- case manager

Driver or Delivery Representative

The driver or delivery representative transports the products to the patient's home and thus must be competent in infusion pump set up, troubleshooting, and the basics of equipment management; proper storage of the products in the home (i.e., which product must go in the refrigerator); infection control procedures; handling of hazardous materials and wastes; confidentiality; advanced directives and responding in emergency situations; identifying patients who may be abused or at nutritional risk; and so forth. It is important to remember that this individual may be the only employee of the home infusion provider who sees and talks to the patient directly. This individual may have to gather information as well as provide information and care to the patient beyond routine delivery services.

Warehouse Supervisor/Technician

The warehouse supervisor/technician is responsible for the coordination and operation of the warehouse and may be responsible for coordinating deliveries, packing medications and supplies for delivery, controlling inventory of drug and supplies, handling returned hazardous materials and wastes, purchasing materials, and managing and maintaining equipment. Sometimes companies have a specially designated equipment management technician who handles the management and maintenance of the pumps, or it may be part of the overall responsibilities of the warehouse supervisor/technician.

Patient Service Representative

The patient service representative is responsible for contacting patients and making sure they have an appropriate inventory of ancillary supplies and medications—in essence, helping the patients coordinate their home inventory of medications and supplies. This individual also serves as the major customer service representative to the patient and may assist in transmitting the patient's desires and requests to other staff in the organization. The patient service representative may also help coordinate deliveries with the warehouse supervisor/technician. This job is less "hands-on" and is generally more of a desk job.

Purchasing Manager

In large organizations, the purchasing manager is responsible for ordering drugs and supplies from wholesalers and manufacturers. This person may also be responsible for negotiating prices and purchasing contracts, and handling drug and product recalls. This responsibility may fall on the warehouse supervisor or pharmacist in smaller organizations.

Billing Clerk/Case Manager

The billing clerk/case manager is responsible for processing bills for home infusion therapy with insurance companies or Medicare carriers (the organizations responsible for paying the bills for Medicare patients). In addition, this individual may be responsible for negotiating prices with insurance company case managers and for verifying a patient's insurance coverage and limits prior to providing care and getting authorization, if needed. This individual may also be responsible for getting initial information from the patient and referral source (physician, hospital, insurance company) to admit the patient to service.

The role of the technician in home infusion therapy can be challenging and varied compared with other practice settings. In addition, it often involves greater latitude for job changes or advancement.

Summary

Home health care is a growing area for health care in the new millennium, and pharmacy practice in this environment is growing with it. Home infusion therapy predominates as a major service in home care that is pharmacy driven. The role of the pharmacist and pharmacy technician in home health care is rich and diverse. Knowledge of new biotech drug therapy, new pump technology, and vascular access devices (catheters) challenges the home infusion therapy practitioner and provides a rewarding career. The constant communication and teamwork involving the patient and health care team that is offered in home care is also professionally rewarding and enhancing. There is little doubt that many pharmacy practitioners will transition into home health care in the coming years, and that home health care will remain an important arena for pharmacy practice in the future.

TEST YOUR KNOWLEDGE

Multiple Choice Questions

1. Home health care as a site for the provision of health care has grown over seventeenfold in the past 34 years and provides services to over
   a. 1.3 million people
   b. 7.2 million people
   c. 10 million people
   d. 17 million people
   e. 31 million people

2. In 1993, home infusion therapy was growing at an annual compounded rate of
   a. 1.4 percent
   b. 7 percent
   c. 13 percent
   d. 38 percent
   e. 156 percent

3. Individuals who are called home health aides are involved in providing which of the following home care services:
   a. home health services
   b. home infusion therapy
   c. home medical equipment
   d. home pharmacy services
   e. personal care and support services

4. Home infusion therapy services involve the provision of home pharmacy services with
   a. home health services
   b. home medical equipment
   c. personal care and support services
   d. clinical respiratory services
   e. occupational therapy

5. The major form of equipment used in home infusion therapy is
   a. oxygen cylinders
   b. ventilators and concentrators
   c. pumps
   d. ostomy supplies
   e. blood glucose monitors

6. Home infusion therapy was made possible through technological improvements in
   a. drugs
   b. syringes
   c. catheters
   d. pumps
   e. sterile environments (e.g., hoods)

7. The types of pharmacies involved in the provision of home infusion therapy include
   a. retail pharmacies
   b. hospital pharmacies
   c. institutional or long-term care pharmacies
   d. HME providers
   e. all of the above

8. The most common form of home infusion therapy is
   a. antibiotics
   b. TPN
   c. pain management
   d. hydration
   e. cancer chemotherapy

9. All of the following are diagnoses for home antibiotic therapy EXCEPT
   a. osteomyelitis
   b. Lyme disease
   c. diabetes
   d. AIDS/HIV infection
   e. sepsis

10. The most complex form of home infusion therapy to compound and admix is
    a. antibiotics
    b. TPN
    c. pain management
    d. hydration
    e. enteral therapy

11. The major differences between pharmaceutical services provided to home care patients and to hospital patients include the following EXCEPT
    a. different pharmacy laws
    b. lack of direct physician involvement
    c. packaging products properly for delivery
    d. expiration dating used
    e. level of sterile technique used

12. The method of pain management in which patients receive a continuous infusion of pain medication and are allowed to periodically bolus themselves on a limited basis is called
    a. pain relief control
    b. patient self-administered therapy
    c. cyclic pain therapy
    d. patient-controlled analgesia
    e. pain self-relief analgesia

13. An example of an elastomeric nonmechanical pump is
    a. Dial-a-Flow
    b. Intermate
    c. Infusaid
    d. CADD-PCA
    e. WalkMed 350

References

ASHP technical assistance bulletin on quality assurance for pharmacy-prepared sterile products. (1993). *American Journal of Hospital Pharmacy, 50,* 2386–2398.

Catania, P. N., & Rosner, M. M. (Eds.). (1994). *Home health care practice* (2nd ed.). Palo Alto, CA: Markets Research.

Conners, R. B., & Winters, R. W. (Eds.). (1995). *Home infusion therapy: Current status and future trends.* Chicago: American Hospital Publishing.

Hicks, W. E. (Ed.). (1999). *Practice standards of ASHP, 1998–99.* Bethesda, MD: American Society of Health-System Pharmacists.

Sterile Preparations-Pharmacy Practice (2000). Chapter 1206 USP 24/NF19.

U.S. Congress, Office of Technology Assessment. *Home drug infusion therapy under Medicare* (OTA-H-509). Washington, DC.

Web Site

National Association for Home Care (NAHC)   www.nahc.org

Long-Term Care

COMPETENCIES

Upon completion of this chapter, the reader should be able to

1. Identify the three different types of long-term care facilities by sponsorship and explain the historical significance of each one.
2. Identify the major source of funding for the long-term care field and describe why the rate structure has such an important effect on services.
3. Differentiate between a service pharmacist and a consultant pharmacist.
4. Describe the supportive role of the pharmacy profession to the nursing profession.

Introduction

Society has struggled with the obligation to care for those who can no longer care for themselves. Historically, this obligation fell to immediate family members or people of the same religion, tribe, or national background. The very earliest institutions had these religious or fraternal philosophies. Individuals not fortunate enough to be taken in by one of these charitable organizations were forced to live on the streets or to seek admission to institutions created by the governing entity (e.g., the county poorhouse, the almshouse, or the local asylum).

In 1965 Congress passed two laws that would have a profound effect on this historical situation. The Medicare and Medicaid programs changed the way America provided for its frail and elderly population. Under Medicare, the elderly were guaranteed health care and, just as importantly, the children of the elderly were absolved of the legal responsibility of paying for care for their parents. The Medicaid legislation guaranteed payment for those deemed to be indigent. Thus a new type of medical welfare was created. With these sound sources of income guaranteed, the growth of institutions willing to provide care mushroomed. Just as social security, a generation earlier, had guaranteed a source of income to the elderly and blind, these two pieces of legislation, commonly referred to as Articles 18 and 19, changed the way care was financed and who would ultimately pay the cost.

Types of Long-Term Care Facilities

The three types of long-term care (LTC) nursing facilities are government sponsored, proprietary, and not-for-profit. The smallest percentage are those institutions run by the government at the federal, state, or county level. These may be veterans' homes and hospitals or county-owned homes run for the benefit of their citizens or some other similar grouping. These are the direct descendents of the poorhouses and almshouses. The second type of nursing home is referred to as proprietary. This type of long-term care facility is by far the most numerous. These are owned by either one person, family, partnership, or corporation. They are run like a business and should make a profit for their investors. The most advanced type of this kind are the large corporations like Beverly Enterprises that are traded on the stock market. The last major type of long-term care facility is referred to as voluntary or not-for-profit. These homes are the direct descendants of those charitable institutions that took care of their own particular followers. The term *voluntary* refers to the composition of the board of directors who serve without personal benefit or inurement, but do so from a wish to benefit society in some fashion. The secondary term, not-for-profit, defines what these institutions do with extra income. Instead of paying a profit or dividend to their shareholders like a for-profit institution rightly does, these facilities are obliged to reinvest the excess revenue back into programs or building improvements for the benefit of the serviced population. These facilities are not obligated to pay taxes and have the ability to raise funds for charitable purposes.

Regulation of Long-Term Care Facilities

All of these facilities are regulated by a massive number of laws, regulations, directives, and government oversight activity. Presently, this micromanagement of the industry shows no signs of lessening. Indeed Centers for Medicare and Medicaid Services (CMS), the former HCFA (Health Care Financing Administration), a federal agency, has taken an extremely active role in driving the survey process which was formally a state function. Predictably, this strict oversight is directly connected to the major role funding from tax dollars plays to fuel this large industry.

Income Sources

Funding for long-term care can be divided conveniently into three categories: (1) tax dollars through Medicare and Medicaid, (2) private pay, and (3) third-party payers.

Medicare and Medicaid

The greatest amount comes from tax dollars through Medicare (e.g., doctors' visits, specialized supplies, limited skilled nursing services) and Medicaid, which is considered the payor of last resort. When all other sources of revenue are exhausted, Medicaid pays for the legitimate costs associated with providing care.

Private Pay

Some revenues come from the private dollar. Basically, the revenue comes from individuals who have assets (wealth) to pay for the care they receive until such time as their resources are low enough to be eligible for Medicaid.

Third-Party Payers

Third-party payers include insurance companies that have sold long-term care policies and, with increasing importance, the managed care companies that negotiate a price for those patients they are obligated to care for. It is most important to note that in the Medicare, Medicaid, and third-party payer programs, payment for services are all-inclusive. The daily rate that is paid must cover all costs of providing adequate care. A large component of providing care is providing the drugs necessary for a quality life situation, which is why long-term care facilities have always been interested in cost containment. Because the drug bill is such an enormous figure—often times equal to the entire annual food budget—long-term care administrators will search out those pharmacists and pharmacy technicians who are dedicated to obtaining the best product and providing the best services for the fewest dollars spent. Although the facility has little effective control over the physician's prescribing habits, pharmacy professionals can often educate physicians about other cost-effective choices.

Population

Who lives in long-term care facilities? For the most part, residents are elderly, ill, and frail individuals who will need increasing care for the rest of their lives. Some specialize in care for children and particular conditions and diseases (e.g., AIDS, cancer). Rehabilitation institutions specialize in short-term stays for those individuals who have the ability to return to life in the larger community. But for the most part, the challenge to those who operate these facilities is the need to balance between rules, regulations, and efficient practice and the great need to recognize these patients as people who need to continue to participate in and enjoy what life has to offer them. Because government policy and funding have created an impetus to admit skilled-care patients, the population of today's nursing home does not resemble the population of 10 or 20 years ago. Today's facilities operate at much the same level of intensity as a small community hospital. Floor staffing in the modern long-term care facility is most commonly a charge nurse, possibly a second nurse on busy shifts, and several certified nursing assistants. Physicians, therapists, and consultants will all be at the facility briefly, but the great bulk of the work is carried out by the nursing staff. A model nursing unit will have 40–45 patients who will receive an average nine prescriptions daily (some drugs given several times a day). This brings the minimum total to about 400 doses daily that the charge nurses must administer (see Appendix A-2).

The challenge for the pharmacist and the pharmacy technician is to communicate the proper information so that the drug achieves the desired effect. Mindful that long-term care facilities care for residents 24 hours a day, 7 days a week, it is probable that many different individuals will perform the same function. The labeling must be clear to avoid misinterpretations by staff members. One popular medication system that is an effective aid for the charge nurse is the unit dose system. In this system, individual pills are packaged in blister packs on a 30-day calendar card so that the nurse can check at any time to verify that the dosage has been given. Nurses are charged with the responsibility of properly administrating medication to the resident. Nurses are taught the "5 rights" of medication administration to ensure accuracy.

1. the right patient
2. the right medication
3. the right dose
4. the right route
5. the right time

The medical staff, in coordination with the pharmacy consultant, should develop policies for an automatic stop order for particular drugs, e.g., antibiotics and steroids. These drugs (and others) require that the patient's drug response be re-evaluated after specific time intervals, e.g., 1 week, 10 days, or 1 month. At that time, a medical decision is made to continue the drug, change the dosage, or discontinue. This is a method to assure the proper monitoring of drug usage.

Any procedure or helpful practice that enables the pharmacist or pharmacy technician to assist the nurse in providing a safe medication delivery system is of great value. The establishment of a policy of automatically discontinuing a medication after a medical staff-approved stop date is another mechanism to ensure potential long-term use of medications be re-evaluated (see Appendix A-1).

Pharmaceutical Personnel in Long-Term Care

There are several types of arrangements by which long-term care facilities obtain the prescriptions for their residents. The larger facilities may have an in-house pharmacy staffed by registered pharmacists and pharmacy technicians. Most small- to moderate-sized facilities, however, find it more feasible to obtain medications from a vendor or service pharmacy. Physicians' orders are transmitted to the off-site store and the filled prescriptions are delivered within a few hours. Drugs are then usually distributed to the units by the RN supervisor and become the responsibility of the charge nurse to properly store and eventually distribute.

The service pharmacies provide an additional service by printing up the MAR (medication administration record) for each resident, which saves the nurse some additional time. They also produce administrative reports as requested. Since prescriptions must be renewed every 30 days in a long-term setting, and since most of the prescriptions are for chronic ailments, it is possible for service pharmacies to forecast, to a large extent, what prescriptions will be repeated. The database maintained by these vendors is increasingly important because the government demands quality assurance activities as well as accurate usage levels for reimbursement issues.

Consultant Pharmacist

Another type of pharmacist is also necessary to the long-term care facility. This is the consultant pharmacist. This person performs the mandated function of monthly reviews of the residents' drug regime and will be watchful for unfavorable interactions or contraindications. This professional reports to the medical director, director of nursing services, administrator, and the attending physicians when a problem has been identified. This consultant also participates in the various committees in the facility such as quality assurance, medical board meetings, and so forth. Occasionally, the consultant pharmacist is asked to provide in-service education for the nursing personnel. The consulting pharmacist is also available to guide the nursing personnel on the safe and legal disposition of unused prescriptions and proper survey preparation.

Emerging Challenges for the Pharmaceutical Professional

Among the growing concerns in the pharmaceutical field, perhaps the most pressing is the sheer number of prescriptions that a typical resident needs. The changing standard of practice in the treatment of heart disease, for example, currently calls for several drugs to be taken to control the condition. This is a typical situation with the treatment of many diseases. This creates a growing problem for the nurse in a long-term care facility. We are rapidly approaching a point, or number, of prescriptions that is so large that it becomes physically difficult, if not impossible, for the elderly resident to ingest. These residents often have difficulty with swallowing or cannot follow instructions. Increasingly, the surveyors are holding nurses to guidelines listed in the package insert. This means that for each prescription, eight ounces of water should be ingested, a certain time must elapse between drugs or between drugs and meals, etc. It falls to the pharmaceutical professionals to develop other means of delivering the medication. Long-acting injections as are used for certain psychotropics, subdermal implants, and transdermal patches are just the beginning of what is the greatest challenge to the delivery of good health care.

Recent legislation now allows hospice providers to serve the dying population in long-term care facilities. Before this change, hospice services were mostly home-based. Hospice personnel have developed expertise in pain management. This area is fast becoming not just a concern for the dying, but for all those patients who could have a better quality of life if they were able to be more comfortable and less controlled by their medical conditions. The pharmaceutical personnel can be of great service by alerting both physician and nursing staff of the benefits of this type of medication.

The complexity of the AIDS/HIV drug regime is another example of "medication overload." The sheer volume of the prescribed treatment plans discourage many patients. The pharmaceutical profession can benefit these patients by improving dosage forms available.

The Future of Pharmacy in Long-Term Care

Pharmacy was probably the first of the caring professions to utilize the computer. Certainly the logic and structure of the pharmacy is well suited to the strengths of the computer. In the future, this natural linkage will become even stronger. With the advent of subacute care in long-term care facilities (with intravenous therapy as well as a completely new spectrum of high-tech drugs), the need for rational administration and continuous quality improvement will grow. As LTC facilities increase their computer sophistication, transmission of information will be rapidly exchanged. On the other end of the spectrum, the healthier elderly will gravitate to the assisted living environment where the direct supervision will be less at a time when the elderly person's ability to comprehend the drug directions may be diminishing. Hence the challenge will be to package, label, and safeguard the product so that it will be used properly for maximum benefit.

Cost containment will increase in importance as the managed health care model becomes more popular. Some experts predict that the managed care model will depend more heavily on drug therapy as opposed to more expensive invasive procedures, while others maintain more drugs will become over-the-counter items, which always presents a challenge for the dispensing pharmacist to be able to predict drug interactions with prescriptions and nonprescription drugs.

Extensive research is being carried out in the use of psychotropic drugs for geriatric (elderly) patients in residences and at home. The target goal is to find effective psychotropic drugs with maximum therapeutic benefits and fewer undesirable side effects, e.g., lethargy, apathy, ataxia, etc. The pharmacist consultant, in conjunction with the medical staff, needs to maintain up-to-date information to provide effective therapy.

Summary

Pharmaceutical care, whether in a community pharmacy, institutional setting, or as part of the growing pharmaceutical clearinghouses, will continue to be a vital service to the care and well-being of the growing elderly population. The challenge will be to provide rational drug therapy that is safe, effective, and affordable.

TEST YOUR KNOWLEDGE

Multiple Choice Questions

1. Legislation that changed the way long-term care was financed was
   a. more individual wealth
   b. Medicare
   c. Medicaid
   d. better social security benefits
   e. both Medicare and Medicaid

2. The newest type of nursing home that was created by this legislation is
   a. voluntary, not-for-profit
   b. governmental
   c. proprietary
   d. hospice
   e. private

3. The most important goal of a long-term care pharmacist is to
   a. fill the prescription as per the doctor's order
   b. write the directions so that no error can be made
   c. help the nursing personnel properly administer the medication by education and support
   d. perform all of the above
   e. perform none of the above

4. Drug regimen reviews on each patient are required
   a. upon admission
   b. upon change of orders
   c. monthly
   d. weekly
   e. never

5. The consultant pharmacist must report errors and discrepancies to
   a. the medical doctor
   b. the director of nursing services
   c. the administrator
   d. all of the above
   e. none of the above

6. Technicians will most probably be responsible for
   a. the packaging of the unit-dose cards
   b. credit on returned drugs
   c. administrative computer duties
   d. all of the above
   e. none of the above

7. Fill in the five "rights" that the nursing personnel follow for proper administration of medications.

   a. _____

   b. _____

   c. _____

   d. _____

   e. _____

8. Managed care companies will probably
   a. use more drug therapy than invasive procedures
   b. become more aggressive in cost-cutting procedures
   c. exercise greater control over doctors' prescribing habits
   d. all of the above
   e. none of the above

9. Elderly populations are not only found in nursing homes, but also
   a. assisted living arrangements
   b. subacute settings
   c. adult day care centers
   d. the community
   e. all of the above

10. To survive in the future, pharmacists and technicians will have to become comfortable with
    a. quality assurance activities
    b. continuous monitoring/risk identification
    c. educational outreach
    d. computerization/information sharing
    e. all of the above

5 Community Pharmacy Practice

COMPETENCIES

Upon completion of this chapter, the reader should be able to

1. Define community pharmacy as a branch of ambulatory care.
2. Discuss the knowledge and skills necessary to practice in the community pharmacy setting.
3. Differentiate between the different practice settings in community pharmacy.
4. Outline the process of preparing a prescription for dispensing.
5. Discuss the role of the pharmacy technician in community pharmacy practice.

Introduction

Community pharmacy is a diverse, dynamic practice environment that is constantly changing. This practice area, which is comprised of several different practice settings, offers many opportunities for the pharmacy practitioner. First and foremost, community pharmacy is a practice environment that requires good people skills and excellent communication because the pharmacy practitioner deals with patients on a daily basis. Pharmacy technicians play a vital role in the community pharmacy, assisting the pharmacist in preparing prescriptions, collecting information from patients, and performing several important non-dispensing functions that will be discussed later in this chapter.

Pharmacists have been at the top of the Gallup poll of most trusted professionals every year, and many people use their community pharmacist as their sole source of health care information. Most people visit their community pharmacy more often than any other health care setting and look to their community pharmacist for information, advice, and counseling. In the community pharmacy, practitioners can recommend a cough and cold remedy in one minute and then help a transplant patient decipher their complex medication regimen in the next minute. Basically, in the community pharmacy, practitioners have to be ready for anything, and every day offers new and exciting opportunities to assist people in improving their health care and quality of life.

Community pharmacy is a branch of ambulatory care practice. **Ambulatory care** simply means that the patients being treated are not hospitalized or institutionalized or that they walk in and out in the same day. Other ambulatory care settings include physicians' offices, clinics, and emergency rooms. Another term for ambulatory care is the outpatient setting. When patients are in the hospital or reside in a long-term care facility, they are referred to as inpatients because they are living, usually temporarily, in the facility. When they are residing at home, they are referred to as outpatients. Community pharmacy is recognized as an outpatient or ambulatory care setting.

There were 2.84 billion prescriptions processed in community pharmacies nationwide in 2000 constituting over 140 billion dollars in sales. That number has increased dramatically over the last few years and is only expected to keep rising. One of the reasons the number of prescriptions is rising is the aging of the population. People are living longer and healthier than ever before. As people age, their requirements for maintenance medications increase and more prescriptions are needed. In addition to the aging of the population, advances in medicine are allowing physicians to treat patients without putting them in the hospital, adding to the numbers of prescriptions processed in the outpatient or community pharmacy setting. More and more medications are available each year, and the more classes of medications discovered, the more prescriptions that will be generated. These factors, along with an increased access to insurance programs, add up to more prescriptions requiring processing in community pharmacies.

Because of the rapid growth in the number of prescriptions, the community pharmacy environment is changing. These changes are necessary to meet the demands of the increasing volume. One change we are witnessing is the increasing role of technology in processing prescriptions. Virtually all community pharmacies utilize computers in the prescription filling process to varying degrees. Besides keeping a computerized patient profile, computers in the pharmacy can be used to screen phone calls and accept refill orders, scan prescriptions to prevent errors, and, in some cases, count the units of medication, fill, and label the vial. Computers are also used to alert the pharmacist to drug interactions and transmit insurance information to a patient's insurance company. In addition to increasing technology, another area that is expanding in community pharmacy is the role of pharmacy technicians. Pharmacists are expanding their role as the drug experts and incorporating more patient care activities into their daily practice. With the increasing complexity of drug regimens, pharmacists need to be spending more time with the patients, counseling and educating them on their disease states and medication therapy. This proves to be a difficult task with the increasing volume of prescriptions we are handling, so technicians in this area are vital to patient care. By performing many of the technical functions in support of the pharmacist, pharmacy technicians are enabling patients to spend more time with the pharmacist, receiving care and information that can help them get the most benefit from their therapy.

Prescription Processing

The primary activity involved in community pharmacy practice is processing prescriptions and delivering them to a patient or caregiver with provision of appropriate drug information. This process remains constant from pharmacy to pharmacy for the most part, with technology and support staff involved in different steps in the process. The process begins when a prescription is presented, either by phone, fax, or in person. The prescription is then entered into the computer and cross-checked with the patients' existing profile. If this is the first time the patients are visiting the pharmacy, additional information needs to be collected from the patients and entered into their record. Once the prescription is entered into the computer, it usually goes on to be processed and filled. Some reasons why it might not progress from this point include lack of refills or authorization for refill, problems with insurance reimbursement, or a clinical problem such as a drug interaction or allergy warning. In all but the last scenario, the pharmacy technician can usually resolve the problem. In the case of a clinical decision, the pharmacist should always be consulted to communicate the problem to the physician and recommend a resolution. Once approved, the prescription is then filled by pulling the drug product from stock, counting the appropriate dosage units or compounding the prescription, placing the product in an appropriate container, and labeling the product. The prescription is then delivered to the patient or caregiver. A pharmacy technician can participate in virtually every step of this process and be a much-welcomed assistant to the pharmacist. However, when a clinical decision needs to be made, such as how to handle an inappropriate dose or drug interaction, the pharmacist is the only person who should ever make those decisions.

Because of the process outlined above, which comprises most of a community pharmacy technician's time, there are certain qualifications that people should possess if they are considering a position as a pharmacy technician in this setting. As was already mentioned, communication and interpersonal skills are a necessity, and potential technicians should pay extraordinary attention to detail because of the nature of their responsibility. Community pharmacies can sometimes be busy, stressful places, and an ability to properly handle these types of situations is crucial. The ability to stay focused among different types of distractions is also necessary. Working in a community pharmacy processing prescriptions also requires knowledge of prescription medications—most importantly their brand and generic names—as well as computer literacy and an understanding of pharmacy billing and third-party (insurance) reimbursement. Many of these skills can be learned through on-the-job training, but formalized training and technician certification programs are making for higher quality personnel.

Types of Community Pharmacies

There are different types of community pharmacies offering varying services to the population they serve. It is helpful to first break down the pharmacies by definition and then discuss the different services each of the types of pharmacies can provide.

Independent pharmacies consist of one to four stores owned and operated by an individual pharmacist or group of individuals. They are not part of a large corporation. They vary greatly in size, volume of prescriptions, and services. Some of the benefits to working for an independent pharmacy would be that there is usually direct access to the owner or main decision-maker, so suggestions can go right to the top. Independent pharmacies are sometimes more likely to specialize in one area of pharmacy, such as surgical supplies or home infusion therapy. These types of services are discussed later in the chapter.

Chain pharmacies also vary in size, volume, and services and can be differentiated from one another based on the setting in which they are housed. Chain drugstores are the most common, and although these stores sell mostly traditional drugstore merchandise, many of them carry a large variety of products. Chain drugstores can be regional, where they only operate stores in one geographical area, or national, with stores spread out all over the country. Examples of national chain drugstores include CVS and Rite-Aid. In addition to chain drugstores, chain pharmacies can be located in supermarkets, and again, be regional or national in scope. Other types of stores that sometimes house chain pharmacies are mass merchandisers like Target, Costco, and K-Mart. So even within chain pharmacy, the settings vary greatly, and the practices can be quite different from place to place.

The services that different types of community pharmacies provide are as diverse as the stores that house them. Usual and customary pharmacy services include prescription processing and basic over-the-counter and general merchandise provision. But the services do not have to end there. Many community pharmacies base the services they provide on the population they serve and the demand in the area they are located.

Surgical Supply

Some community pharmacies provide surgical supplies to patients in their community. This would include durable medical equipment such as knee braces, neck collars, hospital beds, canes, walkers, commodes, and other products. A pharmacy that specializes in durable medical equipment will have a pharmacist and staff that is specially trained to assist patients in choosing the best products, fitting patients for products like braces and orthotic supplies, and obtaining proper reimbursement from insurance providers for these services.

Long-Term Care

Community pharmacies can also provide medications to long-term care facilities in their areas. In addition to providing prescription processing services to the community, they may also have contracts with long-term care facilities to provide their medication for them. Some long-term care facilities, like nursing homes, have their own pharmacies in the building, but many, because of their size or budget, may not. In these cases, the facilities use pharmacies that generally prepare the orders on a daily basis for the inpatients and deliver the medications to the facility. This type of setting combines inpatient and outpatient services into one environment.

Home Infusion

Similar to long-term care provision, some pharmacies provide home care organizations with parenteral medications. These products are prepared in the community pharmacy and then delivered or shipped to the patient's home where a skilled nurse will administer the medication. Home infusion services are discussed in detail in chapter 3 of this textbook.

Specialty Compounding Services

Many community pharmacies across the country specialize in compounding services. Medications that are not readily available in a particular dosage form or in the dose necessary have to be made by a pharmacist. Compounded pharmaceutical products can take the form of oral suspensions or solutions, intravenous admixtures, capsules, topical preparations, or even the unusual, like lollipops. Compounding services are an important part of many community pharmacy services. They are especially useful in special patient populations such as children and veterinary practices. Many times, children will suffer from illnesses that we only have adult medications to treat. In these cases, the medications may only be available as a tablet or capsule or only in a dosage that would far exceed what would be recommended for a child. In these cases, the medication needs to be diluted into a child-appropriate dose and possibly into a dosage form that can be taken by a child who cannot swallow tablets or capsules. In these situations, the pharmacist would prepare a solution or suspension by grinding the available tablets into a powder, adding an appropriate amount of water or other diluent, and then flavoring the preparation to make it palatable. This is just one example of how pharmacists use compounding services to improve the care offered to patients. Veterinary practices also use compounding services on a routine basis. Many veterinarians use human medications to treat their animals. The doses or dosage forms they need are not commercially available. They will then go to a community pharmacy that specializes in compounding veterinary products and use their services to get what they need.

The pharmacy technician offers many different types of services to the compounding pharmacist in the community pharmacy. A technician may be involved in almost any step in the process, from gathering the necessary ingredients to be incorporated to mixing the products together under the supervision of the pharmacist. Some of the skills necessary to participate in compounding services are meticulous attention to detail, properly using equipment necessary to weigh and measure wet and dry ingredients, and knowledge of the metric and apothecary system for weights and measures. Extemporaneous compounding is covered in detail in Chapter 13.

Clinical Services

With the expansion of the pharmacy profession to incorporate more patient care activities into practice, many community pharmacies are offering clinical pharmacy services. Clinical pharmacy has historically been used to describe patient-oriented services in addition to product-oriented services. All pharmacists in the community setting provide clinical services to some degree because any prescription being processed in the pharmacy requires some patient-oriented activity. However, some pharmacies are expanding the types of clinical services they provide and offering a variety of patient education programs, disease-state management services, and medication administration services.

The increasing complexity of many medication therapy regimens requires patients to be well educated about their illnesses and the medications being used to treat them. Pharmacists are an excellent source of this information and many pharmacies offer services to assist patients in managing their illness through patient education. The patient education services offered in community pharmacies usually involve prevalent disease states such as diabetes, asthma, hyperlipidemia, smoking cessation, and hypertension. The pharmacy may offer special counseling sessions with the pharmacist where the patients are taught about their illness, the medications that manage it, and some lifestyle changes they can make to increase their quality of life. This type of program is referred to as **disease state management**. Disease state management is defined as a continuous, coordinated, and evolutionary process that manages and improves the health status of a carefully defined patient population over the entire course of a disease. The patients and pharmacist would meet either on a one-on-one basis or as a group and discuss their disease, monitor their progress, and in many disease management programs, even perform clinical monitoring and make treatment decisions. The results of their regular meetings are usually reported to the patient's physician and the pharmacist is part of that patient's treatment team. Some clinical monitoring that takes place in community pharmacies across the country includes cholesterol testing, blood sugar or diabetes testing, and blood pressure screening and monitoring. These types of services go along with the expansion of pharmacy services to more patient-focused activities.

Another area that many community pharmacists are involved in is immunizations. Over 30 states currently allow pharmacists to administer immunizations, and many community pharmacies have made that a focus of their services. Through a collaborative drug therapy agreement with a physician, a pharmacist is given permission to administer an immunization such as a flu or pneumonia vaccine to patients who meet defined criteria spelled out in the agreement. A **collaborative drug therapy agreement** allows a physician to designate certain responsibilities to a pharmacist. It is a voluntary written agreement between a pharmacist and prescriber that permits expanded authority for the pharmacist, such as the ability to initiate or modify drug therapy or order and perform laboratory tests. It is not limited to the practice of immunizations, and we see these agreements being incorporated into programs for diabetes, cholesterol, and anticoagulant therapy.

Pharmacy technicians can play a vital role in the success of a disease state management program by assisting the pharmacist with the recruitment of patients into the program, managing appointments, maintaining appropriate patient files, and assisting with follow-up. This area of community pharmacy can be especially rewarding because of the impact programs like this can have on a patient's well being.

Summary

In summary, community pharmacy is a diverse, fast-paced environment that requires good interpersonal skills and attention to detail. Pharmacy technicians are becoming an increasingly important part of the expansion of pharmacist services in this area toward patient-focused activities. The role of pharmacy technicians will increase in the future as the volume of prescriptions increases. Community pharmacy can be a tremendously rewarding area of pharmacy practice because practitioners get the opportunity to impact peoples' health care on a daily basis.

TEST YOUR KNOWLEDGE

Multiple Choice Questions

1. Community pharmacy is an example of
   a. inpatient care
   b. ambulatory care
   c. long-term care
   d. acute care

2. There were _____ prescriptions filled in the community pharmacy setting in 2000.
   a. 284,000
   b. 2.84 million
   c. 2.84 billion
   d. 2.84 trillion

3. During the prescription filling process, which of the following activities may a pharmacy technician perform?
   a. taking in the prescription
   b. pulling the product from stock
   c. labeling the prescription container
   d. all of the above

4. A continuous, coordinated, and evolving process that manages and improves the health status of a carefully defined patient population over the entire course of a disease is the definition of which of the following terms:
   a. disease state management
   b. collaborative drug therapy agreement
   c. pharmacy practice
   d. chain pharmacy practice

5. A chain pharmacy is a string of pharmacies that constitutes more than ___ stores owned and operated by the same corporation.
   a. 1
   b. 4
   c. 10
   d. 20

True/False Questions

6. _____ Community pharmacies that specialize in compounding services can further specialize in veterinary medications.

7. _____ A pharmacy technician in the community pharmacy setting should possess good interpersonal skills.

8. _____ A pharmacy technician can make a decision regarding how to handle a drug interaction.

9. _____ A pharmacy technician in the community setting very rarely interacts with the public.

10. _____ The number of prescription processed in the community setting is increasing due to the aging of the population.

References

National Association of Chain Drug Stores, American Pharmacists Association, National Community Pharmacists Association. (1999). *Implementing effective change in meeting the demands of community pharmacy practice in the United States.* Retrieved April 30, 2004, from http://www.nacds.org/user-assets/PDF_files/white_paper_pharmacy.PDF.

Rovers, J. P., Currie, J. D., Hagel, H. P., Mc Donough, R. P., & Sobotka, J. L. (1998). *A practical guide to pharmaceutical care.* Washington, DC: American Pharmaceutical Association.

PART II

The Profession of Pharmacy

Chapter 6: Regulatory Standards in Pharmacy Practice
Chapter 7: Drug Use Control: The Foundation of
            Pharmaceutical Care
Chapter 8: Ethical Considerations for the Pharmacy Technician
Chapter 9: Organizations in Pharmacy

6 Regulatory Standards in Pharmacy Practice

COMPETENCIES

Upon completion of this chapter, the reader should be able to

1. Describe the difference between statutes, rules, regulations, and quasi-legal standards.
2. Identify several federal and state regulatory agencies.
3. Explain the rules, regulations, and reasons for practice standards in health institutions.
4. State the need for the Food, Drug, and Cosmetic Act.
5. Discuss quasi-legal standards that define accepted professional practice.
6. List several requirements of the Controlled Substance Act (CSA).
7. Recognize drugs that fall under regulation of the Controlled Substance Act.
8. State reasons for OSHA regulations.
9. Cite appropriate uses for tax-free alcohol.
10. State several basic components of the Patient's Bill of Rights.

Introduction

Rules and **regulations** are necessary to ensure the orderly and safe functioning of society while protecting and respecting individual prerogatives. No individual or enterprise is without regulation.

Regulations in health care provide for assurance of the safety and welfare of health care recipients, provide for the provision of "minimum standards" of a health care service, and provide standards by which to judge reasonable and prudent practice in a court of law. Additionally, the implementation of new regulations has, overall, a very positive impact on the elevation and expansion of health care services and responsibilities.

Health care institutions are complex entities providing services to every segment of our society. Because of the complexity of hospital services, every department in a health care institution is subject to regulation in some form. The profession of pharmacy—with its direct relationship to the public health, safety, and welfare—is, as such, under the watchful eye of regulatory agencies.

One objective of this chapter is to give the technician an understanding of some federal and state regulatory agencies and the laws, rules, and practice standards affecting institutional pharmacy practice. The other objective is to provide an appreciation of the relationship of these regulatory standards to the specific activities of the pharmacist and the technician in the practice of pharmacy.

Federal and State Statutes

Federal and **state statutes** enacted by a legislative body (Congress or state legislature) outline the conduct of persons or organizations subject to the law. They also enable regulatory agencies to regulate a field pursuant to the mandate of the legislative body.

Two examples of statutes are the federal **Food, Drug, and Cosmetic Act** and the federal **Comprehensive Drug Abuse and Prevention Control Act**.

Rules and Regulations

Rules and regulations are implemental by government agencies at the local, state, and federal levels. For example, regulatory agencies such as the **Food and Drug Administration (FDA)** and the **Drug Enforcement Administration (DEA)** can implement rules and regulations to enforce the Federal Food, Drug and Cosmetic Act and the Comprehensive Drug Abuse and Prevention Control Act, respectively.

Quasi-Legal Standards

Quasi means "similar to." Accepted professional practice standards, standards set by the **Joint Commission on Accreditation of Healthcare Organizations (JCAHO)**, and **U.S. Pharmacopeia (U.S.P.)** guidelines all appear to be "similar to" law, although they are established by semigovernmental or private organizations. These are examples of **quasi-legal standards**—recognized by the federal government and many state governments. They have been sanctioned through statutes and regulations.

Regulatory Agencies and Quasi-Legal Standards

The discussion that follows will illustrate the regulatory agencies' quasi-legal standards and professional practice standards as outlined in the **JCAHO** and **American Society of Health-System Pharmacists (ASHP)** practice standards. To represent the state level, New York regulatory agencies are used as an example.

Federal Versus State Drug-Control Laws

Because federal laws and regulations vary from those of particular states, practicing pharmacists and technicians must learn certain basic rules in order to know where they stand in complying with the law. These rules can be summarized as follows:

1. Pharmacists are equally responsible for compliance with both federal and state laws and respective regulations governing their pharmacy practice.
2. If the federal law or regulation is more stringent than the comparable state law or regulation, or vice versa, the more stringent law or regulation must be followed. In many cases, the state law or regulation is more stringent than its federal counterpart.

State Regulatory Agencies

Every state will have its own unique structure for the regulation of the education, licensing, and discipline of the profession of pharmacy. It should be noted that laws change from state board to state board. For example, some allow technicians to compound IVs, but others do not.

State Board of Pharmacy

In most states, responsibilities of the **state board of pharmacy** are to ensure that the public is well served professionally by pharmacists, and the drugs distributed and dispensed within each state meet standards for purity and potency and are properly labeled.

Other responsibilities include, but are not limited to

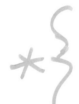

- licensure and registration of pharmacies
- dealing with complaints of professional misconduct
- disciplinary proceedings
- regulations relating to filling and refilling prescriptions (oral and written)
- substitution (generic and therapeutic)
- labeling
- inspections
- poison schedules

Long-Term Care Facilities

A **long-term care facility (LTCF)** is a facility that is planned, staffed, and equipped to accommodate individuals who do not require hospital care, but who are in need of a wide range of medical, nursing, and related health and social services. These services are prescribed by or performed under the supervision of persons licensed to provide such services or care in accordance with the laws of the state in which the facility is located.

The establishment, maintenance, and operation of long-term care facilities is regulated by the states. The majority of the states vest regulatory power in the state health department, although a few states vest power in the state welfare department. Laws and regulations vary from state to state; however, minimum federal standards have been established that must be met in each state. For a long-term care facility to participate in Medicare (Title XVIII) or Medicaid (Title XIX) programs, the facility must comply with the federal Conditions of Participation—Pharmaceutical Services. These regulations are enforced through appropriate state agencies.

The rules governing the handling of pharmaceuticals in long-term care facilities are contained in certain federal laws, the pharmacy practice statutes of the state, and other drug statutes and regulations of the state. Please refer to Chapter 4, "Long-Term Care," for a comprehensive review of this topic.

Federal Regulatory Agencies

An example of a federal regulatory agency is the **Department of the Treasury—Bureau of Alcohol, Tobacco and Firearms**.

Tax-Free Alcohol

In hospitals that use large amounts of **tax-free alcohol**, the hospital pharmacy is normally responsible for procuring, dispensing, storing, and accounting for the tax-free alcohol.

The federal government's philosophy with respect to the use of tax-free ethyl alcohol is that the alcohol will be used only for specific purposes: it will not be used for beverage purposes, is not for resale, and is used in accordance with uses stated on the alcohol permit. If not used according to stated purposes, a tax will be levied for its procurement and subsequent use. In pursuit of this goal, the federal government has devised a number of regulations that mandate specific federal forms be completed by users of tax-free alcohol.

The federal regulatory agency responsible for controlling tax-free alcohol is the Bureau of Alcohol, Tobacco and Firearms (ATF), Department of the Treasury.

Title 27 of the Code of Federal Regulations (CFR) outlines the procedures and the persons eligible for procuring, dispensing, storing, and recovering tax-free alcohol. Tax-free alcohol may be used by hospitals, clinics, blood banks, and sanatoriums for specific research, analysis, or testing.

Tax-free alcohol may be stocked by hospital pharmacies pursuant to applicable federal regulations. These regulations prohibit the sale or distribution of tax-free alcohol to any person off the premises.

There must be adequate storage facilities available for the prevention of unauthorized access to tax-free alcohol. These facilities are to be large enough to hold the maximum quantity of tax-free alcohol that will be on hand at any one time as allowed by the permit.

A bond is required for persons who withdraw more than 1,500 proof gallons of tax-free alcohol per year.

When tax-free alcohol is received, the permittee must account for any loss of contents made in transit. The tax-free alcohol may not be removed from its original packaging unless required by city or state fire code.

Accurate detailed records of all receipts, shipments, usage, destructions, and claims to the withdrawal and use of tax-free alcohol must be kept for easy access by ATF officers. Records must be kept on file for three years after the date of transaction. All records must be kept at the permit premises.

A physical inventory must be made of the tax-free alcohol on a semiannual basis. If a loss is incurred, a claim for allowances must be filed with the regional director.

Taxable Alcohol

Pharmacy departments may have to compound pharmaceutical preparations or fill outpatient prescriptions requiring the use of alcohol, both of which will be used for resale off hospital premises. The alcohol purchased for use in these or similar instances must be alcohol for which appropriate federal and state taxes have been paid. Similarly, alcohol used for beverage purposes within the institution must comply with state law in this regard.

Federal Food, Drug, and Cosmetic Act

The **Federal Food, Drug, and Cosmetic Act** is the federal law (statute) through which the Food and Drug Administration promulgates its rules and regulations. In 1938, Congress enacted the Food, Drug, and Cosmetic Act as an improvement over the initial federal drug control law, the 1906 Pure Food and Drug Act.

The Federal Food, Drug, and Cosmetic Act provides for the following:

- it protects the public health by requiring that only safe, effective, and properly labeled drugs are introduced into commerce
- it protects the public health by requiring the food or cosmetic preparations subject to the act be safe and properly labeled
- it protects the public health by requiring that drugs and medical devices for human use be safe and effective. It requires that drugs and devices conform to government standards or that premarketing government approval for **investigational drugs** or devices be obtained
- it provides that the manufacture, processing, packaging, or holding of drugs comply with "good manufacturing standards" set by the FDA
- it is enforced by the federal Food and Drug Administration (FDA), which promulgates regulations implementing the act
- it requires that over-the-counter (nonprescription) drugs be labeled for safe use by consumers in self-medication
- it provides that dispensing (or distributing) a drug in violation of labeling requirements shall be deemed "misbranding" of the drug
- it provides that a drug containing any filthy, putrid, or decomposed substances or packed or held under unsanitary conditions shall be deemed "adulterated"
- it provides for FDA seizure of drugs misbranded or adulterated

Durham-Humphrey Amendments

The Durham-Humphrey Amendments (enacted in 1951) provided for additional safeguards for prescriptions and over-the-counter drugs.

- They require that prescription drugs (legend drugs) be dispensed to the patient only pursuant to a practitioner's prescription or directly dispensed by the practitioner.
- They provide that the prescription shall ONLY be refilled as authorized by the practitioner.
- They require that oral prescriptions be reduced to writing and filled by the pharmacist.
- They require particular labeling for both prescription drugs and nonprescription drugs.
- They give the FDA broad inspection powers over factories, warehouses, or establishments where drugs, food, devices, or cosmetics are made or processed.
- They provide for limited FDA inspection of pharmacies.
- They provide for the reporting, collection, and evaluation of **adverse drug reactions**.
- They provide for the coordination of **drug recalls** with pharmaceutical manufacturers.
- They provide for the coordination of the **FDA's Drug Quality Reporting System (DQRS)**.

An FDA Regulation

Patient package inserts

FDA regulations require the distribution of **patient package inserts (PPIs)** to each female patient who receives estrogenic or progestational drugs. The PPI, an informational leaflet written for the lay public describing the benefits and risks of each medication, should not be confused with the manufacturer's product insert.

The requirements of the regulation are met if the PPI is provided to the patient before administration of the first dose of the drug and every 30 days thereafter as long as therapy continues. The physician or nurse is responsible for distributing the PPI to inpatients. The pharmacist is responsible for distributing the PPI to outpatients.

Adverse Drug Reactions

One definition of an adverse drug reaction is any unexpected, or unwanted change in a patient's condition that a physician suspects may be due to a drug, that occurs at doses normally used in humans, and that requires treatment, indicates decrease or cessation of therapy with the drug, or suggests that future therapy with the drug carries an unusual risk in the patient.

Most hospitals have a policy that all suspected adverse reactions to drugs will be brought to the attention of the physician, investigated, documented in the patient's chart, and that severe adverse reactions be reported to the FDA.

Upon suspecting that an adverse drug reaction has occurred, the nurse should follow hospital procedure.

1. Alert the prescribing physician that an adverse drug reaction may have occurred and initiate appropriate treatment, if necessary.
2. Record the suspected adverse drug reaction on the patient's chart.
3. Using the hospital's procedures established for reporting an adverse drug reaction, notify the pharmacy of the suspected reaction. The pharmacy will document and review the drug reaction and, where appropriate, pertinent data will be supplied to the Food and Drug Administration on their "MedWatch Form" (Form FDA 3500), as shown in **Figure 6-1**. The back of the form contains advice about voluntary reporting, including important phone numbers, and also functions as a "self-mailer" to the FDA.

Drug Recalls

All drug recalls are voluntary, either manufacturer-initiated or FDA-requested, and the result of reports from the manufacturer or health professionals.

Classes of Recalls

The FDA medical staff determines the health hazard potential of a product (e.g., subpotent labeling errors, adverse drug reactions) and assigns a drug recall classification.

1. *CLASS I*—A situation in which there is a reasonable probability that the use or exposure to a violative product will cause severe adverse health consequences or death.

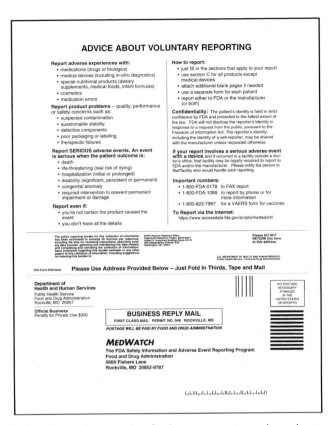

FIGURE 6-1 MedWatch form for voluntary reporting by health professionals of adverse events and product problems *(Courtesy of the Food and Drug Administration)*

2. *CLASS II*—A situation in which the use of or exposure to a violative product may cause temporary or medically reversible adverse health consequences.

3. *CLASS III*—A situation in which the use of or exposure to a violative product is not likely to cause adverse health consequences.

FDA field checks

A post-recall audit is done by the FDA to verify that manufacturers, wholesalers, pharmacists, or customers have received notification about the recall and have taken appropriate action.

Repackaging of Drugs

Repackaging of drugs in a pharmacy requires the use of a repackaging record. A repackaging record must be maintained including the name, strength, lot number, quantity, name of the manufacturer and distributor, the date of repacking, the number of packages prepared, the number of dosage units in each package, the signature of the person performing the repackaging operation, the signature of the pharmacist supervising the repackaging, and such other identifying marks added by the pharmacy for internal record-keeping purposes. In the event of a drug recall, the repackaging record is a source of information referred to in an effort to determine if the recalled drug has been repackaged. Drugs repackaged for in-house use only must have an expiration date 12 months or 50% of the time remaining to the manufacturer's expiration date—whichever is less—from the date of repackaging.

Investigational Drugs

Drugs marketed in this country for either human or animal use must receive the approval of the appropriate bureau of the Food and Drug Administration (FDA). This approval is sought by submission of a New Drug Application (NDA). FDA regulations in effect since 1962 state that to receive approval, the drug must be shown to be both safe and efficacious for the use intended. Since a body of evidence supporting safety and efficacy must be included sometime prior to this approval, the drug must have been actually used by physicians for the conditions named in the application. It is, therefore, during this period of preapproval use that a drug is considered to be investigational. Individuals or pharmaceutical companies desiring to ship or receive drugs that are not covered by an approved NDA must notify the FDA of their intent. This takes the form of an exemption from approved status and is commonly referred to as an investigational new drug (IND) exemption.

Preclinical Studies

Administration of biologically active substances to humans carries unavoidable risk. This risk can be identified through adequate preclinical research. Such research uses animal subjects and establishes the drug's basic biological and toxicological characteristics.

After a new drug's chemical properties and structure are established, biochemical studies are conducted to determine how it is absorbed, distributed, metabolized, and eliminated. This information facilitates projection of animal data to humans and provides the basis for establishing suitable dosage regimens.

Clinical Studies

Phase I studies

Phase I clinical studies represent the first time a new drug is introduced into human beings. Emphasis is now placed on describing the safety of the new agent by defining the pharmacokinetic, toxicological, and pharmacological parameters associated with its use in humans. Such studies should be performed with its use in humans.

Five to twenty participants, with a few serving as a control (placebo) group, are utilized for Phase I clinical trials. Studies with a control group are usually performed double blind (i.e., both the investigator and the subjects are unaware of which drug [active versus placebo] is being administered).

The starting dose of the drug administered to the subjects is less than that expected to show clinical activity; it is also a level considerably below that associated with adverse effects in animals.

In some Phase I studies, drugs known to have high risks associated with their use (e.g., cancer chemotherapeutic agents) are not given to normal subjects but rather to patients who have failed all known effective treatment for the disease.

Phase II studies

Phase II clinical studies are a continuation and expansion of the activities initiated during Phase I trials. Considerable pharmacokinetic and pharmacological data about a drug are generated during Phase I studies, and the relative degree of safety for human use is determined. In Phase II studies, the emphasis shifts toward establishing the activity of the new drug in actual clinical situations. Protocols are developed that specifically address the goals and objectives of the research, the controls and treatments used and the parameters assessed.

Upon completion of Phase II studies, the sponsor reaches a critical crossroad in the life of a new drug. To proceed, evidence of safety and efficacy must be established. Unfavorable outcomes may lead to the abandonment of further research with the drug or to additional preclinical and Phase I work. Favorable results determine whether broad clinical trials are warranted. If an affirmative decision is reached, Phase III studies are initiated.

Phase III studies

The decision to initiate Phase III clinical trials follows a comprehensive review of the preclinical and Phase I and II clinical study results. The need to provide substantial proof of efficacy based on adequate and well controlled clinical investigations is the primary emphasis of Phase III clinical studies. Phase III studies establish the acceptable use of the drug.

Due to the scope of this phase of clinical research, many hundreds of patients may need to be evaluated before meaningful results can be obtained. Therefore, the same study could be conducted in many research centers.

Approval for marketing can be sought only upon completion of all the aforementioned research. To obtain marketing approval, a completed New Drug Application (NDA) form and other materials (e.g., proposed labeling, case report tabulations, drug samples) must be sent to the FDA for review. The response to the NDA submission may be "approved," "approvable" (if certain specified data are provided), or "not approved." The drug may be marketed only upon issuance of an approval letter.

Handling

The procedures for handling investigational drugs are an important part of hospital drug distribution systems. These procedures will naturally reflect the extent to which an institution is involved with research, the resources available, and the particular needs of the hospital. For most community hospitals, the main activities related to investigational drugs will most likely involve the storage, distribution, and control of investigational drugs. In a large teaching hospital, investigational-drug use may result in numerous services and responsibilities requiring full time personnel.

The basic responsibilities of a hospital pharmacy handling investigational drugs are as follows.

- *distribution and control of investigational drugs,* including drug procurement, storage, inventory management, packaging, labeling, distribution, and disposition of unused drugs
- *clinical services,* such as patient education, staff in-service training, and the monitoring and reporting of adverse drug reactions
- *research activities,* such as participating in the preparation or review of research proposals and protocols, assisting in data collection and analysis, serving on the institutional review board (IRB), and conducting pharmaceutical research
- *clinical study management,* which might involve working on study reports to the research sponsor and coordination of study personnel activities

Use of Marketed Products for Unapproved Uses

Physicians often use a marketed drug for an indication or in a manner not in the approved product labeling. In doing so, the physician must have sound evidence or a firm scientific rationale that justifies the intended use. Use of drugs in this fashion is not subject to FDA regulation, nor is it subject to review unless so required by institutional policy as established by a committee within the hospital known as the institutional review board.

Institutional Review Board

The institutional review board (IRB) is a board, committee, or other group formally designated by an institution to review and to approve biomedical research involving human subjects in accordance with FDA regulations. The purpose of IRB review is to ensure that

- risks to subjects are minimized
- risks to subjects are reasonable in relation to anticipated benefits
- informed consent will be sought and documented from each prospective subject or the subject's legally authorized representative
- where appropriate, the research plan makes adequate provision for monitoring the data collected to ensure the safety of subjects
- there are adequate provisions to protect the privacy of subjects and to maintain the confidentiality of data

Orphan Drugs

The Orphan Drug Act was enacted into law in January of 1983. The law provides incentives to drug manufacturers to develop and market **orphan drugs** for the diagnosis, treatment, or prevention of rare diseases or conditions. A rare disease is one that affects less than 200,000 persons in the United States or one that affects more than 200,000 persons, but for which there is no reasonable expectation that the cost of developing the drug and making it available will be recovered from the sales of the drug.

The Controlled Substances Act

The **Controlled Substances Act (CSA)** of 1970 (effective May 1, 1971) is the major federal law regulating the manufacture, distribution, and sale (dispensing/administration) of certain drugs or substances that are subject to or have a potential for abuse or physical or psychological dependence. These drugs or substances are designated as "controlled substances." The law provides a "closed" system for legitimate handlers of these drugs, which should help reduce the widespread diversion of these drugs into the illicit market.

The **Drug Enforcement Administration (DEA)** is the lead federal law-enforcement agency charged with the responsibility for combating controlled substance abuse. The DEA was established July 1, 1973. It resulted from the merger of the Bureau of Narcotics and Dangerous Drugs, the Office for Drug Abuse Law Enforcement, and other drug enforcement agencies. The DEA was established to more effectively combat narcotic and dangerous drug abuse through enforcement and prevention. In carrying out its mission, the DEA cooperates with other federal agencies, foreign as well as state and local governments, private industry, and other organizations.

Schedules of Controlled Drugs

Controlled substances are classified into five schedules.

Schedule I

The controlled substances in Schedule I include drugs having no accepted medical use in the United States and having a high abuse potential. Some of the drugs or substances in Schedule I are heroin, marijuana, LSD, peyote, mescaline, psilocybin, and hallucinogenic substances.

illegal/street drugs

Schedule II

The controlled substances in Schedule II include drugs having a high abuse potential with severe psychic or physical dependence liability. Some drugs in Schedule II are opium, morphine, codeine, hydromorphone (Dilaudid), fentanyl (Duragesic), methadone hydrochloride (Dolophine), meperidine hydrochloride (Demerol), cocaine, and oxymorphone (Numorphan). Also included are amphetamines such as Dexedrine and methylphenidate (Ritalin). Some drugs included in Schedule II are also found in other schedules when combined with other drugs.

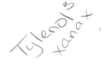
Opium to Ritalin

Schedule III

The controlled substances in Schedule III include drugs having an abuse potential less than those in Schedule I and Schedule II. Some drugs in Schedule III are compounds containing limited quantities of certain narcotic drugs and nonnarcotic drugs (e.g., Tylenol with codeine).

Tylenol 3 xanax

Schedule IV

The controlled substances in Schedule IV include drugs having an abuse potential less than those listed in Schedule III. Some drugs in Schedule IV are phenobarbital, chloral hydrate, chlordiazepoxide (Librium), diazepam (Valium), oxazepam (Serax), clonazepam (Klonopin), lorazepam (Ativan), and Darvocet-N.

Valium

Schedule V

The controlled substances in Schedule V include drugs having an abuse potential less than those listed in Schedule IV. Drugs in Schedule V consist mainly of preparations containing limited quantities of certain narcotic drugs generally for antitussive and antidiarrheal indications.

Robitussin

Some of the drugs in this schedule are Lomotil, Phenergan Expectorant with Codeine, and Robitussin A-C syrup.

Symbols

Each commercial container of a controlled substance is required to have on its label a symbol designating the schedule to which it belongs. The symbols for controlled substances are C-I, C-II, C-III, C-IV, and C-V.

Records and Reports

Hospitals and other health care facilities authorized to purchase, possess, and use controlled substances must keep a number of records both within the pharmacy and at the individual nursing units to ensure appropriate use and control of the controlled substances. These records and reports may include the following:

- an order signed by a person authorized to prescribe, specifying the controlled substance medication for a specifically indicated person
- a separate record at the main point of supply for controlled substances. This shows the type and strength of each drug in the form of a running inventory. The inventory indicates the dates and amounts of such drugs compounded at that site or received from other persons, and their distribution or use.

- a record of authorized requisitions for such drugs for distribution to the nursing units. Such records must indicate receipt at the nursing unit by the signature of a person authorized to control the nursing unit.

With each substock of controlled substances, an administration sheet must be furnished. The administration sheet lists the type of controlled substance, dose, and number of doses furnished to the nursing unit. The sheet also indicates the

- name of the patient
- name of the prescribing physician or practitioner
- date and hour of administration
- quantity of administration
- balance on hand after each administration
- signature of the administering nurse

An entry must be made in the patient's chart to indicate administration of the controlled substance. The entry includes the name of the administering nurse and the date and hour of administration. Partially used doses of controlled substances must have wastage documented by the administering nurse and another nurse as a witness.

Order Forms

Under the Controlled Substances Act, a federal (DEA-222) triplicate order form is necessary for the ordering of controlled substances in Schedules I and II. No charge is made for order forms.

Registration

The Controlled Substances Act exerts its control by way of federal registration of all persons (except the ultimate user or patient) in the legitimate chain of purchase to distribution or dispensing of controlled drugs. Every person or firm who manufactures, distributes, conducts instructional activities with, conducts chemical analysis with, conducts research with, exports, imports, prescribes, administers, or dispenses controlled substances or who proposes to engage in the same must register with the federal Drug Enforcement Administration (DEA) of the U.S. Department of Justice. This registration must be displayed prominently in the pharmacy.

Classification of registrants

Registrants are divided into groups by activities. In New York State for example, hospital pharmacies register as dispensers of nonnarcotic and narcotic Schedule II–V drugs which allows the hospital pharmacy to purchase, stock, and dispense bulk stocks of controlled substances to their respective nursing units. Another example is long-term care facilities that administer controlled drugs to their residents and are registered as "limited dispensers." They can only obtain and administer controlled substances that are patient specific. That is, those controlled drugs that have been dispensed by a licensed pharmacy and have the patient name and directions on the label.

In many cases, state law is much more stringent than federal law and, therefore, will not allow things that would be authorized under federal law. To illustrate, New York State's rules and regulations on controlled substances have several significant differences with federal law and are also stricter than the federal law. For example, all benzodiazepines are classified and handled as Schedule II controlled substances in New York State to curb abuse of these drugs. In addition, all Schedule II controlled substances in New York State require an official NYS prescription, which is purchased from the State of New York.

The dispensing of Schedule II controlled substances requires affixing a warning statement—an orange label containing a caution statement, "Controlled substance, dangerous unless used as directed"—and the federal transfer warning statement, "Caution: Federal law prohibits the transfer of this drug to any person other than the patient for whom it was prescribed."

Lost or Stolen Order Forms

Both federal and state laws have requirements for drug security and regulations for reporting lost or stolen order forms, drug theft, inventory discrepancies, and so forth.

Inventory Requirements

The Controlled Substances Act requires each registrant to make a complete and accurate record of all stocks of controlled substances on hand every two years. The biennial inventory date of May 1 may be changed by the registrant to fit the regular general physical inventory date, so long as the date is no more than six months from the biennial date that would otherwise apply. The inventory must be maintained at the location appearing on the registration certificate for at least two years.

Most pharmacy departments take a physical inventory of their controlled drugs much more frequently than required by federal law. Some departments take controlled drug inventories on a daily basis to ensure appropriate accountability and reconciliation.

Destruction of Controlled Substances

To dispose of any excess or undesired stocks of controlled substances, a pharmacy is required to contact the state Bureau of Controlled Substances or the DEA office for disposal instructions and to request the necessary form(s) [Form 41] from each. The state bureau or the DEA office will advise the registrant of the procedures to be followed.

Federal Hazardous Substances Act

The Federal Hazardous Substances Act was enacted in 1960. The Consumer Product Safety Commission enforces this act.

Poison Prevention Packaging Act

The **Poison Prevention Packaging Act** of 1970 is an amendment to the Hazardous Substances Act. It regulates certain substances defined as household substances. It requires that these substances be packaged for consumer use in "special packaging" that will make it significantly difficult for children under the age of five to open, but not difficult for adults to open.

The "special packaging" is often referred to as "child-resistant containers." One of the main purposes of the act is to extend the special packaging requirements to both prescription and nonprescription drugs.

Special exemptions

Drugs dispensed on prescription or on a medical practitioner's order are exempt from the special packaging requirement if the prescribing doctor specifies a noncomplying container in the order or prescription or if the patient or customer receiving the drug requests a noncomplying container. Another exemption is made for OTC items for elderly or handicapped persons. This exemption allows the manufacturer to market one size of commercial consumer container with noncomplying packaging. But for the exemption to apply, such noncomplying packaging must contain the printed statement, "This package for households without young children." The manufacturer must also market popular sizes of the products in the special packaging as required.

Here is a brief list of substances that are currently required to be sold or dispensed to consumers in the "special packaging."

1. Aspirin-containing preparations must be sold or dispensed to consumers in the special packaging or child-resistant containers.
2. Controlled substances must be dispensed to consumers only in the special packaging or child-resistant containers.
3. Prescription only (legend) drugs for oral human use must be dispensed to the consumer only in child-resistant containers, unless the patient or guardian requests a non-child-resistant container and signs a release to this effect. Exempt from the special packaging requirement for legend drugs is the dispensing of sublingual nitroglycerin preparations and the sublingual and chewable isosorbide dinitrate (Isordil) preparations. These drugs are prescribed for cardiac patients who must be able to quickly get at their medication.

Occupational and Safety Act

The **Occupational and Safety Act of 1970** was passed to assure every working man and woman in the nation safe and healthful working conditions. Under the Occupational and Safety Act, the Occupational Safety and Health Administration (OSHA) was created to decrease hazards in the workplace, to maintain a reporting system for monitoring job-related injuries and illness, and to develop mandatory job safety and health standards.

OSHA is authorized to conduct workplace inspections to determine whether employers are complying with standards issued by the agency for safe and healthful workplaces. Workplace inspections are performed by OSHA compliance safety and health officers.

Hazardous Drugs and Chemicals

An OSHA regulation that became effective May 23, 1988 requires that employees know about the hazards of all chemicals to which they are exposed. The **Hazard Communication Standard (HCS)** is based on the simple concept that employees have both a need and a right to know the hazards and identities of the chemicals to which they are exposed when working. They also need to know what protective measures are available to prevent adverse affects.

The purpose of this standard is to ensure that the hazards of all chemicals are evaluated and that information concerning these hazards is transmitted to affected employees. This transmission of information is to be accomplished by a comprehensive hazard communication program that includes container labeling and other forms of warning, material safety data sheets (MSDS), and employee training.

1. **Written hazard communication program**

Employers must develop and implement a written hazard communications program that includes a list of the hazardous chemicals known to be present by obtaining the appropriate Material Safety Data Sheets (MSDS) for all toxic/hazardous substances in every department.

2. **Material Safety Data Sheets (MSDS)**

   MSDS must be provided by the manufacturer, importer, or distributor for each hazardous chemical used in a workplace. The MSDS must be in English and must contain the following information:

   - chemical and common names
   - if a mixture, chemical and common names of ingredients
   - physical and chemical characteristics, such as flash point and vapor pressure
   - physical hazards, including potential for fire, explosion, and reactivity
   - health hazards, including signs and symptoms of exposure (Both acute and chronic effects should be included.)
   - routes of entry into the body
   - OSHA permissible exposure limit (PEL)
   - precautions for safe handling and use, including hygienic practices and protective measures during repair or maintenance
   - procedures for cleanup of spills and leaks
   - emergency and first aid procedures
   - date of preparation of MSDS or date of latest revision
   - name, address, and telephone number of manufacturer, importer, or distributor.

The employer must maintain copies of the required MSDS for each hazardous chemical in the workplace and ensure that they are readily accessible to employees during each work shift. Alternatively, the employer may subscribe to a service that will fax an MSDS upon request of the employee by calling a toll-free telephone number.

Several OSHA standards and guidelines apply to all departments in health care institutions. Several standards that would relate most specifically to the department of pharmacy and some other departments are as follows.

Air Contaminants

Employees are to be protected from air contaminants and chemicals that could cause injury or illness with regard to potential carcinogenic agents. OSHA published *Guidelines for Cytotoxic (Antineoplastic) Drugs* as a meaningful tool for pharmacy employers and employees handling chemotherapy drugs. The publication provides information regarding personal protective equipment, monitoring, training, and so forth.

Flammable and Combustible Liquids

Appropriate storage containers (e.g., vault, cabinet) must be provided for pharmaceuticals such as alcohol, acetone, and flexible collodion.

Portable fire extinguisher

A sufficient number of portable fire extinguishers of the appropriate type, depending on the hazards in the department, must be available and immediately accessible.

General Concerns about Hazardous Materials

Bulk storage and receiving areas, such as the pharmacy storeroom, must have unobstructed aisles, shelving must be secured to prevent accidental falling, and the area must be kept clean and dry.

Omnibus Budget Reconciliation Act

In adopting the federal **Omnibus Budget Reconciliation Act (OBRA)** of 1990, Congress recognized the escalating pressure to expand social programs, particularly those that impact active older citizens. Senator David Pryor of Arkansas, the principal author and sponsor of OBRA 90, was convinced that the pharmacist could play a key role in improving the effectiveness of drug therapy and reduce the overall costs.

OBRA 90 mandated three main provisions that affect the profession of pharmacy. First, manufacturers are required to provide their best (i.e., lowest) prices, which they offer to any customer, to Medicaid patients by rebating to each state Medicaid agency the differences between their average price and their "best" price. Second, drug-use review and patient counseling is now mandated. Third, the act authorizes government-sponsored demonstration projects relating to the provision of pharmaceutical services.

OBRA 90 requires states to implement regulations consistent with the objectives of the federal law prior to January 1, 1993. In New York State, these regulations took effect on December 4, 1992. States are required to mandate prospective drug-use review, establish programs for retrospective drug-use review, and implement educational programs to rectify problems uncovered as a result of the drug-use review programs. Although the original federal regulations mandate such programs for Medicaid patients only, virtually every state has implemented the new regulations for all patients to ensure all patients a high level of professional service.

Pharmacists are now required to maintain individual patient medication profiles that are expected to contain, in addition to patient demographic information such as name, address, telephone number, gender, and date of birth, information including

- known allergies and drug reactions
- chronic diseases
- a comprehensive list of medications and medical devices and other information appropriate for counseling about the use of prescription and over-the-counter drugs

Utilizing this patient medication profile, pharmacists are expected to conduct a "prospective drug review" before dispensing or delivering a prescription to a patient, or the patient's caregiver, which would include screening for the following:

- therapeutic duplication
- drug-drug interactions, including serious interactions with the over-the-counter drugs
- incorrect drug dosage or duration of treatment
- drug-allergy interactions
- clinical abuse or misuse

After a prospective drug review, regulations require that counseling be provided to each patient and must include all "matters which in the pharmacist's professional judgement, the pharmacist deems significant," including

- the name and description of the medication
- the dosage form, dosage, route of administration, and duration of drug therapy
- special directions and precautions for preparation, administration, and use by the patient

- common severe side effects or adverse effects or interactions that may be encountered, including their avoidance and action required if they occur
- techniques for self-monitoring drug therapy
- proper storage
- prescription refill information
- action to be taken in the event of a missed dose

For mail-order pharmacies, counseling and patient profile information may be conveyed by toll-free, long-distance telephone and is usually patient initiated.

Although any qualified employee of a pharmacy may initiate the offer to have the pharmacist counsel a patient (e.g., technicians), only a pharmacist or a pharmacy intern can provide the actual counseling. The objective of counseling the patient or the patient's caregiver is to improve patient medication compliance, to avoid medication misadventures, and to improve drug therapy outcome.

Pharmacists should note that if a patient refuses to supply information necessary for maintenance of a patient profile, or refuses counseling, the pharmacist may fill a prescription as presented, provided the patient's refusal is documented in the records of the pharmacy. The law, however, expects pharmacists to make a reasonable effort to obtain, record, and maintain the required information. The federal and state regulations use terms such as "counseling," "offer to discuss," and "reasonable effort." These terms mandate that the distribution of printed material and the posting of a sign, alone, do not meet the spirit or letter of the law. Pharmacists are also advised to ensure that physical barriers and other impediments do not exist to discourage patients from receiving professional counseling.

If these regulations are viewed in a positive manner, and as an opportunity to expand and develop a true professional role for pharmacists within the community, the viability of pharmacy practice will be enhanced. The public has need for a readily available professional who will assist them in improving their health care outcomes.

Health Insurance Portability and Accountability Act of 1996

In 1996 Congress passed the **Health Insurance Portability and Accountability Act (HIPAA)**. The purpose of HIPAA is to:

- improve portability and continuity of health insurance coverage in the group and individual markets
- combat waste, fraud, and abuse in health insurance and healthcare delivery
- promote the use of medical savings accounts
- improve access to long-term care services and coverage
- simplify the administration of health insurance.

Within the law, there are two titles: Title I and Title II.

Title I—known as **Insurance Reform**, protects health insurance coverage for workers and their families when they change or lose their jobs.

Title II—known as **Administrative Simplification**, is the act that will fundamentally change the way extended care facilities handle patient information. It aims to improve the efficiency and effectiveness of the American health care system by adopting national standards for electronic healthcare transactions. The law also requires the adoption of security and privacy standards in order to protect personal health care information.

Overview of Administrative Simplification

1.   **Electronic transaction and Code Sets Standards**

The Department of Health and Human Services (HHS) estimates that currently there are about 400 formats for electronic health claims being used in the United States. This lack of standardization minimizes efficiency of the health care system and makes it difficult and expensive to develop and maintain software. HIPAA requires every provider who does business electronically to use standardized health care transaction, code sets, and identifiers. Standardization creates a common language that encourages development of an information system based on the exchange of standard management and financial data using Electronic Data Interchange (EDI). Chain and community pharmacies may use NDC code numbers for the transfer of information relating to drugs and pharmaceuticals.

EDI is an acronym that describes the electronic transfer of information, such as electronic media health claims, in a standard format between trading partners. EDI allows entities within the health care system to exchange medical billing and to process transactions in a manner that is fast and cost effective. EDI can eliminate the inefficiencies of handling paper documents, which will significantly reduce administrative burden, lower operation costs, and improve overall data quality. HHS estimates that these standards will provide a net savings to the health care industry of $29.9 billion over 10 years.

2.   **Health Information Privacy**

Prior to HIPAA, personal health information could be distributed, without either notice or authorization, for reasons that had nothing to do with a patient's medical treatment or health care reimbursement.

Consequently, HIPAA provisions were made to mandate the adoption of Federal privacy protections for individually identifiable health information. These regulations require covered entities to implement standards to protect and guard against the misuse of individually identifiable health information.

Results of Implementation of the HIPAA Regulations

1.   Health plans cannot deny people coverage based on their health status.
2.   Workers who change or lose jobs get better access to health insurance.
3.   Exclusions for preexisting conditions are limited.
4.   Guarantees renewability and availability of health coverage to certain employees and individuals.
5.   Protects and enhances the rights of consumers by providing access to their health information.
6.   Improves the quality of health care in the U.S. by creating national standards to protect an individual's medical records and other personal health information.
7.   Improves the efficiency and effectiveness of health care delivery by providing a national framework for health privacy protection, which will build on the efforts of states, health systems, individual organizations and individuals.

Definitions

HIPAA regulations only apply to "**Covered Entities,**" which include

1.   A health plan that provides or pays the cost of medical care (e.g., group health plan, HMO, Part A or Part B of Medicare, the Medicaid Program)

2. A health care clearinghouse that facilitates procesing of health information from another entity (e.g., billing service)
3. A health care provider of medical or health services (e.g., preventative, diagnostic, or therapeutic services the sale or dispensing of a drug, device or equipment)

Health Information. Any information, whether oral or recorded, including demographic information, created or received by a provider, plan, employer, etc., that relates to the provision of health care of the individual, such that there is a reasonable basis to believe the information can be used to identify the individual.

Protected Health Information (PHI). Prior to HIPAA, personal health information could be distributed for reasons that had nothing to do with a patient's medical treatment or health care reimbursement. PHI includes any individually identifiable health information transmitted or maintained in any form, with the exclusion of employment records.

Business Associate. A person who, on behalf of a covered entity, performs or assists in a function or activity involving the use or disclosure or individually identifiable health information.

Some Preexisting Pharmacy Privacy Requirements

1. **American Pharmaceutical Association Code of Ethics for Pharmacists— Principle 2**
   A pharmacist is dedicated to protecting the dignity of the patient. With a caring attitude and compassionate spirit, a pharmacist focuses on seeing the patient in a private and confidential manner.
2. **American Association of Pharmacy Technicians Code of Ethics for Pharmacy Technicians—Principle VI**
   A pharmacy technician respects and supports the patient's individuality, dignity, and confidentiality.
3. **New York State Regulations on Unprofessional Conduct—Regents Rules 29.1(b)(8)**
   Unprofessional conduct shall include revealing of personally identifiable facts, data, or information obtained in a professional capacity without the prior consent of the patient or client, except as authorized or required by law.

Quasi-Legal Standards

Practice Standards, Guidelines, and Statements

The American Society of Health-System Pharmacists (ASHP) has developed an extensive series of practice standards covering numerous aspects of hospital pharmacy practice. Practice standards provide a basis for evaluation, review, and goal-setting for hospital pharmacy directors and their staff. In a court of law, the practice standards define accepted professional practice and assume quasi-legal status. The system of law in the United States relating to the practice of medicine, pharmacy, and other health professions is based on "reasonable and prudent" practice. Practice standards define reasonable and prudent practice. A practitioner who fails to meet these standards may be found negligent by the courts.

Joint Commission on Accreditation of Healthcare Organizations

No external organization has more impact on hospitals and other health care providers than the **Joint Commission on Accreditation of Healthcare Organizations** or **JCAHO** (often pronounced JAYCO). The Joint Commission was formed in 1951 as a not-for-profit, private, nongovernmental organization by the American College of Physicians, American College of Surgeons, American Hospital Association, American Medical Association, and, later, the American Dental Association for the purpose of improving the quality of health care provided to the public. Representatives of each of the founding organizations sit on the governing body (Board of Commissioners) of the Joint Commission and set policy for the organization. The Joint Commission recently changed its mission to not only address the quality of patient care, but also patient safety.

The Joint Commission achieves its objectives by establishing optimal standards for health care providers. It then evaluates organizations for compliance to these standards through an on-site inspection called a survey and if the organization is in substantial compliance with these standards, awards a certificate of accreditation. To maintain accreditation, the organization is expected to correct any identified deficiencies and be in continuous compliance with the standards. The organization could be surveyed at any time on an unannounced basis, but must be resurveyed at least once every three years.

The Joint Commission currently sets standards and accredits the following types of health care providers:

- hospitals
- home health care agencies
- home infusion providers and home care pharmacies
- long-term care pharmacies
- ambulatory infusion centers
- home medical equipment and home oxygen providers
- ambulatory clinics
- ambulatory surgicenters and office-based surgery practices
- community health centers
- college and prison health care centers
- nursing homes and subacute facilities
- assisted living facilities
- clinical laboratories
- behavioral health organizations
- alcohol and chemical dependency centers
- health care networks
- preferred provider organizations

JCAHO Accreditation

Accreditation is a voluntary process and the organization pays to be surveyed and accredited by the Joint Commission. Currently, over 80% of hospitals are accredited by the Joint Commission, with a significant percentage in other health care areas. So why do health care organizations seek accreditation? First of all, accreditation signifies achievement of a higher level of quality and safety in providing patient care. This brings prestige to the organization, attracting both staff and physicians, and providing a source of pride within the community. Many managed care payors, insurance companies, and HMOs rely on accreditation for determining the quality of a health care provider to contract with. Lack of accreditation can result in the loss of ability to participate in managed care contracts and loss of revenue. Lastly, JCAHO has been granted "deemed status" for participation in Medicare. That means that providers who are accredited by the Joint Commission are "deemed" to meet the Medicare Conditions of Participation and can receive Medicare funding without having separate annual Medicare surveys by state inspectors. Thus, while voluntary in nature, loss of accreditation can not only mean a loss of prestige, but also a loss of significant Medicare and private insurance funding. That is why many hospitals place such importance on preparation for Joint Commission surveys and in adhering to the JCAHO standards.

JCAHO Standards

The Joint Commission provides uniform, nationally recognized standards that define quality patient care. The standards are not minimal, but rather maximally achievable (i.e., not all organizations are in compliance with each standard, but many have demonstrated that they can be). While JCAHO standards require compliance to all applicable laws and regulations, the JCAHO standards often go well above and beyond legal requirements.

In addition, the standards are consensus developed. Expert panels and professional and technical advisory committees representing various professional associations in health care recommend and approve the standards used by JCAHO. Thus, the standards are not developed directly by staff of the Joint Commission, but rather are developed by recognized experts in the health care field. These are published for comment by health care providers before a lengthy approval process and implementation.

The Joint Commission frequently changes its standards, often "raising the bar," in order to get organizations to constantly improve. All standards are published in a Comprehensive Accreditation Manual for each of the major accreditation programs (e.g., hospitals, home care, behavioral health, ambulatory, networks, long-term care), which are provided on a complimentary basis to each organization who has applied for accreditation.

Each standard is a simple sentence followed by an intent statement that more clearly defines the requirements of the standard. In the past, standards and survey processes were designed around departments, such as nursing, pharmacy, dietary, etc. Since 1995, the standards have been designed around important functions performed within the health care organization and involve many departments working together (see **Table 6-1**). Most standards related to pharmacy practice fall within the "Medication Use" section of the "Care of the Patient" chapter. However, other chapters often contain standards pertinent to the pharmacy. For example, the requirement for patient education on medications can be found in the education chapter. In addition, the standards address more than just patient care, addressing good business practices and operations as well. The standards are designed to provide a framework to ask and answer the following questions: Are we doing the right thing? Are we doing the right things well? Is performance being improved as a result? To fulfill the processes that define patient care, collaboration is critical. The design of the Joint Commission standards and survey process allows for effective evaluation of collaboration among health care personnel involved in patient care.

Lastly, the Joint Commission is a strong proponent of the principles of continuous quality improvement or total quality management. This theory requires collection of data to measure, assess, and ultimately improve all processes within

TABLE 6-1   **Functions of Health Care Organizations**

Patient-Focused Functions
- Patient Rights and Organization Ethics
- Assessment of Patients
- Care of Patients
- Education
- Continuum of Care

Organization-Focused Functions
- Improving Organization Performance
- Leadership
- Management of the Environment of Care
- Management of Human Resources
- Management of Information
- Surveillance, Prevention, and Control of Infections

Structures With Functions
- Governance
- Management
- Medical Staff
- Nursing

the organization. Thus decisions are based on data and not gut instinct. The Joint Commission calls this "performance improvement" or "PI." PI forms the cornerstone of all standards. As a result, the performance improvement coordinator of most hospitals is the key person responsible for coordinating the hospital's accreditation preparation efforts.

The JCAHO Survey Process

The survey is conducted by one or more experienced health care professionals who have been specifically trained as surveyors. The size and composition of the survey team and the length of the survey depends on the size of the health care organization being surveyed and the number and types of services provided. Most surveys do not last more than a week, and some last only a day. Most hospitals are surveyed by a physician and a nurse. A hospital administrator may be added to the team if the hospital is large enough. Specialty surveyors in home care, behavioral health, ambulatory, and long-term care may also be assigned. In addition, many surveyors are cross trained to survey multiple areas. Currently, pharmacist surveyors are only used to survey home infusion or home care pharmacy services. The dates of most regular surveys are known well in advance and are posted within the organization.

The Joint Commission surveys and accredits all programs and services for which it has standards. Organizations cannot choose to have only parts of their organization accredited (for example, have their inpatient hospital accredited, but not their emergency room or their home care program). In addition, the Joint Commission surveys all services provided under contract to the organization. Hence, if contracted pharmacy services were utilized by a hospital to replace or supplement its own pharmacy, the contracted pharmacy services would be included in the scope of the survey process as well.

The main components of the survey process include

1. **Opening Conference**

   The survey begins with a brief opening conference with the organization's leadership. The purpose of the conference is to review the agenda, make any last minute adjustments to the agenda, and to explain the upcoming survey process. There is also a daily briefing with leadership each morning to review the findings from the previous day and to set the survey process for the coming day.

2. **Document Review**

   During this session, the surveyors familiarize themselves with the organization while determining if required policies and procedures, protocols, and other documents are present. This review sets the stage for the interactive survey components that follow. Organizations are required to be in compliance not only with applicable laws, regulations, and the Joint Commission standards, but also their own policies and procedures.

3. **Leadership/Strategic Planning Interview**

   Senior leaders of the organization, including administrators, medical staff leaders, nursing leadership, and department heads are interviewed as a group to determine how they work together to perform the various functions of leadership, governance, management, strategic planning, and resource allocation.

4. **Visits to Patient Care Settings**

   This is the longest and most interactive component of the survey process. Surveyors will visit various settings where patient care is performed (for example, in hospitals this may include inpatient units, ambulatory clinics, operating suites, the emergency department, radiology, physician offices). In home care, surveyors actually visit patients in their homes.

   During each visit, patient care provided by staff will be observed. Health care staff, including nurses, pharmacists, social workers, dietitians, and possibly even pharmacy technicians are interviewed along with physicians about their role in patient care and how well they work together. Patients may even be interviewed about the care they receive.

   Staff should be prepared to articulate policy and procedure for patient care activities in which they play a role and the relationship of these policies to the performance of their daily duties. They may be asked to illustrate that role and comment on the care in a specific patient case.

   During a typical inpatient hospital unit visit, the surveyor meets and interviews key unit staff including physicians, nurses, pharmacists, social workers, dietitians, and possibly even pharmacy technicians. Interviews are designed to ensure that caregivers

   - are aware of, and familiar with, established policies and procedures
   - can articulate how those policies and procedures are implemented
   - can relate their execution of policies and procedures to care of individual patients and performance improvement
   - describe how activities for which policies and procedures are not required are performed and meet the intent of the standards

   The surveyor tours the unit to review the overall operation of the unit, including appropriate storage of medications and the availability, placement, and function of life safety equipment and crash carts.

Selected patient records are evaluated in open chart review to determine if patient care documentation is accurate, timely, and complete and that care and services are provided in accordance with the standards. A patient will be selected for interview. Patients will be asked about the care they receive and their caregivers. Related to medication use, patients will be asked if they were informed of their right to pain management, if they were educated about their medications and their use, and if they were told to identify any medication that appeared to look different from what they have received before.

Any hospital with three or more days of survey will receive an "off-shift" visit by a surveyor to evaluate patient care on a particular unit during non-regular shifts (such as 6 PM to 7 AM). Pharmacy services and medication use during these off-shifts will be evaluated.

5. **Function Interviews**

Surveyors devote specific time to meet with a multidisciplinary team of selected caregivers and administrative staff to discuss specific key functions. Although the medication use/nutritional care interview was deleted in 2000, a new medication use interview was added back in 2002. Surveyors will ask specific questions about the medication-use process with emphasis on how the organization has conducted an ongoing proactive evaluation of the medication-use processes used, and what action plans have been developed for improvement in the future.

6. **Record Review**

Surveyors will review a random sample of patient clinical records (for both active and discharged patients) to determine if patient care documentation is accurate, timely, and complete and that care and services are provided in accordance with the standards. In addition, the surveyor will review a random sample of personnel records (including health status files) to determine if the organization is compliant with the management of human resources standards for its staff. Surveyors specifically look for evidence of appropriate hiring process and orientation for new staff and performance appraisals and competence assessment records for existing staff. This activity may be a separate activity or incorporated in other existing activities (e.g., medical record function interview patient care visit). In addition, staff may be asked questions about documentation in these records.

7. **Tour of Facility**

During this activity, the surveyor tours the facility focusing on the management of the environment of care standards, with specific emphasis on having a safe environment including security, fire safety, hazardous material handling, medical equipment use, disaster response, and utility systems. This component often includes a visit to the pharmacy. In addition to evaluating the environment of care standards, surveyors will evaluate inventory control procedures (especially for narcotics) and dispensing and compounding processes, including actual observation of technicians and pharmacists.

8. **Public Information Interview**

The public, including current and former patients as well as current and former employees of the organization, are given an opportunity to meet and talk to the surveyor about any concerns or issues that they have which affect standards compliance. A request for such a meeting must be made prior to the survey. Instructions for requesting such an interview must be posted in the organization for the 30 days prior to the survey. Surveyors gather information during the interview and then investigate any compliance issues afterwards.

9. **Issues Resolution**

   Since many activities on the agenda do not offer the surveyor a lot of time for evaluation, specific time has been set throughout the agenda for the surveyor to go back to any area and evaluate any suspected issues more thoroughly.

10. **Leadership Exit Conference**

    Once the survey process is completed, the surveyors will meet to discuss and integrate their findings. These are inputted into a laptop computer to generate a preliminary report. The report is first discussed with the organization's CEO (chief executive officer) or president and key leadership staff. After which, a leadership exit conference is conducted to formally review the findings of the survey as presented in the preliminary report. Which staff members are in attendance is the decision of the CEO. The organization is given one last opportunity to present evidence of compliance, if not found earlier. In addition, the organization may challenge any finding, and the surveyors will flag it on their report so that it is reviewed by staff at JCAHO headquarters before the final report is generated and sent to the organization. In addition, a summation conference may be held (again, a CEO decision) to briefly summarize the results of the survey to all staff.

It is possible for a technician to be involved in any part of the survey process. However, it is most likely for a pharmacy technician to be involved with the patient care interview process and tour of the pharmacy, if a pharmacy technician is involved at all. It is important for pharmacy technicians to be aware of the pharmacy's policies and procedures and all other hospital policies and procedures that affect them. Technicians should be ready to explain what they do and how they do it. It is extremely important that staff be honest in their answers. Providing false statements or false documentation is treated very seriously. If an organization or any staff member falsifies information on survey, the organization will immediately lose its accreditation and not be able to reapply for a full year. This could result in significant financial hardship to the organization.

JCAHO Survey Results

The surveyor evaluates every standard based on a scoring scale of 1 to 5, with 1 being substantial compliance to the standard, and 5 being no compliance or insufficient compliance to the standard. The exact guidelines for scoring each standard are published in the Comprehensive Accreditation Manual. Any standard with a score of 2 results in what is called a "supplemental recommendation" (formerly called a Type II recommendation). No follow-up is required for supplemental recommendations until the next full survey in three years. Any standard with a score of 3, 4, or 5 results in what is called a "Type I recommendation." Type I recommendations require follow-up by the organization in the form of a written report in anywhere from one to six months following the survey, or another survey is conducted in four to six months. This second survey, known as a focus survey, is one day in length and only looks to see if the organization fixed the problems identified on the full survey. Failure to correct a Type I recommendation after two attempts to do so results in conditional accreditation (a form of probational accreditation). Failure to resolve it after the third attempt results in a loss of accreditation.

Similar standards are grouped into what is called "grid elements." The worst score of any standard within a given grid element determines that grid element's score. A mathematical formula using all grid element scores yields a summary grid score. Accreditation decisions of conditional and nonaccreditation are also based on the number of grid elements with a score of 4 or 5 and the overall summary grid score below a certain number. There are also certain conditions, such as a lack of licensure of key health care professionals, that can automatically result in conditional or nonaccreditation despite other scores.

While the actual final accreditation report of the organization is confidential, the Joint Commission does publicly post a performance report that includes information including the grid element scores, summary grid score, and accreditation decision. These can be found in the quality check section of the Joint Commission's Web site.

The Joint Commission on Accreditation of Healthcare Organizations plays a major role in evaluating health care organizations for their quality of patient care and patient safety. Although accreditation is a voluntary process, it is often critical to the financial success of many types of health care providers, especially hospitals and home care organizations. Most pharmacy technicians will either have no role or a very small role in the accreditation survey process. If technicians are interviewed as part of a survey, they need to be knowledgeable about the policies and procedures that affect their duties and responsibilities and be able to describe their patient care functions to the surveyor. Staff should never hide or lie about anything on the survey, even if they are concerned that it will not make them or their organization look good because there are severe penalties involved. However, there is no need for anxiety or to be scared if a pharmacy technician is asked to be involved. The surveyor is only trying to determine how an organization provides care and is not out to "get" anyone. Surveyors look for bad system problems that are often the fault of no one individual. They do not point out poor performers. The recommendations of surveyors allow the organization to improve its quality and safety of patient care in a nonpunitive environment. For more information about the Joint Commission, check out their web site at www.jcaho.org.

Patient's Bill of Rights

Many states have established a **patient's bill of rights** for hospital and health care institutions. This bill of rights ensures that all patients—inpatients, outpatients, and emergency service patients—are afforded their rights. The hospital's responsibility for assuring patients' rights includes both providing patients with a copy of these rights and providing assistance to patients to understand and exercise their rights.

For the purposes of illustration, the following is an example of the New York State Hospital Patient's Bill of Rights.

Patients' Rights

As a patient in a hospital in New York State, you have the right, consistent with the law, to

- understand and use these rights. If for any reason you do not understand or you need help, the hospital must provide assistance, including an interpreter.
- receive treatments without discrimination as to race, color, religion, sex, national origin, disability, sexual orientation, or source of payment
- receive considerate and respectful care in a clean and safe environment free of unnecessary restraints
- receive emergency care if you need it
- be informed of the name and position of the doctor who will be in charge of your care in the hospital

- know the names, positions, and functions of any hospital staff involved in your care and refuse their treatment, examination, or observation
- a no-smoking room
- receive complete information about your diagnosis, treatment, and prognosis
- receive all the information that you need to give informed consent for any proposed procedure or treatment. This information shall include the possible risks and benefits of the procedure or treatment.
- receive all the information you need to give informed consent for an order not to resuscitate. You also have the right to designate an individual to give this consent for you if you are too ill to do so. If you would like additional information, please ask for a copy of the pamphlet "Do Not Resuscitate Orders—A Guide for Patients and Families."
- refuse treatment and be told what effect this may have on your health
- refuse to take part in research. In deciding whether or not to participate, you have the right to a full explanation.
- privacy while in the hospital and confidentiality of all information and records regarding your care
- participate in all decisions about your treatment and discharge from the hospital. The hospital must provide you with a written discharge plan and written description of how you can appeal your discharge.
- review your medical record without charge. You may obtain a copy of your medical record for which the hospital can charge a reasonable fee. You cannot be denied a copy solely because you cannot afford to pay.
- receive an itemized bill and explanation of all charges
- complain without fear of reprisals about the care and services you are receiving and to have the hospital respond to you and, if you request it, provide a written response. If you are not satisfied with the hospital's response, you can complain to the New York State Department of Health. The hospital must provide you with the health department's telephone number.
- Authorize those family members and other adults who will be given priority to visit consistent with your ability to receive visitors
- make known your wishes in regard to anatomical gifts. You may document your wishes in your health care proxy or on a donor card, available from the hospital.

It is incumbent upon health care workers to be familiar with the bill of rights and to ensure compliance with it.

Summary

There are numerous statutes, rules, regulations, and quasi-legal standards of practice that regulate the pharmacy profession in institutional settings. In many instances, they are minimum standards and requirements that have been established to protect the patient and to ensure safe and effective drug therapy. Pharmacists and technicians should be familiar with and ensure compliance with these standards in their daily activities and responsibilities.

TEST YOUR KNOWLEDGE

Multiple Choice Questions

1. A patient package insert is required to be given to all patients who are taking
   a. steroids
   b. analgesics
   c. estrogenic drugs
   d. vaccines
   e. all of the above

2. Which of the following is considered a controlled substance?
   a. Demerol
   b. morphine
   c. Valium
   d. Phenergan expectorant with codeine
   e. all of the above

3. Regulations affecting pharmacy practice encompass
   a. federal and state statutes
   b. state rules and regulations
   c. CSA regulations
   d. JCAHO standards
   e. all of the above

4. Which of the following is not an approved use of tax-free alcohol?
   a. educational organizations for scientific use
   b. hospitals for medical use
   c. laboratory use for scientific research
   d. beverage purposes
   e. all of the above

5. The Food, Drug and Cosmetic Act encompasses which of the following?
   a. protection of public health
   b. refill authorization of prescription drugs
   c. collection of adverse drug reaction reports
   d. over-the-counter drugs' labeling requirements for safe consumer use
   e. all of the above

   Under Durham-Humphrey Amend.

6. Controlled substances are required by federal law to have appropriate safeguards with their use. Which of the following is not an issue?
   a. inventory requirements
   b. dispensing records and reports
   c. administration of records and reports
   d. storage
   e. patient consent

7. Adverse drug reactions should be reported to the FDA for
   a. documentation
   b. revision of prescribing information
   c. possible drug recall
   d. a possible warning statement
   e. all of the above

8. A Class I recall does not include
   a. voluntary manufacturer initiation
   b. possibility of severe health consequences
   c. FDA initiation
   d. assignment of the drug recall classification by the FDA
   e. any of the above

9. The intent of the Occupational Safety and Health Administration (OSHA) is
    a. to monitor job-related injuries
    b. to develop job safety and health standards
    c. to conduct workplace inspections
    d. to ensure a safe and healthful workplace
    e. all of the above

10. Pharmacy practice standards, guidelines, and statements
    a. define reasonable and prudent practice
    b. establish minimum standards for the profession
    c. are established to protect the patient
    d. ensure safe and effective drug therapy
    e. accomplish all of the above

True/False Questions

11. ___T___ Regulatory agencies stipulate similar goals for pharmaceutical services of both long-term care facilities and hospitals.

12. ___T___ The Poison Prevention Packaging Act of 1970 requires certain substances to be packaged for consumer use in "child-resistant containers."

13. ___T___ The pharmacy standards of the Joint Commission on Accreditation of Healthcare Organizations (JCAHO) provide a quasi-legal standard of practice for the profession.

References

American Society of Health-System Pharmacists. (2003). *Practice standards of the American Society of Health-System Pharmacists.* Bethesda, MD: Author.

Joint Commission of Accreditation of Healthcare Organizations. (2002). *Comprehensive accreditation manual for hospitals.* Oakbrook Terrace, IL: Author.

N.Y.S. Department of Health. Vol. A., chap. III, "Administrative Rules and Regulations," subchapter J, "Controlled Substances," part 80, "Rules and Regulations on Controlled Substances."

University of the State of New York, the New York State Education Department, and the New York State Board of Pharmacy. *Pharmacy Guide to Practice.* Albany, NY.

Relevant Federal Statutes and Regulations

Statutes

Alcohol Tax Law. 26 U.S.C. §§5214, 5217.

Controlled Substances Act of 1970. 21 U.S.C. §§301–392.

Federal Food, Drug, and Cosmetic Act. 21 U.S.C. §§301–392.

Health Maintenance Organization Act of 1973. U.S. Statutes 914.

Narcotic Addict Treatment Act of 1974. U.S. Statutes at Large 124.

Poison Prevention Packaging Act of 1970. U.S. Statutes at Large 1670.

Social Security Amendments of 1965 (Medicare and Medicaid). U.S. Statutes at Large 286.

Regulations

Consumer Product Safety Commission (Poison Prevention Packaging Act). 16 C.F.R. §§1700-1704.

Drug Enforcement Administration. 21 C.F.R. §§1301-1316.

Food and Drug Administration, 21 C.F.R. §§1-1230.

Internal Revenue Service (Alcohol Tax Law). 26 C.F.R. §§213.1-213.176.

Social Security Administration (Medicare); Health Care Financing Administration (Medicaid). Hospitals–20 C.F.R. §405; Skilled Nursing Facilities–20 C.F.R. §405.

Drug Use Control: The Foundation of Pharmaceutical Care

COMPETENCIES

Upon completion of this chapter, the reader should be able to

1. Describe the drug use process.
2. Explain the importance of control in the drug use process.
3. Explain the role of the pharmacist in the drug use process.
4. Explain the role of the pharmacy technician in the drug use process.
5. State the mission of pharmacy practice.
6. Explain pharmaceutical care.
7. Discuss trends in the drug use process and how these trends may affect the roles of the pharmacist and pharmacy technician.

Introduction

Once a drug is approved for use in the United States, a defined process is used to distribute the drug product and make it available for use. This process is organized, complex, and controlled and is called the **drug use process**. Pharmacists and pharmacy technicians are intimately involved in the drug use process, and they are responsible for controlling parts of the process so the drugs are used safely and effectively and not diverted into the wrong hands.

This chapter describes how drugs make their way to the patient after being made by the manufacturer. It will begin with an overview of drug distribution, the self-use of medication, the prescribing, dispensing, and administrating of prescription only medication, and what it means to provide quality drug therapy. The primary focus is on control of the drug use process and how pharmacists and pharmacy technicians exert that control. Lastly, some current issues in the drug use process will be cited.

The Drug Use Process

The drug use process is complex. The drug use process is the system of manufacturing, purchasing, distributing, storing, prescribing, preparing, dispensing, administering, using, controlling, and monitoring drugs and their effects and outcomes (**Figure 7-1**). In short, it is the process of getting a drug to its eventual destination safely, securely, and effectively.

Pharmacy technicians spend most of their time in the buying, storing, preparing, dispensing, and control parts of this process. However, it is important for them to understand the entire drug use process and do what they can to add appropriate control as needed.

Drug Distribution

The United States has the most complex, yet the most efficient, drug distribution system in the world. Automation such as bar coding, computerized inventories, and automated information systems keep the products flowing. As drugs flow through the distribution system, they increase in value.

Drug manufacturers, wholesalers, and retailers are the major firms responsible for the supply and distribution of medication in the United States. **Drug manufacturers** develop and produce the pharmaceutical products. **Drug wholesalers** deliver medication, medical devices and appliances, health and beauty aids, and other products to pharmacies and, with the exception of prescription drugs, to other retailers. **Retailers** (like community pharmacies) deliver these products to the patient.

The Drugs

There are four types of medication: (1) prescription drugs, (2) controlled substances, (3) over-the-counter medication (OTC), and (4) investigational drugs.

Prescription medication

Prescription medication is only made available to the patients when the pharmacist receives a legal prescription from a licensed prescriber. Prescription medication is sometimes called **legend medication.** It is labeled with the Food and Drug Administration's (FDA) required legend, "Caution: Federal law restricts using this medication without a prescription." The FDA has changed the legend to "Rx only" to free up space on the label for other important information that may help decrease errors in use by the patient.

Controlled substances

Controlled substances are also "prescription only products" and are drugs classified by the U.S. Drug Enforcement Agency (DEA) as being addictive or having potential for misuse. These drugs have varying levels of control on their distribution and use based on the drug's addiction liability and potential for abuse. The Comprehensive Drug Abuse Prevention and Control Act of 1970 placed controlled substances into five schedules.

Schedule I. The drug or substance has a high potential for abuse, no currently accepted medical use in treatment in the United States, and there is lack of safety for use of the drug or other substance under medical supervision. Examples of drugs in Schedule I are marijuana, heroin, and LSD (lysergic acid diethylamide).

Schedule II. The drug or other substance has a high potential for abuse, is currently accepted for medical use in treatment in the United States, or has a currently

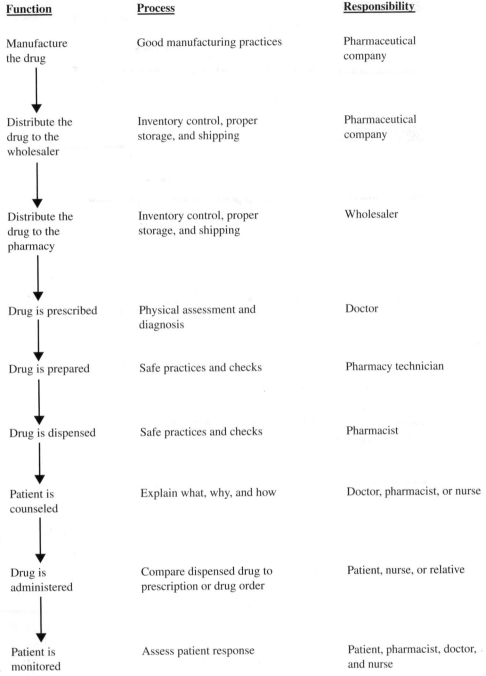

Function	Process	Responsibility
Manufacture the drug	Good manufacturing practices	Pharmaceutical company
Distribute the drug to the wholesaler	Inventory control, proper storage, and shipping	Pharmaceutical company
Distribute the drug to the pharmacy	Inventory control, proper storage, and shipping	Wholesaler
Drug is prescribed	Physical assessment and diagnosis	Doctor
Drug is prepared	Safe practices and checks	Pharmacy technician
Drug is dispensed	Safe practices and checks	Pharmacist
Patient is counseled	Explain what, why, and how	Doctor, pharmacist, or nurse
Drug is administered	Compare dispensed drug to prescription or drug order	Patient, nurse, or relative
Patient is monitored	Assess patient response	Patient, pharmacist, doctor, and nurse

FIGURE 7-1   An Overview of the Drug Use Process.

accepted medical use with severe restrictions. Abuse of the drug or other substance may lead to severe psychological or physical dependence. Examples of drugs in Schedule II are morphine, cocaine, and methadone.

Schedule III. The drug or other substance has a potential for abuse less than the drugs or other substances in schedules I and II, and has a currently accepted medical use in treatment in the United States. Abuse of the drug or other substance may lead to moderate to low physical dependence. Examples of drugs in Schedule III are barbiturates, amphetamines, and codeine.

Schedule IV. The drug or other substance has a low potential for abuse relative to the drugs and other substances in Schedule III and has a currently accepted medical use in treatment in the United States. Abuse of the drug or other substance may lead to limited physical dependence relative to the drugs or other substances in schedule III. Examples of drugs in Schedule IV are stimulants other than amphetamine, tranquilizers such as chlordiazepoxide (like Librium), and diazepam (like Valium).

Schedule V. The drug or other substance has a low potential for abuse relative to the drugs and other substances in schedule IV and has a currently accepted medical use in treatment in the United States. Abuse of the drug or other substance may lead to limited physical or psychological dependence relative to the drugs and other substances in schedule IV. Examples of drugs in Schedule V include codeine when mixed with other ingredients to make a cough syrup and small amounts of opium when mixed with other medicinal ingredients.

Over-the-counter (OTC) drugs

Over-the-counter (OTC) drugs can be sold without a prescription. Some of these drugs may have started out as prescription drugs and converted to OTC status after being found safe. Some OTCs are like prescription only drug products, but have a less active ingredient. Patients seeking an OTC medication for a health problem present a good opportunity for pharmacists to guide and help patients.

Investigational drugs

Investigational drugs are drugs that are being researched and are not yet approved by the FDA for marketing. They are also defined as drugs labeled with the legend, "Caution: New drug, limited by Federal Law to investigational use."

Drugs must travel safely and efficiently from the manufacturer to the pharmacy (all drugs), the doctor (all drugs), nonpharmacy retailer (OTCs), or the researcher (prescription and investigational drugs).

Distribution of Drugs from Pharmaceutical Manufacturers

Most of the pharmaceutical products made by manufacturers go directly to drug wholesalers and to other major distribution centers. Pharmaceutical companies also deliver their products to distribution centers set up by chain pharmacies (e.g., CVS, Rite Aid, Walgreen's), mass merchandisers (e.g., Kmart, Wal-Mart), and grocery store chains that have pharmacies (e.g., Kroger's, Publix).

Although some hospitals can buy directly from the manufacturer, most buy their medication through an arrangement called **group purchasing**. Most hospitals are part of a group of hospitals (e.g., the Catholic Hospital Association, the University Hospital Consortium, the Voluntary Hospitals of America). Pharmaceutical companies ship large quantities of drugs to the buying group warehouses of these hospital groups. The distribution can be similar for most managed care organizations (e.g., Aetna, Cigna, Kaiser Permanente, Prudential).

Distribution of Drugs from Drug Wholesalers

The basic role of the drug wholesaler is to ensure the smooth, safe, and efficient distribution of products to retailers, like community pharmacies (independent, chain, and grocery store), mass merchandisers, hospitals, managed care organizations, and mail-order pharmacies. At the wholesaler, large pallets of drugs delivered from the manufacturer are broken down into smaller units for distribution to pharmacies.

Drug wholesalers (e.g., Amerisource, Bergen Brunswig, Cardinal, McKesson) store products in strategic geographic locations so they can quickly send the products to pharmacies. The Healthcare Distribution Management Association (HDMA) estimates there are 60 wholesale corporations that run 225 distribution centers throughout the United States.

Drug wholesalers are licensed in the state they are located and in the states where they do business. Since most handle controlled substances, they must also have a Drug Enforcement Agency (DEA) license. They are required to adhere to strict storage and handling requirements. They must also ensure the integrity of the medications they deliver. Thus, temperature and humidity must be controlled. They must also protect against diversion (theft of a product).

Drug wholesalers deliver more than 13,000 different pharmaceuticals and biologics and over 15,000 over-the-counter and herbal products, health and beauty aids, medical and hospital supplies, durable medical equipment, and home health care items to 130,000 customers in health care.

Self-Care and the Role of Over-the-Counter Medication

It is important for pharmacists and pharmacy technicians to understand illness and the patient's reaction to it. Seldom do people go to a doctor when they get sick, at least not right away. Most see how they are feeling and how the illness progresses. Some will deny they are ill. Some will seek the advice of family or friends. Still others will take control and seek out as much information as they can about their problem.

Self-Care

People taking a more active role in their health care form a new generation of patients. Documentation of increased interest in self-care is witnessed by the many self-help books, TV programs, newspaper articles, and talk shows covering the topic.

It is difficult to determine what spawned this self-care revolution. However, one reason is obvious—consumers are increasingly self-medicating with nonprescription drugs. The Nonprescription Drug Manufacturers Association has surveyed many consumers to learn about their attitudes about this practice.

- Almost 7 out of 10 consumers prefer to fight symptoms without taking medication, if possible.
- Among consumers, 85% believe it is important to have access to nonprescription medication.
- About 9 out of 10 consumers realize they should take medication only when necessary.
- Of consumers who ended the use of their nonprescription medication, 90% did so because their medical problem or symptoms resolved.
- Even though a medication may be available without a prescription, almost 95% of consumers agreed that care should be taken when using it.
- Nearly 93% of consumers report that they read instructions before taking a nonprescription medication for the first time.

Over-the-Counter (OTC) Medication

Some ill patients, and those who experience a health problem, will find their way to a pharmacy to browse the over-the-counter (OTC) aisle for a cure. Many will try reading the labels of various OTC medications to see if the medication will cure what ails them. Pharmacy technicians should watch for this and alert the pharmacist when they see a patient in the OTC area needing help.

It is fortunate there is a system of self-medication in the United States and that OTC medication can be found everywhere—drugstores, convenience stores, supermarkets, and mass merchandisers. If it were not for this allowance, we would need many more doctors and health care facilities. A recent survey on patient satisfaction with pharmacy services found that patients' highest awareness of OTCs was for cold cures, vitamins, and dental products and that satisfaction was high with these products.

Prescribing Drugs

An important part of the drug use process is how drugs are prescribed. This involves a process that is more complex than most people realize. It starts with a patient's need and the prescriber's—usually a doctor or dentist—willingness to help. In some states, the prescriber might be a doctor's assistant or nurse practitioner; however, these categories of health care workers have limited prescribing privileges. Veterinarians may also prescribe, but only for animals, and certain drugs can be prescribed only by veterinarians and dispensed on the order of a veterinarian.

The Prescription

If the condition warrants a prescribed medication, the drug is ordered using a prescription. A **prescription**—the slang term is script—is an order by a prescriber asking the pharmacist to dispense—prepare, package, and label—specific medication for a patient at a particular time. Before the 1960s, most prescriptions were written using Latin phrases and symbols. Thus doctors and pharmacists needed to know Latin. Although some Latin terms are still used today, most prescriptions are poorly written English that may look like Latin.

The prescription may be written on a prescription blank, which is a piece of paper, usually 4 inches by 6 inches, preprinted with terms, lines, and space to write information. However, there is no legal requirement the information be on such a form—it can be on any piece of paper, even a restaurant napkin. In fact, there is no requirement the prescription be written by the prescriber at all. Most prescriptions can be provided to the pharmacist orally. The prescribers should document in their records the medication that was ordered for the patient. The pharmacist, on receiving an oral prescription from a prescriber, must, under legal requirement, immediately record the prescription in writing. In most states, pharmacy technicians are not permitted to take oral orders.

Parts of a prescription
A model prescription can be seen in **Figure 7-2**. The legal requirements for a prescription vary from state to state. However, there are eight essential components of every prescription.

1. *Date*. The prescription should be dated the same day it is written or ordered by the doctor. It should be presented to the pharmacist within a reasonable time of seeing the doctor.
2. *Name and Address of Patient*. It is important to identify the patient properly. Initials should be turned into names to keep from confusing the patient with someone else. All names should be correctly spelled. An address and tele-

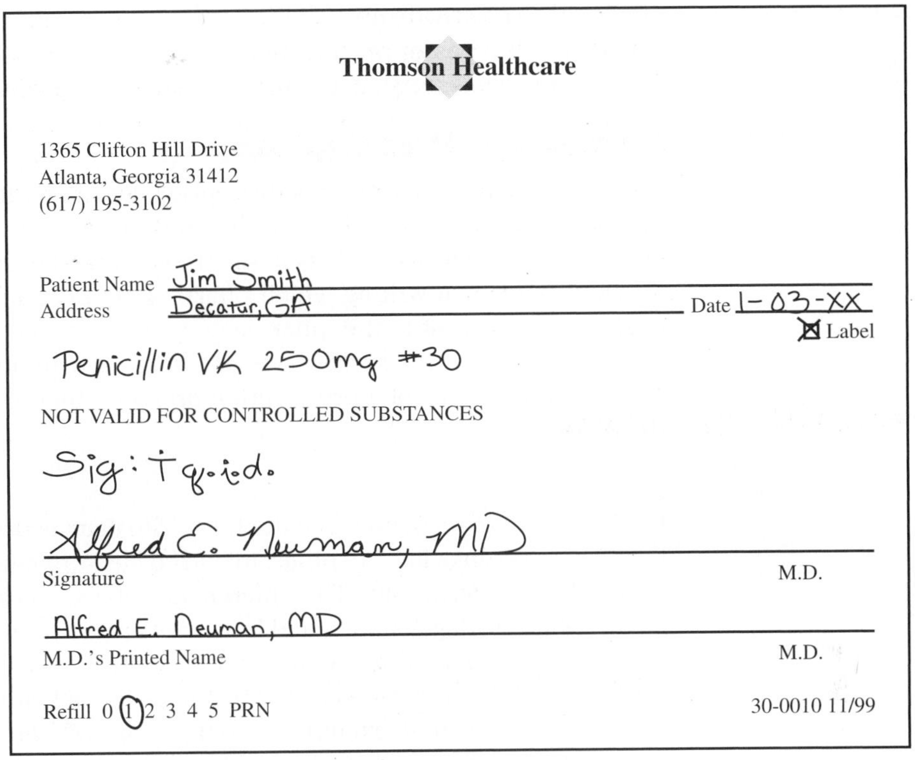

Thomson Healthcare

1365 Clifton Hill Drive
Atlanta, Georgia 31412
(617) 195-3102

Patient Name Jim Smith
Address Decatur, GA Date 1-03-XX
☒ Label

Penicillin VK 250mg #30

NOT VALID FOR CONTROLLED SUBSTANCES

Sig: T q.i.d.

Alfred E. Neuman, MD
Signature M.D.

Alfred E. Neuman, MD
M.D.'s Printed Name M.D.

Refill 0 (1) 2 3 4 5 PRN 30-0010 11/99

FIGURE 7-2 An Example of a Prescription (the Rx).

phone number is important in case it becomes necessary to contact the patient at a later time. Age and gender are other important information that can be gathered in the pharmacy.

3. *Superscription*. The "Rx" symbol is the superscription that heads the introduction to the prescribed medication. Rx in Latin means "recipe."
4. *Inscription*. This part of the prescription contains the name, strength, and quantity of medication to be prepared.
5. *Subscription*. This section may include any special instructions or directions to the pharmacist about the method of preparation and dispensing.
6. *Signatura*. This section of the prescription is usually shortened "Sig." In Latin, the signatura means "take." The "Sig" is the directions to be typed on the label of the prescription container. If safe, the pharmacist must put the medication to be taken at one time and the number of times a day on the prescription label, as directed by the prescriber. However, the pharmacist may add directions to the label that help in taking the medication correctly. Other information added to the label may be the medication's lot number and expiration date.
7. *Refill Information*. It is important for patients to know if their medication can be refilled without returning to the prescriber. If there is no refill, it is preferable to put this on the label.
8. *Signature, Address, and Registry Number of the Prescriber*. The prescription must be signed by the prescriber. The signature and address of the prescriber authenticates the prescription. If the prescription is a narcotic or controlled substance, the doctor needs to add his or her DEA registry number. There are other requirements for narcotic and other controlled substance prescriptions that are beyond the scope of this book.

Types of prescriptions

There are all types of prescriptions—new ones, refills, trade name, generic, narcotics, controlled substances, and compounded (prepared in the pharmacy).

Writing the Prescription

The writing of the inscription, subscription, and signatura is filled with specific terminology and often uses Latin terms and apothecary, avoirdupois, or the more standard metric measure. This is why most patients cannot read them, or it is because of poor handwriting which pharmacists become masters at reading. However, when in doubt, the pharmacy technician must always check with the pharmacist. Pharmacy technicians are working within the law if they prepare the label. All ingredients of a prescription prepared by the technician are checked by the pharmacist.

Drug orders

It is important to recognize that doctors write **drug orders** for patients in organized health care settings like hospitals, managed care organizations, and nursing homes rather than prescriptions. The differences between a drug order and prescription are in definition, legal status, and how they are written.

A drug order is a medication order, written to a pharmacist by a legal prescriber, for an inpatient—assigned to a bed—of an institution. A drug order has legal requirements that exempt it from having all the information needed on a prescription, but it needs to have information beyond a prescription, like the patient's location (e.g., room number). An example of a drug order can be seen in **Figure 7-3**.

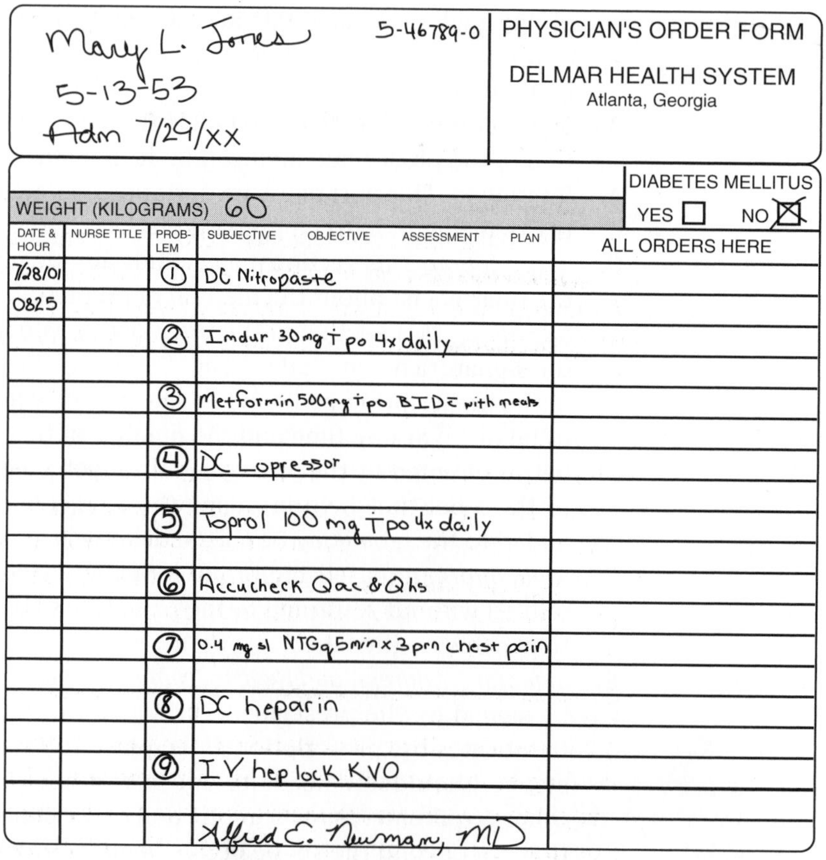

				PHYSICIAN'S ORDER FORM
Mary L. Jones 5-46789-0 5-13-53 Adm 7/29/xx				DELMAR HEALTH SYSTEM Atlanta, Georgia

					DIABETES MELLITUS
WEIGHT (KILOGRAMS) 60					YES ☐ NO ☒
DATE & HOUR	NURSE TITLE	PROB-LEM	SUBJECTIVE OBJECTIVE ASSESSMENT PLAN		ALL ORDERS HERE
7/28/01 0825		①	DC Nitropaste		
		②	Imdur 30mg ↑ po 4x daily		
		③	Metformin 500mg ↑ po BID c̄ with meals		
		④	DC Lopressor		
		⑤	Toprol 100 mg ↑ po 4x daily		
		⑥	Accucheck Qac & Qhs		
		⑦	0.4 mg sl NTG q 5min x 3 prn chest pain		
		⑧	DC heparin		
		⑨	IV hep lock KVO		
			Alfred E. Newman, MD		

FIGURE 7-3 An Example of a Drug Order.

When prescribing drugs in an organized health care setting, the doctor normally must prescribe only those drugs found in the organization's formulary. A **formulary** is a listing of drugs of choice, as determined by relative drug product safety, efficacy, and effectiveness, and information about each drug, approved by the medical staff of that organization, for use within the organization.

Drug Samples

Sometimes a patient may receive a sample of the medication or a sample of the medication and a prescription for the medication. These drug samples are small quantities of the drugs supplied to the doctor, usually by sales representatives of drug companies. The idea behind samples is for the patient to try the medication to see if it works and is tolerated before having their prescription filled (slang for dispensed) at a pharmacy.

Pharmacists, and some regulators, like state boards of pharmacy, health departments, and the Joint Committee on Accreditation of Healthcare Organizations (JCAHO), frown on samples. This is because of lack of control over samples and, even though they are dated, they sometimes go out-of-date before they are given to patients. In addition, some doctors feel they may become biased toward a certain drug or start using the most expensive drugs if they are provided samples. Therefore, some doctors refuse to use them.

Dispensing

Once patients receive a prescription, they will decide whether or not to take the prescription to a pharmacist to be filled. Surprisingly, some patients do not have their prescription filled. If patients decide they would like the prescription filled, they need to select a pharmacy.

Types of Retail Pharmacies

Independent community pharmacies

Patients have various choices where their prescription will be filled. Independent community pharmacies are owned and managed by a pharmacist (a sole ownership) or a pharmacist with other pharmacists or non-pharmacists (a partnership). Independent community pharmacies were the first pharmacies in the United States and, for many years, the only pharmacies. An example would be a pharmacy named "Carr's Pharmacy."

Chain store pharmacies

Chain store pharmacies are usually owned and managed by large companies. However, there are a few, small, usually pharmacist family-owned, local chains. Chain pharmacies are run according to corporate policy, and most of the people in upper management who oversee the operations of pharmacies in the company are not pharmacists. Examples of chain store pharmacies are CVS, Eckerd Drug, Rite Aid, and Walgreens.

Mass merchandiser pharmacies

Mass merchandiser pharmacies are owned by large corporations and managed according to the procedures of the corporations. Like chain pharmacies, most of the people in upper management who oversee the operation of pharmacies in the corporation are not pharmacists. Examples of mass merchandiser pharmacies are Kmart and Wal-Mart.

Food store pharmacies

Food store pharmacies are found within grocery store chains. They try to appeal to the "one-stop shoppers." Like chain and mass merchandise pharmacies, these pharmacies are owned by large corporations. The people within the corporation who have control over the operations of pharmacies may not be pharmacists. Examples of food store pharmacies are Albertson's, Kroger's, and Publix. Registered pharmacists are always responsible for direct pharmacy services to the customer.

Mail order pharmacies

Mail order pharmacies can be divided into two categories: those affiliated with large pharmacy benefits management (PBM) companies and smaller, independent operations. PBMs are employed by employers, or the insurers of employers, to manage and handle pharmacy claims.

Mail order pharmacies accept new prescriptions from patients through the mail, fill the prescriptions, and send them back through the mail to the patients. Refills for medication are requested by telephone, e-mail, or postcard.

A 1996 survey showed that 7% of patients buy their medication from mail order pharmacies. Eighty-seven percent of mail order users were "very satisfied" or "extremely satisfied" with the service. About 75% believed the prices they paid were lower than a community pharmacy would charge. Ninety percent (90%) of the prescriptions were for refills versus 46% of prescriptions refills brought into a community pharmacy. Nearly half (46%) of mail order customers were 55 years old or older.

Sometimes the mail order pharmacy is located in a state other than the state where the patient lives. The lack of one-on-one contact with a pharmacist and the delay in receiving medication are the main reasons people do not use mail order pharmacies. Examples of mail order pharmacies are those associated with the American Association of Retired Persons (AARP) and the PBM Medco Health Solutions.

Outpatient pharmacies in hospitals

Some larger hospitals have outpatient pharmacies within the hospital, usually close to the entrance, the clinics, or emergency room. These pharmacies dispense medication to ambulatory patients. These pharmacies fill prescriptions written by doctors on the hospital staff. They also dispense the first filling of a new prescription for a patient being discharged from the hospital and prescriptions for employees of the hospital.

Internet pharmacies

Recently some Internet or cyber-pharmacies have emerged. The first question about these is usually "Are they legal?" They are if they are licensed in the state where they are located and in the states where they are doing business. These pharmacies run much like mail order pharmacies, but with a few new wrinkles. Some Internet pharmacies are establishing personal contact between pharmacists and patients via e-mail. They are also using patient profiles, offering OTC sales, and providing a wide choice of delivery options including mail, express delivery, or pick up at an affiliated retail pharmacy. Examples of Internet pharmacy services are Drugstore.com, Planet-Rx, and Soma.com.

The Dispensing Process

The dispensing of medication, a prescription, is an organized process. Most patients have never been behind a prescription counter to see what takes place. It is much more than "count and pour" (the medication) and "lick and stick" (the label). Here are the recommended steps in dispensing a prescription.

- Accept the prescription and establish the pharmacist-patient relationship.
- Review the prescription and patient information.
- Review the patient's medication profile.
- Review the insurance coverage.
- Retrieve the drug or ingredients from storage.
- Prepare or compound (making) the medication.
- Label the container.
- Check and dispense the medication and label.
- Counsel the patients about their medication.

Drug Distribution in Organized Health Care Settings

Although some organized health care settings, like hospitals, have outpatient pharmacies that dispense medication on the order of a prescription for its ambulatory patients, most of the medication dispensed is for inpatients.

There are three primary systems for distributing drugs in hospitals and other organized health care settings: floor stock, unit-dose, and centralized IV admixtures.

Floor Stock

Medication can be stored on the patient care units in the form of **floor stock**; however, this is not recommended. If this is done, medication should be limited. The caution on storing medication in this manner is due to safety. Floor stock offers more opportunity for error because there is no check and balance system to avoid mistakes. The nurse can go to floor stock where the medication is stored, usually on a shelf or in a drawer, take out what is needed, and provide it directly to the patient.

The most common drugs in floor stock are narcotics which are always under lock and key with strict counting needs, various intravenous solutions (IVs), and emergency drugs (usually in a kit). Some patient care units, like the emergency room (ER), intensive care units (ICUs), the operating room (OR), and recovery room (RR), have more floor stock than others.

Unit-Dose

The second method of drug distribution is called unit-dose. A **unit-dose** is a dose dispensed from the pharmacy that is ready to be given to the patient, which means that no further dosage preparation, calculation, or manipulation is required. Unit-dose systems are safer because there is less opportunity for error and there is a built-in check and balance system.

In the unit-dose system of medication distribution, there are two medication drawers for each patient. One drawer is in the pharmacy being filled, while the other is on the patient care unit being used by the nurse to give medication to that patient. Each drawer is usually divided into two sections: one for regularly scheduled medication and the other for PRN (as needed) medication. The pharmacy places enough medication for the patient for the next shift (7 AM to 3 PM, 3 PM to 11 PM, or 11 PM to 7 AM), or next 24-hour period. At the end of the shift or 24-hour period, the drawers are exchanged.

The built-in check and balance system in the unit-dose system is based on three sets of medication records—the doctor's orders in the patient's record, the patient's pharmacy profile, and the nursing Kardex.

The pharmacy receives a copy of the patient's medication orders. Ideally, pharmacy technicians, rather than pharmacists, enter the medication orders into the patient's profile which is part of the pharmacy computer system. If the hospital has a total information system, the orders flow directly from the doctor's electronic orders into an electronic version of the patient's pharmacy profile in the computer system. On the patient care unit, the unit clerk transcribes (copies) the medication orders into the nursing Kardex (a card for each patient in a folder). The nurse must check and initial these transcriptions. The nurse uses the Kardex as a reminder of what, when, and to whom to administer medication. In an automated system, the nurse receives a printed list showing what to administer, to whom, and at what time.

There are three sets of medication records for each patient—the physician's order, the pharmacy patient profile, and the nursing Kardex. They should be identical. The best procedure for checking a patient's unit dose drawer is for the pharmacist to check the contents of the drawer against the nursing Kardex rather than the pharmacy patient profile from which the drawer was filled. If the drawer is not correct, one of three things happened: (1) the drawer was filled wrong, (2) there was a computer entry error made in the pharmacy, or (3) there was a transcription error made between the doctor's order and the nursing Kardex. Which error occurred? The answer can be found by checking the doctor's order in the patient's record.

IV Admixtures

The third drug distribution system is for IV admixtures. **IV admixtures** are intravenous (IV) solutions to which medication is added. Such medication is administered to patients intravenously (into their vein) and must be sterile (i.e., free of anything that can cause infection, including germs such as bacteria, viruses, and fungi). The technique of adding medication to IV solutions should be done carefully and under ideal aseptic conditions. For years, nurses prepared the IV solution on the patient care unit, a place full of germs. If this is still allowed in the hospital, there must be a policy on how nurses should do this.

It is now recommended by ASHP and JCAHO standards that IV admixtures be prepared in the pharmacy using aseptic (germ free) technique and a laminar flow hood. A laminar flow hood is a sterile work area with positive pressure airflow that filters the air. Pharmacists and pharmacy technicians are trained to prepare IV admixtures properly and should be recertified on how to do this. Once the IV admixtures are prepared, preferably by a pharmacy technician rather than a pharmacist, they should be checked by a pharmacist. When an IV additive solution is contaminated during preparation, the bacteria grows quickly with time and temperature. Therefore, IV additive solutions should be prepared just before they are needed and refrigerated between the time they are prepared and the time they are used. Delivery of IV admixtures to the patient care units is usually done by a courier or a pneumatic tube system.

Drug preparation and distribution can be done from a large central pharmacy (66% of hospitals) or from a central pharmacy and smaller, decentralized satellite pharmacies (34% of hospitals). Decentralized pharmacies are located in strategic locations in the hospital and serve several patient care units. Central pharmacies are more efficient, need less inventory, and use less personnel. The advantages of decentralized, satellite pharmacies are faster service, more service, and more opportunity for staff pharmacists to deliver pharmaceutical care on the floors.

Medication Use in the United States

According to a recent national survey, over half (51%) of American adults take two or more medications each day. In addition, almost half of Americans (46%) take at least one prescription medication each day, while more than a quarter (28%) take multiple prescription medications daily.

Rates of prescription medication use are highest among older Americans. Seventy-nine percent of those 65 years old or older reported taking one prescription medication each day compared with 63% of respondents age 55 to 64, 52% of respondents age 45 to 54, and 28% of respondents age 44 years or younger. Americans age 65 or over who take prescription medications take an average of four each day.

Among respondents who reported use of a prescription medication within the past week, the majority (61%) indicated the medication was for a long-term health condition such as cardiac, thyroid, or hypertension. Twenty-four percent said they are treating a recurring health problem, while 10% indicated they are treating a short-term, acute health condition.

U.S. pharmaceutical sales in 1998 were estimated at $102.5 billion, a 12% increase over 1997. When diagnostics and over-the-counter (OTC) products were included, that figure reached $128 billion. Besides increasing use, there are more products available. In the early 1960s, there were 650 products. Today there are over 10,000 products available.

More than $18 billion of OTCs are sold yearly in the traditional pharmacy outlets like independent and chain pharmacies. This number is much higher if non-traditional retail outlets are considered. Some of this growth is because of more people taking an interest in self-care, and some is because of the FDA switching some "prescription only" products to OTC status. In the ASHP patient survey, nearly two-thirds of the respondents reported taking an average of two nonprescription medications in the past week. Nearly one-third indicated they take an average of two nonprescription medications each day.

Besides increased OTC sales in the United States, the use of alternative medicines like herbal supplements, megavitamins, and other nontraditional cures is increasing dramatically. Between 1990 and 1997, the use of herbal medicines rose from 2.5% to 12.1%, for megavitamins from 2.4% to 5.5%, and for folk cures from 0.2% to 4.2%. Overall, 4 out of 10 Americans are trying alternative health treatments. In the ASHP survey, greater than one-third (39%) of respondents reported taking an average of four herbal supplements and vitamins in the past week. More than one-third (40%) reported taking an average of two herbal supplements or vitamins each day.

In addition to more medication being taken, there has been a shift of where patients are buying their medication. Although every community pharmacy is filling more prescriptions, the two fastest growing are mail order and food stores pharmacies, and the slowest growing are independent community pharmacies. In fact, there is some concern that the independent corner drugstore may not be able to survive much longer.

Medication Administration

Patients usually receive medication one of three ways: (1) self-administration, (2) administration from a friend or relative, or (3) administration from a nurse.

Self-administration is the way most medication is taken. It may also be the most dangerous. Unless the doctor, nurse, or pharmacist counsels the patient on taking the medication, the chances of the patient taking it correctly decrease. The patient should understand the name of the medication, what it is for, and what to expect from it. Most importantly, the patient needs to understand how to take the medication correctly. Does taking one tablet three times a day mean three times during the waking hours or spread out every eight hours? Does it need to be taken with water or can it be taken with fruit juice or milk? Can patients stop taking the medication when they feel better or do they need to take it until it is all gone? If they miss a dose, should they take twice as much next time? How should the medication be stored? What about side effects?

Medication managed by a friend or relative is needed when the patient is sick and at home. This method of medication administration may be safer than self-administration. Most people are more careful when being responsible for others. They also tend to ask more questions and are afraid to do anything wrong. Friends and relatives also are better at giving the medication on a schedule or reminding the patient when the medication is due.

Nurse-administered medication is the most accurate method of administering medications. Nurses know medication and how to give it, and if they do not, they have been trained to find out. Nurses pride themselves on this important role. They also have developed ways to administer the medication to the most ornery patient or youngest child.

No matter who gives the medication, it is easy to make an error like forgetting to give it, giving the wrong drug, giving too much or too little, or giving it at the wrong time. This is unfortunate since so much effort went into making an appointment, seeing the doctor, getting a diagnosis and a prescription, and getting the prescription filled. Not taking the medication properly can result in an extended illness, going back to the doctor, having an adverse reaction, or possibly having to go to the emergency room or hospital. All of this results in more time and expense.

Compliance with Taking the Medication as Prescribed

The problem

Some people never get their prescription filled or, if it is called in to the pharmacist, never pick it up. How big of a problem is this? One study looking at this problem in community pharmacies found that about 2% of people never picked up their prescription. This translates into 40 million prescriptions not picked up and $1 billion in lost sales. Reasons cited for this problem were recovery (39%), having a similar drug at home (35%), did not feel they needed it (34%), and do not like taking medication.

The problem of unclaimed prescriptions is also a problem for outpatient pharmacies in hospitals. A 1995 study showed that 1.6% of patients did not pick up their medication. One proposed solution to this problem is to call the patient to remind them their medication is ready for pickup.

Even if a person has a prescription filled, it does not mean they will take it as prescribed. Either forgetting or purposely not taking medication as prescribed is called **noncompliance**.

Noncompliance is a big problem. There are various means of discovery rates of medication compliance, such as urine tests, serum tests, pill counts, patient interviews, and record reviews. As reported in the literature, rates of noncompliance with prescribed therapy vary between 15% and 93%. The variance is explained by different patient populations, the category of drugs, how often the medication is prescribed each day, and by differences in study design. Medication compliance rates vary significantly for several disease states.

The underlying problems associated with medication noncompliance are patient actions (decisions and behaviors). Patients decide whether to take a medication and how often. Reasons for patients not taking their medication or not taking it as prescribed include cost, feeling better, side effects, not realizing the importance, and forgetting.

The cost

The cost of medication noncompliance is high in lives lost, time lost, and added care needed. It has been estimated that 125,000 Americans die each year simply because they fail to take their medication as prescribed. Equally disturbing are the unnecessary hundreds of thousands of extra hospital admissions because of medication noncompliance. In one study, 36 of 89 medication-related admissions were related to medication noncompliance. Of these, 54% were because of intentional noncompliance. The cost was $2,150 for each admission in 1990.

Another study examined the records of seven patients not taking their medication as prescribed. More than $14,000 was spent on outpatient visits, hospital days, and emergency room visits over one year as a direct result of medication noncompliance.

There is also the cost of time, such as having to stay home or leave work or school to seek medical attention. The estimated cost is a loss of 20 million workdays a year or about 1.5 billion dollars in lost earnings. The annual economic cost of medication noncompliance in the United States is estimated to be more than $100 billion dollars.

Solutions

Many groups of people, like doctors, nurses, pharmacists, the American Association of Retired People (AARP), the Task Force for Compliance, and the National Council on Patient Information and Education (NCPIE), have been working on the problem of medication noncompliance. A lot has been learned and more still needs to be done. Each patient not taking medication as prescribed has a different reason or set of reasons for not being in compliance. Thus the solution for getting the patient to be compliant will differ from one patient to the next.

Pharmacy technicians should learn methods to discover if there has been noncompliance and alert the pharmacist of this problem. Once it has been determined there is a noncompliance problem, the pharmacist should try to find out why. The most common issues are cost, other needs, fear of the medication not working or causing adverse effects, or forgetfulness.

The most effective way to improve medication compliance is by understanding why the patient is not taking the medication as prescribed and then using a combination of methods specifically designed to address the patient's reasons for not being compliant. Doing this is not only in the patient's best interest, but also in the pharmacist's best interest both clinically and economically. Unfilled prescriptions and prescriptions not refilled produce an estimated loss of 100 million prescriptions valued at $1.2 billion yearly.

Pharmaceutical Care

The pharmacy profession has decided the mission of pharmacy practice is to help patients make the best use of their medication. To do this, pharmacists need to get out from behind their counters and out of the hospital pharmacy and be in direct contact with patients. In other words, pharmacists needs to be more concerned about patients than about drug products. This idea is called pharmaceutical care.

> "Pharmaceutical care is defined as the functions performed by a pharmacist in ensuring the optimal use of medications to achieve specific outcomes that improve a patient's quality of life; further, the pharmacist accepts responsibility for outcomes that ensue from his or her actions, which occur in collaboration with patients and other health-care colleagues." (Kier & Pathak, 1991)

This definition was later revised to: The mission of the pharmacist is to provide pharmaceutical care. Pharmaceutical care is the direct, responsible provision of medication-related care for the purpose of achieving definite outcomes that improve a patient's quality of life.

A newer definition of pharmaceutical care was developed in 1997:

A practice in which the practitioner takes responsibility for a patient's drug-related needs and is held accountable for this commitment.

There continues to be controversy about the name *pharmaceutical care*. Some pharmacists—mostly community pharmacists—feel the word *pharmaceutical* should be replaced with the words *pharmacy* or *pharmacist* in *pharmaceutical care* (i.e., pharmacy care or pharmacist care). The rationale is that the word *pharmaceutical* is too closely associated with drug products, and by calling it pharmaceutical care, anyone can provide it. The expression *pharmacy* or *pharmacist care* avoids these problems. However, most professional pharmacy organizations and schools of pharmacy are still using the original term *pharmaceutical care*.

The Elements of Pharmaceutical Care

Regardless of which definition of pharmaceutical care is used, each definition encompasses six general principles or elements.

1. *Responsible provision of care.* The pharmacist should accept responsibility for the patient.
2. *Direct provision of care.* Pharmaceutical care is directly provided to patients. This means the pharmacist must be in direct contact with patients. They must see and talk with patients.
3. *Caring.* This virtue, a key characteristic among nurses and doctors, has been the most understated virtue of pharmacy. It is the centerpiece of pharmaceutical care.
4. *Achieving positive outcomes.* There are several positive, clinical outcomes that can occur because of taking medication: cure of disease, elimination or decline of a patient's symptoms, arresting or slowing of a disease process, or preventing a disease or a symptom.

   There are also negative outcomes from taking medication: the medication fails to work as expected, there are nagging side effects, or there are adverse drug reactions that cause moderate patient morbidity, a life-threatening or permanent disability, or death.

   Besides clinical outcomes, there are also economic (cost) and humanistic outcomes (functional status, quality of life, and patient satisfaction). Under pharmaceutical care, it is the pharmacists' responsibility to do everything they can to achieve positive patient outcomes and avoid the negative effects of taking medication.

5. *Improving the patient's quality of life*. Everyone has a certain, measurable quality of life. Under the pharmaceutical care model of delivering care, the pharmacist must, with the patient and the doctor, set reasonable treatment goals for each drug prescribed that will improve the patient's functioning and health-related quality of life.

6. *Resolution of medication-related problems*. The task of pharmaceutical care is to resolve medication-related problems. **Medication-related problems (MRPs)** are undesirable events a patient experiences that involve (or are suspected of involving) drug therapy and that actually (or potentially) interfere with a desired patient outcome.

Pharmaceutical care involves identifying potential and actual MRPs, resolving actual MRPs, and preventing potential MRPs. There are eight MRPs.

1. *Needed drug therapy*. The patient has a medical condition that requires the introduction of new or added drug therapy.

2. *Unnecessary drug therapy*. The patient is taking drug therapy that is unnecessary given his or her present condition.

3. *Use of wrong drug*. The patient has a medical condition for which the wrong drug is being taken.

4. *Dosage is too low*. The patient has a medical condition for which too little of the correct drug is being taken.

5. *Dosage is too high*. The patient has a medical condition for which too much of the correct drug is being taken.

6. *An adverse drug reaction*. The patient has a medical condition because of an adverse drug reaction or event.

7. *Not receiving the drug*. The patient has a medical condition for which the patient needs, but is not receiving, the drug.

8. *Drug interaction*. The patient has a medical condition and there is a drug-drug, drug-food, or drug-laboratory test interaction.

Quality Drug Therapy

There is much more to being a pharmacist than making sure the patient receives the drug prescribed and doing what you can do to make sure the drug is taken as prescribed. Today pharmacists are trained to help each patient receive quality drug therapy. Quality drug therapy is safe, effective, timely, and cost-effective drug therapy delivered with care.

Pharmacists used to fill prescriptions written by doctors and were not allowed to question whether the drug prescribed was the best drug for the patient. This has changed for various reasons. First, the drugs are getting more complex, more potent, and there are more of them. Second, doctors cannot know everything about every drug. Third, the clinical education of the pharmacist has expanded. And fourth, the scope of practice and legal duty of the pharmacist to help and protect the patient has expanded.

A doctor prescribes a drug based on what he or she knows and considers is best. A pharmacist may see the patient differently, may know information the doctor does not know about the drug, or knows about other drugs that may benefit the patient. Thus if the pharmacist thinks the patient may benefit from changing the prescribed drug—its dose, route of administration, or dosage form, or changing to another drug—he or she is obligated to call the doctor and discuss it.

Pharmacy technicians should look for problems in prescriptions and drug orders to bring to the attention of the pharmacist. This helps the pharmacist and helps protect the patient from harm.

Medication Safety and Drug Misadventures

Although medication can be wonderful, helping to cure an illness, or helping a patient feel better, it also has the potential for harm. When there is harm from medication, these events are called drug misadventures.

Side Effects

All drugs have side effects. **Side effects** are known, usually minor, annoying effects of the drug experienced by most people taking the drug. An example is the drowsiness associated with some antihistamine drugs used for treating hay fever symptoms. Since side effects are expected, minor events, they are not a drug misadventure per se.

Adverse Drug Reactions

Some drugs can cause more dangerous conditions called adverse drug reactions. **Adverse drug reactions** are unwanted, more serious, adverse effects of the drug that are not experienced by every patient taking the drug.

Allergic Drug Reactions

Patients allergic to a drug or an ingredient in the medication, even a color dye, can experience drug reactions that can vary from a minor annoyance to a life threat. It is critical that every pharmacy, patient profile, and computer system contain information on each patient's allergies.

Drug-Drug Interactions

Some drugs interact with other drugs, or interact with food or drinks the patient is taking. One drug can make another drug inactive or overactive. The outcome of a drug interaction can range from a minor inconvenience to death. Pharmacists must be vigilant about detecting and stopping these interactions from occurring.

Medication Errors

Medication errors rarely occur when considering the millions of prescriptions and doses of medication patients receive yearly. The incidence is a fraction of a percent. However, this is meaningless if the error occurs to you or someone you love. Therefore, the public has zero tolerance for medication errors. That means pharmacists and pharmacy technicians have to be accurate all the time and there is no room for errors.

Pharmacists have built good check and balance systems—a safety net—for detecting medication errors before they harm patients. However, medication errors occasionally occur within the drug use process. These errors are usually the result of a medication system failure rather than the failure of one person.

As a group, adverse drug reactions, allergic drug reactions, drug-drug interactions, and medication errors are called drug misadventures or adverse drug events.

Control of the Drug Use Process

The drug use process is extensive and complex. It is also designed with many checks and balances to keep patients from experiencing a preventable drug misadventure. At the center of this control is the pharmacist and pharmacy technician. Laws, rules and regulations, accreditation policies, and pharmacy tradition have given the pharmacist this important responsibility. Although pharmacists have accepted this responsibility, and they are up to the task, they cannot do it alone. They need the help of pharmacy technicians, other health professionals, and patients who will take responsibility for their own health.

Current Issues in the Drug Use Process

The Rising Number of Prescriptions and Limited Numbers of Pharmacists

The number of prescriptions filled each year is rising at an unprecedented rate. This rise is because of increased demand and better drugs. The large, baby boom generation will soon be reaching 65 years old, and these individuals will need more medication as they get older. At the same time, the pharmacy profession is being stretched. A shortage of pharmacists is becoming clear because of expanded roles for pharmacists and an increased use of medication.

The profession's response has been to start 10 more schools of pharmacy. However, from all suggestions, this may not be enough. To meet the demand and to preserve or expand the pharmacist's clinical role, pharmacy will need to better use pharmacy technicians, reorganize pharmacies to be more efficient, and increase the use of pharmacy automation and information technology.

Pharmacy Automation

Pharmacy departments are slowly moving to maximize the automation available for charting, packaging, labeling, and dispensing medications. The cost of current equipment is high and the skills needed must be learned. This is an area where pharmacy technicians can excel. The pharmacist's time can be better utilized in patient care if the technicians can ensure an efficient drug distribution system.

Summary

The drug use process is a complex process that involves manufacture, distribution, prescribing, preparation, storing, dispensing, administering, monitoring, and review of drugs and their use. The process is controlled and at the center of this control are various checks and balances, regulations, and the pharmacist and pharmacy technician. Even with control, the system is not perfect and thus needs constant attention and improvement.

Note: Much of what has been written in this chapter has been reprinted with permission from *Pharmacy: What It Is and How it Works*. Copyright CRC Press, Boca Raton, Florida.

TEST YOUR KNOWLEDGE

Multiple Choice Questions

1. The societal purpose of pharmacy practice is to
   a. dispense medication
   b. provide drug information
   c. help people make the best use of their medication
   d. prepare drugs

2. The drug use process is
   a. when people abuse drugs
   b. methods used to prepare drugs
   c. steps involved in getting drugs to their final destination
   d. how drugs are managed

3. What is drug use control?
   a. any method used to reduce the improper use of a drug
   b. federal drug enforcement regulations
   c. a method to accurately measure who uses drugs
   d. FDA manufacturing rules

4. Why is control needed in the drug use process?
   a. to protect patients from harm
   b. to satisfy FDA requirements
   c. to keep drugs from being illegally diverted
   d. both A and C

5. Which of the following is not a drug use control method?
   a. formulary
   b. laws, rules, and regulations
   c. policies and procedures
   d. all of the above

6. Which of the following is not considered a medication misadventure?
   a. errors
   b. adverse reactions
   c. side effects
   d. drug interaction

7. What primary duty do pharmacists perform for society?
   a. prepare medication for patients
   b. help patients use their medication safely
   c. supply drugs
   d. price the prescription accurately

8. Pharmacy technicians will legally perform their duties as long as they
   a. check everything they do in the pharmacy
   b. read all labels at least three times before dispensing the drug
   c. have all labels and products checked by the pharmacist
   d. are certified

9. A major change that is transforming pharmacy into a true clinical profession is
   a. the use of automation
   b. the use of more pharmacy technicians
   c. pharmaceutical care
   d. all of the above

10. How will the changes in question nine affect pharmacy technicians?
   a. They will be more involved in running automation.
   b. They will be doing higher level functions.
   c. They may need more education.
   d. All of the above.

References

American Pharmacists Association. (2000). *Handbook of non-prescription drugs*. Washington, DC: Author.

Anonymous. (1996). No-show customers cost community pharmacies $1 billion annually. *American Journal of Health-System Pharmacists, 53*, 1236, 1239–1240.

Bauman, A. E., Craig, A. R., & Dunsmore, J. (1989). Removing barriers to effective self-management of asthma. *Patient Education and Counseling, 14*, 217–226.

Bentley, J. P., Wilkin, N. E., & McCaffrey, D. J. (1999). Examining compliance from the patient's perspective. *Drug Topics, 143*(14), 58–67.

Berg, J. S., Dischler, J., Wagner, D. J. (1993). Medication compliance: Healthcare problem. *The Annals of Pharmacotherapy, 27*, S5–S19, S21–S22.

Bloom, B. S. (1988). The medical, social, and economic implications of disease. In W. van Eimeren & B. Horisberger (eds.), *Socioeconomic evaluation of drug therapy*. New York, NY: Springer-Verlag.

Brodie, D. C. (1967). Drug-use control: Keystone to pharmaceutical service. *Drug Intelligence, 1*, 63–65.

Clark, I. T. (1991). Improving compliance and increasing control of hypertension: Needs of special hypertensive populations. *American Heart Journal, 121*, 664–669.

Col, N., Fanale, J. E., & Kronholm, P. (1990). The role of medication noncompliance and adverse drug reactions in hospitalizations of the elderly. *Archives of Internal Medicine, 150*, 841–845.

Eisenberg, D. M., Davis, R. B., & Ettner, S. L. (1998). Trends in alternative medicine use in the United States, 1990–1997. *Journal of the American Medical Association, 280*, 1569–1575.

Goselin, R. A., & Robbins, J. (1999). *Inside pharmacy: The anatomy of a profession*. Lancaster, PA: Technomic Publishing Company, Inc.

Hamilton, W. R., & Hopkins, U. K. (1997). Survey of unclaimed prescriptions in a community pharmacy. *Journal of the American Pharmaceutical Association, 37*, 341–345.

Healthcare Distribution Management Association. (2001). Healthcare product distribution: a primer. Retrieved August 5, 2001, from www.healthcaredistribution.org.

Hemminki, E., Brambilla, D. J., McKinlay, S. M., & Posner, J. G. (1991). Use of estrogens among middle-aged Massachusetts women. *Drug Intelligence and Clinical Pharmacy, 25*, 418–423.

Japsen, B. (2001, January 26). Saying yes to free drug samples raises concern. *Atlanta Journal*.

Joglekar, M., Mohanaruban, K., Bayer, A. J., & Pathy, M. S. J. (1988). Can old people on oral anticoagulants be safely managed as out-patients? *Postgraduate Medicine, 64*, 775–777.

Jones, E. F., & Forrest, J. D. (1992). Contraceptive failure rates based on the 1988 NSFG. *Family Planning Perspective, 24*, 12–19.

Kelly, W. N. (1999). Drug use control: The foundation of pharmaceutical care. In *Pharmacy practice for technicians* (2nd ed.). Clifton Park, NY: Delmar Learning.

Kier, K. L., & Pathak, D. S. (1991). Drug-usage evaluation: Traditional versus outcome-based approaches. *Topics in Hospital Pharmacy Management, 11*, 9–15.

Kirking, M. H., Zaleon, C. R., & Kirking, D. (1995). Unclaimed prescriptions at a university hospital's ambulatory care pharmacy. *American Journal of Health-System Pharmacy, 52*, 490–495.

Leppik, I. E. (1990). How to get patients with epilepsy to take their medication. The problem of noncompliance. *Postgraduate Medicine, 88*, 253–256.

Martin, E. W. (1971). The Prescription. In *Dispensing of medication* (7th ed.). Easton, PA: Mack Publishing Company.

Nagasawa, M., Smith, M. C., & Barnes, J. H. (1990). Meta-analysis of correlates of diabetes patients' compliance with prescribed medications. *Diabetes Education, 16*, 192–200.

National Pharmaceutical Council, Inc. (1996). *Pharmaceutical benefits under state medical assistance programs.* Reston, VA: Author.

New ASHP survey unveils snapshot of medication use in U.S. American Society of Health-System Pharmacists. Bethesda, MD. Press Release of January 18, 2001.

Nonprescription Drug Manufacturers Association (1992). *Self-medication in the '90's: Practices and perceptions.* Washington, DC: Author.

Ortho Biotech, Inc. (1999). *1999 retail pharmacy digest: measuring customer satisfaction.* Raritan, NJ: Author.

Powell, B. J., Penick, E. C., & Liskow, B. I. (1986). Lithium compliance in alcoholic males: A six month follow up study. *Addictive Behaviors, 11*, 135–140.

Robbins, J. (1987). Forgetful patient: High cost of improper medication compliance. *US Pharmacist 12*, 40–44.

Rosman, A. W., & Sawyer, W. T. (1988). Population-based drug use evaluation. *Topics in Hospital Pharmacy Management, 8*, 76–91.

Rovelli, M., Palmeri, D., Vossler, E. (1989). Noncompliance in organ transplant recipients. *Transplantation Proceedings, 21*, 833–834.

Rucker, T. D. (1987). Prescribed medications: System control or therapeutic roulette? In *Control aspects of biomedical engineering.* International Federation of Automatic Control. New York: Oxford.

Salek, M. S., & Sclar, D. A. (1992). *Medication compliance: The pharmacist's pivotal role.* Kalamazoo, MI: The Upjohn Company.

Sloan, N. E., Peroutka, J. A., & Morgan, D. E. (1994). Influencing prescribing practices and associated outcomes utilizing the drug use evaluation process. *Topics in Hospital Pharmacy Management, 14*, 1–12.

Smith, M. (1985). The cost of noncompliance and the capacity of improved compliance to reduce health care expenditures. In *Improving medication compliance.* Reston, VA: National Pharmaceutical Council.

The National Council on Patient Information and Education (NCPIE). (1995). Prescription medicine compliance: A review of the baseline of knowledge. Washington, DC: Author.

The Task Force for Compliance. (April 1994). Noncompliance with medications. Baltimore, MD: Author.

8 Ethical Considerations for the Pharmacy Technician

COMPETENCIES

Upon completion of this chapter, the reader should be able to

1. List the six ethical principles available to resolve an ethical dilemma.
2. Reflect upon the concepts present in the *Code of Ethics for Pharmacy Technicians*.
3. Identify, prospectively, practice situations where ethical dilemmas may occur.
4. Detect the presence of an ethical dilemma and sort through alternative responses.

Introduction

This chapter focuses on ethical challenges faced by practitioners, pharmacists, and pharmacy technicians, in our changing health care environment with the adoption of the pharmaceutical care standard. It provides guidance on how to approach an ethical dilemma, presents six ethical principles that may be applied to face these dilemmas, and describes the nature and importance of ethical codes of behavior. Technicians are reminded of the responsibilities and risks imposed on them both by state governments and the pharmacy profession the pharmacists they assist. Practical considerations are raised in the areas of drug distribution and patient communication, and the tools provided should assist pharmacy technicians in making sound ethical evaluations. Final ethical choices regarding drug therapy resides with the pharmacist.

The Changing Health Care Environment

American society and our health care system are evolving in unexpected, challenging, and sometimes disturbing ways. Diversity and mobility are the norms of existence, not the exception. Scientific and medical discoveries and advances present a health care environment that can produce unprecedented results, but at ever-increasing costs. Federal and state government and third-party payors dominate our health care delivery system and frequently decide what treatment is given or how to distribute lessening resources, shifting decision-making from the traditional physician-patient environment to a corporate model. Globalization, computerization, and Internet use provide patients a broader reach and outlook yet disconnect them and their activities from the local neighborhood that formed the basis of their personal and professional interactions. While individuals and society are more dependent on business, financial, and religious institutions for their well-being, recent scandals present disturbing ethical concerns about organizational leadership and make us question whether the trust we have placed in these institutions and their leaders is misguided and unwarranted.

Pharmacy practice is not immune to change. Practitioners are challenged to keep current with numerous drug therapy advances while facing an informed and more assertive patient population that seeks active participation in its treatment. Pharmaceutical manufacturers produce new classes of drugs and new delivery systems that benefit patients. However, some are merely "me too" drugs that just provide more expensive, not better, care. Some drug companies offer financial incentives to doctors, pharmacists, and allied health professionals to prescribe or recommend particular drugs or to switch patients from one medication to another, whether or not this activity is in the best interest of the patient or falls within the context of "pharmaceutical care."

Pharmaceutical Care

Providing a patient with quality pharmaceutical care is now the basic standard for pharmacy practice. "**Pharmaceutical care**" as defined by Hepler and Strand is "the direct, responsible provision of medication-related care for the purpose of achieving definite outcomes that improve a patient's quality of life." Pharmacy education has adopted pharmaceutical care as its endpoint and developed PharmD curricula to implement its adoption. Pharmaceutical practitioners are under pressure to maximize use of their resources to meet this standard and recognize the need for trained assistants to lessen the pharmacist's burden in drug distribution. Pharmacy technicians are vital partners in the delivery of pharmaceutical care to the patient population.

The Role of the Pharmacy Technician

According to the ASHP's "White Paper on Pharmacy Technicians," a **pharmacy technician** is "an individual working in a pharmacy, who, under the supervision of a licensed pharmacist, assists in pharmacy activities that do not require the professional judgement of the pharmacist." They are employed in a variety of settings: hospitals, community pharmacies, mail-order pharmacies, long-term care facilities, and home health care and they assist pharmacists to manage drug distribution and paperwork and enable the pharmacist to concentrate on providing direct patient care. Pharmacists depend on the technician's expertise to facilitate expansion of their professional scope of practice, and technicians are central to maintaining pharmacy's professional stability and growth by performing duties that do not require the professional skills and judgement of a licensed pharmacist. Pharmacy technicians must therefore share the pharmacist's ethical commitment to safe medication use.

Technician training can be based on a structured educational program or provided on-the-job. Activities may include collecting and organizing information to assist pharmacists in patient care, developing and managing medication distribution and control systems. On a state-by-state basis, limitations are placed on technician responsibility and authority by the level of recognition they receive (registration, certification, or licensure) and whether or not they have their own scope of practice. *The NABP Survey of Pharmacy Law (2001)* indicates that 26 states currently register, certify, license, or enroll pharmacy technicians. In the other states, health care personnel are performing the activities of the technician but may not receive specific recognition or regulation by a licensing agency. Most states play a direct role in regulating pharmacy technician practice and in determining scope of practice. Communications with the prescriber, including refill authorization, preparation of the label as well as the medication, entering the prescription into the computer system or patient information into the profile, and medication preparation, including compounding and reconstituting of oral liquids, are all activities the state may delegate to the technician. There are other technician issues decided state-by-state: the level and type of training, continuing education requirements, and whether or not they can review the work of other technicians. Health care personnel acting as pharmacy technicians in states that do not certify, register, or license and do not have the title, legally derive their power to act from the pharmacist and the pharmacist's scope of practice act. Thus their limitations on practice and ethical considerations must flow directly from the pharmacist they assist.

Those pharmacy technicians recognized separately by a state must still coordinate their activities and ethical conduct with pharmacists, though they are separately responsible for their behavior legally and morally.

Codes of Professional Behavior

Self-discipline and self-regulation are essential components of professional behavior. Ethical codes set standards and responsibilities among members of a group and govern interactions with other organizations, patients, clients, colleagues, and society. Codes declare to all the collective conscience of the group involved and the norms of professional behavior they value. They usually focus on dealing honestly with patients, suppliers, and competitors, respecting individual autonomy, recognizing the right to make informed decisions, maintaining confidentiality, and promoting just and effective use of resources. The first medical code was the *Hippocratic Oath*, which dates back to the fifth century BC.

The aftermath of World War II and its unethical excesses encouraged the World Medical Association to adopt the *Geneva Convention of Medical Ethics*, followed by the *Nuremberg Code*, suggesting guidelines for human experimentation and the need for voluntary consent of a patient. Later, the World Medical Association adopted the *Declaration of Helsinki*, emphasizing the importance of informed consent and full disclosure to the patient.

Health care professional groups and organizations acknowledge the need to declare to the public they serve the values they deem important and by which they wish to be judged. Albert Jonsen believes that professionalism should focus on honesty, integrity, respect for patients, a commitment to patients' welfare, a compassionate regard for patients, and dedication to maintaining competency in knowledge and technical skills. Professional organizations recognize that codes make explicit the primary goals and values of the group, and individuals who join make a moral commitment to uphold the values and obligations expressed. The codes may also focus on inspirational ideals, serve as a statement of organizational principles, and provide rules to govern behavior. When these codes are created and ratified by the membership of a professional organization or the profession itself, they have more societal impact than if they are imposed by the leadership of the organization with little or no member input or acceptance.

The Code of Ethics for Pharmacy Technicians

The *Code of Ethics for Pharmacy Technicians* was drafted by the American Association of Pharmacy Technicians in 1996 to deal with the particular duties and responsibilities of technicians. The code has most relevance for technicians who are members of the organization, but also has persuasive impact on all pharmacy technicians regardless of professional affiliation or work environment. The principles expressed in the technician's code include assisting pharmacists in providing the best care for patients based on the moral guidelines expressed in the pharmacist's code, supporting honesty and integrity, maintaining competence, knowledge, and expertise, respecting patient confidentiality, avoiding activities that bring discredit to the profession, and meeting standards required by law.

Those pharmacy technicians not separately licensed, registered, or certified serve as agents of a pharmacist and therefore are bound by the principles of the American Pharmaceutical Association's *Code of Ethics for Pharmacists* because their professional activities derive from the pharmacist's responsibilities.

The Pharmacist's Code of Ethics

The pharmacist's code has evolved over the years and reflects behavioral guidelines for pharmacy practice as it exists today. Its principles are designed to guide pharmacists in their relationships with patients, health professionals, and society including helping patients achieve optimum benefit from medications while maintaining their trust, being caring, compassionate and discreet, respecting a patient's autonomy and dignity, acting with honesty and integrity, maintaining professional competence, respecting the beliefs and values of colleagues, and allocating health resources in a fair and just manner. A copy of the code is shown in **Figure 8-1**. Pharmacists also have an oath, similar to the *Hippocratic Oath*, which is taken voluntarily by many practitioners and declares values that parallel those expressed in the *Code of Ethics*.

Ethical Decision-Making

Organizations and professional associations cannot carry out their policies as a group but instead rely on individual members to implement the standards they have adopted. Identifying an ethical question, or facing an ethical dilemma, is done by an individual and the actions taken are primarily based on individual moral assumptions or beliefs.

Ethics is the study of precepts or principles used to assist us in making the correct choice when faced with alternative possibilities for action in a moral situation. Lowenthal and Meth believe it is a "process that resolves dilemmas and judges the appropriateness of one's behavior in situations where a protocol cannot be applied." Practitioners are encouraged to do the right thing, as if all issues are clearly delineated, focusing on right versus wrong or good versus evil. We rarely face such clear-cut situations. In reality, we encounter ethical dilemmas and are challenged to come up with an acceptable response. An ethical dilemma is a difficult moral problem involving two or more mutually exclusive and morally equal courses of action. We are often asked to choose between the better of two imperfectly acceptable alternatives or the lesser of two objectionable ones.

American Pharmaceutical Association
Code of Ethics for Pharmacists (1994)

Preamble. Pharmacists are health professionals who assist individuals in making the best use of medications. This Code, prepared and supported by pharmacists, is intended to state publicly the principles that form the fundamental basis of the roles and responsibilities of pharmacists. These principles, based on moral obligations and virtues, are established to guide pharmacists in relationships with patients, health professionals, and society.

I. A pharmacist respects the covenantal relationship between the patient and pharmacist.

Considering the patient-pharmacist relationship as a covenant means that a pharmacist has moral obligations in response to the gift of trust received from society. In return for this gift, a pharmacist promises to help individuals achieve optimum benefit from their medications, to be committed to their welfare, and to maintain their trust.

II. A pharmacist promotes the good of every patient in a caring, compassionate, and confidential manner.

A pharmacist places concern for the well-being of the patient at the center of professional practice. In doing so, a pharmacist considers needs stated by the patient as well as those defined by health science. A pharmacist is dedicated to protecting the dignity of the patient. With a caring attitude and a compassionate spirit, a pharmacist focuses on serving the patient in a private and confidential manner.

III. A pharmacist respects the autonomy and dignity of each patient.

A pharmacist promotes the right of self-determination and recognizes individual self-worth by encouraging patients to participate in decisions about their health. A pharmacist communicates with patients in terms that are understandable. In all cases, a pharmacist respects personal and cultural differences among patients.

IV. A pharmacist acts with honesty and integrity in professional relationships.

A pharmacist has a duty to tell the truth and to act with conviction of conscience. A pharmacist avoids discriminatory practices, behavior or work conditions that impair professional judgment, and actions that compromise dedication to the best interests of patients.

V. A pharmacist maintains professional competence.

A pharmacist has a duty to maintain knowledge and abilities as new medications, devices, and technologies become available and as health information advances.

VI. A pharmacist respects the values and abilities of colleagues and other health professionals.

When appropriate, a pharmacist asks for the consultation of colleagues or other health professionals or refers the patient. A pharmacist acknowledges that colleagues and other health professionals may differ in the beliefs and values they apply to the care of the patient.

VII. A pharmacist serves individual, community, and societal needs.

The primary obligation of a pharmacist is to individual patients. However, the obligations of a pharmacist may at times extend beyond the individual to the community and society. In these situations, the pharmacist recognizes the responsibilities that accompany these obligations and acts accordingly.

VIII. A pharmacist seeks justice in the distribution of health resources.

When health resources are allocated, a pharmacist is fair and equitable, balancing the needs of patients and society.

Source: American Pharmaceutical Association website,
www.aphanet.org/pharmcare/ethics.html

FIGURE 8-1 Code of Ethics for Pharmacists *(adopted by the membership of the American Pharmacists Association, then the American Pharmaceutical Association, October 27, 1994).*

The methods we use to determine the correctness of our actions are imprecise and when placed within a health care setting, have a complexity and impact beyond our personal concerns. How then do you handle conflict, make the choices you must, and live with the consequences as health care practitioners and as individuals? Amy Haddad and her fellow authors suggest that "we utilize ethical judgement skills and apply ethical principles based on our personal and professional value system and the needs of our society and the patient." It is hoped we will be able to recognize when a dilemma exists, define the elements of the dilemma, develop alternative solutions, act on the appropriate solution, and evaluate the outcome.

Ethical Principles

Ethicists do not agree on the number of distinct ethical principles used to solve dilemmas. A consensus recognizes the following six: honesty, promise-keeping, nonmaleficence, beneficence, autonomy, and justice.

The principle of honesty deals with our obligation to tell the truth in our dealings with others. However, are we bound to do this totally, in every situation, or are there circumstances when it is in no one's best interest to "tell the truth, the whole truth, and nothing but the truth"?

Moral people have an obligation to keep the promises they make. However, sometimes even with the best of intentions, we may make promises we are unable to fulfill because circumstances change or the ability to comply is no longer within our control. Does promise-keeping require us to blindly continue with a promise, no matter the cost to ourselves or others?

Under the principle of nonmaleficence we are obliged to "do no harm" to others, but many people will grudgingly engage in behavior that harms one person, particularly a stranger, if it defends or protects others, particularly family members or friends.

Beneficence requires that we act in a positive way in our dealings with others; that we "do good." It also mandates preventing harm to others if it is in our power.

Autonomy supports the concept that people have the right to live their lives as they see fit. Exercise of autonomy is limited where the rights of one person come in conflict with the rights of another. How do you draw this line?

Justice or equality recognizes the belief that all people should receive respect and that benefits conferred on one individual should be available to all. However, it does not require that all people be treated exactly alike all the time.

Recognizing the presence of these principles in a challenging moral situation may simplify the handling of the situation. However, the use of these principles to solve ethical dilemmas is complicated when the situation faced presents two or more of them in conflict. You must determine which principle is dominant in your value system, or which will do the most good, or do the least harm, and act accordingly. You have a moral imperative to follow your conscience, regardless of the consequences.

The Decision-Making Process

When an ethical issue arises in a practice setting, try to understand all the implications of your actions before you act. Following these simple steps may help lessen negative impacts that arise from the decisions you make.

- Look at the ethical issue in the broadest context. Who is involved? Who will it affect? What are my options?

■ Decide if you are just faced with an ethical question or are dealing with an ethical dilemma, which may have negative consequences regardless of the actions you take.

■ If you are facing a dilemma, determine the alternative responses you may make to the situation.

■ Look at the risks involved for each response for patients, yourself, your organization or employer, your profession, and society.

■ Assess the benefits derived to each group for each alternative.

■ Identify the ethical principles present in the situation; see if any are in conflict and determine which principle is most important.

■ Make your behavioral decision based on knowledge and evidence, not emotion.

■ Afterward, evaluate the consequences of your actions and determine if you would repeat the choice you made.

Realize there will always be unintended consequences to your actions. Just because you make the "right" decision does not mean you will not have to deal with personal, professional, and legal fallout.

Practical Application

Practice situations that may be a source of ethical conflict fall into two general categories: those related to the drug distribution system and those involving communication with patients, their families, and other health professionals.

Drug distribution issues

■ What do you do when you feel the prescription presented by the patient seems not only inappropriate based on the information you possess, but potentially harmful? Are you less concerned if the prescription, while inappropriate, is neither harmful nor beneficial?

■ How do you handle the patient who asks for a few pills to tide them over until they get a new prescription? Does it matter how long the patient has been your customer or that the drug involved is habit-forming?

■ Do you dispense a controlled medication to a patient you suspect has a substance abuse problem?

■ When is it necessary to confront or report a colleague you believe is diverting drugs?

■ If you are approached by a medical retailer to participate in a patient "switch" to their generic drug in return for financial compensation, how do you respond?

■ Should you do something if the drug prescribed is not approved for use with the patient's disease?

■ Is it important to make sure patient information gathered in the dispensing function is made available to others only on a "need to know" basis?

■ If you are asked to prepare a medication whose use contradicts your personal beliefs, ethically or religiously, do you refuse?

These are some of the drug distribution scenarios that pharmacists and pharmacy technicians may have to face and work through.

Communication issues

Communication scenarios can also present ethical challenges. Patient involvement and consent to treatment is one of the most basic tenets of modern health care. The patient should know what medications he or she is taking, what the side effects may be, what the prognosis is, and what alternative treatments or medications are available.

Everyone agrees patients must provide health professionals with "informed consent." The characteristics of informed consent include shared decision-making between the patient and his or her provider based on mutual respect and good communication. Good communication requires adequate disclosure of the nature of an intervention, its risks, and its benefits. Ethical questions arise as to how much information is enough, how much is too much, where to draw the line, and who should be making these determinations.

Respecting the patient's privacy and maintaining confidentiality are other ethical minefields for pharmacists and pharmacy technicians. It is essential that the patient trust health care providers to ensure patient will continue treatment. This is particularly true when patients are vulnerable because of their age (e.g., the elderly, a minor child) or their disease state (e.g., AIDS, mental illness, sexually transmitted disease). Intentional or unintentional disclosure of information may have a negative impact on patients, their employment status, their finances, or their personal relationships. However, health professionals also have responsibilities to protect the society they serve. How do you distinguish between these competing health needs? Does your answer differ based on the nature of the disease the patient possesses? Can you contemplate a set of circumstances where you would feel it necessary to keep health information on a child from a parent, or information on a husband from a wife?

There are also ethical dilemmas that cross both categories.

- If a prescriber asks you to incorrectly label a prescription because he does not want the patient to know the nature of the medication or that she is receiving a placebo, how do you respond?
- When a patient asks what a drug is used for, do you assume that the prescriber has not communicated with the patient on the medication and tell the patient everything you know without contacting the prescriber?
- What is your responsibility to your patients and your profession when it becomes clear that a colleague is no longer functioning well or acting in a competent manner? Do you tell someone? Do you report your colleague anonymously?
- A medication mistake is made with a patient and you discover it after the patient has left. How far do you have to go to rectify the situation? Should you admit the mistake up front and if you do, to whom should you admit the mistake?

We are sure you can easily supply more examples of practice situations where ethical questions are raised and ethical dilemmas faced. You will notice that we did not supply the answers. That is your job. We have given you some suggestions on the principles to consider and the ways to approach a dilemma. But in the end, it is your value system that will determine your response.

Risk/Benefit Response

Let us remind you that any decision brings with it the risk of being judged wrong and having to face the consequences of your actions. Accepting responsibility for your decisions is central to acting professionally. Do not be surprised or caught off guard by one of the examples we have raised. Assess your value system and ask yourself what you would do before being faced with the situation. Be prepared.

The extent to which a pharmacy technician may directly experience these situations is dependent on the scope of practice recognized in the state and the relationship the technician has with the pharmacist he or she assists. If you made ethical mistakes in the past, it is important to analyze retrospectively what you did and why you did it so you do not repeat the behavior.

As the pharmacist becomes more and more involved in providing pharmaceutical care to patients in all practice settings and the need for medications continues to expand, the role of the pharmacy technician will expand and the nature of ethical dilemmas they face will change. Be ready to meet the challenge.

Summary

Because of the changing nature of the health care environment and the emergence of pharmaceutical care as the standard for pharmacy practice, pharmacy technicians and pharmacists are facing ethical challenges not previously anticipated. This chapter provides the information and the tools to deal with the ethical dilemmas that may arise in both the drug distribution and patient care arenas. The six ethical principles and the two codes of ethics present a starting point for your quest to seek solutions to these dilemmas, to minimize risk to your patients and yourself, and to provide the public the benefits of pharmaceutical care.

TEST YOUR KNOWLEDGE

Multiple Choice Questions

1. Pharmaceutical care
   a. focuses on medication outcomes that improve the quality of a patient's life
   b. is of no concern to a pharmacy technician
   c. is only a pharmacy practice issue, not a pharmaceutical education issue
   d. has yet to be accepted as a standard of pharmacy practice

2. Pharmacy technicians
   a. are licensed by all states
   b. all have the same scope of practice
   c. are meant to assist pharmacists in their practice
   d. do not have ethical obligations to the patient population

3. The earliest known example of an ethical code in medicine was
   a. *The Nuremberg Code*
   b. *The Hippocratic Oath*
   c. *The Declaration of Helsinki*
   d. *The Geneva Convention of Medical Ethics*

4. The *Code of Ethics for Pharmacy Technicians*
   a. has direct application to the activities of all pharmacy assistants
   b. has direct application to the activities of all pharmacy technicians
   c. has direct application to the activities of all pharmacists
   d. has direct application to the activities of members of the American Association of Pharmacy Technicians

5. Pick the statement which is false.
    a. Ethical principles help us make choices between moral alternatives.
    b. Ethical dilemmas always present clear-cut choices between right and wrong.
    c. Our ethical choices sometimes force us to select the lesser of two evils.
    d. Personal and professional values have a place in the ethical decision-making process.

6. The principle of beneficence means
    a. you can do harm
    b. you should do good
    c. you should treat everyone equally
    d. you should let people do what they want

7. The ethical decision making process
    a. can be a complex, time-consuming activity
    b. takes no time or thought
    c. never has any unintended consequences
    d. is free of risk

8. Ethical conflicts in the drug distribution system may include
    a. intentional disclosure of patient information in violation of patient confidentiality
    b. dispensing a controlled substance to a patient you believe has a drug abuse problem
    c. not getting "informed consent"
    d. releasing patient information under a public health initiative

9. Ethical conflicts in the patient communication area may include
    a. finding a colleague who may be diverting drugs
    b. being asked to prepare a medication whose purpose conflicts with your religious beliefs
    c. being asked by a husband about his wife's medication and its purpose
    d. being asked by a patient to supply a few pills to tide them over

10. Facing ethical dilemmas
    a. will bring about the same result in every person
    b. will always make you pleased with the results of your decisions
    c. will never subject you to professional or legal consequences
    d. will always be a personal and professional challenge

References

American Society of Health-System Pharmacists. (1996). White paper on pharmacy technicians. *American Journal of Health-System Pharmacy, 53,* 1991–1994.

Haddad, A. M., Kaatz, B., McCart, G., McCarthy, R. L., Pink, L. A., & Richardson, J. (1993). Report of the ethics course content committee: Curricular guidelines for pharmacy education. *American Journal of Pharmacy Education, 57,* 34S–43S.

Hepler, C. D., & Strand, L. M. (1990). Opportunities and responsibilities in pharmaceutical care. *American Journal of Health-System Pharmacy, 47,* 533–543.

Jonsen, A. R. (2002). *Clinical ethics.* New York: McGraw-Hill.

Lowenthal, W., & Meth, H. (1993). The continuous review of courses: A system for maintaining curricular effectiveness. *American Journal of Pharmacy Education, 57,* 134–139.

National Association of Boards of Pharmacy. (2001). Status of pharmacy technicians. In *Survey of Pharmacy Law.* Park Ridge: Author

Strandberg, K. (2002). *Essentials of law and ethics for pharmacy technicians.* Boca Raton: CRC Press.

Web Site

American Pharmacists Association www.aphanet.org

9 Organizations in Pharmacy

COMPETENCIES

Upon completion and review of this chapter, the student should be able to

1. Identify the major groups in pharmacy that have specialized associations.
2. Describe the two major issues that have brought about the formation of national pharmacy organizations.
3. Explain the historical aspects and identify the first college of pharmacy founded in the United States.
4. Discuss the early problems associated with the issue of drug quality in this country.
5. Match the acronyms to the full names of the various pharmacy associations.

Introduction

One of the characteristics of a profession is the organization of the membership into professional associations. Associations act through the collective voice of the members to set standards of practice and conduct for the profession. If the quantity rather than the quality of associations were an indicator of professionalism, pharmacy would certainly be near the top of the list. One of pharmacy's strengths—its diversity of practice environments and opportunities—is also one of its weaknesses. Each group of practitioners formed national associations (and numerous state and local associations) to further their professional objectives. Independent owner pharmacists, hospital pharmacists, long-term care pharmacists, academic pharmacists, and many other groups have formed into associations, each with its own distinctive name and set of initials or acronym. Selected pharmacy and pharmacy technician organizations and their web site addresses are listed in **Table 9-1**.

The goal of this chapter is to familiarize the reader with pharmacy associations and the important role they play in the profession in the United States. Finally, the professional journals that function as the voice of the various associations will be listed.

Historical Development

Two major issues caused the formation of the first local and national pharmacy associations in the United States: the development of educational standards for practice and the quality of drugs available to the pharmacist for use in preparing prescriptions.

TABLE 9-1   Pharmacy and Pharmacy Technician Associations

AACP	American Association of Colleges of Pharmacy www.aacp.org
AAPS	American Association of Pharmaceutical Scientists www.aapspharmaceutical.com
AAPT	American Association of Pharmacy Technicians www.pharmacytechnician.com
ACCP	American College of Clinical Pharmacy www.accp.com
ACPE	American Council on Pharmaceutical Education www.acpe-arcredit.org
AMCP	Academy of Managed Care Pharmacy www.amcp.org
APhA	American Pharmacists Association www.aphanet.org
ASCP	American Society of Consultant Pharmacists www.ascp.com
ASHP	American Society of Health System Pharmacists www.ashp.com
NABP	National Association of Boards of Pharmacy www.nabp.org
NACDS	National Association of Chain Drug Stores www.nacds.org
NCPA	National Community Pharmacists Association www.ncpanet.org
NPTA	National Pharmacy Technician Association www.pharmacytechnician.org
PTCB	Pharmacy Technician Certification Board www.ptcb.org
PTEC	Pharmacy Technician Educators Council

The first issue—education—has continued to be a primary concern of all pharmacy associations, since it affects both future and current practitioners. The formation of the Philadelphia College of Pharmacy in 1821, the first formal educational program in pharmacy, was one result of the organization of the first professional association of pharmacy. Additionally, the Philadelphia College of Pharmacy inspected drugs for quality and acted to arbitrate disputes between members of the college. Following the lead of Philadelphia pharmacists, other associations or colleges of pharmacy were formed in Boston, New York, Baltimore, Cincinnati, and St. Louis. Formal educational programs were not provided in the early years by these other "colleges," but eventually each evolved into a true college of pharmacy, providing a regular curriculum leading to education of pharmacy practitioners.

The issue of drug quality was an important concern to the early practitioners of pharmacy and medicine in the United States, because the drugs available to the physicians and pharmacists of the nineteenth and early twentieth centuries were mostly of natural origin. These animal and vegetable preparations were often imported into the United States. There was no U.S. pharmaceutical industry. The pharmacist would utilize these crude drugs to prepare the medications prescribed by the physician. Because these animal and vegetable products were so costly, it was not uncommon for drug merchants to adulterate (dilute) the desired material with worthless plant or animal by-products. The early pharmacy associations provided inspection committees to examine these imported materials. They also lobbied vigorously for governmental inspection at the major ports of entry. It was not until 1906, with the passage of the Food and Drug Act, that the federal government became involved with ensuring drug quality and purity.

Drug production and drug quality are still a major concern of pharmacy professional associations because of the many sources of drug products now available. The FDA Medical Products Reporting Program, MedWatch, provides a mechanism for health professionals to report drug-product quality problems to the FFDA, and conversely, for the FDA to provide regular feedback to the health care community about safety issues involving medical products. The MedWatch program is supported by over 140 organizations, including all major organizations in pharmacy.

Organizations or associations are a way of life for Americans. The American Society of Association Executives is the national association representing over 10,000 association members serving more than 287 million persons and companies.

Although there are many organizations in pharmacy, some are of greater importance to the pharmacy technician. These include the ASHP, formed in 1942, which now has almost 30,000 members. Housed in its new quarters in suburban Washington, it has an annual budget of $28 million.

The American Pharmacists Association (APhA) is 150 years old and today has a membership of almost 50,000. APhA provides continuing education programs for pharmacists and technicians. APhA has been the birthplace for many pharmacy associations.

The training and recognition of pharmacy technicians in the United States has been a slowly evolving process which began in the mid-1960s. In this country, however, pharmacists over the years have engaged assistance to carry out ancillary tasks to expedite the preparation and dispensing of medication. European pharmacies, on the other hand, have a history of long-established and recognized pharmacy technician education programs. The first textbook specific to pharmacy technician education was published by Mosby Publishers in 1968 and authored by Durgin and Hanan. Formal technician training programs were established in that same era by Mercy Medical Centre in Long Island, New York, and in the Rhode Island Hospital in that state. Throughout the country, formal and informal programs were emerging to better train technicians who were already on the job. In 1979 the American Association of Pharmacy Technicians (AAPT) was formed. In 1983 the ASHP accredited the first pharmacy technician training program at Thomas Jefferson Hospital in Philadelphia.

National Associations of Pharmacists and Pharmacy Technicians

The first national association of U.S. pharmacists was the American Pharmaceutical Association (APhA). The APhA is now known as American Pharmacists Association. Formed in Philadelphia in 1852, APhA has grown into the largest of the national associations in pharmacy, with approximately fifty thousand members. The original objectives of the association, written over 100 years ago, addressed the major concerns of the profession then and surprisingly the major concerns now. They are improvement and regulation of drug supply and quality, inter- and intraprofessional relations, improvement of the scientific knowledge base of the profession and dissemination of that new knowledge through publication, educational standards for practice of the profession, restriction of drug-dispensing functions, and creation of ethical standards of practice. APhA supports voluntary certification of technicians by the pharmacy profession but opposes licensure, registration, or certification by state law or regulation.

In addition to being the first national professional pharmacy association, APhA is also considered to be the "parent" of many other pharmacy associations. The American Society of Health System Pharmacists (ASHP), the National Community

Pharmacists Association (NCPA), the American College of Apothecaries (ACA), the American Association of Colleges of Pharmacy (AACP) and the American Association of Pharmaceutical Scientists were all initiated by special interest groups originally a part of APhA.

APhA is organized into three academies: the Academy of Pharmacy Practice and Management (APPM), the Academy of Pharmaceutical Research (APRS), and the Academy of Student of Pharmacy (ASP). APhA also has a research foundation and a political action committee (PAC). APhA cofounded the Pharmacy Technician Certification Board (PTCB) with ASHP, the Illinois Council of Health-System Pharmacists, and the Michigan Pharmacists Association. The PTCB office is located within the APhA association building. PTCB offers certification and recertification exams several times each year. Information on certification exam contents and process are available on the PTCB Web site. As of January 2004, there were more than 157,000 certified pharmacy technicians (CPhTs).

APhA was also responsible for the formation of the Board of Pharmaceutical Specialties (BPS) in 1976 with the following responsibilities:

- recognize specialties in pharmacy practice
- set standards for certification and recertification
- objectively evaluate individuals seeking certification and recertification
- serve as a source of information and coordinating agency for pharmacy specialties

The American Society of Health-System Pharmacists (ASHP) is a 30,000 member professional association that represents pharmacists who practice in hospitals and other components of the health care system. ASHP currently focuses its programs and resources on a set of 10 practice domains, including acute care, ambulatory care, clinical specialists, home care, long-term care, chronic care, managed care, new practitioners, pharmacy practice management, and technicians. ASHP was founded at the 1942 meeting of APhA, and from its founding until 1972, membership in the parent organization (APhA) was required for membership in ASHP. ASHP has been a vigorous proponent of the role of the pharmacist as the drug-use control expert in organized health care settings. ASHP has taken strong positions regarding education of pharmacists and technicians and has accrediting standards for pharmacy residencies designed for pharmacy graduates, and for pharmacy technician training programs.

Education has been a hallmark for all organizations in pharmacy, but APhA and ASHP have been exceptionally strong. APhA now provides a framework for specialty certification of pharmacists. Their annual meeting is well organized and of benefit to pharmacists and technicians as well as to the industry.

ASHP holds two large meetings annually. The annual meeting, like the one at APhA, provides general education. The midyear clinical meeting provides a forum for pharmacists and technicians, but also has special educational programming for clinical specialists.

The National Community Pharmacists Association (NCPA), formerly the National Association of Retail Druggists (NARD), developed from the parent APhA's Section on Commercial Interests as an independent organization in 1898. NCPA has strongly represented the interests of the independent pharmacy owner since its inception and has championed the independent practice alternative to students of pharmacy. In 1991 NCPA created the National Home Infusion Association (NHIA). A special focus of NCPA has been the training and certification of pharmacists in various areas of "pharmacist care" through the National Institute for Pharmacist Care

Outcomes (NIPCO). NCPA also supports a Management Institute that provides information, training, and resources to improve pharmacy management. NCPA has a reputation for being a vigorous defender of the independent owner's rights on Capitol Hill. NCPA lobbied for over a decade for legislation to make armed robbery a federal offense. The NCPA PAC was also the first in pharmacy and has the slogan "Get into politics or get out of pharmacy."

The American Society of Consultant Pharmacists (ASCP) is an organization for pharmacists who provide drug therapy management services and medication distribution to older adults and others with chronic illness. ASCP provides the health care practitioners with a particular interest in the geriatric patient with education and resources to improve their practice skills. Health professionals, other than pharmacists, are eligible to become members of ASCP.

The Academy of Managed Care Pharmacy (AMCP) is a professional association of pharmacists and associates who serve patients in the managed health care system environment. The goals of AMCP, ASHP, and APhA often overlap, and multiple memberships in these associations is not uncommon.

The American College of Clinical Pharmacy (ACCP) consists primarily of Pharm.D. clinical practitioners and faculty members. Its stated mission is to facilitate the creation, transmission, and application of new knowledge in the science of pharmacotherapy.

The American College of Apothecaries (ACA) is a small, selective association of community-based practitioners. Membership is granted only if the practitioners and their pharmacy complies with certain standards of professional service and appearance. Dual membership in APhA is required.

In addition to APhA and ASHP, there are two professional associations expressly for pharmacy technicians, the American Association of Pharmacy Technicians (AAPT) and the National Pharmacy Technician Association (NPTA). Both associations hold annual meetings during the summer months and provide their members with access to educational services.

The Pharmacy Technician Certification Board (PTCB) was established in January 1995 through the efforts of APhA, ASHP, the Illinois Council of Health-System Pharmacists (ICHP), and the Michigan Pharmacists Association (MPA). It provides a voluntary mechanism for a national certification program.

PTCB offers the certification examination several times each year. To be eligible to take the examination, the candidate must have a high school diploma or GED. The cost for the application fee is currently $120. Recertification and continuing education are required by the board. As of January 1997, more than 18,000 technicians are certified. These individuals make up a valued group and are a powerful contribution to the mission of pharmacy.

The Pharmacy Technician Educators Council (PTEC) usually meets jointly with the American Association of Colleges of Pharmacy (AACP) at the AACP annual meeting. Members include faculty members of formal technician training programs most often associated with community colleges.

Other Associations

Many other national associations in pharmacy represent special segments of the profession. These are presented here with a brief description of their membership and mission.

The National Association of Chain Drug Stores (NACDS) is an organization of corporations, generally represented by their chief executive officers, many of whom are not pharmacists. The title is misleading because NACDS represents a variety of businesses, not only chain or multioutlet pharmacies. Grocery chains, department stores, and a variety of discount outlets that have pharmacies belong to NACDS. The strength of this organization lies in its size and large financial capabilities. Chains are the largest employer of practicing pharmacists. While nonpharmacy merchandising has been a large concern of NACDS, recent consumer trends have suggested that chains pay more attention to the pharmacy department and the employee pharmacist. The Food Marketing Institute (FMI) represents the food retailing business (supermarkets). Supermarket-located pharmacies are the most rapidly growing sector of retail pharmacy and FMI has a division of programs for this segment of the industry.

The American Association of Colleges of Pharmacy (AACP) is an organization of pharmacy colleges and schools. Representation of deans and faculty members is accomplished through membership on their respective councils, which have equal representation in the House of Delegates. The AACP is primarily concerned with educational issues, such as curricula and teaching methodology. AACP members approved a four-year professional curriculum leading to the doctor of pharmacy degree (PharmD) as the single entry-level degree for pharmacy in July 1992. Because a minimum of two years of preprofessional education is required for entry into the professional degree program, the PharmD degree is often and erroneously referred to as a six-year degree program. Presently, more than 50% of all students entering the professional degree program have more than two years preprofessional higher education. No final implementation date was set for implementation of the curriculum. The AACP adopted a policy of supportive personnel (pharmacy technicians), which states that the training of such personnel be based on sound educational principles. The AACP also recommended that its member schools offer their assistance for the development of those objectives.

The American Council on Pharmaceutical Education (ACPE) is the independent, government-recognized accrediting agency of degree and continuing education programs in pharmacy. Formed in 1932 through the efforts of APhA, AACP, and the National Association of Boards of Pharmacy (NABP), the ACPE has, through its representative membership, proposed and published the standards that schools must meet to obtain accreditation. Criteria such as budget, governance, faculty quality and quantity, admission standards, physical facilities, library, curricula, and student achievement are all considered during the accreditation process. Accreditation is voluntary, but inasmuch as all states require graduation from an accredited school of pharmacy as a prerequisite of licensure, an unaccredited program could not survive. Accreditation is also needed to qualify for a variety of state and federal financial aid programs.

The National Association of Boards of Pharmacy (NABP) is an organization of the members of the individual state boards of pharmacy which are generally charged with the licensure of pharmacies and pharmacists and, in many states, with inspection and law enforcement activities. The NABP, since its inception in 1904, has worked to standardize the requirements for pharmacist licensure while maintaining the posture of individual states' rights. Through its efforts, reciprocity—transfer of licensure among most states—has been facilitated and a national licensing exam for pharmacists, the NABPLEX, is used as a major part of all but several states' licensing examinations. The NABP makes available the North American Pharmacist Licensure Exam (NABPLEX), the Multi-State Pharmacy Jurisprudence Exam, and the Foreign Pharmacy Graduate Equivalency Exam to assist state pharmacy boards in their evaluation of candidates for pharmacy licensure.

Association Publications

One of the first actions of a professional association is the publication of a journal for the dissemination of scientific and professional information for the membership and the profession. The founders of the Philadelphia College of Pharmacy were responsible for the publication of the first American pharmacy journal, the *Journal of the Philadelphia College of Pharmacy,* in 1825. In 1835 the title was changed to the *American Journal of Pharmacy* and has been published continually to this day. Since that initial effort, the many national associations of pharmacy have continued and expanded on this effort, each with its own journal and newsletter (**Table 9-2**). In addition, several associations—most notably APhA and the ASHP—have produced publications providing pharmacists and other health professionals with needed drug information, such as the *Handbook of Nonprescription Drugs* and the *American Hospital Formulary Service.* The ASHP also publishes the *International Pharmaceutical Abstracts,* which is a semimonthly abstracting service of the world's pharmaceutical literature.

TABLE 9-2

Organizational Publications

AACP	*American Journal of Pharmaceutical Education*
AAPS	*Pharmaceutical Research; AAPS PharmSci*
AMCP	*Journal of American Pharmacists Association; Pharmacy Today*
APhA	*American Journal of Health-System Pharmacists*
ASCP	*America's Pharmacist*
ASHP	*The Consultant Pharmacist*
NCPA	*Journal of Managed Care Pharmacy*
NPTA	*Today's Technician*

Summary

There are a number of professional organizations that meet the specialty needs of their membership.

Organizations represent members practicing in community, chain, hospital, consulting, and clinical pharmacy practice. Colleges of pharmacy, accrediting agencies, state boards of pharmacy, wholesalers, and more comprise additional specialty membership groups in pharmacy practice.

The various organizations in pharmacy link together pharmacists who are engaged in the numerous aspects of the profession. As a result, all pharmacists have the opportunity to enter the mainstream of the constantly evolving growth and development of the profession of pharmacy.

TEST YOUR KNOWLEDGE

Multiple Choice Questions

1. An identifying characteristic of a profession is
   a. the organization of the membership into professional associations
   b. that all members agree on all professional policies regarding education and other important matters
   c. that all members have the same professional, academic degree
   d. that financial objectives are of primary importance

2. The major issues that gave us the first national association of pharmacists were
   a. educational programs required
   b. means of expanding profitability
   c. quality and purity of drugs
   d. a and c
   e. a, b, and c

True/False Questions

3. ___T___ An organization represents the special interests of the membership.

4. ___T___ The American Society of Health-System Pharmacists has taken a strong position regarding education of pharmacists and technicians.

5. ___T___ The National Community Pharmacists Association (NCPA) represents the interests of independent retail pharmacy owners.

Matching Questions

6. __C__ ASHP   a. open to all pharmacists

7. __b__ NCPA   b. independent community retail pharmacists

8. __a__ AACP   c. hospital pharmacists

9. __d__ APhA   d. pharmacy educators

10. __e__ PTEC   e. pharmacy technicians

References

Flanagan, M. E. (1995). Voluntary technician certification program reflects changes in practice. *American Pharmacy, NS35*(5), 18–23.

Murer, M. M. (1996). Technician certification leads to recognition, better patient care. *Journal of the American Pharmaceutical Association, NS36,* 514–520.

Smith, J. E. (1995). The national voluntary certification of pharmacy technicians. *American Journal of Health System Pharmacy, 52,* 2026–2029.

PART

III Professional Aspects of Pharmacy Technology

Chapter 10: The Prescription, Terminology, and Medical Abbreviations

Chapter 11: Pharmaceutical Dosage Forms

Chapter 12: Pharmaceutical Calculations

Chapter 13: Extemporaneous Compounding

Chapter 14: Parenteral Compounding

Chapter 15: Administration of Medications

Chapter 16: Drug Information Centers

Chapter 17: Drug Distribution Systems

Chapter 18: Infection Control and Prevention in the Pharmacy

The Prescription, Terminology, and Medical Abbreviations

COMPETENCIES

Upon completion of this chapter, the reader should be able to

1. Recognize word elements and be able to define and be aware of word element combinations in medical terminology.
2. Define commonly used medical terminology and abbreviations.
3. Graphically illustrate apothecary symbols.
4. Identify drugs by both the brand/trade names and generic names.
5. Differentiate "look-alike" and "sound-alike" drugs.
6. Identify the various parts of a prescription.

Introduction

Pharmacists and technicians both are exposed to a myriad of terms and abbreviations in the daily practice of institutional pharmacy. Not all of the terms, symbols, or abbreviations included in this chapter pertain solely to pharmacy, but technicians should be acquainted with these and other terms to carry out their duties effectively.

This chapter is divided as follows:

1. common word elements
2. common medical terms
3. abbreviations
4. commonly used apothecary symbols
5. brand/trade names and generic names
6. look-alike and sound-alike drugs
7. the prescription

Common Word Elements

Medical terminology is a combination of word elements. For example, bradycardia means a slowing of the heartbeat. The word was created by combining the word elements of the prefix "brady-", which means slow, and the suffix "-cardia", which means heart. This list of commonly used word elements should enable the technician to understand and create many acceptable medical terms. (*Note:* Elements followed by a hyphen are prefixes; elements preceded by a hyphen are suffixes.)

a(n)-	an absence, not	micr(o)-	small
aden(o)-	gland	morph(o)-	shape, form
adipo-	fat	my(o)-	muscle
-algia	pain	myel(o)-	bone marrow, spinal cord
ante-	before		
anti-	against	nas(o)-	nose
arthro-	joint	necr(o)-	dead
aur(i)-	ear	nephr(o)-	kidney
brady-	slow	-oma	tumor
-cardi(a)	heart action	ophthalm(o)-	eye
-cele	tumor, hernia	os, oste(o)-	bone
chole-	bile, gall	-osis	disease process
-cid(e)	kill	-ostomy	surgical opening
col(i), (o)-	colon	ot(o)-	ear
cop(o)-	vagina	path(o)-	disease
cyst(i), (o)-	sac, bladder	phleb(o)-	vein
dermat-	skin	-plasty	forming, shaping
-ectomy	excision	-plegia	paralysis
eu-	well, normal	pneum(o)-	lung, air
gluc(o)-	sweet, sugar	pod(o)-	foot
hem(o)-, hema-, hemat(o)-	blood	poly-	many
		post-	after
hemi-	half	procto(o)-	anus, rectum
hepat(o)-	liver	pulm(o)-	lung
hyper-	above	recto-	backward, behind
hypo-	below	rhin(o)-	nose
infra-	beneath	-rrhea	flow
inter-	between	super-	over, above (amount)
intra-	within		
-itis	inflammation	supra-	above (position)
lith(o)-	stone	tachy-	rapid
macr(o)-	large, long	thora(o)-	chest
mal-	abnormal	ur(o)-	urine, urological
mast(o)-	breast	vesic(o)-	bladder

Common Medical Terms

accelerated care unit (ACU) Separate unit in the hospital where patients are prepared to better care for themselves and their condition after being discharged from the hospital.

acidosis Acid/base imbalance causing the blood and body tissues to become excessively acidic.

acute A severe condition rising rapidly to a peak and then subsiding.

additive (parenteral) An addition of an active ingredient to a solution that is intended for intravenous administration or irrigation.

alkalosis Acid/base imbalance causing the blood and body tissues to become excessively alkaline or basic.

allergen An agent that provokes the symptoms of an allergy.

allergy An abnormal reaction to a substance, situation, or physical state.

ambulatory patient A patient who is able to walk and is not restricted to bed.

amphetamine A stimulant drug; also known as uppers, bam, bennies, browns, bumblebee, butterflies.

anabolic agent A substance that builds up tissue protein.

anabolism The body process during which proteins are synthesized and tissues are formed.

analgesic A substance that relieves pain.

anaphylaxis A hypersensitivity reaction that is immediate, shock-like, and possibly fatal.

anesthetic A drug used to decrease sensation.

aneurysm A dilation or bulging out of a blood vessel wall.

antepartum Before the onset of childbirth.

antibiotic A substance that is able to kill or inhibit the growth of bacteria or other microorganisms.

anticoagulant A drug that prevents or delays coagulation or clotting of blood; a "blood thinner."

antiflatulent A drug that facilitates expulsion of gas from the GI tract.

antigen An agent that stimulates antibody formation.

antineoplastic A substance that prevents the development or spread of tumor cells.

antipruritic A drug that relieves itch.

antipyretic A drug that reduces fever.

antiseptic An agent that inhibits the growth of microorganisms, but does not necessarily kill them.

antitoxin A specific agent neutralizing a poison or toxin.

antitussive A drug used for the relief of cough.

arrhythmia An abnormal, irregular heartbeat.

arteriosclerosis Hardening of the arteries.

arthritis Inflammation of joints.

ascites Accumulation of fluid within the abdominal cavity.

aseptic technique A method of preparation that will prevent contamination of a site (e.g., wound) or product (e.g., IV admixture).

atherosclerosis Lipid (fat) deposits in large and medium size arteries.

atonic Weak tone or absence of tone.

bactericide An agent capable of killing bacterias.

bacteriostat An agent that inhibits the growth of bacteria.

benign Not malignant or invasive.

biopsy Excision of a small piece of tissue for diagnostic purposes.

blood urea nitrogen (BUN) An indication of kidney function.

bradycardia Slow heart rate.

buccal Between the gum and cheek.

calibration A method of standardizing a measuring device.

carcinogen Any substance that causes cancer.

catabolism The breakdown of body proteins.

cathartic A drug used to produce evacuation of the bowel.

central service An area in the hospital where general sterilization procedures are performed; serves as a storage facility for various types of equipment.

chemotherapy Treatment of a condition with drugs. Currently used in reference to the treatment of cancer.

chronic Of long duration or frequent recurrence.

coagulation Blood-clotting process.

cocaine A topical anesthetic; also known as coke, crack, snow, blow, white horse, 8-ball.

colostomy Creation of an opening into the colon through the abdominal wall.

compliance Act of adhering to prescribed directions.

congestive heart failure (CHF) Failure or diminished ability of the heart to pump an adequate blood supply to the rest of the body.

crack An illicit, pure form of cocaine, usually smoked in a pipe.

creatinine clearance A measure of renal function.

decongestant A drug used to open the air passages of the nose and lungs.

decubitus ulcer A bedsore.

deoxyribonucleic acid (DNA) A double-stranded structure that is the molecular basis of heredity.

diabetes mellitus A chronic disease affecting carbohydrate metabolism.

diagnosis The identification of a disease from its signs and symptoms.

diastolic pressure The force exerted by the blood on the blood vessels when the ventricles of the heart are in a state of rest before systole.

diluent An agent that dilutes or reconstitutes a solution or mixture.

diuretic A drug used to increase urinary output; "water pill."

electrocardiogram A graphic record of the heart's action by electronic measurement.

electroencephalogram A tracing or electronic recording of brain waves.

embolism A traveling blood clot that may deposit in a vessel and obstruct flow through that vessel.

emergency room A hospital unit where patients are treated for conditions that require immediate attention.

equivalent weight The gram molecular weight divided by the highest valent ion in the molecule.

erythrocyte A red blood cell.

estrogen A hormone that produces secondary sex characteristics in the female.

etiology The cause(s) of a disease.

expectorant A drug that promotes the secretion and excretion of mucus from the lungs and trachea.

febrile Body temperature above normal.

fibrillation Rapid, ineffectual heartbeat.

floor stock Medications that are routinely kept on the nursing unit.

gastric Pertaining to the stomach.

generic drug name The nonproprietary (non-brand) name of a drug.

glucose tolerance test A test for diabetes based on the ability of the liver to store glycogen.

hemorrhage Severe bleeding.

hemostat An agent used to arrest hemorrhage.

hepatitis Inflammation of the liver.

heroin An illicit drug derived from morphine; also known as brown sugar, salt, horse.

hyperalimentation Intravenous feeding; total parenteral nutrition (TPN).

hypertension High blood pressure.

hypnotic A drug used to induce sleep.

hypotension Low blood pressure.

immunity Resistance to infection.

incubation The period between exposure to an infective disease process and the symptoms of infection.

infection The successful invasion of the body by pathogenic organisms.

inflammation The condition characterized by pain, heat, redness, and swelling.

infusion The slow injection of a solution into a vein, subcutaneous tissue, or other tissue.

injection The act of forcing a liquid medication into the blood or body.

inpatient A patient who requires the use of a hospital bed and is registered in the hospital to receive medical or surgical care.

intensive care unit (ICU) A hospital where the patient receives constant and vigilant attention.

intradermal Situated or applied within the skin.

intrathecal Within the subdural space of the spinal cord.

intramuscular Within the muscle.

iontophoresis Introduction of medication into the tissue by means of an electric current.

jaundice Yellow appearance of skin and mucous membranes resulting from the deposition of bile pigment.

laboratory A hospital department where chemical or biological testing is performed for the purpose of aiding diagnosis.

leukemia A disease characterized by an extremely high white blood cell count.

lozenge A small, medicated or flavored disk intended to be dissolved in the mouth.

LSD **L**ys**e**rgic acid **d**iethylamide, a hallucinogen; also known as beast, black sunshine, the chief.

MAO inhibitors A class of drugs that act as antidepressants by inhibiting the enzyme **m**ono**a**mine **o**xidase.

malignant A type of tumor that invades healthy tissue and becomes progressively worse.

marijuana Substance, from hemp, that has an effect on mood, perception, and psychomotor coordination; also known as sinse, weed, herb, grass, dope, reefer, maryjane.

mastectomy Removal of the breast.

medication administration record (MAR) A record maintained by the nursing staff containing information about the patient's medication and its frequency of administration.

meninges The membrane that surrounds the brain and spinal cord.

meningitis Inflammation of the meninges.

metabolism The process by which an organism converts food to energy needed for anabolism.

metastasis The spread of disease from one organ to another.

milliequivalent (mEq) One-thousandth of an equivalent weight.

miotic A drug that causes constriction of the pupil.

mnemonic code An abbreviation used in computerized medication order entry.

morgue A place where a corpse is kept until released for burial.

mucolytic A substance that liquifies, dissolves, or digests mucus.

mydriatic An agent that dilates the pupil of the eye.

myocardial infarction (MI) Injury to the heart muscle (myocardium) due to inadequate oxygen supply caused by the occlusion of a coronary artery.

narcotic A drug that is habit forming and addictive and produces relief from pain.

nephritis Inflammation of the nephron.

nephron Functional unit of the kidney.

obstructive jaundice Jaundice that results from an impediment to the flow of bile from the liver to the duodenum.

occlusion Blockage of a blood vessel.

operating room A unit in the hospital where major surgical procedures are performed.

outpatient department An area of the hospital where various medical services are provided to patients who do not require a hospital bed (outpatients).

oxytocic An agent that causes uterine contractions.

palliative A treatment that provides relief but no cure for a condition.

parenteral solution Sterile solutions intended for subcutaneous, intramuscular, or intravenous injection.

pathogen Any disease-producing organism.

pathology That branch of medicine concerned with the essential nature of disease, especially the structural and functional changes in tissues caused by the disease process.

patient medication profile A record kept in the pharmacy of patient data and current drug therapy. It contains such information as initiation and discontinuation of medication orders and dosage form and strength. It also indicates any allergies, diagnosis, or other information pertinent to drug therapy.

PCP Phencyclidine, a hallucinogen; also known as busy bee, buzz, zombie.

pertussis Whooping cough; an acute infectious disease of the respiratory tract.

pH A measurement of acidity or alkalinity.

pharmaceutics The science of drug-delivery systems.

pharmacist A person licensed to dispense medication and to counsel on drug therapy.

pharmacogenetics The study of the relationship between heredity and response to drugs.

pharmacognosy The study of therapeutic agents derived from natural sources (e.g., plants).

pharmacokinetics The study of bodily absorption, distribution, metabolism, and excretion of drugs.

pharmacology The study of the action of drugs on the body.

pharmacotherapeutics Pertaining to the use of drugs in the prevention or treatment of disease.

pharmacy, contemporary A health service concerning itself with the knowledge of drugs and their effects on the body.

pharmacy intern A person obtaining practical experience and training in pharmacy to meet the requirements of the state board of pharmacy for licensure as a pharmacist.

pharmacy resident A graduate from an accredited pharmacy school enrolled in a program designed to develop expert skills in pharmacy practice.

pharmacy technician Support personnel with education and training that allows performance of select tasks as delegated by the supervising pharmacist.

pharmacy, traditional The art and science of compounding and dispensing medications.

phlebitis Inflammation of the veins.

physical therapy (PT) Physical manipulation for the purpose of rehabilitation.

plasma The fluid portion of the blood in which the blood cells are suspended.

postpartum Occuring after childbirth or delivery.

prognosis The expected outcome of the course of the disease.

pulmonary Pertaining to the lungs.

purified protein derivative (PPD) Product used as a skin test for tuberculosis antibodies.

radiation therapy The use of X-rays in the treatment of a disease.

radiology (X-ray) department An area of the hospital where diagnosis and treatment are performed using X-rays, radioisotopes, and other similar methods.

radiopharmacy A branch of pharmacy dealing with radioactive diagnostics.

recovery room (RR) Area in the hospital where patients are monitored and treated immediately after leaving the operating room.

renal Pertaining to the kidney.

respiration The breathing process.

ribonucleic acid (RNA) A single-stranded structure that is the molecular basis for protein synthesis.

rubella German measles.

sedative A drug used to allay anxiety and excitement; often used to help a patient sleep.

serum The clear fluid of the blood separated from solid parts.

signs Objective bodily evidence of distress found by physical examination.

solvent A substance used to dissolve another substance.

sterilization The act or process of rendering sterile; the complete destruction of microorganisms by heat or bactericidal compounds.

styptic An agent that stops or slows bleeding by contracting blood vessels when applied locally.

subcutaneous Under the skin.

sublingual Under the tongue.

symptom Subjective evidence of a disease; evidence of disease as perceived by the patient.

syncope   Fainting; a transient loss of consciousness due to inadequate blood flow to the brain.

syndrome   A group of signs and symptoms that characterize a particular abnormality.

synergism   A joint action of agents in which the total effect of the combination is greater than the sum of their individual independent effects.

systolic   The force exerted by the blood when the ventricles are in a state of contraction.

tachycardia   Rapid heart rate.

telephone order   An order for a drug or other form of treatment that is given over the phone to an authorized receiver by an authorized prescriber.

testosterone   A hormone that produces secondary sex characteristics in the male.

toxic   A toxin that has been detoxified by moderate heat and chemical treatment that retains its antigenicity.

toxin, bacterial   A noxious or poisonous product that causes the formation of antibodies called antitoxins.

trachea   Windpipe.

tracheotomy   An incision into the trachea.

tranquilizer   A drug to relieve anxiety or agitation.

urticaria   Eruption or rash associated with severe itching.

vaccine   Any material that produces active immunization in the formation of antibodies.

valence   Those electrons that are associated with bonds between elements.

vasconstriction   Narrowing of blood vessels.

vasodilation   Relaxation of smooth muscles of the vascular system that produces dilation of the blood vessel.

ventricular fibrillation   Rapid ineffectual action of the ventricle of the heart.

verbal order   An order for a drug or other treatment that is given verbally to an authorized receiver by an authorized prescriber.

vertigo   A sensation the patient experiences that the external world is revolving around the patient; dizziness.

virus   A submicroscopic agent of infectious disease that is capable of reproduction.

viscosity   An expression of the resistance of a fluid to flow.

vitamin   A general term for a number of organic substances that occur in many foods in small amounts required for normal growth and maintenance of life.

written order   An order for a drug or other form of treatment that is written on the appropriate form by an authorized prescriber.

Common Medical/Pharmacy Abbreviations and Terminology

a, ante	before
aa	of equal parts
ac	before meals
ad (*)	right ear
ad lib	as much as desired
ADI	American Drug Index
adm	admission
ADR	adverse drug reaction
Af, a fib	atrial fibrillation; rapid, ineffectual atrial heart rate
AHFS	American Hospital Formulary Service
AIDS	acquired immunodeficiency syndrome
alb	albumin
am	morning
amb	ambulatory
amt	amount
anabolism	protein synthesis
anaphylaxis	hypersensitivity reaction
ANDA	Abbreviated New Drug Application
antitussive	cough reliever
APAP	acetaminophen
APT	Association of Pharmacy Technicians
APhA	American Pharmacists Association
ARC	AIDS-related complex
aq	aqueous
as (*)	left ear
ASA	aspirin
ASHP	American Society of Health-Systems Pharmacists
au (*)	both ears
AZT	azidothymidine, zidovudine
BBVD	bloodborne viral disease
bid	twice daily
biw	twice weekly
BM	bowel movement
BMR	basal metabolic rate
BP	blood pressure
BUN	blood urea nitrogen; a kidney function test

c	with	ECT or EST	electroconvulsive therapy
Ca	calcium	EEG	electroencephalogram
CAD	coronary artery disease	embolism	traveling blood clot
caps	capsules	ENT	ear, nose, and throat
CAT	computerized axial tomography	ER	emergency room
cath	catheter	FBS	fasting blood sugar
CBC	complete blood count	FDA	Food and Drug Administration
CC	chief complaint	febrile	elevated body temperature
cc (*)	cubic centimeter (milliliter)	fuo	fever of unknown origin
CCU	coronary care unit	g, gm	gram
CDC	Centers for Disease Control and Prevention	GI	gastrointestinal
		gr	grain
CHF	congestive heart failure	gtt	drop
Cl	chloride	GU	genitourinary
cm	centimeter	GYN	gynecology
CNS	central nervous system	h, hr	hour
CO_2	carbon dioxide	H_2O	water
COPD	chronic obstructive pulmonary disease	Hct	hematocrit
		Hgb	hemoglobin
CPR	cardiopulmonary resuscitation	HIV	human immunodeficiency virus
C&S	culture and sensitivity	H&P	history and physical
CQI	continuing quality improvement	hs (*)	hour of sleep, bedtime
CSF	cerebrospinal fluid	hx	history
CTU	cardiac transition unit	ICU	intensive care unit
CV	cardiovascular	ILL	international unit
CVA	cerebral vascular accident (stroke)	IM	intramuscular
CVP	central venous pressure	IND	investigational new drug
dc, d/c (*)	discontinue	INH	isoniazid
DEA	Drug Enforcement Agency	I & O	intake and output
decubitus	bedsore	IV	intravenous
DIC	Drug Information Center	IVPB	intravenous piggyback; small volume parenteral
diag	diagnosis		
Disp	dispense	IVSS	intravenous soluset; small volume parenteral
DTD	let such doses be given		
DM	diabetes mellitus; disease affecting carbohydrate metabolism	JCAHO	Joint Commission for Accreditation of Healthcare Organizations
DME	durable medical equipment	K	potassium
DNA	deoxyribonucleic acid	KCl	potassium chloride
DO	doctor of osteopathy	kg	kilogram
DPT	diphtheria, pertussis, tetanus vaccine	kvo	keep vein open
		l	liter
DRG	diagnosis related group	lb	pound
D5W	dextrose 5% in water	LPN	licensed practical nurse
D5/0.33	dextrose 5% in 0.33% sodium chloride	LR	lactated Ringer's solution
		mcg, ug	microgram
D5/0.45	dextrose 5% in 0.45% sodium chloride	MD	medical doctor
		mEq	milliequivalent
D5/0.9	dextrose 5% in 0.9% sodium chloride	Mg	magnesium
DRL	dextrose 5% in Ringer's lactate	MI	myocardial infarction
DR	delivery room	ml	milliliter
dx	diagnosis	MOM	milk of magnesia
ECG or EKG	electrocardiogram	ms	morphine sulfate, multiple sclerosis

mvi	multivitamin	qhs (*)	every bedtime
NARD	National Association of Retail Druggists	qid (*)	four times daily
		qod (*)	every other day
Na	sodium	qs	quantity sufficient
NDA	new drug application	rbc	red blood cell; erythrocyte
NF	National Formulary	RL	Ringer's lactate
ngt	nasogastric tube	RN	registered nurse
non rep (nr)	do not repeat	RNA	ribonucleic acid
NPH	neutral protamine Hagedorn insulin	r/o	rule out
npo	nothing by mouth	rt, R	right
NS	normal saline; 0.9% sodium chloride	Rx	prescription
NSAID	nonsteroidal anti-inflammatory drug	s	without
NTG	nitroglycerin	sc, sub Q (*)	subcutaneous
n/v	nausea/vomiting	SDS	same day surgery
O_2	oxygen	sig	let it be imprinted, label
OB	obstetrics	sl	sublingual
od (*)	right eye	sos	if necessary
oob	out of bed	ss	half; sliding scale
OPD	outpatient department	SSE	soap suds enema
OR	operating room	SSKI	saturated solution of potassium iodide
os	left eye		
ostomy	surgical opening	stat	immediately and once only
ou	both eyes	STD	sexually transmitted disease
p	after	syncope	fainting
PA	physician's assistant	tab(s)	tablet(s)
PACU	post anesthesia care unit (recovery room)	TB	tuberculosis
		tid	three times daily
pathogen	disease-causing organism	tiw (*)	three times weekly
pb	piggyback	thrombus	blood clot
pc	after meals	t.o.	telephone order
PDR	*Physicians' Desk Reference*	TPN	total parenteral nutrition
pH	hydrogen ion concentration	tr	tincture
PharmD	doctor of pharmacy	TWE	tap water enema
PID	pelvic inflammatory disease	U (*)	unit
pm	afternoon, evening	ug (*)	microgram
PMU	pain management unit	ung	ointment
po	by mouth	USP	United States Pharmacopoeia
PPD	purified protein derivative	USPDI	United States Pharmacopoeia Drug Information
premi	premature		
prep	prepare for	ut dict, ud	as directed
prn	as needed	UTI	urinary tract infection
PT	physical therapy	VA	Veteran's Administration
PVC	premature ventricular contraction	V fib	ventricular fibrillation; rapid ineffective ventricular heart rate
PZI	protamine zinc insulin		
q	each, every	vertigo	dizziness
QA	quality assurance	vs	vital signs
qam	every morning	vss	vital signs stable
qd (*)	daily	WBC	white blood cell count; leukocyte
q_h	every _ hour(s)	WDWN	well-developed, well-nourished

Commonly Used Apothecary Symbols

ℨ (*)	drachm, teaspoonful
℥	ounce
℥ss	half ounce, tablespoon
m (*)	minim
=	equal
♀	female
♂	male
>	greater than
<	less than
↑	elevated, increased
↓	depressed, decreased
%	percent
°	degree
Δ	change

Not all symbols and abbreviations are absolute; many of them have more than one meaning when used in different contexts. When in doubt, the technician should consult the registered pharmacist on duty.

*Error-prone abbreviations, symbols, and dose designations that have contributed to medication errors. See Chapter 27, "Preventing and Managing Medication Errors," for the rationale of their misinterpretation.

Brand/Trade Names and Generic Names

The following section lists the brand/trade names of commonly used medications and their corresponding generic names. This list does not contain every drug available. The technician is advised to become familiar with the appropriate texts that contain this information.

Brand	**Generic**
Achromycin	tetracycline
Actifed	triprolidine/pseudoephedrine
Activase	alteplase, TPA
Adalat	nifedipine
Advil	ibuprofen
Afrin	oxymetazoline
Aldomet	methyldopa
Alternagel	concentrated aluminum hydroxide
Amoxil	amoxicillin
Amphojel	aluminum hydroxide
Ancef	cefazolin
Antivert	meclizine
Apresoline	hydralazine
Aricept	donepezil
Artane	trihexyphenidyl
Atarax	hydroxyzine
Ativan	lorazepam
Auralgan	antipyrine/benzocaine

Brand	Generic
Axid	nizatidine
Bactrim	trimethoprim sulfate/sulfamethoxazole
Benadryl	diphenhydramine
Bentyl	dicyclomine
Biaxin	clarithromycin
Brethine	terbutaline sulfate
Buspar	buspirone
Calan	verapamil
Capoten	captopril
Carafate	sucralfate
Cardizem	diltiazem
Cardura	doxazosin mesylate
Catapres	clonidine
Ceclor	cefaclor
Cefotan	cefotetan
Chlor-Trimeton	chlorpheniramine
Cipro	ciprofloxacin
Claritin	loratadine
Cleocin	clindamycin diphenhydramine
Cogentin	benztropine
Colace	docusate sodium
Compazine	prochlorperazine
Corgard	nadolol
Coumadin	warfarin
Cozaar	losartan
Cytotec	misoprostol
Decadron	dexamethasone
Deltasone	prednisone
Demerol	meperidine
Depakene	valproic acid
Depakote	divalproex sodium
Desyrel	trazodone
Diabinese	chlorpropamide
DiaBeta	glyburide
Diamox	acetazolamide
Diflucan	fluconazole
Dilantin	phenytoin
Dimetapp	brompheniramine/phenylpropanolamine
Ditropan	oxybutynin
Dramamine	dimenhydrinate
Dulcolax	bisacodyl
Duragesic	fentanyl
Dyazide	triamterene/hydrochlorothiazide
E.E.S.	erythromycin ethylsuccinate
Effexor	venlafaxine
Elavil	amitriptyline
Ery-Tab	erythromycin base
Flagyl	metronidazole
Floxin	ofloxacin
Fortaz	ceftazidime
Fragmin	dalteparin

Brand	Generic
Fungizone	amphotericin B
Garamycin	gentamicin sulfate
Glucotrol	glipizide
Halcion	triazolam
Haldol	haloperidol
Hexadrol	dexamethasone
Hydrodiuril	hydrochlorothiazide
Hytrin	terazosin
Ilosone	erythromycin estolate
Ilotycin	erythromycin base
Imdur	isosorbide mononitrate
Inderal	propranolol
Indocin	indomethacin
Isoptin	verapamil
Keflex	cephalexin
Kefzol	cefazolin
Kenalog	triamcinolone
Klonopin	clonazepam
Kwell	lindane
Lanoxin	digoxin
Lasix	furosemide
Levaquin	levofloxacin
Levothroid	levothyroxine
Lipitor	atorvastatin
Lopid	gemfibrozil
Lopressor	metoprolol
Lotrimin	clotrimazole
Lovenox	enoxaparin
Luvox	fluvoxamine
Mefoxin	cefoxitin
Mellaril	thioridazine
Micronase	glyburide
Minipress	prazosin
Motrin	ibuprofen
Mycelex	clotrimazole
Mycostatin	nystatin
Mylicon	simethicone
Naprosyn	naproxen sodium
Nebcin	tobramycin
Neurontin	gabapentin
Nizoral	ketoconazole
Norvasc	amlodipine
Oretic	hydrochlorthiazide
Paxil	paroxetine
Pepcid	famotidine
Phenergan	promethazine
Plavix	clopidogrel
Prilosec	omeprazole
Prinivil	lisinopril
Procan SR	procainamide sustained release
Procardia	nifedipine

Brand	Generic
Pronestyl	procainamide
Prozac	fluoxetine
Proventil	albuterol
Reglan	metoclopramide
Retrovir	zidovudine
Robinul	glycopyrrolate
Robitussin	guaifenesin
Rocephin	ceftriaxone
Rufen	ibuprofen
Septra	trimethoprim sulfate/sulfamethoxazole
Sorbitrate	isosorbide dinitrate
Stadol	butorphanol
Synthroid	levothyroxine
Tagamet	cimetidine
Tazicef	ceftazidime
Tazidime	ceftazidime
Tegretol	carbamazepine
Tenormin	atenolol
Theo-Dur	theophylline sustained release
Thorazine	chlorpromazine
Tobrex	tobramycin
Tofranil	imipramine
Toprol XL	metoprolol extended release
Trental	pentoxifylline
Trilafon	perphenazine
Trovan	trovafloxacin
Tylenol	acetaminophen
Ultram	tramadol
Vanceril	beclomethasone
Vasotec	enalapril
Ventolin	albuterol
Vibramycin	doxycycline
Vistaril	hydroxyzine
Xanax	alprazolam
Zantac	ranitidine
Zestril	lisinopril
Zithromax	azithromycin
Zocor	simvastatin
Zoloft	sertraline
Zovirax	acyclovir
Zyloprim	allopurinol

Common Look-Alike and Sound-Alike Drug Names

The following list contains names of some drugs that are easily mistaken for each other due to similar pronunciation or spelling. This list serves as a warning. It cannot replace proper care in reading medication orders. For a more comprehensive list of sound-alike drug names, see Appendix D.

acetazolamide	acetohexamide	diphenhydramine	dimenhydrinate
albuterol	atenolol	enalapril	Anafranil
Aldomet	Aldoril	flurbiprofen	fenoprofen
alprazolam	lorazepam	Gantrisin	Gantanol
Alupent	Atrovent	glipizide	glyburide
amiodarone	amrinone	Hycodan	Hycomine
amitriptyline	nortriptyline	Hycodan	Vicodin
Amoxil	Amcill	Hydralazine	hydroxyzine
Apresazide	Apresoline	Inderal	Isordil
Atarax	Ativan	Indocin	Minocin
atenolol	timolol	Lioresal	lisinopril
bacitracin	Bactroban	Lovenox	Luvox
Catapres	Cataflam	Orinase	Ornade
cefotaxime	cefoxitin	Prilosec	Prozac
chlorpromazine	promethazine	quinine	quinidine
clonidine	Klonopin	terbutaline	tolbutamide
Cordarone	Corvert	tolazamide	tolbutamide
desipramine	imipramine	Trimox	Diamox
digitoxin	digoxin	Vasosulf	Velosef
Dynapen	Dynacin	Xanax	Zantac

Adapted from "Look-Alike and Sound-Alike Drug Names" by N. M. Davis, M. R. Cohen, and B. Teplisky, 1992, *Hospital Pharmacy, 27,* pp. 96–106.

The Prescription

A prescription is an order for a medication or treatment issued by a physician or other properly licensed medical practitioner. The prescription specifies a medication, a dose, and frequency of use for a specific patient. Prescriptions are usually written on a preprinted form containing the prescriber's name, address, telephone number, and other pertinent information. There are blank spaces for the practitioner to handwrite or type information about the patient, medication desired, and directions for use. Legal requirements for specific information vary from state to state. Information generally found on prescriptions is:

- prescriber information and signature
- patient information
- date prescription was written
- rx (meaning "take thou," "you take," or recipe)
- the inscription—medication prescribed
- the subscription—dispensing instructions for the pharmacist (e.g., quantity)
- the signa, or sig—directions for use for the patient

TEST YOUR KNOWLEDGE

Multiple Choice Questions

1. An erythrocyte is
   a. a red blood cell
   b. a white blood cell
   c. a platelet
   d. a thrombocyte
   e. a leucocyte

2. Fibrillation is a synonym for
   a. a flutter of the left ventricle
   b. a spasm of the myocardium
   c. rapid ineffectual heartbeat
   d. trembling of the fingers
   e. difficulty in breathing

3. A test for kidney function is
   a. CBC
   b. CHF
   c. KFT
   d. BUN
   e. EKG

4. Diabetes mellitus affects
   a. protein metabolism
   b. carbohydrate metabolism
   c. purine metabolism
   d. lipid metabolism
   e. all of the above

5. A bedsore is known as
   a. an abscess
   b. a bulus
   c. a decubitus ulcer
   d. a laceration
   e. dermatitis

6. A traveling blood clot is
   a. an embolism
   b. a thrombus
   c. a hematoid
   d. all of the above
   e. none of the above

7. A pathogen is
   a. a bacillus
   b. a virus
   c. a carcinogen
   d. a septic substance
   e. any disease-producing organism

8. Syncope is a synonym for
   a. fainting
   b. ataxia
   c. dizziness
   d. fatigue
   e. coma

9. Vertigo is another name for
   a. fainting
   b. ataxia
   c. dizziness
   d. fatigue
   e. coma

10. An ostomy is
    a. a disease process
    b. an excision
    c. a surgical opening
    d. an incision
    e. a plastic repair

Matching Questions

11. _____ anaphylaxis   a. protein synthesis

12. _____ anabolism   b. resistant to infection

13. _____ antitussive   c. hypersensitivity reaction

14. _____ immunity   d. temperature above normal

15. _____ febrile   e. cough reliever

Matching II

16. _____ inscription   f. dispensing instructions to the pharmacist

17. _____ signa   g. recipe

18. _____ date   h. patient instructions

19. _____ Rx   i. the medication

20. _____ subscription   j. when the prescription was written

References

Davis, N. M., Cohen, M. R., & Teplisky, B. (1992). Look-alike and sound-alike drug names. *Hospital Pharmacy, 27*, 96–106.

Dorland's Illustrated Medical Dictionary. (2003). Philadelphia: Elsevier Science.

Mason, R. (1978). Medical terminology. In Durgin, Hanan, & Ward (Eds.), *Pharmacy Technician's Manual* (2nd ed.). St. Louis: C.V. Mosby Co.

Pharmaceutical Dosage Forms

COMPETENCIES

Upon completion of this chapter, the reader should be able to

1. Explain the different interpretations of "dosage form" by the patient, by members of the health care team, and by pharmacists.
2. List four physiochemical properties of a drug.
3. Name four formulation aids used in the preparation of a given dosage form.
4. Describe the advantages and disadvantages of the major classes of pharmaceutical dosage forms—namely liquids, solids, and aerosols.
5. Differentiate the characteristics of a solution and a suspension.
6. List five desirable qualities for an external suspension.
7. Name and define four solid dosage forms currently in use.
8. Explain the differences between compressed tablets, sublingual or buccal tablets, and multiple compressed tablets.
9. Describe an oral osmotic (OROS) drug dosage design and give an example.
10. Outline five advantages of the transdermal patch.

Introduction

A **dosage form** is a system or device for delivering a drug to the biological system. Drugs are defined as chemicals of synthetic, semisynthetic, natural, or biological origin that interact with human or animal biological systems resulting in an action that may either be intended to prevent, cure, or reduce ill effects in the human or animal body or to detect disease-causing manifestations. In actual practice, a pure drug is seldom used. What is generally administered to obtain the desired effect is the drug product, that is, the active ingredient (drug) combined with inert or physiologically inactive materials to produce a dosage form.

The term "dosage form" means different things to different people. To a patient, for instance, the term signifies the gross physical or pharmaceutical form in which the drug is made available for administration or use (e.g., tablet, capsule, **solution**, injection, **ointment**). To the members of the health care team, the dosage form of a drug is a drug-delivery system. Any alteration in the system will be expected to alter the delivery rate and the total amount of drug delivered to the site of action.

The pharmacist, however, uses the term "dosage form" in a more comprehensive manner to include the physiochemical properties of the drug itself (e.g., particle size, salt form, **polymorphic state**, dissolution characteristics) and the nature and quantities of various formulation aids used in the preparation of the given dosage form (e.g., diluents, excipients, additives, preservatives).

Classification

Because of the diverse nature, mode of action, and route of administration, dosage forms may be classified in several different ways. The major classes of pharmaceutical dosage forms may be broadly categorized as liquid, solid, and miscellaneous.

Liquid Dosage Forms

It is well known that biological responses are elicited by the **molecular form** of the drug. Thus, no matter in what dosage form (solid, liquid, or gas) a drug is administered, the action at the molecular level involves interaction of biological constituents with the individual molecules of the drug. Therefore, for a drug to elicit the desired response, it has to be present in the form of a molecular dispersion (solution) at the site of action. Thus liquid dosage forms are often the dosage form of choice for the following reasons:

- They are effective more quickly than a solid dosage form because the solid form will have to undergo **dissolution** after administration.
- They are easier to swallow (especially for pediatric and geriatric patients) than solid dosage forms.
- Certain substances can be given only in a liquid form because either the character of the remedy or the large dose makes administration in any other form inconvenient.
- Certain chemical substances may cause pain (e.g., potassium iodide and bromide) or gastric irritation (e.g., aspirin) when administered in a solid state.
- Uniformity and flexibility of dosage are easily obtained in liquid dosage forms.
- Liquid forms are the dosage forms of choice in certain types of pathological conditions in which absorption of particular ions is dependent on dissolution and the absorption environment is deficient in effecting dissolution. For example, a liquid dosage form provides calcium ions in an absorbable form in patients who lack acidity to dissolve calcium carbonate powder.

Liquid dosage forms also have the following disadvantages:

- They are liable to undergo deterioration and loss of potency much faster than solid dosage forms.
- They present many flavoring and sweetening problems.
- Many instances of incompatibility arise because of interaction between dissolved substances.
- In the absence of proper **preservatives**, liquids provide excellent media for bacterial and mold growth.
- The presence of preservatives may present problems of a diverse nature.
- Inaccuracy in various doses may arise due to the patient measuring the dose with a household device (e.g., a teaspoon).

■ Oral liquid dosage forms are bulkier to carry than oral solid dosage forms and necessitate the use of a measuring device (e.g., a teaspoon).

■ Many interactions arise because of changes in solubility produced by solvent alterations.

The two major classes of liquid pharmaceutical dosage forms are (1) those containing soluble matter, and (2) those containing insoluble matter.

Liquid dosage forms containing soluble matter

Liquid dosage forms containing soluble matter—true solutions—consist of one or several soluble substances (solute) dissolved in a solvent (usually water). The solute may be solid, liquid, or gas and the solvent may be any water-miscible (**hydrophilic**) liquid. Hydrophilic solvents are preferred because such a solvent system is miscible with body fluids.

Some of the potential problems that one should be aware of in dealing with the solution dosage forms are described next.

Solvent system. Most drugs, being weak organic acids or weak organic bases, possess sufficient solubility in organic solvents (e.g., alcohol), but lack adequate water solubility. Solutions of such drugs are generally made using a blend (mixture) of solvents. Products intended for oral administration usually utilize a **hydroalcoholic** solvent system, sometimes containing more than 20% alcohol (e.g., elixirs). A mixture of such a product with another product using only water as the solvent or dilution of the product with water is likely to cause precipitation of the poorly water-soluble compound.

pH change. In some instances, it is desirable not to use a hydroalcoholic solvent system. In such cases, the manufacturer uses a salt form of the drug that, unlike the drug itself, possesses good water solubility. For acidic drugs, the salt form is generally the sodium salt; for basic drugs, the commonly used forms are the hydrochloride or the sulfate. Since the conjugate entity of these salts is a strong acid or strong base, the pH of the resulting solution is far removed from neutrality. Although dilution of these solutions with water does not pose any problems, one must be careful if two such solutions are mixed. For example, a solution containing the hydrochloride of one drug when mixed with a solution containing the sodium salt of another drug is likely to result in the precipitation of both drugs because the hydrochloride and sodium moieties of the two drugs will neutralize each other, resulting in poorly water-soluble, weakly basic, and weakly acidic drugs.

Buffer system. A number of drug solutions are stable within a given pH range. To ensure maximum stability and a longer shelf life of such solutions, a **buffer** system is used to maintain the pH of such solutions within the range of optimal stability. Dilution of a drug product's solution that has been formulated with a buffer system is likely to alter the pH of the solution and possibly reduce the buffer capacity.

Liquid dosage forms containing insoluble matter

To derive some or all of the advantages of administering a liquid dosage form, insoluble solutes may be suspended in a vehicle. Two common dosage forms are **suspensions** and **emulsions**.

Suspensions. Suspensions consist of a two-phase system in which the internal (dispersed) phase is solid and the external phase is liquid. The dispersed solid is generally in a state of fine subdivision, having a particle size that may approach colloidal dimensions. The liquid phase in most pharmaceutical suspensions is aqueous. A suspension formulation may be preferred over the administration of the solute as a solid dosage form because the solid may have poor solubility. When formulated as a suspension, the solid will generally show a better rate of solubility because of improved wetting of the drug particles and increased surface area.

Pharmaceutical suspensions may be classified into three groups: (1) orally administered mixtures, (2) externally applied lotions, and (3) injectable preparations.

Orally administered mixtures may supply insoluble and often distasteful substances in a pleasant-tasting form. Examples of oral suspensions are the oral antibiotic syrups, which normally contain 250–500 mg of the solid material per 5 mL of suspension. The concentration of the suspended material may be greater in the case of pediatric drops or in antacid and **radiopaque** suspensions.

Externally applied **lotions** provide dermatological materials in a form that is convenient and suitable for application to the skin. The concentration of the dispersed phase in such formulations may exceed 20% (e.g., calamine lotion).

Injectable preparations provide an insoluble drug in a form suitable for intramuscular administration. Such preparations contain from 0.5% to 30% of solid particles and are generally of low viscosity since viscosity affects the ease of injection. Particle size is another significant factor since it affects the availability of the drug, especially in depot therapy (e.g., Procaine Penicillin G). However, injectable preparations are formulated with a relatively minute particle size of the solute so as to enable the suspension to pass through the needle of the syringe.

An acceptable suspension possesses the following desirable qualities:

1. The suspended material should not settle rapidly. The particles that do settle down must be readily redispersed into a uniform mixture (suspension) when the container is shaken.
2. The suspension must not be too viscous, but should pour freely from the orifice of the bottle or through a syringe needle.
3. In the case of suspensions intended for external application (e.g., a lotion), the product
    - must be fluid enough to spread easily over the affected area
    - must not be so mobile that it runs off the surface of application
    - should dry quickly after application to the affected area
    - should provide an elastic protective film that will not rub off easily
    - should have an acceptable color and odor

Gels and jellies. Gels and jellies are also two-phase systems of a solid and a liquid. However, they differ from true suspensions because in these preparations it is difficult to distinguish between the external phase and the internal phase. The particles of the solid phase are interlinked like irregular meshwork; thus, the liquid partly surrounds the interconnected solid particles and is partly occluded by them (e.g., lidocaine gel).

Emulsions. Emulsions consist of a heterogeneous system of at least one immiscible liquid intimately dispersed into another in the form of droplets, whose diameters, in general, range from about 0.1 to 10 micrometers. The system is stabilized by the presence of an **emulsifying agent**, the choice of which is governed by the composition of the emulsion and the route of administration of the emulsion. Either the dispersed phase or the continuous phase may range in consistency from that of a mobile liquid (emulsions and lotions of relatively low viscosity) to a semisolid.

Emulsions are considered to be dispersions of oil or water. When an oil or any oily substance is the dispersed phase, the emulsion is called an oil-in-water (o/w) emulsion. When water is the dispersed phase, the emulsion is called a water-in-oil (w/o) emulsion. More recent in its origin is a third type of emulsion described as a microemulsion or transparent emulsion. The transparent emulsions possess the property of transparency because of the very small particle size (generally 0.05 micrometer or less) of the dispersed phase (e.g., Haley's M.O.).

Medicinal emulsions for oral administration are usually of the o/w type and require the use of o/w emulsifying agents (e.g., synthetic nonionic surface active agents, acacia, tragacanth, gelatin). An o/w emulsion is a convenient means of orally administering water-insoluble liquids, especially those that have an unpleasant taste or odor. Because the oil globules are completely surrounded by an aqueous **medium**, the taste of the oil is almost completely masked and the odor is also markedly suppressed. Also, it has been observed that some oil-soluble compounds (e.g., some of the vitamins) are absorbed more completely when emulsified than when administered orally as an oily solution because, in an emulsion, a large surface area of the oily solution (provided by the oil droplets) is made available for contact at the absorption site. Similarly, the use of intravenous emulsions has been studied as a means of maintaining debilitated patients who are unable to assimilate materials administered orally. Radiopaque emulsions have found application as diagnostic agents in X-ray examinations.

Emulsions intended for external application may be o/w or w/o type. Oil-in-water emulsions for external use offer the advantage of being water-washable and nonstaining. In the preparation of such emulsions, the following emulsifying agents (in addition to the ones already mentioned) are used: triethanolamine stearate, sodium lauryl sulfate, and monovalent soaps (e.g., sodium oleate). The water-in-oil emulsions, which are used almost exclusively for external application, contain one or several of the following emulsifying agents: polyvalent soaps (e.g., calcium palmitate), synthetic nonionic sorbitan esters, wool fat, and cholesterol.

In the pharmaceutical and cosmetic products for external use, emulsification is widely used to formulate dermatological and cosmetic lotions and creams that have a better patient acceptability. For example, in the formulation of foam-producing aerosol products, the **propellant** forms the dispersed liquid phase within the container which vaporizes when the emulsion is discharged from the container.

Because emulsions are heterogeneous in nature, they present stability problems. An improper selection of the emulsifying agent, either in quality or in quantity, may lead to separation of the emulsion during storage. By shaking the container, the emulsion may reform (creaming) or not reform at all (breaking). Caution must be exercised when an emulsion is to be diluted or mixed with another liquid. An emulsion may be diluted only with a liquid that is miscible with the external phase. Also, dilution of an emulsion may dilute the concentration of the emulsifying agent leading to creaming or breaking of the emulsion. If the dilution is done with a liquid that possesses characteristics different from those of the external phase of the emulsion, the emulsion can break. The same is true when an emulsion is mixed with another liquid. When two emulsions are mixed, another factor that must be considered is the nature of the emulsifying agent in the two emulsions. If one emulsion contains an **anionic** emulsifying agent and the other contains a **cationic** agent, the mixture will tend to produce interaction between the emulsifying agents and both emulsions may break.

A simple method to determine the type of emulsion (o/w or w/o) is to dilute the emulsion with an equal quantity of water and shake the container. An o/w emulsion will dilute with water, but a w/o emulsion will not dilute.

Solid Dosage Forms

Solid dosage forms in current use include powders, granules, capsules, and tablets. Powders and granules constitute a very small portion of the solid dosage forms dispensed today. Capsules and tablets have gained popularity because they are

- easy to package, transport, store, and dispense
- convenient for self-medication
- largely devoid of taste and odor
- more stable than other solid dosage forms
- predivided dosage forms and, therefore, provide an accurate dose
- especially suited for those drugs that are not stable in liquid form and, therefore, provide a longer shelf life for such drugs
- more suited for the formulation of sustained and delayed release of medication because controlled-release techniques are generally more applicable to solid than to liquid dosage forms

Powders

Powders have certain inherent advantages. For example, they give the physician free choice of drugs, dose, and bulk; they permit the administration of large "bulk" of medicinals; and they may be administered as a suspension if the patient has difficulty swallowing a tablet or capsule. However, powders are not the dosage form of choice for drugs that have an unpleasant taste or are not stable when exposed to the atmosphere.

Powders are prescribed for both internal and external use. When intended for internal use, powders may be prescribed as bulk, dispersible, or divided powders. Powders prescribed for external use are dispensed as dusting powders.

Bulk powders are supplied as multidose preparations, the dose being measured by the patient. This dosage form is used for drugs having a large dose and low toxicity because of the variation in dose weight inherent in domestic methods of measurement (e.g., with a household teaspoon). Also, such measurements are volumetric and the dose weight will vary with the bulk **density** of the powder and the degree of fill, depending on whether level or heaped measures are used.

Antacids are frequently prescribed in this manner. They contain substances such as aluminum hydroxide, calcium or magnesium carbonate, magnesium trisilicate, and sodium bicarbonate.

Bulk powders may also be used as antiseptics or cleansing agents for a body cavity. For example, dentifrices generally contain a soap or detergent and a mild abrasive. Similarly, douche powders are products that are completely soluble and are most commonly intended for vaginal use, although they may be formulated for nasal, otic, or ophthalmic use.

Dispersible powders are readily wetted by water to form an extemporaneous suspension for oral administration. The quantity contained in a dispersible powder may be enough for a single dose or may contain a sufficient amount to last two to three days. It is important that the formulation is such that the powder settles slowly and that foam is not produced. If a wetting agent is used, it must be relatively free from any toxicity.

Dispersible powders are used for substances that are unstable in the presence of water, and, therefore, cannot be formulated as liquid dosage forms.

Divided powders are dispensed in individual doses. To achieve accuracy, each dose is individually weighed, transferred to a powder paper, and the powder paper is folded. Divided powders containing **hygroscopic** and **volatile** drugs are stored in waxed paper, then double wrapped with a bond paper to improve the appearance of the completed powder. They may also be dispensed in metal foils, small heat-seal plastic bags, or other containers.

Dusting powders are locally applied nontoxic preparations that are intended to have no **systemic** action. They are dispensed in a very fine state of subdivision to enhance effectiveness and minimize irritation. Commercial dusting powders are available in sifter-top cans, sterile envelopes, or pressure aerosols. Foot powders, talcum powders, and antiperspirants available as pressure aerosols are generally more expensive than those marketed in other containers, but they offer the advantage of protection from air, moisture, and contamination, as well as convenience of application.

Absorbent powders are intended to absorb excretions on the surface of the skin from superficial infections. They usually contain starch, often with zinc oxide, kaolin, or talc.

Antifungal substances, such as salicylic acid and zinc undecylenate, are applied as powders diluted with starch, kaolin, or talc. Insecticides, such as chlorophenothane and benzene hexachloride, are incorporated in dusting powders for the destruction of lice, fleas, ticks, and so forth.

Granules

Granules are small, irregular particles. They are used as effervescent granules or they may be marketed for therapeutic purposes.

The effervescent granules contain sodium bicarbonate and either citric acid, tartaric acid, or sodium biphosphate in addition to the active ingredients. On solution in water, carbon dioxide is released as a result of the acid-base reaction causing effervescence, which serves to mask the taste of salty and bitter medications. Laxative salts, such as magnesium and sodium sulfate, are frequently formulated as effervescent granules.

Capsules

Capsules are solid dosage forms in which the drug is enclosed in a "shell" of a suitable form of gelatin. Upon administration, the gelatin shell dissolves in 10 to 20 minutes, releasing the drug. Since the shell usually does not dissolve completely, capsules should not be used for very soluble compounds such as potassium or calcium chloride, potassium bromide, or ammonium chloride. In these cases, when the partly dissolved capsule comes in contact with the stomach wall, the concentrated solution may cause localized irritation and gastric distress.

Capsules may be made of hard or soft gelatin. Hard capsules are generally used for dry powders. The contents may range from 50 mg to 1 gm per capsule. Some manufacturers prefer to seal their capsules to prevent the loss of drug because of accidental opening or to discourage easy removal of the contents. Soft capsules, also known as "soft shell" or "soluble elastic" capsules, are a one-piece construction with the liquid fill material literally wrapped inside a sealed, gelatin matrix. The contents of the soft capsule range from 1 to 480 minims. The capsule may be spherical (pearls) or ovoid (globules) in shape.

Hard capsules are two-piece capsules manufactured as empty shells. The contents are filled in the capsules mechanically or manually after the capsule shells are manufactured. Soft capsules are filled with the contents during their manufacture. They cannot be filled after the soft capsules have been manufactured.

Tablets

Tablets are solid pharmaceutical dosage forms prepared either by compressing or by molding. They are the most popular of all the medicinal preparations intended for oral use. They offer the advantages of accuracy and compactness of dosage, portability, convenience of administration, and blandness of taste.

Although most frequently discoid in form, tablets may be round, oval, oblong, cylindrical, or triangular. Manufacturers generally add a colorant to a tablet formulation either for identification or for aesthetic purposes. Some tablets are scored so that they may be easily broken in halves or quarters. However, sustained-action tablets should never be broken or crushed unless directed by the manufacturer because the technology used in such tablets may not warrant their breaking or crushing. A majority of tablet dosage forms are embossed with the name of the manufacturer or tablet code number. Depending on their method of production, tablets are classified as molded or compressed.

Molded tablets were originally made from moist materials on a triturate mold, but are now usually made by compression on a tablet machine. Such tablets must be completely and rapidly soluble. Three types are common.

1. *Hypodermic tablet (HT)*. These were meant to be placed in the barrel of the hypodermic syringe where they must dissolve in less than 10 seconds. They are not presently used in clinical practice.
2. *Dispensing tablets (DT)*. These are designed solely to provide an accurate quantity of a potent drug for use in compounding another form, such as capsules, powders, and solutions. They are never intended for administration in their original form.
3. *Tablet triturates (TT)*. These contain a potent drug (usually one part) and a suitable diluent (usually nine parts), such as lactose.

Compressed tablets are formed by compression and are made from powdered, crystalline, or granular material alone or in combination with binders, disintegrants, lubricants, and fillers.

The three major methods of preparing compressed tablets are described as wet granulation, dry granulation, and direct compression. For those materials that do not lend themselves to direct compression, the formulation is first granulated (wet or dry) and then compressed. The basic steps involved in the preparation of tablets by granulation are as follows:

Wet Granulation	Dry Granulation
Weighing	Weighing
Preblending	Preblending
Granulation	**Milling**
Drying	Blending
Milling	Compression
Blending	
Compression	

Whereas wet granulation is the most common method of preparing compressed tablets, dry granulation is preferred for heat- and moisture-sensitive drugs.

Among the various types of compressed tablets available in the market, the following six are most common:

1. *Standard compressed tablets (CT)*. These are the conventional tablets we are all familiar with and are compressed on a tablet machine.

2. *Enteric-coated tablets (ECT).* These are compressed tablets coated with substances that resist solution in gastric fluid, but release the medication in the intestinal tract.

3. *Sugar-coated tablets (SCT).* These are tablets containing a sugar coating. Sugar coating is used to cover the objectionable taste or odor of medicinals and to protect sensitive materials subject to deterioration due to light, air, oxygen, etc. However, sugar is a hygroscopic substance and the coating operation is very time-consuming.

4. *Film-coated tablets (FCT).* These are tablets covered with a thin film of a water-soluble material. Such coverings impart the same general characteristics as a sugar coating and the coating operation is relatively simple, less time-consuming, and economical.

5. *Sublingual or buccal tablets (ST).* These are tablets intended to be inserted below the tongue or in the buccal pouch where the active ingredient may be directly absorbed through the mucosa.

6. *Multiple compressed tablets (MCT).* These are tablets made by more than one compression cycle. Layered tablets are prepared by compressing additional tablet granulation on a previously compressed tablet. Press-coated tablets are prepared by compressing another layer around a preformed compressed tablet.

Miscellaneous tablets are those that are specially formulated or intended for a specific function. Two common types include the following:

1. *Chewable tablets.* These are compressed tablets that are to be chewed rather than swallowed.

2. *Delayed- or sustained-action tablets.* These are special formulations of tablets in which the active ingredient is either released at a constant rate for prolonged periods or the release is delayed. These products are also variously described as "timed release," "long acting," "prolonged action," or some similar term implying an extended period of action for a given drug. **Table 11-1** lists some of the terms that have been used synonymously in recent years.

It should be mentioned that the USP recognizes and defines the term "modified release" to embody the terms in common use today. The definition of "modified release" includes those dosage forms for which the drug-release characteristics (i.e., time and location of release) are chosen to accomplish convenience or therapeutic objectives that are not offered by conventional dosage forms such as solutions, ointments, or dissolving dosage forms. The two types of modified-release dosage forms are (1) extended release—one that allows at least a twofold reduction in dosing frequency as compared with conventional dosage forms—and (2) delayed release—one that releases the drug at a time other than promptly after administration.

1. *Lozenges.* Also known as troches or pastilles, these are discoid-shaped solids containing the medicinal agent in a suitable flavored base, meant to be placed in the mouth where they slowly dissolve, liberating the active ingredient.

2. *Pellets.* As used now, the term signifies small cylinders meant to be implanted, usually **subcutaneously**, for prolonged and continuous absorption of potent hormones, such as testosterone or estradiol.

Miscellaneous Dosage Forms

The dosage forms considered under this section have been classified miscellaneous for the sake of convenience. The properties associated with these dosage

TABLE 11-1
Alphabetical Listing of Some Names Associated with Oral Sustained-Release Dosage Forms

Constant release	Prolonged action
Continuous action	Prolonged release
Continuous release	Protracted release
Controlled action	Repeat action
Controlled release	Repository
Delayed absorption	Retard
Delayed action	Slow acting
Delayed release	Slowly acting
Depot	Slow release
Extended action	Sustained action
Extended release	Sustained release
Gradual release	Sustained release depot
Long acting	Timed coat
Long lasting	Timed disintegration
Long-term release	Timed release
Programmed release	

forms are either unique to them or represent a combination of the properties of solid and liquid dosage forms.

Aerosols

Aerosols are systems consisting of a suspension of fine solid or liquid particles in air or gas. Aerosols may be classified as either pharmaceutical aerosols or medicinal aerosols.

Pharmaceutical aerosols are intended for topical administration or for administration into one of the body cavities, such as the ear, eye, rectum, or vagina.

Medicinal aerosols are intended both for local action in the nasal areas, the throat, and the lungs and for prompt systemic effect when absorbed into the bloodstream (e.g., from lungs—inhalation or aerosol therapy).

Aerosols offer convenience and ease of application. If the product is packaged under sterile conditions, sterility can be maintained without danger of contamination. The use of aerosols eliminates the irritation produced by the mechanical application of a medicinal, especially over an abraded area. Medication can also be applied to areas that are difficult to reach otherwise.

Inhalation therapy avoids the trauma of injections and the decomposition of orally administered drugs in the gastrointestinal tract.

Because the particle size of therapeutic aerosols affects their clinical usefulness, it is essential that the aerosol dosage form be formulated with the most effective particle size. For example, particles larger than 30 nm are most likely to be deposited in the trachea; those 10–30 nm may reach the terminal bronchiole; those 3–10 nm may reach the alveolar duct; those 1–3 nm may reach the alveolar sac; and particles less than 0.5 nm in size may reach the alveolar sac and be exhaled.

Isotonic solutions

Body fluids, including blood and **lacrimal fluids**, have an osmotic pressure identical to that of a 0.9 percent solution of sodium chloride. Thus, a 0.9 percent solution of sodium chloride is said to be **iso-osmotic** with physiological fluids. The term *iso-osmotic,* which is a physical term comparing the osmotic pressure, is used interchangeably with the term **isotonic**, which means "having the same tone." A solution is isotonic with a living cell if there is no net gain or loss of water by the cell, or other change in the cell, when in contact with that solution. A solution that is iso-osmotic may not necessarily be isotonic. For example, a solution of boric acid is iso-osmotic with blood and lacrimal fluid, but is isotonic only with lacrimal fluids. It causes hemolysis of red blood cells because the molecules of boric acid pass freely through the erythrocyte membrane regardless of concentration.

When dealing with isotonic solutions, caution must be exercised because any alteration in the composition of the solution (e.g., dilution) may affect the tonicity of the solution.

Ointments and pastes

Ointments and pastes are semisolid preparations used mainly for local application to skin or mucous membrane. They may be classified according to the relationship of water to the composition of the base used to prepare the ointment or paste.

Absorption bases, although essentially **anhydrous** in nature, absorb water. However, they are insoluble in water and are not water washable.

Emulsion bases are of two types. Water-in-oil emulsion bases contain water in the internal phase and oil in the external phase. Thus they are insoluble in water. They absorb water, but are not water washable. Oil-in-water emulsion bases contain oil in the internal phase and water in the external phase. Thus they are water washable.

Oleaginous bases are insoluble in water, do not contain or absorb water, and are not water washable.

Water-soluble bases may be essentially anhydrous or they may contain water. In either case, they absorb water to the point of solubility. Thus they are water soluble and water washable.

Suppositories

Suppositories are solid unit dosage forms intended for the application of medication to any of several body orifices, namely the rectum, vagina, or urethra. These dosage forms may exhibit their therapeutic activity locally or systematically, either by melting at body temperature or by dissolving in the aqueous secretions of the mucous membrane. Suppositories intended for administration via the vagina or the urethra are sometimes referred to as "inserts," particularly when made by compression as a specially shaped tablet. Melting or dissolution of suppositories in the secretions of the cavity usually releases the medication over a prolonged period. Commonly used suppository bases can be oleaginous (e.g., cocoa butter or theobroma oil, synthetic triglyceride mixtures), water soluble (e.g., glycerinated gelatin, polyethylene glycol polymers), or hydrophilic (e.g., polyethylene sorbitan monostearate, polyoxyl 40 stearate).

Rectal suppositories for adults are usually 2.5–3.5 cm long, weigh about 2 gm each, and have a tapered shape. The largest diameter is 1.2–1.3 cm, usually tapered to about 6–7 mm. For pediatric use, the diameter and the length is less, with reduction of weight to about 1 gm.

Vaginal suppositories vary in shape from globular or ovoid to modified conical shapes. They weigh from 3–5 gm and are used primarily for local effects.

Urethral suppositories, like vaginal suppositories, are primarily used for local action. These are slender rods, from 3–5 mm in diameter, and range in length from 60–75 mm for the female urethra and from 100–150 mm for the male urethra. Although somewhat flexible, urethral suppositories are firm enough for insertion.

Gastrointestinal System

The gastrointestinal therapeutic system (GITS) is based on Alza Corporation's OROS (oralosmosis) design. This dosage form resembles an ordinary tablet, but the characteristics of drug release and drug delivery are very different.

The system consists of an osmotic drug-containing core surrounded by a semi-permeable polymer membrane that is pierced by a small, laser-drilled delivery orifice. Upon ingestion of the dosage form, water is osmotically drawn through the membrane from the gastrointestinal tract at a constant and controlled rate, thereby creating a drug solution inside the tablet. The influx of water pushes the drug solution out of the orifice at a constant rate.

The first product marketed in this country based on this technology is Ciba-Geigy's Acutrim, an over-the-counter appetite suppressant. Administered once daily, this dosage form delivers 20 mg of phenylpropanolamine initially and then 55 mg released osmotically for approximately 16 hours.

Ocular System

Topical application of drugs to the eye is common for eye disorders. The most pre-scribed ocular dosage form is the traditional eyedrop solution. But the eyedrop is not an efficient drug-delivery system because the greater part of the 1 to 2 drops (50–100 microliters) is squeezed out of the eye by the first blink following adminis-tration. The residual volume mixes with the lacrimal fluid (about 7–8 microliters), becomes diluted, and is drained away by the nasolacrimal drainage system until the solution volume returns to the normal tear volume of 7–8 microliters. The initial drainage results in the loss of about 75% to 80% of the administered dose within five minutes of instillation. Then drainage stops and the residual dose declines slowly.

The efficiency of an ophthalmic drug delivery system can be greatly improved by prolonging its contact with the corneal surface. To achieve this purpose, sus-pensions of drug particles in pharmaceutical vehicles are prepared, viscosity-enhancing agents such as methylcellulose are added to the eyedrop preparation, or the drug is provided as an ointment.

Recently, drug-presoaked hydrogel-type contact lenses have been shown to prolong the drug-eye contact time. The Bionite lens, for example, is inserted into the eye after being presoaked in the drug solution. Similarly, sauflon hydrophilic contact lenses are manufactured from a vinyl pyrrolidone acrylic copolymer of high water content. These contact lenses have been shown to improve the deliv-ery of fluorescein, phenylephrine, pilocarpine, chloramphenicol, and tetracycline.

The new generation of drug dispersing ocular inserts consists of a medicated core matrix confined within a pair of flexible, transparent, biocompatible, and tear-insoluble polymer membranes that provide the required degree of permeability for the drug. When the insert is placed in the conjunctival cul-de-sac between the sclera of the eyeball and the lower lid, the drug is continuously released by diffu-sion through the membrane as a result of solvation in the lacrimal fluid.

Alza Corporation's Ocusert System is a pilocarpine core reservoir sandwiched between two sheets of transparent, **lipophilic**, rate-controlling membranes. When placed in the cul-de-sac, the pilocarpine molecules penetrate through the rate-controlling membranes. This controlled pilocarpine-releasing therapeutic system has several advantages over the conventional eyedrop solution. It provides better patient compliance, less frequent dosing, around-the-clock protection for four to seven days, fewer ocular and systemic side effects, possible delay in the **refractory** state, and a significantly smaller dose of pilocarpine for the effective management of **intraocular** pressure in the treatment of glaucoma. The administration of one Ocusert Pilo-20 insert, for example, delivers a daily dose of only 0.4–0.5 mg compared with the 4–8 mg provided by the instillation of 1 to 2 drops of the conventional 2% pilocarpine solution administered four times a day.

Transdermal System

The **transdermal** system is an innovation that employs the skin as a portal of drug entry into the systemic circulation. Using the **percutaneous** route instead of the more conventional oral, parenteral, pulmonary, or rectal routes, this technique is designed to provide systemic therapy for acute or chronic conditions that do not involve the skin.

Among the most popular and intriguing percutaneously administered drug-delivery systems is the transdermal patch. The advantages of this system include convenience, uninterrupted therapy, better patient compliance, accurate drug dosage, and regulation of drug concentration. The patch is formulated to deliver a constant, controlled dose of the drug through the intact skin, where it enters directly into the bloodstream. These delivery systems have a backing layer, a drug reservoir, a membrane, and an adhesive layer that incorporates a priming dose of the drug.

Nitroglycerin is available in various forms—sublingual, oral, intravenous injection, topical ointment, and transdermal preparations (**Table 11-2**). The popular transdermal preparations of nitroglycerin are Ciba-Geigy's Transderm-Nitro, Searle's Nitrodisc, and Key's Nitro-Dur.

All nitroglycerin transdermal patches are designed to be applied to the upper arm or chest to provide the drug for 24 hours. Although these patches can be applied anywhere on the body except the distal parts of the extremities, most patients have a tendency to apply these near the thorax, perhaps on the assumption that the medication for the heart should be placed near the heart. Manufacturers do recommend, however, that each patch should be applied at a site different from that used the previous day to avoid irritation.

Transderm-Scop, a scopolamine-containing transdermal delivery system marketed by Ciba-Geigy, is a circular, flat, tan disc, about 2 mm thick and the size of a dime. Each disc contains 1–5 mg of scopolamine and is programmed to deliver

TABLE 11-2   Comparison of Nitroglycerine Dosage Forms

Dosage Form	Dose	Antianginal Effect	
		Onset	Duration
Intravenous	Variable	Minutes	Minutes
Sublingual	0.15–0.6 mg every 30 min	2 minutes	up to 30 minutes
Oral, timed release	2.5–9.0 mg twice daily	1/2–1 hour	8–9 hours
Topical ointment (2%, 15 mg/in.)	1–2 in. every 4 hours	30 minutes	3 hours
Transdermal	1 patch every 12–24 hours	30 minutes	20–24 hours

0.5 mg of scopolamine over three days. According to Ciba, this delivery system is more effective than the conventional oral dose, which has been reported to cause excessively rapid heartbeat, confusion, and hallucination. The patch works best when placed behind the ear on a hairless site, delivering scopolamine through intact skin directly into the bloodstream for three days.

Other drugs available as transdermal patches include hormone preparations and nicotine (for smoking cessation).

Summary

In recent years, the pharmaceutical industry has made significant progress in the development and manufacture of dosage forms. The new concepts of bioavailability have made it possible to prepare more efficient delivery systems. The latest developments include such dosage forms as the transdermal delivery system (TDS) popularly known as the "patch," the osmotic pump, and the insulin pump. In the future, one can expect dosage forms containing optimal amounts of active ingredients to provide maximal therapeutic benefits, thus markedly reducing or completely eliminating the side effects of therapeutic agents.

TEST YOUR KNOWLEDGE

Multiple Choice Questions

1. Drugs are defined as chemicals of
   a. natural origin
   b. synthetic origin
   c. semisynthetic origin
   d. biological origin
   e. all of above

2. Which of the following is not a drug dosage form?
   a. brew
   b. tablet
   c. solution
   d. injection
   e. ointment

3. Drug formulation aides include
   a. diluents
   b. excipients
   c. additives
   d. preservatives
   e. all of the above

4. For a drug to elicit the desired response, it is required at the site of action to be in the form of
   a. a hydrosolvent
   b. a molecular dispersion
   c. an isotonic solution
   d. a soluble gel
   e. an acidic vehicle

5. A soluble substance is called
   a. a solvent
   b. a solubilizer
   c. a solute
   d. a solution
   e. none of the above

6. Medicinal emulsions for oral administration are usually
   a. o/w type
   b. w/o type

7. Which of the following is not a solid dosage form?
   a. powder
   b. capsule
   c. gel
   d. granule
   e. tablet

8. Antifungal substances are applied as powders that may be diluted with
   a. starch
   b. kaolin
   c. talc
   d. a and c
   e. a, b, and c

9. The most prescribed ocular dosage form is
   a. eyedrop solution
   b. ophthalmic ointments
   c. drug-presoaked hydrogel-type contact lens
   d. ocular inserts
   e. core reservoirs in lipophilic membranes

10. Advantage(s) of transdermal patches include
   a. convenience
   b. uninterrupted therapy
   c. better patient compliance
   d. regulation of drug concentration
   e. all of the above

True/False Questions

11. _____ In actual practice, a "pure" drug is seldom used.

12. _____ Liquid dosage forms are rarely the drug of choice.

13. _____ In an acceptable suspension, the particles never settle down.

14. _____ Emulsions contain at least one immiscible liquid.

15. _____ Tablets should never be chewed before swallowing.

Matching Questions

16. _____ medicinal aerosols

17. _____ transdermal patches

18. _____ bionite lens

19. _____ lozenges

20. _____ pellets

a. slowly dissolved in the mouth

b. implanted subcutaneously

c. inhaled through nose or mouth

d. applied to the skin

e. inserted into the eye

12 Pharmaceutical Calculations

COMPETENCIES

Upon completion of this chapter, the reader should be able to

1. Interpret a medication order accurately.
2. Convert quantities stated in apothecary units to their equivalent units in the metric system.
3. Convert quantities stated in metric or apothecary units to other units within those systems (e.g., g to mg).
4. Set up valid proportions to perform calculations required in administering medications.
5. Calculate quantities to be administered when ordered in fractional doses.
6. Calculate safe dosages for infants and children.
7. Calculate dosages for individual patients given the patient's weight and/or height and the recommended dose.
8. Perform calculations necessary for the infusion of IV medications.
9. List five steps to decrease errors in interpreting the strength of drugs from the written order.

Introduction

It is common practice in hospitals today for the pharmacist to calculate and prepare the drug dosage form for administration to the patient. Often the drug is provided in a unit-dose package. However, this practice does not relieve the nurse from the legal and professional responsibility of ensuring that the patient receives the right dose of the right medication at the right time in the right manner. This chapter will review the necessary calculations involved in the safe administration of drugs to the patient.

Interpreting the Drug Order

The welfare of the patient necessitates proper interpretation of the medication order. If any doubt exists, or if a particular order appears unusual, it is the nurse's responsibility to check with the physician or the pharmacist.

Abbreviations derived from Latin are often used by physicians and pharmacists in writing and preparing drug orders. Refer to **Tables 12-1 through 12-5** for common abbreviations. The technician must be able to interpret these abbreviations correctly when they are encountered in the drug order. Some examples of drug orders encountered in practice include the following:

EXAMPLE 1

Caps. Diphenhydramine (Benadryl) 25 mg q4h po
Interpretation: Give the patient one 25 mg capsule by mouth every 4 hours.

TABLE 12-1

Amount/Dosage

Abbreviation	Latin Derivation	English
Gal	congius	gallon
cc		cubic centimeter
g	gramma	gram
gr	granum	grain
gtt	gutta	drop(s)
lb	libra	pound
m	minimum	minim
mL		milliliter
no	numerus	number
qs	quatum sufficit	quantity sufficient
ss	semis	one-half
ℨ	drachma	dram
℥	unica	ounce

TABLE 12-2

Preparations

Abbreviation	Latin Derivation	English
cap	capsula	capsule
elix	elixir	elixir
EC		enteric coated
ext	extractum	extract
fl	fluidus	fluid
pil	pilula	pill
sol	solutio	solution
supp	suppositorium	suppository
susp		suspension
syr	syrupus	syrup
tab	tabella	tablet
tr	tinctura	tincture
ung	unguentum	ointment

EXAMPLE 2

Elixir Acetaminophen (Elixir Tylenol) gtts 20 tid pc and hs po
Interpretation: Give 20 drops of elixir acetaminophen by mouth three times a day after meals and 20 drops by mouth at bedtime.

EXAMPLE 3

100 mg Demerol IM stat. 50 mg q4h prn pain
Interpretation: Give 100 mg of Demerol intramuscularly immediately, then give 50 mg of Demerol intramuscularly not more often than every 4 hours prn.

The abbreviation "prn" can often be a source of trouble if not interpreted carefully. In the order described in the last example, the medication (Demerol) can be administered if the dosing interval of at least 4 hours is maintained. The nurse

TABLE 12-3

Routes

Abbreviation	Latin Derivation	English
ID		intradermal
IM		intramuscular
IV		intravenous
IVPB		intravenous piggyback
OD (*)	oculus dexter	right eye
OS	oculus sinister	left eye
OU	oculo utro	both eyes
AD (*)	auricula dexter	right ear
AS (*)	auricula sinister	left ear
AU (*)	auriculi utro	both ears
po	per os	by mouth
sc (*)	sub cutis	subcutaneous
sl	sub lingual	sublingual
GT		gastrostomy
NG		nasogastric
NJ		nasojejunal

*Error-prone abbreviations that have contributed to medication errors. See Chapter 27 for the rationale of their misinterpretation.

TABLE 12-4

Special Instructions

Abbreviation	Latin Derivation	English
aa	ana	of each
ad lib	ad libitum	as desired
c̄	cum	with
dil	dilutus	dilute
per	per	through or by
R$_x$	recipe	take
s̄	sine	without
stat	statim	immediately

TABLE 12-5

Times

Abbreviation	Latin Derivation	English
ā	ante	before
ac	ante cibum	before meals
am	ante meridian	before noon
bid	bis in die	twice a day
h	hora	hour
hs (*)	hora somni	hour of sleep or at bedtime
noct	noctis	night
o	omnis	every
od (*)	omni die	every day
oh	omni hora	every hour
p	post	after
pc	post cibum	after meals
pm	post meridian	after noon
prn	pro re nata	whenever necessary
q	quaque	every
qd (*)	quaque die	every day
qh (q3h, etc.)	quaque hora	every hour (3, 4, etc.)
qid (*)	quarter in die	4 times a day
sos	si opus sit	if necessary (one dose only)
tid	ter in die	3 times a day

*Error-prone abbreviations that have contributed to medication errors. See Chapter 27 for the rationale of their misinterpretation.

TABLE 12-6

Values of Single Roman Numbers

Roman Numerals		Value
s̄s̄	=	½
I or i	=	1
V or v	=	5
X or x	=	10
L or l	=	50
C or c	=	100
D or d	=	500
M or m	=	1000

assesses the patient's need for the Demerol to control pain or the patient requests the medication, and it may be administered if it has been four hours or more since the previous injection.

Most prescriptions are written in the metric system; however, the apothecary system using Roman numerals is still used by some prescribers through force of habit. A few of the most common Roman numerals are shown in **Table 12-6**.

Ratio and Proportion

Nearly every problem that arises in calculations involving medication can be broken down to simple ratio and proportion. Developing skill in setting up ratios and proportions will be an invaluable aid to the nurse in solving medication problems quickly and accurately.

Ratio

A ratio is the relationship of two quantities. It may be expressed in the form 1:10 or 1:2500, or it may be expressed as a fraction—1/10 or 1/2500. The ratio expression 1:10 or 1/10 can be read as one in ten, one-tenth, or one part in ten parts.

EXAMPLE 4

For every twenty students there is one teacher. The ratio of teachers to students is 1 in 20 or 1:20 or 1/20.

Proportion

A proportion is formed by using two ratios which are equal. For example, $1/2 = 5/10$. When two ratios or fractions are equal, their cross product is also equal. The cross product is obtained by multiplying the denominator of one ratio by the numerator of the other, as follows:

$$\frac{1}{2} \diagdown\!\!\!\!\diagup \frac{5}{10} = 2 \times 5 = 10 \times 1$$

The cross products are equal: $10 = 10$. Therefore, the ratio 1/2 is equal to the ratio 5/10.

Does $1/4 = 3/12$?

$$\frac{1}{4} \diagdown\!\!\!\!\diagup \frac{3}{12} = \frac{12}{12}$$

The cross products are equal: $12 = 12$. Therefore, 1/4 is equal to 3/12.

This characteristic of proportions is very useful in solving problems that arise in drug administration. If any three of the values of a proportion are known, the fourth value can be determined.

EXAMPLE 5

The prescriber orders 20 mg IM of a drug for a patient. The drug is available in a 10 mL vial which contains 50 mg of drug. How many milliliters will be needed to supply the dose of 20 mg?

SOLUTION

Three things are known from the statement of the problem.

1. 10 mL vial on hand
2. 50 mg of drug in the 10 mL vial
3. 20 mg is the desired dose

A ratio can be stated for the drug on hand.

$$\frac{10\ \text{mL}}{50\ \text{mg}} \text{ reduced to lowest terms} = \frac{1\ \text{mL}}{5\ \text{mg}}$$

A ratio can also be stated for the required dosage.

$$\frac{x \text{ mL}}{20 \text{ mg}}$$

Thus the proportion is

$$\frac{1 \text{ mL}}{5 \text{ mg}} = \frac{x \text{ mL}}{20 \text{ mg}}$$

Note in the proportion that the units are labeled and like units are located in the same position in each fraction or ratio (1 mL is opposite × mL and 5 mg is opposite 20 mg). It is important to label the parts of the proportion correctly. Note that the answer label is always the label with the "x."

Important: Three conditions must be met when using ratio and proportion.

1. The numerators must have the same units.
2. The denominators must have the same units.
3. Three of the four parts must be known.

To solve the last example, simply find the cross product and solve for the unknown (x).

$$\frac{1 \text{mL}}{5 \text{ mg}} = \frac{x \text{ mL}}{20 \text{ mg}}$$

$$5 \times x; = 1 \times 20$$

$$5x = 20$$

$$x = 4 \text{ mL (20 divided by 5)}$$

Therefore, 4 mL of the solution contains 20 mg of drug.

It is helpful to note that a proportion is similar to the way we think logically: if this is so, then that will follow. Problems can be analyzed with the if-then approach.

In the last example, we could say IF we have 10 mL containing 50 mg of drug, THEN x mL of solution will contain 20 mg of drug.

$$\underset{\text{IF}}{\frac{10 \text{ mL}}{50 \text{ mg}}} \text{ or } \underset{}{\frac{1 \text{ mL}}{5 \text{ mg}}} = \underset{\text{THEN}}{\frac{x \text{ mL}}{20 \text{ mg}}}$$

Remember that the first ratio of a proportion is always formed from the quantity and strength (concentration) of the drug on hand.

EXAMPLE 6

Ampicillin oral suspension contains 250 mg of the drug in each 5 mL. How many milliliters would be measured into a medication syringe to obtain a dose of 75 mg of ampicillin?

SOLUTION

1. Set up the proportion beginning with the drug on hand.

$$\underset{\text{IF}}{\frac{5 \text{ mL}}{250 \text{ mg}}} = \underset{\text{THEN}}{\frac{x \text{ mL}}{75 \text{ mg}}}$$

2. Then cross multiply.

$$250(x) = 5(75)$$
$$250(x) = 375$$
$$x = 1.5 \text{ mL}$$

PRACTICE PROBLEMS

Solve the following problems by setting up the proportion and finding the unknown quantity. Answers are at the end of the chapter.

1. Elixir of digoxin contains 50 micrograms (mcg) of digoxin in each milliliter. How many micrograms of the drug are in 0.3 mL of the elixir?
2. Lugol's solution contains 50 mg of iodine per milliliter. How many milligrams of iodine are in 0.3 mL of the solution?
3. Elixir of diphenhydramine (elixir of Benadryl) contains 12.5 mg per 5 mL (teaspoonful). How many milliliters are needed to provide 30 mg of the drug?
4. The physician orders 2.5 mg of theophylline to be administered orally to a pediatric patient. If elixir of theophylline contains 80 mg of theophylline per tablespoonful (15 mL), how many milliliters of the elixir should be administered?
5. A vial contains 250 mg of tetracycline HCl in a total of 2 mL of solution. How many milligrams of tetracycline HCl are contained in 0.6 mL of this solution?

Conversion Between Systems of Measurement

Before reviewing the types of calculations used in determining medication dosages, it is necessary to examine conversions between systems of measurement. It was mentioned previously that nearly all medication orders today are written using the metric system. However, some orders will be written using apothecary notation. The technician must be able to convert from the apothecary system to the metric system and from one unit to another unit within both systems.

Conversion between systems requires the use of approximate weight and measure equivalents. The key word here is "approximate." The approximate values are not *exact* equivalents. For example, 1 g = 15 gr approximately = 15.432 gr exactly. The pharmacist uses the exact equivalents in compounding medications. In calculations involving dosages, however, it is not necessary to use exact equivalents. In fact, since the exact equivalents involve many decimal places and fractional numbers, their use could lead to awkward calculations with an increase in errors. Thus the approximate equivalents are used in calculations for medication dosages. Approximate equivalents are used in the examples and problems in the remainder of this chapter. For example, 30 milliliters (mL) = 1 fluid ounce (fl oz) in all calculations. Similarly, 1 gram (g) = 15 grains (gr).

Review of the Metric System

The three basic units of the metric system are the meter (length), the gram (weight), and the liter (volume). Only the units of weight and volume are considered in this chapter. Multiples or parts of these basic units are named by adding a prefix. Each prefix has a numerical value, as shown in **Table 12-7**.

TABLE 12-7

Metric Prefixes

Small Units	Large Units
deci = 0.1	deka = 10
centi = 0.01	hecto = 100
milli = 0.001	kilo = 1000
micro = 0.000001	mega = 1,000,000
nano = 0.000000001	

TABLE 12-8

Common Metric Abbreviations

Measure	Abbreviation
nanogram	ng
microgram	mcg
milligram	mg
gram	g
kilogram	kg
milliliter	mL
deciliter	dL
liter	L
millimeter	mm
centimeter	cm
meter	m
kilometer	km

Examples of the use of the metric prefixes are as follows:

- 1 milliliter (mL) = 1/1000 liter = 0.001 L
- 1 milligram (mg) = 1/1000 gram = 0.001 g
- 1 microgram (mcg) = 1/1,000,000 gram = 0.000001 g
- 1 nanogram (ng) = 1/1,000,000,000 gram = 0.000000001 g
- 1 kilogram (kg) = 1000 times 1 gram = 1000 g
- 1 deciliter (dL) = 1/10 liter = 0.1 L

Table 12-8 shows examples of common metric abbreviations.

Liter
The liter is the basic unit of volume used to measure liquids in the metric system. It is equal to 1000 cubic centimeters of water. One cubic centimeter is considered equivalent to one milliliter (mL); thus 1 liter (L) = 1000 milliliters (mL).

Gram
The gram is the basic unit of weight in the metric system. The gram is defined as the weight of one cubic centimeter of distilled water at 4°C.

Conversions

Using Table 12-7, the following values can be determined:

- 1000 g = 1 kg
- 1000 mg = 1 g
- 1000 ng = 1 mcg
- 1000 mcg = 1 mg
- 1000 mL = 1 L
- 100 mL = 1 dL

Two rules apply to conversions within the metric system.

- *Rule 1.* To convert a smaller quantity to a larger denomination, move the decimal point to the left.
  —Smaller to larger (S to L) = Right to left (R to L)
    Smaller ⟶ Larger
    Right ⟶ Left
    Example:
    1000 mcg ⟶ 1 mg
- *Rule 2.* To convert a quantity to a smaller denomination, move the decimal point to the right.
  —Larger to smaller (L to S) = Left to right (L to R)
    Larger ⟶ Smaller
    Left ⟶ Right
    Example:
    1 g ⟶ 1000 mg

Note that the two Ls are on the same side in each rule.

EXAMPLE 7

Convert 22 g to milligrams.

SOLUTION

The change is from larger to smaller with a difference of 1000 between the units. The rule in this case is: Larger to smaller (L to S) = Left to right (L to R).

Because the difference is 1000 between grams and milligrams, the decimal point is moved three places to the right. Thus, 22 g = 22,000 mg.

EXAMPLE 8

Convert 150 mL to liters.

SOLUTION

In changing from milliliters to liters, the change is from smaller to larger (S to L), with a difference of 1000 between the units (1000 mL = 1 L). Therefore, move the decimal point from right to left (R to L). Because there is a difference of 1000 between the units, move the decimal point three places to the left. Thus 150 mL = 0.15 L.

PRACTICE PROBLEMS

6. 2000 mg = _____ g
7. 50 g = _____ mg
8. 2 L = _____ mL
9. 230 ng = _____ mcg

10. 250 mg = _____ g
11. 2.5 kg = _____ g
12. 0.5 L = _____ mL
13. 1.5 L = _____ dL
14. 20 mg = _____ g
15. 0.7 mg = _____ mcg

Apothecary System of Weights

The apothecary system of weights is based upon the grain (gr), which is the smallest unit in the system. The origin of the grain is uncertain, but it is believed that at one time solids were measured by using grains of wheat as the standard.

In practice, the technician will seldom see apothecary units of weight with the exception of the grain, which is still commonly used in ordering medications such as nitroglycerin (1/100 gr, 1/150 gr), atropine sulfate (1/200 gr, 1/150 gr), codeine sulfate (1/8 gr, 1/4 gr, 1/2 gr, 1 gr), and morphine sulfate (1/6 gr, 1/8 gr, 1/2 gr). To convert grains to metric units, the following approximate equivalent is used:

$$15 \text{ grains} = 1 \text{ gram}$$

EXAMPLE 9

Convert 4 grains to grams.

SOLUTION

$$\frac{15 \text{gr}}{1 \text{ g}} = \frac{4 \text{ gr}}{x \text{g}}$$

$$x = 0.27 \text{ g}$$

Apothecary System of Volume (Liquid) Measure

The apothecary liquid measures are the same as the avoirdupois measures that we use daily, such as ounces, pints, and quarts. The smallest unit of volume in the apothecary system is the minim ($\mathfrak{m}$). The minim should *not* be confused with the drop because they are not equivalent. The size of a drop varies with the properties of the liquid being dispensed or measured. **Table 12-9** shows the common units of liquid measure in the apothecary system.

Apothecary System Notation

In the apothecary system, the unit is written first, followed by the quantity. For small numbers, lowercase Roman numerals are used. Arabic numbers are commonly used for large numbers (i.e., greater than 40). **Table 12-10** shows examples of apothecary system notation.

Converting From the Apothecary System to the Metric System

The use of tabular information is helpful in converting between the systems of weights and measures. Many conversions, however, can be readily made by use of two important equivalents and the ratio and proportion method.

The equivalents are:

$$15 \text{ gr} = 1 \text{ g}$$

$$\mathfrak{m} \, 16 = 1 \text{ mL}$$

TABLE 12-9

Liquid Measure in the Apothecary System

Measure		Equivalent
60 minims (m)	=	1 fluid dram (fl dr or fl ʒ)*
8 fluid drams (fl dr)	=	1 fluid ounce (fl oz or fl ʒ) = 480 minims (m)
16 fluid ounces	=	1 pint (pt)
2 pints	=	1 quart (qt) = 32 fluid ounces (fl oz)
4 quarts	=	1 gallon = 128 fluid ounces

*The fluid dram sign (ʒ) is often used by physicians to represent 1 teaspoonful or 5 mL. The apothecary symbol for one-half fluid ounce or 1 tablespoonful is ʒ s̄s. When this appears in the directions for use (Signa), it is read as 1 tablespoonful or 15 mL.

TABLE 12-10

Apothecary Notation

Quantity	Notation
1/10 grain	gr 1/10
1 grain	gr i
1½ grains	gr is̄s
10 grains	gr x
15 minims	m XV
150 minims	m 150
2½ ounces	ʒ iis̄s

EXAMPLE 10

The physician orders 7 1/2 grains of aminophylline po for a patient. On hand are aminophylline tablets 500 mg. How many tablets are required for one dose?

SOLUTION

First the physician's order must be converted to a metric unit, or the strength of the tablets on hand must be converted to an apothecary unit. It is preferable to convert to metric units in all cases.

Setting up the proportion gives:

$$\text{IF} \qquad \text{THEN}$$
$$\frac{1\text{ g}}{15\text{ gr}} = \frac{x\text{ g}}{7.5\text{ gr}}$$

Cross multiplying:

$$15x = 7.5$$
$$x = 0.5\text{ g (500 mg)}$$

Thus the 7 1/2 gr ordered by the physician is equal to one of the 500 mg tablets on hand. The dose is 1 tablet of 500 mg aminophylline (7 1/2 gr aminophylline).

EXAMPLE 11

How many milligrams of nitroglycerin are in one 1/150 gr tablet of the drug?

SOLUTION

This problem requires conversion from the apothecary system to the metric system. Use the equivalent 1 g = 15 gr. The proportion is:

$$\begin{array}{cc} \text{IF} & \text{THEN} \\[6pt] \dfrac{1\ g}{15\ gr} & = \dfrac{x\ g}{1/150\ gr} \end{array}$$

Cross multiplying:

$$15x = 1/150 = .0067$$
$$x = 0.0004\ g = 0.4\ mg$$

Remember, when converting in the metric form from larger to smaller, the decimal point moves left to right.

PRACTICE PROBLEMS

16. 6 pints   = _____ fluid ounces
17. 17 g   = _____ gr
18. 26 quarts   = _____ gallons
19. 200 minims = _____ fluid ounces
20. 65 grains   = _____ g
21. 3 gallons   = _____ pints

Calculation of Fractional Doses

Nurses encounter fractional or partial medication dosages frequently because physicians often order medication for a patient in a strength that differs from the strength of the preparation on hand.

The ratio and proportion method can be used to solve all problems of fractional dosages. The concentration of the medication on hand forms the IF ratio of the proportion.

EXAMPLE 12

The physician orders 1 million units of penicillin G for a patient. The penicillin G on hand is available as a solution containing 250,000 units/mL.

SOLUTION

Find the strength of the product on hand. This expression forms the IF ratio of the proportion:

$$\begin{array}{cc} \text{IF} & \text{THEN} \\[6pt] \dfrac{250,000\ units}{1\ mL} & = \text{_____} \end{array}$$

Place the number of units wanted in the THEN ratio and solve for the unknown x.

$$\text{IF} \qquad \text{THEN}$$
$$\frac{250,000 \text{ units}}{1 \text{ mL}} = \frac{1,000,000 \text{ units}}{x \text{ mL}}$$
$$250,000x = 1,000,000$$
$$x = 4 \text{ mL}$$

Remember to label all parts of the proportion carefully with the appropriate units.

EXAMPLE 13

The physician orders 250 mcg of cyanocobalamin (vitamin B_{12}) IM daily. The vitamin B_{12} on hand is labeled 1000 mcg/mL. How many milliliters should be given to the patient?

SOLUTION

The concentration of B_{12} on hand is 1000 mcg/mL. Therefore, the IF ratio is:

$$\frac{1000 \text{ mcg}}{1 \text{ mL}}$$

Placing the number of micrograms needed opposite the micrograms of the IF ratio results in:

$$\text{IF} \qquad \text{THEN}$$
$$\frac{1000 \text{ mcg}}{1 \text{ mL}} = \frac{250 \text{ mcg}}{x \text{ ML}}$$

Solving for x yields:

$$x = 0.25 \text{ mL}$$

To supply 250 mcg of vitamin B_{12} requires 0.25 mL.

EXAMPLE 14

A patient is to be given 25 mg of diphenhydramine (Benadryl) po. The Benadryl is available as elixir of Benadryl 12.5 mg/5 mL. How many milliliters should be given to the patient?

SOLUTION

$$\text{IF} \qquad \text{THEN}$$
$$\frac{12.5 \text{ mg}}{5 \text{ mL}} = \frac{25 \text{ mg}}{x \text{ mL}}$$
$$x = \frac{125}{12.5}$$
$$x = 10 \text{ mL}$$

EXAMPLE 15

A medication order calls for 750 mg of calcium lactate to be given tid po. On hand are tablets of calcium lactate 0.5 g. How many tablets should be given for each dose?

SOLUTION

Note: When using ratio and proportion the units must be alike. Grams cannot be used in a proportion with milligrams. Therefore, in this example the grams must be converted to milligrams or the 750 mg converted to grams. Changing the grams to milligrams yields:

$$0.5 \text{ g} = 500 \text{ mg}$$

Remember: Larger to smaller = Left to right. A 1000 difference means moving the decimal point three places to the right.

$$\text{IF} \qquad \text{THEN}$$
$$\frac{500 \text{ mg}}{1 \text{ tab}} = \frac{750 \text{ mg}}{x \text{ tab}}$$
$$x = 1.5 \text{ or } 1\tfrac{1}{2} \text{ tablets}$$

PRACTICE PROBLEMS

22. A patient is to receive a 100 mg dose of gentamicin. On hand is a vial containing 80 mg/mL of the drug. How many milliliters should be given to the patient?
23. A multiple dose vial of a penicillin G potassium solution contains 100,000 units per milliliter. How many milliliters of this solution must be administered to a patient who requires a 750,000 unit dose?
24. A physician orders 30 mg of Demerol IM for a patient. How many milliliters of a Demerol solution containing 100 mg/mL must be given to the patient?
25. The nurse is asked to administer an intramuscular dose of 45 mcg of an investigational drug. How many milliliters must be withdrawn from a vial containing 20 mcg/mL of the drug?
26. A pediatric patient is to be given a 70 mg dose of Dilantin by administering an oral suspension containing 50 mg of Dilantin per 5 mL. How many milliliters of the suspension must be administered?

Calculation of Dosages Based on Weight

The recommended dosages of drugs are often expressed in the literature as a number of milligrams per unit of body weight per unit of time (refer to package inserts or the *Physicians' Desk Reference*). Such dosage expressions are commonly used in depicting pediatric doses. For example, the recommended dose for a drug might be 5 mg/kg/24 hours. This information can be utilized by the pharmacist to

- calculate the dose for a given patient; and
- check on doses ordered that are suspected to be significant over- or underdoses.

EXAMPLE 16

The physician orders Mintezol tablets for a 110-pound child. The recommended dosage for Mintezol is 20 mg/kg per dose. How many 500 mg tablets of Mintezol should be given to this patient for each dose?

SOLUTION

1. Since the dose provided is based on a kilogram weight, convert the patient's weight to kilograms by proportion.

$$1 \text{ kg} = 2.2 \text{ lb}$$

$$\frac{1 \text{ kg}}{2.2 \text{ lb}} = \frac{x \text{ kg}}{110 \text{ lb}}$$

$$x = 50 \text{ kg}$$

2. Calculate the total daily dose using the recommended dosage information: 20 mg/kg. This is interpreted as, "For each kilogram of body weight, give 20 mg of the drug."

$$\frac{20 \text{ mg}}{1 \text{ kg}} = \frac{x \text{ mg}}{50 \text{ kg}}$$

$$x = 1000 \text{ mg}$$

3. Calculate the number of tablets needed to supply 1000 mg per dose. The concentration of tablets on hand = 500 mg/tablet.

$$\frac{500 \text{ mg}}{1 \text{ tab}} = \frac{1000 \text{ mg}}{x \text{ tab}}$$

$$x = 2 \text{ tablets per dose}$$

EXAMPLE 17

The recommended dose of meperidine (Demerol) is 6 mg/kg/24 h for pain. It is given in divided doses every 4 to 6 hours. How many milliliters of Demerol injection (50 mg/mL) should be administered to a 33-pound child as a single dose every 6 hours?

SOLUTION

1. Calculate the daily dose for a 33-pound child.

$$\frac{6 \text{ mg}}{1 \text{ kg (2.2 lb)}} = \frac{x \text{ mg}}{33 \text{ lb}}$$

By inserting the conversion unit 2.2 lb for 1 kg in the ratio, there is no need to do a separate calculation of the number of kilograms in 33 pounds.

$$x = 90 \text{ mg of Demerol per day (24 hours)}$$

2. Calculate the number of milliliters of Demerol injection (50 mg/mL) needed for the total daily dose.

$$\frac{50 \text{ mg}}{1 \text{ mL}} = \frac{90 \text{ mg}}{x \text{ mL}}$$

$$50x = 90$$

$$x = 1.8 \text{ mL every 24 hours}$$

3. Calculate the number of milliliters to be given every 6 hours.

$$\frac{1.8 \text{ mL}}{24 \text{ h}} = \frac{x \text{ mL}}{6 \text{ h}}$$

$$24x = 10.8$$

$$x = 0.45 \text{ mL}$$

PRACTICE PROBLEMS

27. The recommended dose of cefamandole nafate (Mandol) for a pediatric patient is 50 mg/kg/day. How many milligrams must be given daily to a 60-pound child?
28. Acyclovir (Zovirax) is administered in a dose of 15 mg/kg/day. How many milligrams of the drug must be administered daily to a 175-pound adult?
29. The recommended dose for methotrexate is 2.5 mg/kg every 14 days. How many milligrams of this drug must be administered to a 125-pound adult for each dose?
30. Chlorpromazine HCl is to be administered in a dose of 0.25 mg/lb. How many milligrams of this drug must be administered to an 85-kilogram patient?
31. A recommended dose for the administration of streptomycin sulfate is 10 mg/lb/day. How many milligrams of this drug must be administered daily to a 63-kilogram adult?

Pediatric Dosage Calculations

When the manufacturer's recommended dosage is not available to determine dosages for children, the nomogram is the most accurate method to use. The nomogram is a chart that uses the weight and height (size) of the patient to estimate his or her body surface area (BSA) in square meters (m^2). This body surface area is then placed in a ratio with the body surface area of an average adult ($1.73 m^2$). The formula used with the nomogram method is:

$$\text{Child's dose} = \frac{\text{Child's body surface area in } m^2}{1.73 \ m^2 \ (\text{BSA of average adult})} \times \text{Adult dose}$$

To determine the child's BSA, the weight and height of the child must be known. The nomogram scales contain both metric (kg, cm) and avoirdupois (lb, inches) values for height and weight. Thus, the BSA can be determined for pounds and inches or kilograms and centimeters without making conversions.

Appendix C of this text contains the nomogram "Body Surface Area of Children." Note the three columns labeled height, body surface area, and weight. Also note that the height and weight scales show both metric and avoirdupois values.

To determine the body surface area, a ruler or straightedge is needed. (A piece of paper or cardboard can be used if there is at least one even, straight edge.) The following steps demonstrate the use of the nomogram.

1. Determine the height and weight of the patient. This information may be given in metric values (e.g., height = 84 cm, weight = 12 kg) or in avoirdupois values: height = 33.5 inches, weight = 26.5 pounds. Mixed values can also be used: height = 85 cm, weight = 26.5 pounds.
2. Place the straightedge on the nomogram connecting the two points on the height and weight scales that represent the patient's values. Assume the patient is a child weighing 26.5 pounds and standing 33.5 inches tall. Then 26.5 pounds on the weight scale and 33.5 inches on the height scale are connected using the straightedge.
3. Where the straightedge crosses the center column (body surface area) a reading is taken. This value is the body surface area in square meters for the patient. In our example, BSA = 0.52 m^2.

   Note: The three scales are divided into five divisions between the major numbered sections, which vary in value as the scales are ascended. To interpret the value of the divisions, take the difference between the two numbers and divide by 5.

For example, on the kg scale between 5 kg and 6 kg there is a difference of 1, so each division between 5 and 6 is 0.2 kg (1 divided by 5). Between 1.5 kg and 2 kg, the difference is 0.5. Therefore, each division between 1.5 and 2 kg is 0.1 kg (0.5 divided by 5).

4. Substitute the BSA value in the formula to calculate the dosage for the child. For example, if the dose of aminophylline is 500 mg for an adult, what is the dose for a child with a calculated BSA of 0.52 m²?

$$\frac{\text{Child's}}{\text{dose}} = \frac{\text{BSA of child in m}^2}{1.73 \text{ m}^2 \text{ (BSA of average child)}} \times \frac{\text{Adult}}{\text{dose}}$$

Therefore,

$$= \frac{0.52 \text{ m}^2}{1.73 \text{ m}^2} \times 500 \text{ mg}$$

$$= 0.3 \times 500 \text{ mg}$$

$$= 150 \text{ mg of aminophylline}$$

With practice, the nurse can become proficient in using the nomogram and will find it a useful tool for calculating dosages.

PRACTICE PROBLEMS

Solve the following problems using the nomogram in Appendix H.

32. Find the BSA for the following children.
    a. 9 pounds, 23 inches BSA   = _____ m²
    b. 3.2 kg, 50 cm BSA   = _____ m²
    c. 15 kg, 40 inches BSA   = _____ m²
33. The adult dose of methyldopa (Aldomet) is 250 mg. What is the dose for the child in problem 32-c?
34. If the adult dose of furosemide (Lasix) is 40 mg, what is the dose for a child whose BSA is 0.53 m²?
35. An adult dose of theophylline is 400 mg. What is the dose for a child who weighs 25 kg and who has a height of 105 cm?
36. If the adult dose of diazepam (Valium) is 10 mg, what is the dose for an 18-pound child with a height of 27 inches?

Calculations Involving Intravenous Administration

Pharmacists are often required to determine the flow rates for intravenous infusions, to calculate the volume of fluids administered over a period of time, and to control the total volume of fluids administered to the patient during a stated period of time. The calculations necessary to perform these tasks can all be accomplished by the use of ratio and proportion.

Chapter 14 provides information on the techniques involved in IV administration, the equipment used, and the documentation to be prepared by the nurse administering IV solutions. The calculations required for IV administration are detailed in the following sections.

Calculating the Rate of IV Administration

When the physician orders intravenous solutions to run for a stated number of hours, the pharmacist may have to compute the number of drops per minute to comply with the order.

To calculate the flow rate using the ratio and proportion method, three steps are required. One must determine

1. the number of milliliters the patient will receive per hour,
2. the number of milliliters the patient will receive per minute, and
3. the number of drops per minute that will equal the number of milliliters computed in step 2. The drop rate specified for the IV set being used must be considered in this step. The drop rate is expressed as a ratio of drops per mL (gtt/mL).

EXAMPLE 18

The physician orders 3000 mL of dextrose 5% in water (D5W) IV over a 24-hour period. If the IV set is calibrated to deliver 15 drops per milliliter, how many drops must be administered per minute?

SOLUTION

1. Calculate mL/hr.

$$\frac{3000 \text{ mL}}{24 \text{ hr}} = \frac{x \text{ mL}}{1 \text{ hr}}$$

$$x = 125 \text{ mL/hr or}$$

$$= 125 \text{ mL/60 min}$$

2. Calculate mL/min.

$$\frac{125 \text{ mL}}{60 \text{ min}} = \frac{x \text{ mL}}{1 \text{ min}}$$

$$x = 2 \text{ mL/min (approx.)}$$

3. Calculate gtt/min using the drop rate per minute of the IV set.
   IV set drop rate = 15 drops/mL

$$\frac{15 \text{ gtt}}{1 \text{ mL}} = \frac{x \text{ gtt}}{2 \text{ mL (amt needed/min)}}$$

$$x = 30 \text{ gtt/min}$$

EXAMPLE 19

The physician orders 1.5 L of lactated Ringer's solution to be administered over a 12-hour period. The IV set is calibrated to deliver 10 gtt/mL. How many drops per minute should the patient receive?

SOLUTION

1. Determine the number of milliliters to be administered in 1 hour. Since the answer requested is in milliliter units, first convert liter quantity to milliliters.

$$1.5 \text{ L} = 1500 \text{ mL}$$

$$\frac{1500 \text{ mL}}{12 \text{ hr}} = \frac{x \text{ mL}}{1 \text{ hr}}$$

$$x = 125 \text{ mL/hr or}$$

$$= 125 \text{ mL/60 min}$$

2. Calculate the number of milliliters per minute.

$$\frac{125\text{mL}}{60\text{ min}} = \frac{\text{x mL}}{1\text{ min}}$$

$$\text{x} = 2\text{ mL/min (approx.)}$$

3. Calculate the number of drops per minute.

$$\text{IV set drop rate} = 10\text{ gtt/mL}$$

$$\frac{10\text{ gtt}}{1\text{ mL}} = \frac{\text{x gtt}}{2\text{ mL}}$$

$$\text{x} = 20\text{ gtt/min}$$

The following example shows how to calculate the time required to administer an IV solution when the volume and flow rate are known.

EXAMPLE 20

How long will it take to complete an IV infusion of 1.5 L of D5W being administered at the rate of 45 drops/minute? The IV set is calibrated to deliver 15 drops/mL. This problem is a variation of the flow rate problem considered earlier.

SOLUTION

1. Determine the number of milliliters/minute being infused.

$$\text{Drop rate of IV set} = \frac{15\text{ gtt}}{1\text{ mL}} = \frac{45\text{ gtt}}{\text{x mL}}$$

$$15\text{x} = 45$$

$$\text{x} = 3\text{ mL/min}$$

2. Calculate the number of milliliters/hour.

$$3\text{ mL/min} \times 60\text{ min/hr} = 180\text{ mL/hr}$$

3. Calculate the number of hours required to administer the total volume of the solution. If 180 mL are delivered each hour, then how many hours are required to administer 1500 mL (1.5 L)?

$$\frac{180\text{ mL}}{1\text{ hr}} = \frac{1500\text{ mL}}{\text{x hr}}$$

$$180\text{x} = 1500$$

$$\text{x} = 8.3\text{ hours, or 8 hours 20 minutes}$$

PRACTICE PROBLEMS

37. The physician orders 1200 mL of D5W solution to be administered over a 10-hour period. The IV set is calibrated to deliver 18 gtt/mL. How many drops per minute should the patient receive?

38. A patient is to receive 150 mL of an IV infusion over a period of 4 hours. The IV set is calibrated to deliver 15 gtt/mL. How many drops per minute should the patient receive? (Round off answer to nearest whole drop.)

39. An IV infusion containing 750 mL is to be administered at a drop rate of 40 gtt/min. The IV set is calibrated to deliver 20 gtt/mL. How long will it take to administer the entire infusion?

40. A nurse wishes to administer 1200 mL of an IV infusion at a rate of 45 gtt/min. The IV set is calibrated to deliver 15 gtt/mL. How long will it take to administer the entire infusion?

41. The physician orders 100 mL of a drug solution to be administered at a rate of 20 gtt/min. The IV set is calibrated to deliver 12 gtt/mL. How long will it take to administer the entire infusion?

Calculations Involving Piggyback IV Infusion

The physician may order medications to be run piggyback with the IV electrolyte fluids. The medications are usually dissolved in 50 or 100 mL of an IV solution and run for 1 hour through the open IV line. The flow rate for these piggyback infusions is calibrated the same way as the rate for the regular IV solutions.

EXAMPLE 21

An IV piggyback of cefazolin sodium (Ancef, Kefzol) 500 mg in 100 mL/hour is ordered. The piggyback IV set is calibrated to deliver 10 gtt/mL. How many drops/minute should be administered?

SOLUTION

1. The entire 100 mL is to be infused in 1 hour. Calculate the number of milliliters/minute.

$$\frac{100 \text{ mL}}{60 \text{ min}} = \frac{x \text{ mL}}{1 \text{ min}}$$
$$60x = 100$$
$$x = 1.7 \text{ mL/min}$$

2. Calculate the flow rate.

$$\text{Drop rate} = \frac{10 \text{ gtt}}{1 \text{ min}} = \frac{x \text{ gtt}}{1.7 \text{ mL}}$$
$$x = 17 \text{ gtt/min}$$

The volume of the piggyback and the time of its administration must be accounted for in calculating the daily fluid requirements of the patient. In Example 21, assume that the patient is to have a total of 2000 mL of electrolyte solution administered in 24 hours, and that cefazolin sodium 500 mg in 100 mL/hr is ordered q.i.d. The number of milliliters per day and the times of the piggyback infusion must be subtracted from the daily fluid requirement.

$$\begin{aligned}
\text{cefazolin 100 mL q.i.d.} &= 100 \times 4 = 400 \text{ mL} \\
\text{Run 1 hour} \times 4 &= 4 \text{ hr} \\
\text{Daily requirement} &= 2000 \text{ mL in 24 hours} \\
\text{Subtract piggyback} &= -400 \text{ mL in 4 hours} \\
&= 1600 \text{ mL in 20 hours}
\end{aligned}$$

Calculate the flow rate based on 1600 mL over a 20-hour period to administer the correct amount of fluid to the patient.

EXAMPLE 22

The medication order indicates that the patient is to have a maximum of 2000 mL of IV fluids in 24 hours. In addition, the patient is to receive **gentamicin** 50 mg in 100 mL

D5W over 30 minutes q8h. The IV set is calibrated to deliver 10 gtt/mL. How many drops/minute should the piggybacks be run and how many drops/minute should the IV solution D5W be administered between piggybacks to keep the vein open?

SOLUTION

1. Calculate the total volume of the piggyback solutions and the total hours they run. Order calls for 100 mL over 30 minutes q8h (q8h = 3 doses in 24 hours).

$$100 \text{ mL} \times 3 \ = \ 300 \text{ mL total}$$
$$30 \text{ min} \times 3 \ = \ 90 \text{ min or } 1.5 \text{ hr}$$

2. Subtract these totals from the daily total of IV fluid.

$$2000 \text{ mL} - 300 \text{ mL} \ = \ 1700 \text{ mL}$$
$$24 \text{ hr} - 1.5 \text{ hr} \ = \ 22.5 \text{ hr}$$

3. Calculate the flow rate for the D5W to be used between the three piggybacks using the adjusted totals.

$$\frac{1700 \text{ mL}}{22.5 \text{ hr}} \ = \ \frac{75 \times \text{mL/hr}}{1 \text{ hr}}$$
$$75 \text{ mL hr} \div 60 \ = \ 1.25 \text{ mL/min}$$

Using a drop rate of 10 gtt/mL, we have

$$\frac{10 \text{ gtt}}{1 \text{ mL}} \ = \ \frac{\times \text{ gtt}}{1.25 \text{ mL}}$$

$$x = 12.5 \text{ or } 12 \text{ drops/min}$$

4. The piggyback calculation is as follows:

$$100 \text{ mL} \ = \ 30 \text{ min}$$
$$100 \text{ mL} \div 30 = 3.3 \text{ mL/min}$$
$$\text{Drop set calibration} = 10 \text{ gtt/mL}$$
$$\frac{10 \text{ gtt}}{1 \text{ mL}} \ = \ \frac{\times \text{ gtt}}{3.3 \text{ mL}}$$
$$x = 33 \text{ drops/minute}$$

Will deliver 100 mL of gentamicin solution in 30 minutes.

PRACTICE PROBLEMS

42. An IV piggyback of lincomycin containing 1 g of drug in 100 mL is to be infused over 1 hour. The IV set is calibrated to deliver 15 gtt/mL. How many drops/minute should be administered?

43. An IV piggyback of pentamidine isethionate (Pentam-300) containing 300 mg of drug in 150 mL of D5W is to be infused over 1 hour. The IV set is calibrated to deliver 20 gtt/mL. How many drops/minute should be administered?

44. An IV piggyback of enalapril maleate (Vasotec IV) containing 10 mg of drug in 50 mL of 0.9% sodium chloride injection is to be infused over 30 minutes. The IV set is calibrated to deliver 15 gtt/mL. How many drops/minute should be administered?

Calculations Related to Solutions

Solutions are formed in two ways: (1) by dissolving a solid called the *solute* in a liquid called the *solvent,* or (2) by mixing two liquids together to form a solution. An example of the first way is adding salt to water to make a normal saline solution. Mixing Zephiran Chloride solution with water to make an antiseptic wash is an example of the second way.

Percentage Solutions

Many solutions are available in or are prepared to a specified percentage strength. To produce a solution of the desired strength, it is necessary to calculate the exact amount of drug to be added to a specific volume of liquid. Although most solutions are prepared by the pharmacist if they are not commercially available, the nurse must understand the concept of percentage to interpret medication labels.

Percentage is defined as the number of parts per hundred and is expressed as follows:

$$\frac{\text{No. of parts} \ \times \ 100}{100 \text{ parts}} = \text{Percentage (\%)}$$

To calculate the percentage of active ingredient in a solution, the amount of active ingredient in grams is divided by the total volume of the solution. To convert the result to a percentage, it is multiplied by 100.

Problems in percentage solutions are generally concerned with three types of percentages: weight to volume, weight to weight, and volume to volume. Weight to volume percentage (W/V%) is defined as the number of grams of solute in 100 mL of solution. Typical W/V% examples include the following:

■ 1 L of D5W, which contains 5 g of dextrose in each 100 mL of solution
■ a 1/4% solution of pilocarpine HCl, which contains 1/4 g (0.25 g) of pilocarpine HCl in each 100 mL of solution

EXAMPLE 23

What is the weight to volume percentage (W/V%) of sodium chloride (solid solute) in normal saline solution if 9 g of the salt are dissolved in 1000 mL of water?

SOLUTION

$$\frac{\text{Amount of salt in grams: 9 g}}{\text{Total volume of solution: 1000 mL}} \times 100 = 0.9\%$$

Weight to weight percentage (W/W%) is defined as the number of grams of solute in 100 g of a solid preparation. *Note:* Some W/W% solutions are used primarily in laboratory work. Concentrated hydrochloric and sulfuric acids are two examples of weight to weight percentage solutions. Typical W/W% examples include the following:

■ a 10% ointment of zinc oxide, which contains 10 g of zinc oxide in each 100 g of ointment
■ hydrocortisone cream 1/2%, which has 1/2 g (0.5 g) of hydrocortisone in each 100 g of cream

The third form of percentage is volume to volume (V/V%), which is defined as the number of milliliters of solute in each 100 mL of solution. Examples of this form include the following:

■ rubbing alcohol 70%, which contains 70 mL of absolute alcohol in each 100 mL of the solution
■ a 2% solution of phenol, which contains 2 mL of liquified phenol in each 100 mL of solution

When the type of percentage is not stated, assume that for solutions of a solid in a liquid the percentage is W/V, for solutions of a liquid in a liquid the percentage is V/V, and for mixtures of two solids the percentage is W/W.

Prevention of Medication Errors

Medication errors fall into several categories, such as omitting the dose, administering the wrong dose, administering an extra dose, administering an unordered drug, administering by the wrong route, and administering at the wrong time. Here we will consider the errors that occur when the drug order is misinterpreted. Very often, the way the amounts are expressed in the original order for weights, volumes, and units can cause interpretational errors.

For instance, writing .5 instead of 0.5 can result in a tenfold error if the decimal point is missed. In general, the following rules should be followed in transcribing orders.

■ Never leave a decimal point naked. Always place a zero before a decimal expression less than one. Example: 0.2, 0.5.
■ Never place a decimal point and zero after a whole number, because the decimal may not be seen and result in a tenfold overdose. Example: 2.0 mg read as 20 mg by mistake. The correct way is to write 2 mg.
■ Avoid using decimals when whole numbers can be used as alternatives. Example: 0.5 g should be expressed as 500 mg and 0.4 mg should be expressed as 400 mcg.
■ When possible, use the metric system rather than grains, drams, or minims.
■ Always spell out the word *units*. The abbreviation "U" for unit can be mistaken for a zero. Example: 10 U interpreted as 100 units. The better way is to write out 10 units.
■ Error-prone abbreviations that have contributed to medication errors are noted throughout the chapter with an asterisk (*). See Chapter 27 for the rationale of their misinterpretation.

SUGGESTED ACTIVITIES

■ Visit a pharmacy, ask to see the prescription balance and examine the apothecary and metric weights. Compare the 1 g weight with the 1 gr weight. Check the size of the 10 mg, 50 mg, and 500 mg weights.
■ Examine a number of medication orders from past weeks. See how many orders violated the principles listed in the section on prevention of medication errors.
■ Examine the labels of some foodstuffs for sodium content (usually listed in milligrams). Calculate the percentage of sodium in the products.

- Using the manufacturer's suggested dosage information found in the package insert for a drug, calculate the dose for several patients who have been taking the drug. Compare the prescribed dose with the calculated dose.
- Prepare a chart of flow rates for the most commonly ordered IV volumes and times of administration. Use the calibrated flow rate of your institution's IV sets.
- Using the information on the label, compare the alcohol content of various cough syrups by calculating the number of milliliters of alcohol present in 5 mL of each preparation.

ANSWERS TO PRACTICE PROBLEMS

1. 15 mcg
2. 15 mg
3. 12 mL
4. 0.46 mL
5. 75 mg
6. 2.0 g
7. 50,000 mg
8. 2000 mL
9. 0.23 mg
10. 0.25 g
11. 2500 g
12. 500 mL

13. 15 dL
14. 0.02 g
15. 700 mcg
16. 96 fluid ounces
17. 255 gr
18. 6.5 gal
19. 0.42 fluid ounces
20. 4.33 g
21. 24 pints
22. 1.25 mL
23. 7.5 mL
24. 0.3 mL

25. 2.25 mL
26. 7 mL
27. 1364 mg
28. 1193 mg
29. 142 mg
30. 47 mg
31. 1386 mg
32. a. 0.25 m^2
   b. 0.198 m^2
   c. 0.65 m^2
33. 94 mg
34. 12.25 mg

35. 190 mg (BSA = 0.82)
36. 2.14 mg (BSA = 0.37)
37. 36 drops/minute
38. 9 drops/minute
39. 6.25 hr (375 min)
40. 6.67 hr (400 min)
41. 1 hr (60 min)
42. 25 drops/minute
43. 50 drops/minute
44. 25 drops/minute

Summary

Accuracy in pharmaceutical calculations is one of the most critical and most important functions in the profession of pharmacy. Every dosage calculation should always be double-checked by a pharmacist. Pharmacists frequently double-check each other in this important matter. Life and death can hinge on a proper or improper dose being administered. Emergency situations or other life-threatening situations are never an excuse for undue haste and lack of sufficient double-checks. Care and vigilance are required whenever drug doses or formulations are calculated.

References

Carr, D. S. (1989). New strategies for avoiding medication errors. *Nursing 89, 19* (8), 39–45.

Daniels, J. M., & Smith, L. M. (1990). Clinical calculations. *Nursing 90, 20* (7), 78–79.

Davis, N. M., & Cohen, M. R. (1981). *Medication errors.* Philadelphia: G. F. Stockley.

Deglin, J., & Mull, V. L. (1989). Dosage calculations. *Nursing 89, 19* (9), 100–102.

Hyams, P. A. (1990). Hospital drug quiz. *Nursing 90, 20* (1), 77.

McCaffery, M., & Beebe, A. (1989). Giving narcotics for pain: The secrets to giving equianalgesic doses. *Nursing 89, 19* (10), 161–165.

Morris, L. L. (1989). Dosage calculation charts. *Critical Care Nurse, 9* (5), 92–94.

Richardson, L. I., & Knight Richardson, J. (1994). *The mathematics of drugs and solutions with clinical applications* (5th ed.). New York: McGraw-Hill.

Stoklosa, M. J., & Ansel, H. C. (2001). *Pharmaceutical calculations* (11th ed.). Philadelphia: Lea and Febiger.

Wolf, Z. R. (1989). Medication errors and nursing responsibility. *Holistic Nursing Practice, 4* (1), 8–17.

13 Extemporaneous Compounding

COMPETENCIES

Upon completion of this chapter, the reader should be able to

1. Define a Class A prescription balance, a counter balance, and a solution balance.
2. Describe what is meant by extemporaneous compounding.
3. Explain the circumstances that may require the extemporaneous compounding of a drug dosage form.
4. Outline the steps required to accurately weigh a pharmaceutical ingredient.
5. Describe the meaning of the term "geometric dilution."
6. Explain the difference between a solution and a suspension; an ointment and a cream.
7. Describe the process of levigation.
8. List some of the steps involved in the process of compounding suppositories.
9. Give an example of the ingredients found in an enteral solution.
10. List the essential equipment used in the compounding process.

Introduction

This chapter will familiarize students with terminology, equipment, and principles of **extemporaneous compounding** and their role in providing this service. The student should understand this to be an introduction to compounding; experience is needed to develop this valuable skill. While it is beyond the scope of this chapter to review all types of compounding, the most common and relevant practices are reviewed. The student is referred to compounding textbooks for more detailed knowledge.

Extemporaneous compounding is a true pharmaceutical service, not simply the redistribution of a commercially available commodity. This service requires a specialized knowledge of physical and chemical properties of drugs and their vehicles. This knowledge is based on sound scientific principles; however, the practice is closer to an art.

Extemporaneous compounding may be defined as the timely preparation of a drug product according to a physician's prescription, a drug formula, or a recipe in which the amounts of the ingredients are calculated to meet the needs of a particular patient or group of patients.

Although demand is less, the need for extemporaneous preparations continues. Extemporaneous pharmaceutical compounding is among the most exciting, challenging, and rapidly expanding areas in pharmacy today. Practically every medical discipline incorporates these dosage forms in their everyday practice. Many pharmaceutical products are either no longer produced or for some reason become temporarily unavailable. Many commercially available products are in dosage forms which may not be convenient for dosing a specific patient. These are some of the challenges that are overcome by modern compounding techniques. Veterinary medicine, sports medicine, ophthalmology, and pain management have opened up vast new areas for the compounder. The compounding of sterile products such as ophthalmics, injectables, and IV, when done following proper procedure, is both very challenging and professionally rewarding. With the development of modern equipment and devices, the properly equipped compounding pharmacy is capable of delivering the highest quality specialty dosage forms.

Equipment

Traditional Equipment

The tools of pharmaceutical practice are those used to measure, transfer, transform, and handle medications in any way desired. Those involved in nonsterile compounding are classic and every pharmacy technician should be familiar with their proper handling.

Every pharmacy is required to have a **Class A prescription balance (Figure 13-1)**. Class A balances have a sensitivity requirement of 6 mg. A scale's sensitivity is the smallest weight required to move the indicator at least one degree. A typical Class A torsion balance can weigh quantities up to 120 g.

A **solution balance** is a single pan instrument with an unequal arm that acts as a compound lever. These balances are less accurate than Class A balances, but are useful for measuring large masses with a weighing capacity of about 20 kg.

Counter balances are double-pan balances also capable of weighing large quantities, but again are not intended for small weights, having a sensitivity of 100 mg and a limit of about 5 kg.

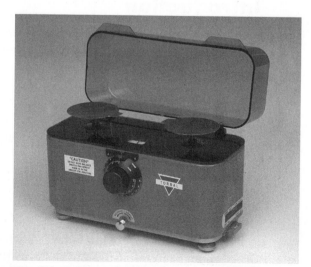

FIGURE 13-1   The Class A prescription balance, required in every pharmacy, has a scale sensitivity of 6 mg to 120 g.

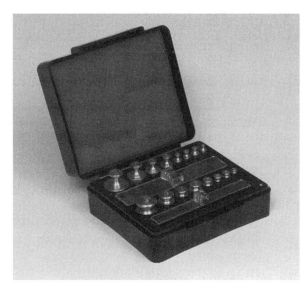

FIGURE 13-2 Pharmaceutical weights should be corrosion resistant and handled with forceps.

Weights used with the balances should be of good quality and stored well. It is preferred weights be made of corrosion-resistant metals such as brass (**Figure 13-2**). Metric weight sets are commonly available in a range of from less than 1 g to 50 g. Always use forceps to transfer the weights and take care not to drop them. Keep the weights covered in their original case when not in use.

Spatulas (**Figure 13-3**) are used to transfer solid ingredients to weighing pans. They are the preferred mixing instruments with semisolid dosage forms, such as ointments and creams. These are available in stainless steel and hard rubber or plastic. Care must be used with materials that corrode metals such as iodine, salts of mercury, or tannins. Use rubber spatulas for these agents. Check that spatulas are clean and have indented edges.

Weighing papers, preferably nonabsorbable paraffined glassine paper, should always be used to weigh powders and other solid and semisolid pharmaceuticals to prevent contamination or damage to the weighing pans. For small amounts of powders, the paper should be creased diagonally from each corner and then flattened and placed on the pans. This ensures a collection trough in the paper. Discard the paper after each product to prevent contamination.

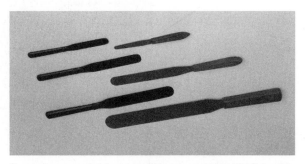

FIGURE 13-3 Spatulas, available in stainless steel and hard rubber or plastic, are used to transfer solid ingredients to weighing pans.

Weighing Techniques

The critical first step in any pharmaceutical dispensing is the selection of the proper drug and dose. Qualitative and quantitative accuracy is the hallmark of our profession. Technicians given the responsibilities of compounding must learn the skills and work carefully under the supervision of a pharmacist.

Prior to weighing with a Class A balance, the technician should gather and organize all materials in a level, well-lighted, draft-free area. The balance should be leveled by adjusting the thumbscrew at the base of the legs until the pointer rests at zero. Place weighing papers on each pan and adjust balance again if necessary. The beam weight should be all the way to the left and set at zero. When equilibrium is reached, the balance is arrested in place by a lock screw. The desired weights are placed in the right pan using forceps. The desired material is placed on the left pan using a spatula. When weighing less than a gram, one may wish to shift the weight beam to the appropriate weight. The balance is carefully unlocked to observe the movement of the pointer, which will shift to the side with the greater weight. Relock the balance and use a spatula to subtract or add material being weighed. This process is repeated until equilibrium is reached and the indicator is at the zero point. The balance is then locked, the lid closed, and the lock released one final time to verify the equilibrium. The weight should be checked by a pharmacist. If it is correct, the material can be removed from the balance in the cradle of the folded weighing paper. Weights should be checked three times: when selected, when resting on the pan, and when returned to the kit.

When weighing, we must keep in mind the sensitivities and limitations of the balance used.

Essential equipment that technicians must be familiar with include the mortar and pestle, commonly available in three types: glass (**Figure 13-4**); wedgewood; and porcelain (**Figure 13-5**), which is quite similar to wedgewood in use and appearance. Wedgewood and porcelain mortars are relatively coarse and are used to grind (**triturate**) crystals and large particles into fine powders. Both are earthenware and are somewhat porous and will easily stain. Glass mortars are preferable for mixing liquids and semisoft dosage forms.

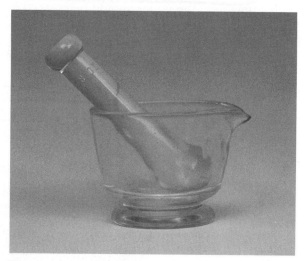

FIGURE 13-4 Glass mortar and pestle is preferable for mixing liquids and semisoft dosage forms.

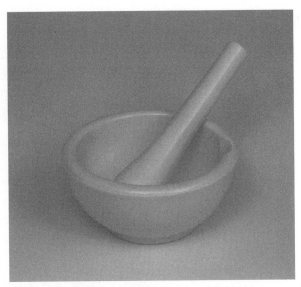

FIGURE 13-5 Porcelain mortar and pestle is used for trituration of crystals and large particles.

When mixing ingredients, always place the most potent drug, which is usually the smallest amount, into the mortar first. Then add an equal amount of the next most potent ingredient and mix thoroughly. This process is repeated until all ingredients are added. Because each addition is approximately equal to the amount in the mortar, the process is called geometric dilution.

Ointment slabs are ground glass plates, often square or rectangular, that provide a hard, nonabsorbable surface for mixing compounds. When combining creams and ointments, we use the spatula to spread the material, using a shearing force to mix ingredients. Some pharmacists use disposable, nonabsorbent parchment paper to cover the work area, which is not as durable as the ointment slabs, but saves time in cleaning.

Accurately measuring liquids is an essential skill technicians must master. Equipment consists of conical **graduates** (**Figure 13-6**), cylindrical graduates (**Figure 13-7**), and syringes. Beakers are generally not accurate enough for prescription work.

Conical graduates are the easiest to use with wide mouths and narrow bases and are the easiest to clean. Liquids may be stirred in them with the aid of a

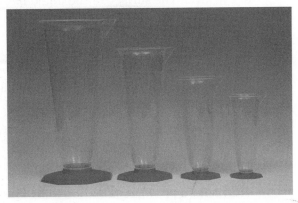

FIGURE 13-6 Conical graduates have a wide mouth and a narrow base.

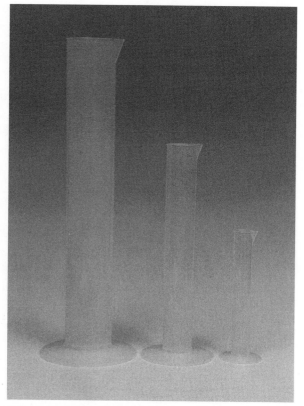

FIGURE 13-7 Cylindrical graduates provide greater accuracy for measuring.

stirring rod. As the diameter of the graduate increases, the accuracy of the measurement decreases. This design makes the narrow-diameter cylindrical graduates preferable when greater accuracy is desired. Graduates are available in sizes ranging from 10 mL to 4000 mL. When selecting a graduate, always choose the smallest graduate capable of containing the volume to be measured. Avoid measurements of volumes that are below 20 percent of the capacity of the graduate because the accuracy is unacceptable. For example, a 100 mL graduate cannot accurately measure volumes below 20 mL. When measuring small volumes, such as 30 mL and less, it is often preferable to use a syringe. Disposable plastic injectable and oral syringes are readily available in all pharmacies and have essentially replaced the use of smaller-sized graduates.

When measuring liquids in a graduate, it is important that the reading be done at eye level. The surface of the liquid has a concave or crescent shape that bulges downward, called the **meniscus**. When measuring liquids, the correct reading is the mark at the bottom of the meniscus.

Most graduates are marked "TD" (to deliver). They are calibrated to compensate for the excess of fluid that adheres to the surface after emptying the graduate. Caution must be used to differentiate this from older glassware marked "TC" (to contain) or errors in accuracy will result. Keep in mind that even "TD" glassware will retain excessive amounts of viscous liquids if not drained completely. Essentially no liquid should remain in the graduate after emptying.

Modern Equipment

The modern pharmacy compounding labs are equipped with digital electronic balances. These balances greatly increase the ease and accuracy of the weighing process. These balances do away entirely with the need for the counter weights that had been used with the earlier torsion balanaces. Because they are self-leveling and self-calibrating, they remove a great deal of potential error and stress from the weighing process. They allow for greater accuracy and improved record-keeping due to their ability to be interfaced with printers and computer software programs that enable a record of weights and calibrations to be retained. The more sophisticated software programs will actually enable the weights to be applied directly to log the formula being prepared.

Electronic balances will vary based upon their purpose. Bulk balances are used to weigh quantities greater than 1 g. Standard prescription balances are accurate to 1 mg, while analytical balances have the ability to be accurate to 0.001 mg.

Since chemicals are never weighed directly onto the table of the balance, different receptacles are used to contain the chemicals being weighed. The most common receptacles have been glassine weigh papers; however, most compounders now use different types of weigh boats. Weigh boats come in several shapes, sizes, and materials depending on their use. Some have an octagonal shape, allowing several chemicals to be weighed into the same weigh boat into separate corners, making the process more efficient. Electronic balances allow this process because they can be reset to a zero reading, which is known as taring, with each chemical added. A formula with six chemicals can be weighed into one weigh boat by taring the balance after each chemical has been weighed. Weigh boats also allow chemicals to be transported more efficiently from the balance to the processing area.

The recent development of the mini-ointment mill has added a whole new dimension to semisolid compounding. The ointment mill allows solid ingredients to be incorporated into cream, gel, and ointment bases by milling the active ingredients to minute particle size and efficiently incorporating and dispersing the active ingredient throughout the base. This process is similar to methods used in the commercial manufacture of creams, gels, and ointments and enhances the effect of the active ingredients in the base. The old method of using the ointment tile or pad along with geometric dilution, although effective, could not result in the same particle size and distribution of active ingredient. The ointment mill also allows a greater concentration of active ingredient to be incorporated into the base. When making an ointment or cream using the mill, the active ingredient is usually combined with a small amount of the base in the weigh boat. This combination is milled while increasing amounts of the base are added. The final product is evenly dispersed and smooth to the touch.

The electronic mortar and pestle (EMP) is a modern, motorized piece of equipment used to combine multiple ingredients into ointment, gel, and cream bases. It is far more efficient than using a hand-operated mortar and pestle for many reasons. Its rapid rotation allows for greater dispersion of ingredients. The more elaborate EMPs can have computer controls. The electronic mortar and pestle saves processing time because not only can it be set to operate by itself, but is able to produce a large quantity of product in one single operation. Many finished products are both mixed and blended in their final dispensing container, thus reducing handling and preserving the purity of the final product. The newest of the EMPs allows the mixing of up to 500 g of finished product.

Today basic compounding equipment will always include a combination thermostatically controlled hot plate and magnetic spinner. This combination allows semisolids and liquids to be heated and stirred at the same time. It also allows the heating of viscous liquids without burning. A magnetic stirring rod is placed in the bottom of the holding vessel and it is spun by a magnet within the hot plate. The speed of the stirring rod is controlled by a rheostat.

New pressure-driven tube heat-sealers and tube-filling devices allow the compounder to package creams, gels, and ointments in collapsible plastic tubes and seal them in much the way a manufacturer would. The final product is elegantly presented. In instances where products must be packaged in metal tubes, modern crimping devices allow a professional-looking seal to be applied. The most popular tube sizes range from 3 g to 120 g. Tubes can also be filled from the large-size electronic mortar and pestle jar or by using special tube-filling devices.

Homogenizers are used to both reduce particle size of active ingredients and disperse and emulsify them into suspensions, emulsions, and low viscosity lotions. Homogenizers are necessary in the compounding of sterile suspensions in ophthalmics and sterile injectables where particle size and dispersion are critical to the efficacy of the dosage at the site of use.

Compounding Principles

Liquids

Liquids are probably the most common form of compounded medications. Extemporaneous, nonsterile compounds most often involve solutions and suspensions, whereas emulsions and lotions are less popular. Solutions are clear liquids in which the drug is completely dissolved. The simplest compound solution involves the addition of a drug in liquid form to a vehicle such as water or syrup. This involves careful liquid measurement of the drug, using graduates or syringes, and then dilution to the final volume desired. Gentle shaking effects thorough dispersion of additives.

Solids

When solids are required in solution, they must be carefully weighed, using a prescription balance. Most solids dissolve readily in the solvent, but others require intervention. Some solids may be reduced in size by grinding in a mortar to increase dissolution rates. Other times, the vehicle is heated to enhance dissolution, but care must be used since some drugs decompose at higher temperatures. Dissolution of a solute may require vigorous shaking or stirring.

Suspensions

Suspensions are liquid preparations of drugs containing finely divided drug particles distributed uniformly throughout the vehicle. Suspensions appear cloudy in nature and shaking is often required to resuspend drug particles that have settled. Depending on particle size, some suspensions settle so rapidly that a uniform dispersion cannot be maintained long enough for an accurate dose to be withdrawn. Such preparations require a **suspending agent**, a thickening agent that gives some structure to a suspension. Typical agents are carboxymethylcellulose, methylcellulose, bentonite, tragacanth, and others. Some suspending agents may bind the drug, limiting availability, so these agents should not be used indiscriminately. While some solid drugs may be added directly to a suspending vehicle, some agents need to be "wetted" first. That is, the powder to be added is first mixed with a wetting agent such as alcohol or glycerin in a mortar with a pestle. This displaces the air from the particles of the solid and allows them to mix more readily with a suspending vehicle. Next, the vehicle is added in portions and mixed with mortar and pestle until a uniform mixture results. This mixture is then blended into the remaining vehicle. The mortar and pestle can be rinsed with small portions of the vehicle and added until the final volume is reached. Suspensions should be dispensed in tight, light-resistant containers that contain enough air space for adequate shaking. The bottle should contain the auxiliary label "Shake well." Refrigeration may be used to slow separation.

Ointments and Creams

These two semisolid external dosage forms are still popular choices for extemporaneous compounds and share common preparation techniques. Ointments are oil based in nature, whereas creams are water based. Given the commercial availability of unmedicated cream and ointment bases, their preparation is more of historic interest, but we will focus on the addition of drugs to these bases. In the simplest cases, physicians often desire the combined effects of two or more ointments or creams in a specified proportion. This usually involves the thorough mechanical mixing of the weighed bases on an ointment slab using a spatula until a uniform preparation has been obtained. Using the spatula, transfer the material into an ointment jar just big enough for the final volume. When filling the ointment jar, use the spatula to bleed out air pockets. Tapping the jar on the countertop will settle the contents. Wipe any excess material from the outside of the jar, including the cap screw threads. Cover the jar and label appropriately.

Drugs in powder or crystal form, such as salicylic acid, precipitated sulfur, or hydrocortisone, are often prescribed to be mixed into cream or ointment bases. Large particles should be reduced to fine powder with a mortar and pestle. The ointment base may be placed on one side of the working area, with the powders to be incorporated on the other. Using a spatula, mix a small portion of powder with a portion of the base on an ointment slab. Repeat this until all powder is incorporated into the base and a uniform product is produced.

Occasionally, the direct mixture method results in a gritty product with poorly dispensed clumps of powder that fail to blend in despite vigorous mixing. Here it is desirable first to reduce the particle size of the powder by levigating it. **Levigation** is the mixing of powder with a vehicle in which it is insoluble to produce a smooth dispersion of the drug. The dispersion is then mixed with the base. When using ointments, mineral oil is a good levigating agent. When working with creams, glycerin or water can often be used.

Transdermal Gels

Ointments and creams are used to introduce and maintain the presence of drugs to the body topically. Their effectiveness is usually limited to the drug's ability to pass through the skin barriers. Transdermal gels are able to disrupt the lipid layers of the stratum corneum of the skin without damaging it the way harsher agents can. The most popular form of transdermal gel is the pleuronic lecithin organogel or PLO gel. PLO allows the medication to slip through the stratum corneum into systemic circulation via dermal-epidermal blood flow. PLO gels are used in all disciplines of compounding. These gels are extremely effective for the delivery of pain management drugs to local sites with excellent results and decreased liver absorbtion. Combinations of localized pain trigger receptor agonists (i.e., drugs that block pain) can be incorporated into a single gel and applied with excellent results. These gels have many positive uses. They are used in veterinary medicine to allow ease in dosing. Cats, which can be difficult to medicate, will respond extremely well to PLO gels administered to the pinna or inner flap of the ear. They can also be used to deliver drugs to pediatric patients who might otherwise be difficult to dose. A good example of this is the dosing of the drug Secretin to treat autism. It replaces the need for daily injections and the absorption is equivalent.

These gels are easily compounded using the ointment mill or the EMP. The active ingredient is dissolved in a solvent and combined with isopropyl palmitate and Pleuronic-127. They are then blended and mixed to allow the formation of small emulsion units called micelles, which transport the drug across the skin barrier.

There are many other new forms of gels, such as aqueous gels, which are water miscible and easily washable and act as very effective carriers for drugs across the skin barrier. Though not every drug can be introduced in gel form and the expiration dating of gels is usually less than six months, they have proved to be a valuable tool for compounding.

Troches, Lollipops, and Gummy Bears

Pharmacists had always compounded pastilles and troches by using a hand-rolling technique. They incorporated certain types of drugs into a candy base and were able to produce a hard disc- or barrel-shaped troche or pastille that would be placed in the cheek and allowed to dissolve. Modern compounders are able to produce troches that can contain a much wider array of active ingredients and can be sugar free and elegantly colored and flavored. The advent of the troche mold allows the active ingredient to be calculated and combined in to a premeasured amount of base to make a much more uniform product. There are many troche bases, such as soft, chewy, and hard, which allows for greater flexibility in dosing. The different bases are used to adjust the time that the drug takes to be absorbed along with adapting to the personal preference of the patient. The recent development of lollipop molds now allow medication to be incorporated in this very attractive and fun dosage form. Actiq, which is a commercial pain medication with the active ingredient fentanyl, started out as a custom-compounded product. It was designed to allow the pleasant dosing of a narcotic analgesic to both children and hospice patients. Lollipops are a good dosage form for ease of compliance. As with troches, they can be made sugar free and in literally 101 flavor combinations.

Gummy Bears are another dosage form used to deliver medication to children. The same base is used in their formulation as is used for soft troches. The base is melted and the active ingredient, suspending agents, sweetener, and choice of flavors are combined and introduced into a pre-calibrated mold. Children particularly like this dosage form.

Flavoring

The development of modern flavoring techniques, along with a multitude of different flavors, sweeteners and flavoring vehicles, has added a great deal of flexibility to modern compounding. There are flavors that are either oil soluble or water soluble. There are powdered flavorings that can be added to dry bulk powders for veterinary use, such as apple flavor for horses. There are specific flavors for either level of pH balance. There are flavors to enhance most dosage forms. The development of more sweetening products now allows the compounder to make a greater assortment of sugar-free products. Flavoring is very important in medication dosing compliance. Very bitter drugs can be made more palatable. Dosage forms can be changed, for example, tablets can be pulverized, suspended, and flavored, creating a different dosage form of the same drug. This is especially useful in dosing children and also those patients who have difficulty swallowing. Commercially available liquid products can be flavor enhanced to make them taste better. Prescriptions can be flavored for animals based on preference. Cats like tuna fish, while dogs like liver flavor. Small birds like tutti-fruitti. Hundreds of bases, flavors, and flavor combinations are now available.

Suppositories

Suppositories are solid dosage forms intended for insertion into body orifices, predominantly rectal or vaginal, where they melt or dissolve to release their active ingredients. Extemporaneous manufacture of suppositories remains a vital art today for several reasons. Industrial manufacturers market relatively few products in suppository form in this country, in part because rectal administration is not socially popular. So although the products are limited, there is a subgroup of patients who cannot tolerate oral medications, but who also are not candidates for parenteral drug therapy.

Suppositories must be manufactured so that they remain solid at room or refrigerated temperatures, yet melt readily at body temperature—a fine line indeed. This process is accomplished by using special bases, such as cocoa butter or polyethylene glycol. Polyethylene glycols are available in various molecular weight ranges. Those of 200, 400, or 600 are liquids; those over 1000 are solid and waxlike. Often, combinations of liquid (low molecular weight) and solid polyethylene glycol are used to achieve a suppository that melts as desired. By increasing the waxy portion of the blend, we gain a suppository that melts more slowly and provides more sustained action.

To prepare suppositories, the base material is melted and the active ingredients are added. The material is poured into molds and chilled until congealed. Then they are removed from the mold.

Most modern compounding labs will tend to use disposable suppository strip molds (**Figure 13-8**). These are pre-calibrated to the specific bases, are easier to fill and dispense, and can be heat-sealed to present a far more elegant and professional-looking product. Modern compounders melt the base by placing it in the beaker with a magnetic stirrer at the bottom, then heating on an electric hot plate with a stirrer. The mixture must be allowed to cool almost to the point of congealing so as not to melt the plastic molds and also to properly fill the mold cavity.

Suppositories (both commercial and extemporaneous sources) are still commonly used to deliver analgesics, hormones, antiemetics, laxatives, and vaginal anti-infectives.

Capsules

Extemporaneous capsule manufacturing remains a popular means of providing unusual (and often low) doses of oral medication. The student may recall that commercially available capsules cannot be divided. Tablets can only be reliably broken

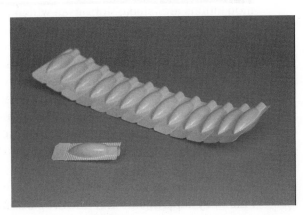

FIGURE 13-8 Suppository molds.

in quarters at best and usually only halves. A typical situation for capsule compounding may be when a drug is only available in 50 mg tablets or capsules, but the prescribing physician desires 12.5 mg doses, or what would amount to a one-quarter dose. If crushed, the resulting powder would be too small to handle accurately. To facilitate measuring, first dilute the crushed tablet (or emptied capsule) with inactive filler and measure a portion containing the desired amount. Select empty, hard gelatin capsules available in eight sizes, with 000 the largest and 5 the smallest. In general, the smallest capsule capable of containing the final volume is used because patients often have difficulty swallowing large capsules. To fill each capsule, place the powder on a tile or paper and press the body of the capsule repeatedly into the powder until it is filled. Be careful not to touch the powder with your fingers. This is called the punch method of capsule filling. Place the cap onto the body and weigh the result, using an empty capsule the same size as the **tare**. Adjust the weight, if needed, by adding or removing powder. To keep the capsule clean during the process, the compounder may wear rubber gloves or finger cots. Since some material is lost in the process, always calculate a little extra material to compensate for this loss.

In this example, we select a #3 capsule and set the final weight at 200 mg. To make 10 capsules, we need three 50 mg tablets, which would produce twelve doses in theory. Twelve doses of 200 mg requires 2400 mg of final powder. Three tablets might weigh 700 mg, to which we would add 1700 mg of diluent, such as lactose powder, by trituration. We would pack 200 mg of this powder into each capsule to yield the 12.5 mg dose.

The use of capsule-filling machines can greatly facilitate the process of filling capsules. These machines vary from a strictly manual to a highly automated process. The use of a machine requires the prior development of a formulation that will deliver a given dose of a drug in a pre-calculated volume of powder. As such, they are useful for manufacturing batches of a standard formula.

The machines require the loading of capsules into a molded plate. The capsule bodies may be separated by hand or by an automated process, leaving the capsule openings aligned with the surface of the plate. The formulated powder is poured over the plate and spreaders are used to fill the capsules. The capsules are then closed by hand or by an automated process. The machine is inverted to release the filled capsules.

The machines are useful for filling many capsules in a timely manner because they are designed to fill from 50–300 capsules with each operation.

Lotions

Lotions are liquid preparations intended for external application. The most common lotions are "shake" lotions in which insoluble substances are dispersed by agitation. Often gums or other agents are used as suspending agents to prevent rapid settling of suspended particles. To prepare shake lotions, place the measured powders of the formula into a mortar and triturate until well blended. Slowly add a liquid levigating agent and triturate to form a smooth paste, free of gritty particles. Add the vehicle in small portions with continued trituration. After roughly two-thirds of the vehicle has been added, transfer the solution to a graduated vessel and rinse the mortar with remaining vehicle to bring the lotion to its final volume. Transfer this to a well-sealed bottle and label "Shake well."

Enteral Preparations

Pharmacy departments may also prepare enteral nutrition products. Although enteral literally means "in the intestine," the term is commonly used to mean a refined liquid diet often administered by nasogastric tube to patients unable to eat solid foods.

Preparation of enteral products usually involves simple dissolution of powdered material in a blender, following package directions. But at times there is a need for varied dilutions of feedings to match a patient's clinical state. We use pharmaceutical calculations to prepare a 2/3- or 3/4-strength formula. For example, suppose a package of powdered dietary supplement is normally diluted to 500 mL. To prepare a 2/3-strength enteral formula, we divide 500 mL by 2/3 to yield 750 mL. Each packet should be dissolved to 750 mL to yield the more diluted 2/3 mixture required.

At times, these oral feedings are supplemented with additional electrolytes, such as sodium chloride or potassium chloride. The student may be required to convert weight in milligrams to milliequivalents (mEq).

It is important to use clean equipment, precise measurement, and proper packaging, labeling, and storage of these products. They often require refrigeration after preparation and each product has a recommended expiration period.

As the student readily learns, there are quite a few pharmaceutical skills involved in the proper preparation and dispensing of enteral products.

Sterile Compounding, On-Site Sterility, and Pyrogen Testing

Many compounding labs are equipped to prepare sterile compounds including ophthalmic drops and ointments, injectable solutions and suspensions, and intravenous drugs. This is an area of practice where many drugs must be prepared near to the time of actual use due to the instability of the final products. Great care must be taken to ensure the integrity of these compounds. The products must be prepared in a sterile environment. Special equipment is required to prepare these compounds. The creation of new on-site testing for selective impurities and sterility allows for the proper compounding of the products. Pyrogens are dead cell particles which can cause fever if allowed to exist in the sterile product. They are easily prevented by proper technique and can now be easily tested on-site prior to the release of the drug to the patient. One such test is Pyro-Test. This test can give a final result within one hour of preparation. Sterility can also be verified by the use of similar on-site tests, such as Q-Test. These tests are designed to use only minute volumes of the finished product. There are also products that test the accuracy of the person performing these procedures. Periodic testing of personnel is necessary to maintain the standard of the compounding facility. Most responsible compounders will send a specified percentage of their products for outside testing to ensure the integrity of their procedures.

Sterilization

It is vital when talking about sterilization to understand the concept of maintaining the integrity of the pharmaceutical product to be dispensed. Proper sterilization techniques start with using betadine scrub to wash hands and nails thoroughly under the sink for several minutes before applying gloves, arm sleeves, hairnet, and lab coat to ensure aseptic procedure is intact. Technicians can spread microorganisms into the hood by wearing jewelry, coughing, sneezing (not wearing a mask), or loose facial hair. No food, beverages, or gum should be allowed in the sterile area. The hood should always be cleaned properly with alcohol after each compounded prescription is completed. There are four methods of sterilization we will discuss in this chapter: thermal, chemical, filtration, and radiation.

There are two types of thermal sterilization: moist heat and dry heat. Moist heat is used to coagulate the protein contained in microorganisms. Dry heat causes death by oxidation. Microorganisms need protein to survive and thermal sterilization prevents this organism from surviving. Moist heat sterilization is performed in an autoclave, which uses steam under pressure for a specified period of time. Dry sterilization is performed in an oven between 140°C to 260°C to kill spores and other microorganisms. This method of sterilization is preferred for products such as mineral oil, paraffin, and zinc oxide.

Chemical sterilization uses chemical agents to prevent microorganism proliferation. The most common chemical agent used in this process is ethylene oxide. This chemical only requires a temperature of 54°C for approximately 4 to 16 hours and can be used for rubber and plastic items. This type of sterilization can never be used in IV solutions due to possible chemical reactions.

Filtration, aside from being the easiest, is the most often used form of sterilization in most pharmacies. In order for a filter to prevent passage of all bacteria, it must be no more than 0.22 microns in size. Filters are used for IV, IM and ophthalmic preparations since heat and chemicals often damage these solutions. Filter sizes range from 0.025 to 14 microns. The smallest of bacteria can be eliminated using a 0.22-micron filter. This filter is widely used as a standard in a majority of compounding procedures.

Radiation is a form of sterilization normally used in hospitals, laboratories and large institutions. This method is largely used to sterilize hospital supplies, vitamins, antibiotics, steroids, plastic syringes, and needles.

Most pharmacies will prepare sterile products in either a horizontal or vertical airflow hood; each provides a class 100 clean environment. The horizontal laminar flow hood consists of three major components: a pre-filter, a HEPA filter, and the work surface. The horizontal hood blows clean air from the back of the hood to the front, maintaining a clean area within three inches of its outside boundaries. The constant airflow through the HEPA filter prevents all particles greater than 0.3 microns in size from entering the sterile area. The vertical airflow hood sends the sterile filtered air from the top of the cabinet to the base and recirculates within the cabinet. It is a closed system which better protects the person performing operations within the clean barrier. Vertical flow hoods can be used for those products toxic to humans and the environment, such as chemotherapeutic drugs. Both types of hoods must be cleaned before each operation with the proper chemical compounds. A more detailed and thorough discussion of laminar airflow hoods is presented in Chapter 14.

Labeling of Finished Products and Record-Keeping

Extemporaneous products should be labeled with neat, well-designed labels, in accordance with hospital policy. Outpatient prescription labels must contain all information required by state and local laws. Labels should be typed and affixed with adhesive tape to protect the label. Auxiliary labels should be affixed if applicable.

The label should contain the ingredients and proportions of the compounded prescription. If a master compounding form was used, the internally assigned lot number should appear on the label.

In general, no specific expiration date can be assigned to an extemporaneous compound unless the institution has a policy for assigning reasonable expiration dates. Even with such a policy, some judgment is needed on the part of the supervising pharmacist. It may suffice to list the date of preparation on the label.

Accurate record-keeping is essential in extemporaneous compounding. Master formula records (**Figure 13-9**) are excellent sources for both directions for compounding and uniform record-keeping. When using a master form, record all lot

EXTEMPORANEOUS PREPARATION
GENTIAN VIOLET 10%

MATERIALS
- 1 glass flask 600ml
- Absolute alcohol 300ml
- Gentian Violet 30gm
- Stirring rod
- 1 oz. amber dropper bottle

LABEL
- Gentian violet solution
- 10% W/V
- In 95% absolute alcohol
- Volume: 300 ml
- Control # _____
- Tech/R.Ph. _____ Exp. date _____

Procedure
1. Clean all materials to be used and rinse with absolute alcohol.
2. Weigh out 30 gram gentian violet and have pharmacist check it.
3. Measure out 300ml absolute alcohol and have pharmacist check it.
4. In glass flask, dissolve the gentian violet in the absolute alcohol. Stir well until in solution.
5. Measure out 30ml and put in 1 oz. glass amber dropper bottle.
6. Have pharmacist check label.
7. Put label on product.
8. Have pharmacist check final product.

Date Prepared	Control #	Ingredients	Mft. & Lot #	Amt. Used	Check by R.Ph	Expiration Date of Prod. Made	Quant. Prep.	Sample Label	Tech.

FIGURE 13-9 Master formula record.

number information on the form and use the internal lot number on the prescription label. These master records also contain the amount of ingredients used, initials of the preparer and the pharmacist who checked the finished product, and all measurements. All work sheets should be filed as permanent records.

With single extemporaneous compounds without master records, such as those involving outpatient prescriptions, the lot numbers and manufacturers of the ingredients can be recorded on the prescription.

Cleaning Equipment

Cleaning the equipment is as important as the preparation and labeling of the product. It should not be overlooked. Improperly cleaned equipment can contaminate the next preparation and be dangerous to the patient. Cleaning is sometimes not as simple as washing dishes because oily residues, such as ointments, often must be dissolved. Proper cleaning may require a rinse with organic solvents such as alcohols or acetate to facilitate removal. When working with these volatile solvents, the student must be aware of their flammable nature as well as the risk of inhaling fumes. Although these fumes are generally safe for limited exposure, care must be taken to wash solvents down the drain with cold water to limit exposure. Occupational safety data sheets should be available in every pharmacy, outlining the hazards of each substance.

Summary

Bulk compounding by pharmacy technicians should be viewed as a challenge and a rewarding skill. The student can readily appreciate the necessity of competence in other aspects of pharmacy such as calculation, dose forms, and pharmaceutical terminology. The responsibility of bulk compounding should not and will not be required of technicians who are not trained or not competent with these skills. Any bulk compounding must be done only under close supervision of a licensed pharmacist, and in some states, must be done only via master manufacturing records.

Bulk compounding is a difficult art to master, but it is one of the most rewarding. It remains one service no other health care profession can provide.

TEST YOUR KNOWLEDGE

Multiple Choice Questions

1. The concave surface of a liquid in a graduate is called the
   a. sight line
   b. metric point
   c. meniscus
   d. tare

2. Clear liquids in which drugs are completely dissolved are called
   a. suspensions
   b. emulsions
   c. lotions
   d. solutions

3. The hazards of using organic solvents are
   a. their flammability
   b. toxic fumes
   c. their explosive nature
   d. a and b
   e. all of the above

4. Which product would yield the greatest volume? A packet of external nutrition/supplement diluted to
   a. full strength
   b. 3/4 strength
   c. 2/3 strength

5. A master formula record should contain
   a. directions for compounding
   b. a record of lot numbers
   c. the initials of preparer and checking pharmacist
   d. the amount of ingredients used
   e. all of the above

True/False Questions

6. _T_   Extemporaneous compounding has increased in demand in modern pharmaceutical practice.

7. _F_   Class A prescription balances, solution balances, and counter balances are quite similar and can be used interchangeably for any weighing needs of a pharmacy.

8. _F_   A semisolid external dosage form with an oily base is called a cream.

9. _T_   A levigating agent would be added to a suspension to reduce the rate of settling.

10. _F_   Suppositories are only intended for rectal use.

11. _T_   When selecting capsules, the higher the size number, the smaller the capsule.

12. _T_   Lotions are most commonly prepared using a mortar and pestle.

References

Ansel, H. H. (1972). *Introduction to pharmaceutical dosage forms.* Philadelphia: Lea & Febiger.

Gennaro, A. R. (Ed.). (1990). *Remington's pharmaceutical sciences* (18th ed.). Easton, PA: Mack Publishing Co.

Parrot, E. L. (1970). *Pharmaceutical technology.* Minneapolis, MN: Burgess Publishing Co.

Shrewsburg, R. (2001). *Applied pharmaceutics in contemporary compounding.* Englewood, CO: Morton Publishing Co.

14 Parenteral Compounding

COMPETENCIES

After completion of this chapter, the reader should be able to

1. Outline the major reasons for administering injectable drug products.
2. Define common injectable routes of administration.
3. Describe three characteristics of parenteral products.
4. Define a sterile product.
5. Explain the concept of laminar airflow.
6. Define the technician's role in parenteral admixture services.
7. Describe safety considerations related to handling parenteral products.

Introduction

Parenteral **compounding** services have become an increasingly important aspect of hospital pharmacy practice. Advances in medical technology, new drug products, and other changes in the health care environment all contribute to the need for these services. Parenteral products in the form of injectable drugs have been estimated to account for as much as 40% of all drugs administered in hospitals. Additionally, there is an increasing use of parenterals in the home health care setting. Many hospitals and home care agencies are providing these services. The pharmacy technician is an integral part of the production of parenteral products, both in hospitals and in the home care industry. This chapter will discuss various aspects of parenteral products and the technician's role in parenteral compounding.

Background

The term *parenteral* is associated with drugs administered by injection. The discussion of parenteral compounding in this chapter will emphasize injectable products, but the same general principles apply to all sterile products.

The extent of parenteral compounding varies considerably among institutions. Nevertheless, all such services share a common goal of providing accurately prepared, sterile products for use by or administration to patients.

Injectable drug products may be administered by several routes and for many reasons. Administration of a drug by injection may be necessary for patients who are unable or unwilling to take medications by mouth. Some drugs, such as insulin, cannot be given orally because they will be destroyed in the gastrointestinal tract. Others must be given by injection for rapid and/or continued action. Many diagnostic tests involve the injection of dyes or radioactive drugs. These are only a few of the many reasons for administrating injectable drugs.

An extremely important consideration with injectables is that, regardless of the route of administration, all bypass one of the major body defense mechanisms—the skin. When intact, the skin prevents the entry of microorganisms into the circulation. For this reason, the necessity of providing a sterile product and using proper techniques in administering it cannot be overemphasized. Quality assurance must be maintained from the point of manufacture, through the pharmacy parenteral admixture service, to the administration of the parenteral product.

Routes of Administration

There are a number of different routes by which injectable drugs can be administered. The route chosen will depend on the characteristics of the drug to be administered, the type of effect desired, and the intended site of action.

Some of the more common routes of administration are outlined here.

- **Intradermal (ID)**—injected within the skin, just below the surface, usually used for diagnostic tests and certain vaccines. The volume does not exceed 0.1 ml.
- **Subcutaneous (SC)**—injected deeper than ID administration, into the loose tissue layer beneath the skin. Volumes of up to 1 ml may be given. This route provides for a more rapid onset of action and shorter duration than intramuscular.
- **Intramuscular (IM)**—injected into a muscle mass, usually the deltoid (upper arm) or the gluteus (buttocks). Volumes of up to 5 ml may be given, depending on the size of the muscle mass. IM injections have a slower onset of action and a longer duration than SC injections.
- **Intravenous (IV)**—injected directly into a vein. Large volumes may be given by this route, which is useful for very rapid onset of action or for medications that cannot be given by other routes.
- **Intracardiac (IC)**—injected within one of the chambers of the heart, usually used only in emergency situations such as cardiopulmonary resuscitation.
- **Intra-arterial (IA)**—injected directly into an artery. This injection is a risky procedure that may result in a spasm of the artery and the stoppage of circulation in the area. This route is sometimes used for cancer chemotherapy to deliver medication directly to the desired site of action (such as the liver).
- **Intrathecal (IT)**—injected into the spinal fluid. Preservative-free drugs must be used because many preservatives can damage the nervous system. Some antibiotics and chemotherapy agents are administered by this route to achieve satisfactory concentrations in the brain or cerebrospinal fluid.

Characteristics of Parenteral Products

All parenteral products must be manufactured or prepared under conditions that ensure sterility and freedom from particulate matter. The word *sterile* indicates there are no living microorganisms present. A product is either sterile or unsterile—there is no in-between. Sterility can be achieved through heat, gas, or filtration methods. The method used will depend on the physical characteristics of the product to be sterilized. The use of moist heat under pressure (autoclaving) is the most commonly used method. The use of gamma radiation to sterilize some empty IV containers and other accessories has also been employed. During extemporaneous preparation, the use of proper **aseptic** technique is essential to maintain the sterility of the products being used.

In addition to being sterile, injectable products must also be pyrogen free. Pyrogens are products of microbial metabolism and cause symptoms of fever and chills when injected into a patient. Proper treatment of water and equipment used during manufacturing and the use of nonpyrogenic equipment (such as syringes) are necessary to prevent introduction of pyrogens into the final product.

Parenteral products must also be free from the presence of particulate matter. Particulate matter consists of undissolved substances that are unintentionally present in parenteral solutions. Examples of such substances are glass, rubber, cloth or cotton fibers, metal, and plastic. Undissolved particles may be present in suspensions; however, the particles are active ingredients, not contaminants.

Particulate matter in injectables, especially in IV products, could cause inflammation of the vein (phlebitis) or could harm the patient by lodging in small blood vessels and blocking blood flow. For this reason, suspensions cannot be administered by the intravenous route. The use of proper techniques and procedures during manufacturing and compounding, and careful visual observation, are essential in preventing particulate contamination.

Intravenous Products

Intravenous products comprise the majority of parenteral preparations in the pharmacy. Because such products are administered directly into the bloodstream, a number of special considerations are involved. Such concerns as drug compatibilities and rates of administration are particularly important.

Drug compatibilities are of concern with IV solutions. Incompatibilities often manifest themselves as a precipitation or crystallization, which could have disastrous consequences if either entered the patient's circulation. Not all incompatibilities are visible, however. A drug may be deactivated or lose a significant amount of its potency without being apparent on visual examination. Incompatibilities may occur between two or more drugs or additives or between a drug and the solution in which it is mixed.

The stability of drugs in solution is also an important consideration. Because drugs prepared in a parenteral admixture service are usually made in advance of when they are to be administered, the stability must be known and the product prepared accordingly. Such information is usually available from several sources, including the package insert. One factor that often affects stability is the concentration of the drug in solution. As a general rule, the more concentrated the solution, the less stable it is. In addition, the temperature at which the finished product is stored may significantly affect its stability. Many products are more stable under refrigeration, while some are more stable at room temperature.

The pharmacist, using available reference sources, will determine the compatibilities and stabilities of parenteral admixtures. Drugs should never be mixed without knowing and checking this information.

Osmolality is a characteristic that results from the number of dissolved particles in the solution. Blood has an osmolality of approximately 300 milliosmoles (mOsm). Intravenous solutions that have osmolality values of 300 are said to be isotonic. Solutions that have osmolality values of greater (hypertonic) or less than (hypotonic) 300 may cause damage to red blood cells, pain, and tissue irritation. The greater the deviation from 300 mOsm, the more pronounced these reactions will be. At times, it may be necessary to administer hypertonic or hypotonic solutions— usually slowly and through large, free-flowing veins to minimize the reactions.

Another important characteristic is the pH of the solution. The pH is a measure of the acidity or alkalinity of a product. On the pH scale, which ranges from 1 to 14, a number less than 7 means the product is acidic. A number greater than 7 indicates alkalinity. The farther the number is from 7, the more acidic or alkaline the product is. The pH is important both for the physiological effects on the patient and for additive compatibilities. Some drugs will be incompatibile in a particular solution due to the effects of pH.

Types of IV Solutions

Intravenous solutions are classified as small-volume parenterals (SVPs) or large-volume parenterals (LVPs). A large-volume parenteral is a solution of 100 ml or more. LVPs are primarily used to provide fluid, electrolytes, and nutrients to the patient. Small-volume parenterals, on the other hand, are usually 100 ml or less and are primarily used as vehicles for delivering medications. IV containers are available in plastic or glass (**Figure 14-1**).

Solutions flow from the containers to the patient by means of an IV administration set (**Figure 14-2**). For solution to flow from a glass container, air must be able to enter the container as fluid flows out. Air enters through a vent located in the administration set. Flexible plastic containers do not require venting because the container collapses as fluid flows out of it.

Plastic containers offer many advantages over glass, such as being lightweight and unbreakable. Plastic containers made of polyvinyl chloride (PVC) may sometimes interact with medications. Certain medications have a tendency to adsorb or "stick to" PVC, making less drug available to the patient (e.g., nitroglycerin). In addition, the plasticizer (DEHP) may leach into some products (e.g., fat emulsion). The consequences of such **leaching** to the patient are not clear. Polyolefin and non-DEHP vinyl IV containers are available that provide the benefits of flexible plastic

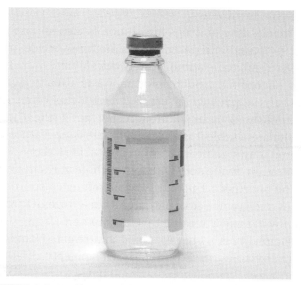
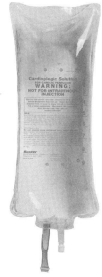

FIGURE 14-1   Types of IV containers (A) glass, (B) flexible plastic bag (*Courtesy of Baxter Healthcare Corporation*).

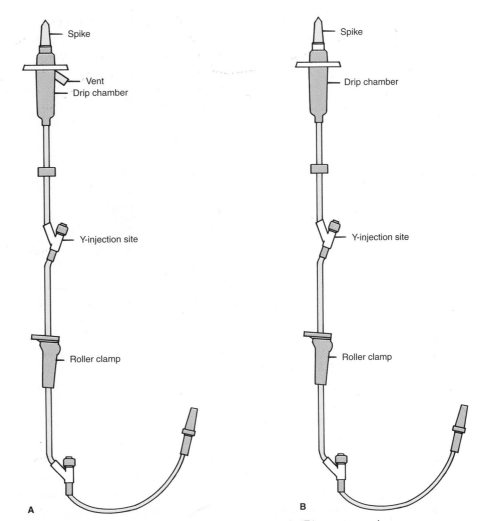

FIGURE 14-2 IV administration sets (A) vented, (B) nonvented.

without the drawbacks of PVC. There is no plasticizer to leach into solution and less possibility of drug adsorption with these products.

The administration of IV medications may be accomplished in one of three ways: IV push, infusion, or **piggyback**.

IV push involves the injection of a relatively small volume of drug by means of a needle and syringe. This type of injection, sometimes referred to as a bolus, may be administered directly into a vein or into the tubing of a running IV solution. This technique is usually used when a very rapid effect is desired.

The IV administration of a large amount of fluid over a prolonged time period is known as an infusion. Infusions may be used to supply the patient with fluid, nutrients, and medications.

With the piggyback method, medications in small amounts of fluid (usually 50 to 100 ml) are infused into the tubing of a running IV solution (primary IV). The piggyback solution is contained in a minibag or bottle (see **Figure 14-3**) and is typically infused over a period of 30 to 60 minutes.

Another method of delivering IV piggyback medications involves the use of syringes instead of piggyback containers. A syringe containing medication is mounted on a syringe pump which expels the contents of the syringe over a specific time period.

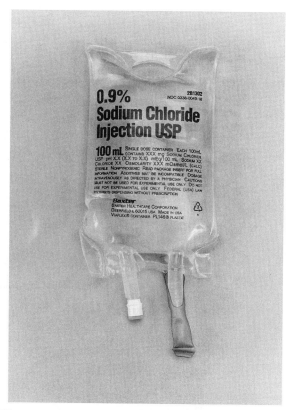

FIGURE 14-3   Plastic piggyback bag *(Courtesy of Baxter Healthcare Corporation).*

In some instances, a patient may not have a primary IV solution, yet must receive piggyback medications. Patients may then receive a heparin lock, which is a short tube inserted into a vein. When a piggyback is not infusing through it, the heparin lock is filled with a heparin solution or sodium chloride solution so that blood does not clot and block the tube.

Preparation of Parenteral Products

Laminar Airflow Hoods

The preparation of parenteral products requires strict adherence to aseptic technique. Aseptic technique involves the preparation and handling of sterile products in a way that prevents contamination by microorganisms. Contamination can occur from the environment in which the product is prepared, as well as from the person preparing it. The best way to reduce the environmental effects is to control the work area in such a way as to produce a *clean* work area. Laminar airflow hoods, when properly operated, are very effective at providing a clean area; however, using poor technique can easily cancel the benefits of laminar airflow.

Laminar airflow hoods provide filtered air that flows through the hood in straight, parallel lines. The air is filtered through a **high-efficiency particulate air (HEPA) filter** that removes 99.97% of all particles larger than 0.3 μm in size. Essentially, this filter is able to remove all microbial contaminants and particulate matter. The air flows at a sufficient velocity to keep a work area free from contamination. The airflow may be in either a vertical or a horizontal direction. In a hori-

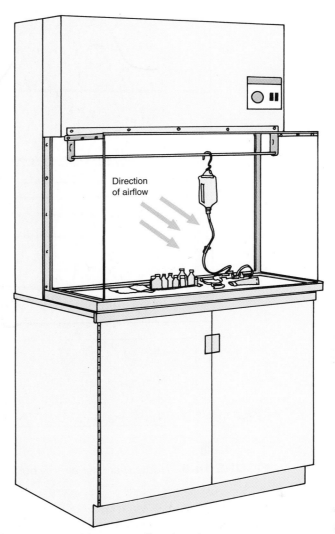

Direction
of airflow

FIGURE 14-4 Horizontal laminar airflow hood.

zontal hood, the HEPA filter is located at the back of the hood, and air flows to the front (as shown in **Figure 14-4**). In a vertical hood, airflow passes through a HEPA filter located at the top and is drawn out the bottom through grates (**Figure 14-5**). Unlike the horizontal hood, the vertical hood allows protection for the operator because the airflow is contained within the hood (**Figure 14-6**).

The type of vertical flow hood most commonly used in the pharmacy is the class II hood, divided into the following types:

Type A hoods recirculate a portion of the air (after first passing through a HEPA filter) within the hood and exhaust a portion of this air back into the parenterals room.

Type B1 hoods exhaust *most* of the contaminated air through a duct to the outside atmosphere. This air first passes through a HEPA filter.

Type B2 hoods exhaust *all* of the contaminated air to the outside atmosphere after passing through a HEPA filter. Air is not recirculated within the hood or returned to the parenterals room atmosphere.

Type B3 hoods utilize recycled air within the hood. All exhaust air is discharged to the outside atmosphere. Type A hoods may be converted to type B3 hoods.

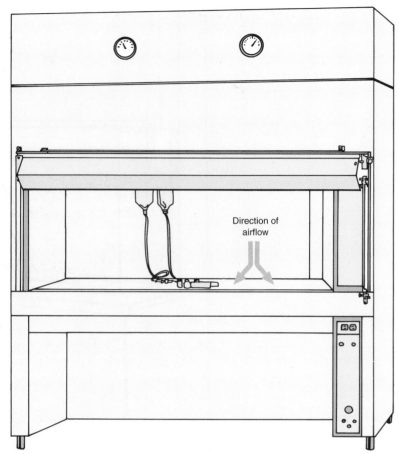

FIGURE 14-5   Vertical laminar airflow hood.

Laminar airflow hoods of all types need to be properly cleaned and maintained to ensure their ability to provide a clean work area. Hoods are usually cleaned several times during the course of a day. Appropriate antimicrobial solutions such as 70% isopropyl alcohol or solutions of povidone-iodine are frequently used for disinfection. Care should be taken when cleaning class II hoods with alcohol. Excessive use of alcohol in hoods where the air is recirculated (type A, B1, and B3) may result in a buildup of alcohol vapors in the hood.

Many pharmacies will run their laminar airflow hoods continuously. If the hood has been turned off, it must be allowed to run for 30 minutes before preparing IV admixtures. The inside of the hood must be thoroughly cleaned with alcohol or another disinfectant. Cleaning is performed using long, side-to-side motions starting at the back of the hood and working forward. Cleaning should be done before and after preparing a series of admixtures and if there is a spill in the hood.

Class II hoods that are used in the preparation of hazardous drugs (e.g., cytotoxic drugs) should be decontaminated regularly by using a high pH stainless steel cleaner. The use of aerosol cleaners, although convenient, should be avoided to prevent damage to the HEPA filter and accumulation of aerosol propellants in the hood.

All laminar airflow hoods must be certified on a regular basis to ensure their proper functioning. Inspection occurs annually for horizontal hoods and every six months for class II hoods.

Good aseptic technique is essential to maximize the benefits of a laminar airflow hood. It is important to remember, however, that laminar airflow can be eas-

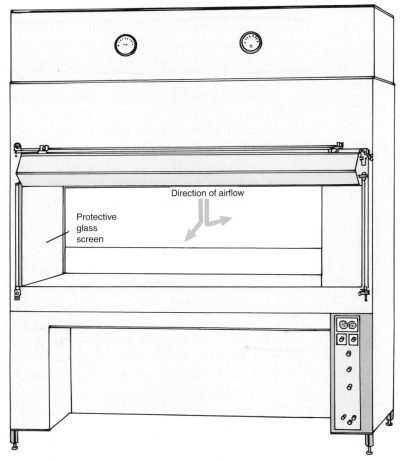

FIGURE 14-6 This vertical laminar airflow hood protects the operators.

ily disrupted. Such disruptions increase the risk of contamination. Sneezing, coughing, and even talking directly into a laminar airflow hood can disrupt the airflow sufficiently to contaminate the work area. Breezes from an open door or window, or sudden, rapid hand movements within the hood, can also disrupt the airflow.

When preparing parenteral products, several steps are critical to follow. First and foremost is proper handwashing with a suitable antimicrobial cleanser, such as chlorhexidine gluconate or povidone-iodine. Careful attention to scrubbing hands and arms up to the elbow is vital. Jewelry should not be worn on the hands and arms. Hands must be rewashed when returning from outside the parenterals area or if there is any possibility that they have been contaminated. Some institutions require gowning and the use of gloves. Unfortunately, gloves may give a false sense of security. It is important to remember that gloves are not a substitute for proper handwashing. The warm, moist environment created by wearing gloves can create ideal conditions for microorganisms to grow. Failure to properly wash the hands can increase the potential for microbial contamination. In addition, gloves can become contaminated as easily as ungloved hands. Any gloves or gowns worn inside the parenterals area must be removed when leaving the area to prevent contamination upon returning.

Before preparing any products, all necessary materials should be gathered. Those needed for each product should be placed in the hood in a manner that does not obstruct the clean airflow. Solutions and additives must be checked for expiration dates and freedom from particulate matter. The outer containers should be cleaned of dust and wiped or sprayed with alcohol prior to being placed in the hood. Plastic solution containers should be squeezed to check for leaks. There must be no items inside the hood that are not used in preparing the product (e.g., labels, papers).

Work performed in the hood area should be done in the center of it. There must be no obstruction between the HEPA filter and the product being prepared. In a horizontal hood, work must be done at least six inches inside it. The airflow at the outer six inches of the hood is subject to many disturbances and, therefore, may be contaminated. With a vertical hood, the viewing screen must be lowered to its proper position, since this acts to contain the airflow within the hood, provide proper laminar airflow, and protect the user.

Ampules and Vials

Drugs and other additives to IV solutions are packaged in ampules or vials. They are available either in liquid form or as sterile solids or powders. Sterile solids must be reconstituted with a suitable solution (diluent) before addition to the IV fluid. Ampules are sealed glass containers with an elongated neck that must be snapped off. Most ampules are weakened around the base of the neck for easy breaking. Such ampules can be recognized by a colored band around the base of the neck. If the ampule is not weakened, it may be necessary to score it with a file to prevent shattering of the top. A filter needle or straw should be used when withdrawing the contents of an ampule. These products have a 5-micron filter incorporated in them to remove any particulate matter which may fall into the ampule when opened. The filter needle or straw is removed and replaced with a regular needle before injecting the drug into the solution.

Vials are made of glass or plastic and have a rubber stopper through which a needle is inserted to withdraw or add to the contents. Care must be taken not to force excessive air into the vial since this can lead to aerosolizing of the contents into the air, or in extreme cases, bursting of the vial. When withdrawing solution from a vial, an equal volume of air is usually drawn up in the syringe and injected into the vial before withdrawing the contents. Some medications are packaged under pressure or may produce gas (and therefore pressure) upon reconstitution. In these situations, air should *not* be injected into the vial before withdrawing the drug. Vials may be labeled for single use or multiple dose use. Multidose products contain a preservative to inhibit microbial contamination after the vial has been opened, and may be withdrawn from more than once. Single-use vials do not contain preservatives and should be discarded after use.

Some manufacturers supply antibiotics in powder form in oversized vials or bags. These minibottle or minibag containers typically have a 100 ml capacity and the drug is reconstituted using a suitable diluent. In addition, each container is equipped with its own hanger so that it can be hung as a piggyback container. The advantage to this type of system is that the drugs are ready for use once they are reconstituted and do not have to be transferred to another container. Large-scale preparation is facilitated by manufacturers' piggyback containers.

Working with Needles and Syringes

Needles and syringes are used for virtually all parenteral product preparation. Syringes consist of a barrel and a plunger (**Figure 14-7**). They range in capacity from 0.3 ml to 60 ml. Volumes are marked along the barrel. Needles range in size from

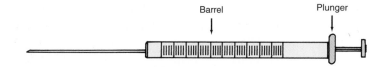

FIGURE 14-7   Syringe—barrel and plunger

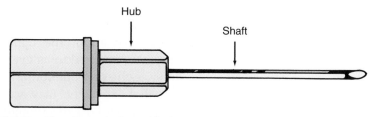

FIGURE 14-8   Needle—shaft and hub.

3/8 inch to 3½ inches or longer and consist of a shaft and a hub (**Figure 14-8**). The thickness of the needle is represented by gauge size, with 29 gauge being the finest and 13 gauge the thickest. Needles of 26 to 29 gauge are most commonly used for subcutaneous and intradermal injections. Larger gauge needles (18 to 25) are used for intramuscular injections.

In preparing parenteral products, the gauge of the needle used should be the smallest practical size. If a large gauge needle is used, there is a risk of **coring** when injecting into a vial or IV container. Coring occurs when a needle rips a piece of the vial stopper at the injection site. This piece then falls into the container and creates a situation of particulate matter contamination.

Safety Considerations

There are a number of safety considerations involved in preparing parenteral products, including opening the glass ampules, various effects of the medications, and needle sticks.

Opening Glass Ampules

The process of opening a glass ampule presents risks related to broken glass. If proper technique is not used, the ampule may shatter and cut the fingers or hand. In addition, glass splinters may be thrown from the ampule when opened. These splinters could strike the eye when working in a horizontal laminar airflow hood. To reduce the risk of shattering the ampule, it is essential that it not be forced open. Most ampules have a weak spot that can be located by rotating the ampule slightly if it does not snap open with moderate pressure. It is also useful to wrap an alcohol wipe around the top of the ampule when opening to provide some protection to the fingers if the ampule shatters and to reduce the possibility of glass splinters becoming airborne.

Local and Systemic Effects of Medications

Medications may be absorbed into the body through the skin and by inhalation, thus resulting in undesirable effects when significant exposure occurs. Such effects may be localized (confined to the site of exposure, such as the skin), or systemic (within the body). An example of a local effect would be a rash or redness. An example of a systemic effect would be low blood pressure from exposure to nitroglycerin.

It is extremely important to take precautions to avoid undue exposure to medications. Anyone suffering from allergies to particular medications should wear gloves and work in a vertical laminar airflow hood when handling these products. Any medication spilled on the skin should be washed off immediately. Proper technique is vital to avoid unnecessary exposure to medications.

There is much concern about the handling of, and exposure to, cancer chemotherapy agents (also referred to as cytotoxic drugs). Some of these agents have been shown to have the potential of producing serious adverse effects. It is not clear, however, to what extent this may occur from exposure in the workplace. Therefore, it is important to follow recommended procedures for handling these substances.

In January 1986, the federal Occupational Safety and Health Administration (OSHA) released recommendations on safe handling of cytotoxic drugs by health care personnel. The American Society of Health-System Pharmacists (ASHP) has subsequently released technical assistance bulletins on handling cytotoxic and hazardous drugs, which incorporate these recommendations and those of other agencies and organizations. Technicians must be aware of these recommendations and strictly follow the procedures established at their place of employment.

It is possible to be exposed to hazardous drugs in various ways. According to the ASHP, "This exposure may be through the inadvertent ingestion of the drug on foodstuffs (e.g., workers' lunches), inhalation of drug dusts or droplets, or direct skin contact." The danger is due not only to the *immediate* effects of a toxic drug, but also to how much exposure occurs over time. In other words, the effects may be cumulative. Long-term exposure *may* produce serious effects such as cancer, impaired fertility, and organ damage, although this has not been proven. Clearly, preventing unintended exposure to these substances is essential.

The ASHP has established four goals for handling hazardous drugs.

1. Protect and secure packages of hazardous drugs.
2. Inform and educate all involved personnel about hazardous drugs and train them in the safe handling procedures relevant to their responsibilities.
3. Do not let the drugs escape from containers when they are manipulated (i.e., dissolved, transferred, administered, or discarded).
4. Eliminate the possibility of inadvertent ingestion or inhalation and direct skin or eye contact with the drugs.

Proper procedures must be in place and *followed* to prevent inadvertent exposure to cytotoxic drugs. This includes the use of appropriate equipment (e.g., vertical laminar airflow hoods, gowns, gloves) and appropriate storage and disposal of these agents. While the consequences of exposure to cytotoxic drugs remain unclear, reducing the possibility of such exposure is an essential goal of all involved.

Needle Sticks

It is easy to accidentally stick oneself with a needle in an IV admixture area. It is, however, relatively easy to avoid such occurrences. Although the needles used within the pharmacy should normally be "clean" (i.e., not contaminated by blood from another person), needle sticks are a cause of concern. The site of injury may become infected, the resulting bleeding may contaminate other products, and there may be adverse reactions caused by exposure to any drug contained in the needle.

Needle sticks can be avoided by working carefully and not rushing when preparing parenteral products. Re-capping of needles should be avoided when possible since this is often a source of needle sticks. If it is necessary to re-cap a needle, extra care must be taken. Finally, never reach into a disposal box (sharps container) or attempt to pack down discarded syringes in these boxes. Do not fill the sharps containers more than three-fourths full.

Role of the Technician

The technician is a vital part of a parenteral admixture program. The exact role that a technician plays will vary among states because of differences in pharmacy laws. In addition, as mentioned, the degree to which parenteral admixture services are provided varies considerably among different institutions. However, technicians generally are responsible for the following:

- preparing labels and sorting computer-generated labels
- maintaining proper stock and supplies in the parenterals area
- assembling drugs and solutions to be used for admixtures
- reconstituting manufacturers' piggyback vials and additives
- preparing IV admixtures under a pharmacist's supervision
- assigning lot numbers and maintaining appropriate records for batch preparations
- preparing prefilled syringes
- preparing parenteral nutrition base solutions
- labeling completed admixtures
- delivering completed admixtures to appropriate areas
- maintaining workload statistics
- maintaining dispensing records and patient charges
- ensuring that all needles, syringes, and chemotherapy are properly discarded
- ensuring that no stock is outdated or deteriorated
- ensuring that medications are appropriately stored (refrigerator, freezer)
- maintaining the parenterals area in a neat and orderly manner

Summary

The parenterals technician must be a meticulous, motivated person. The preparation of parenteral products is a high-risk activity. Due to the nature of the products prepared, any errors or improper preparations have the potential to cause harm to the patient. The technician must work with the pharmacist, who is responsible for checking and supervising all the technician's activities. Quality and accuracy must never be compromised. All work must be carried out in a diligent, professional manner. The technician is a key player in the functioning of a pharmacy parenterals admixture service.

TEST YOUR KNOWLEDGE

Multiple Choice Questions

1. Injectable medications account for what percentage of all drugs administered in the hospital?
   a. 40%
   b. 50%
   c. 80%
   d. 30%
   e. 20%

2. Drugs are given by injection when
   a. the patient is unable to take oral medication
   b. the patient refuses to take oral medication
   c. there is a need for rapid drug action
   d. the drug may be destroyed in the gastrointestinal tract
   e. all of the above

3. The most important characteristic of an injectable solution is
   a. color
   b. viscosity
   c. dispersability
   d. sterility
   e. fluidity

4. A drug can be sterilized by
   a. moist heat
   b. gas
   c. filtration
   d. none of the above
   e. all of the above

5. Pyrogenic contamination may cause the patient to have
   a. fever
   b. chills
   c. infection
   d. a and b
   e. a and c

6. Particulate matter in an intravenous solution may
   a. cause phlebitis
   b. cause dermatitis
   c. block blood flow in small blood vessels
   d. rupture a blood vessel
   e. all of the above

7. To maintain an aseptic work environment, the technician should
   a. thoroughly wash hands
   b. wear gloves
   c. wear a clean gown
   d. wear a face mask
   e. do all of the above

8. Solution osmolality is a characteristic that results from
   a. the degree of acidity
   b. the degree of alkalinity
   c. a neutral pH
   d. the number of dissolved particles
   e. the number of undissolved particles

9. Intravenous solutions may be administered as
   a. infusions
   b. bolus
   c. piggyback
   d. saddleback
   e. a, b, and c

10. Vertical laminar airflow hoods
    a. should not be used to prepare cytotoxic drugs
    b. protect the operator from hazardous drugs
    c. do not require cleaning
    d. are not used in hospitals
    e. none of the above

True/False Questions

11. __T__ As a general rule, the more concentrated the solution, the less stable it is.

12. __F__ There is no need to be concerned about exposure to cytotoxic drugs.

13. __F__ Intramuscular, intravenous, and subcutaneous routes of injection are interchangeable.

14. __T F__ Visual inspection of parenteral products ensures that the drug is safe and stable.

15. __T__ The pH of a sterile solution can affect both stability and compatibility.

Matching Questions

16. __b__ intradermal
17. __g__ subcutaneous
18. __d__ intramuscular
19. __a__ intravenous
20. __f__ intra-arterial
21. __c__ intrathecal
22. __e__ intracardiac

a. used for large volume injection
b. injected within the skin
c. injected into the spinal fluid
d. common injection sites are the gluteus and deltoid
e. injected into a chamber of the heart
f. injected into a major artery
g. injected into the loose tissue layer below the skin

References

American Society of Health-Systems Pharmacists (2004). ASHP technical assistance bulletin on handling cytotoxic and hazardous drugs. *Practice Standards of ASHP.*

American Society of Health-Systems Pharmacists (2004). ASHP technical assistance bulletin on quality assurance for pharmacy-prepared sterile products. *Practice Standards of ASHP.*

Hunt, M. L., Jr. (1995). *Training manual for intravenous admixture personnel* (5th ed.). Chicago: Precept Press.

Turco, S., & King, R. E. (Eds.). (1994). *Sterile dosage forms* (4th ed.). Philadelphia: Lea & Febiger.

15 Administration of Medications

COMPETENCIES

Upon completion of this chapter, the reader should be able to

1. Specify the drug information that should be reviewed by the health care practitioner prior to administering a drug to a patient.

2. Describe the clinical and technical concerns required for administering medications by the following routes: oral, topical, rectal, vaginal, intraocular, intranasal, into the ear.

3. Identify five methods in which the person administering medications can reduce medication errors.

4. Discuss the characteristics and professional concerns of a drug administrator or drug technician.

5. Differentiate the directions that should be given to a patient receiving a buccal tablet and a gelatin capsule.

6. Differentiate labeling requirements between internal and external drug preparations.

7. List five situations in which a drug is discontinued or drug administration is interrupted.

8. Describe the procedure to be followed if a patient states, "I cannot swallow that large tablet."

9. Discuss some causes of medication errors. Explain the universal policy to be observed if a medication error is detected.

10. List the requirements for each health care practitioner who accepts the responsibility for the administration of medications.

Introduction

This chapter focuses on the clinical, professional, and technical aspects of medication administration. While policies and procedures vary from institution to institution (and the institution's policy takes precedence over what is written here), the person who administers medications must always respect the dignity, privacy, safety, and autonomy of the patient. Patient cooperation is essential to the administration of most forms of medications. Even those patients who appear comatose, confused, or otherwise compromised should have the proposed procedure explained to them. Each health care practitioner who accepts the responsibility for the administration of medications must become familiar with the patient population, the institution's policies concerning medications, the approved methods of medication administration, the formulary and other resources that are available for reference and information, and the institution's expectations of the person who administers medications. All are very serious responsibilities.

Medication Orders

Drug administration is initiated with the physician's (prescriber's) order. No drug is given to a patient without physician authorization. There are a number of different kinds of medication orders. Orders written in the chart at the time of admission, which may be subsequently increased, decreased, or deleted, are the most common type of medication orders. Another type of drug order is a verbal order that may be given by the physician to a nurse or pharmacist, usually via the phone, when an emergency or unusual circumstance arises. Prior to initiation, verbal orders should be repeated to the prescriber. Verbal orders are always reduced to writing in the patient's chart, signed by the order taker, and cosigned by the physician on the next visit to the hospital. Verbal orders should be cosigned by the physician within 24 hours or as specified by hospital policy. Medication orders are also written on transfer and discharge of patients and with changes in the patient's condition or required medical therapy.

STAT orders are orders for drugs that should be immediately administered. The immediacy relates to the patient's condition such as the need for pain relief, experiencing clinical distress, or a drug or allergic reaction. The person administering drugs always gives top priority to making sure the patient receives a STAT drug in timely fashion. Orders written by the physician to be given to the patient only if required by the patient's condition are prn (pro re nata) orders. One-time orders are written for specific circumstances such as patient sedation for a test or procedure. Standing orders sometimes accompany a patient on admission to the hospital or are the printed drug regimens prescribed by the physician or a physician group to treat particular conditions (e.g., women who are admitted to the obstetrical unit preceding childbirth). These orders may be prewritten and signed by the physician or stamped on the chart with the physician's signature. Medication orders may also be included in physician, unit, or patient-specific protocols, pathways, and standards of care.

Hospital policy may permit drug orders to be written by persons other than medical physicians, including **physician assistants**, clinical nurse practitioners, dentists, **podiatrists**, and pharmacists. These policies must be known and observed.

Information Needed on Drug Orders

To properly administer a drug, the following information is needed for each drug order:

- patient's full name, room number, bed number, and other identifiers required by hospital policy (e.g., medical record numbers, ID barcodes)
- name of drug (clearly written), dosage strength (e.g., 10 mg), dosage schedule (e.g., q.d., STAT, t.i.d.)
- route of administration (e.g., sublingual, subcutaneous, instill in left eye)
- length of time drug is to be given (e.g., for 24 hours, 1 week, length of hospital stay, as needed)
- prescriber's signature

The drug order is entered into the patient's medication order forms (this can be done by hand or as part of a computerized physician order entry (CPOE) system) and transmitted to the pharmacy to be filled. Illegibility of handwritten physician orders has been identified as a key contributor to medication errors, which is leading to the development and implementation of CPOE systems. The person who administers the drug verifies the label on the drug by comparing it with the order on the patient's medication record. Computerized medication systems are being used more and provide additional levels of automated checking—drug order to patient to drug being administered. A rule of thumb—never administer a medication without checking it three times against the order or medication administration record (MAR). Leave all medications fully labeled in their unit dose packages until you are at the bedside. The last check just prior to administration is the most important because it is your last chance to pick up an error.

The Medication Administrator or Medication Technician

The person who will administer drugs to the patient should be in good health, free of communicable infections (e.g., a head cold, a sore throat, an open lesion). This is of importance for both the patient and the drug administrator. Patients are susceptible to **nosocomial** infections (infections incurred in the hospital). Often the patient is weak, has had surgery or radiation therapy, and the immune system may be compromised for these or other reasons (e.g., aging process, malnutrition). The drug administrator who is at a low physical ebb due to exhaustion or poor health is more likely to make a drug administration error than a person who is well, alert, and fully attentive. In addition, a drug administrator (e.g., nurse, pharmacist, technician) who is in poor health is more apt to pick up an infection from a patient. It is important for any person who gives direct patient care to ensure and maintain good health through proper nutrition, exercise, and healthy living habits. In case of an upper respiratory infection or other indisposition, the drug administrator should inform the supervisor for a change of assignment away from direct patient care for the duration of the illness. Personal protective devices to ensure standard precautions for bloodborne disease transmission will be used during medication delivery as required. If the patient is in isolation due to an infectious, transmittable disease, the drug administrator should follow hospital policy regarding protection. In all events, persons who are about to administer drugs should thoroughly wash their hands before handling any drugs and rewash the hands between patients when hospital policy or aseptic technique requires it. Handwashing is the single most effective infection control measure.

The **medication technician** or **medication administrator** should appreciate the responsibility inherent in the role. This person should be knowledgeable about the responsibilities of the other members of the health team regarding drug administration and communicate effectively with them. The medication technician should always give priority to patient care, treating each patient with dignity and professional concern regardless of physical or mental impairment, lifestyle orientation, religious beliefs, or cultural background. It is necessary that the medication technician be totally familiar with the policies and procedures that prevail in a particular hospital and always know the physician, nurse, or pharmacist to whom he or she directly reports. Any unusual physical or emotional change noted by the technician during medication rounds should be immediately reported to the charge nurse. Professional confidentiality regarding any patient in the technician's care is of prime importance. Patients have, at all times, a right to have personal matters respected and held in confidence. Technicians should report to work dressed in professional attire, with name identification badge, in keeping with the dignity of the position and the respect they should expect from others.

Administration of the Drug

Prior to drug administration, the medication technician should become familiar with the following information regarding the drug:

- general and special uses or indications
- usual dose or dosage range
- special precautions (e.g., do not give with food, observe patient for rash)
- side effects that may occur
- foods or other drugs that should not be given with the drug
- time when onset of action is expected

By reviewing this information before administering the drug, mistakes and errors can be avoided and the patient's wellbeing better ensured. Hospital policy will indicate how involved the medication technician becomes in providing this information to the patient. Generally, the registered nurse or the pharmacist has the responsibility to answer drug information questions and to counsel the patient on proper drug use.

Patient Rights

Nearly every patient in the hospital will receive drugs during the stay. Each patient is entitled to the "five rights" for safe, appropriate drug administration. Drug rights of the patient include the right drug, right dose, right route (or right dosage form), right time, and right patient. These rights should be memorized and checked prior to each drug administration.

The right patient

The first right requirement is to verify that the right patient is the one to receive the drug. The patient should be addressed by his or her name and then the patient identification armband should be checked. Just addressing the person by name is not sufficient. Persons may respond positively, even if they have not clearly heard their name due to distractions, deafness, or language barriers. Beds are often shifted to different positions in the room, so identifying a person as the patient in room 120 bed 3 is insufficient information and may be misleading. Computerized medication systems that utilize barcoding or other methods of patient identification are being implemented by hospitals. Before administering any medication, the patient's identification must be verified and compared to the actual medication order or medication profile.

The right drug

The right drug is verified by checking the physician's (prescriber's) order sheet and the nurse's (or pharmacist's) drug administration form, drug Cardex, or drug summary on computer profile. Thousands of drugs are available and many sound alike, are spelled alike, and look alike. Abbreviation of drug names has become a risky practice and many hospitals are limiting or eliminating the use of medication abbreviations entirely as a risk reduction strategy. One or two letters in a name can mean an entirely different drug. The prescriber must be contacted if there are any questions or doubts concerning the order. Most drugs used in hospitals today are in unit-dose packages. The name is clearly visible on each drug dosage form.

Labels should be checked three times before the drug is administered. The Institute for Safe Medication Practices (ISMP) has identified top high-risk drugs. These are medications that have been involved frequently in serious errors. Examples include insulin and chemotherapy. It is important to follow your hospitals special safety precautions when administering these high-alert drugs.

The right dose

Accurate **dosage strength** is critical to beneficial drug administration. Giving the wrong strength, particularly to children or infants, can be and has been fatal. The right dose is further checked with special care given to decimal points. A zero before the decimal, called a "leading decimal," (e.g., 0.1 mg) should be noted. Care should be taken if there is a zero after the decimal, called a "trailing zero," which can be misleading and can be misread, leading to a 10 times greater dosage error (e.g., 1.0 is one, not ten). Orders for units must always be written out. The abbreviation "u" for units can be misread as a "10" and lead to a 10 times greater dosage error.

Proper dosage strength should never be presumed by anyone in the prescribing, dispensing, or administering process. Physicians must clearly indicate the desired strength on the medication order, pharmacists are expected to further verify dosage to be sure it is within appropriate therapeutic limits, and nurses are expected to further check that the dosage strength ordered by the physician was accurately dispensed by the pharmacist or pharmacy technician. After the drug and dosage strength has gone through these three checkpoints, the last checkpoint resides with the person who administers the drug to the patient. If any dosage changes have been made along the way, the change should be clearly indicated on the patient's chart and other medication records. Children, the elderly, and patients with impaired liver and kidney function are at the greatest risk of adverse drug events related to medication dosage.

The right route/dosage form

In addition to ensuring that the right drug in the right strength has been selected, it is important to check and be sure that the drug is given by the right route in the right dosage form. Drugs come in many different dosage forms. Liquids come as solutions, tinctures, suspensions, syrups, and elixirs. Oral solid dosage forms come as **tablets**, gelatin **capsules, caplets, enteric-coated tablets, extended-release capsules**, sublingual tablets, and buccal tablets. External preparations include creams, ointments, and lotions. Some medications in ointment form contain potent active ingredients. The length of the ointment strip must be carefully measured by the drug administrator. Injectable medications must be carefully checked to be sure whether the injection should be administered by intramuscular, intravenous, subcutaneous, or other route of administration. Drop-type drugs must be checked and used only as indicated for the eye, ear, or nose. There are many suppository dosage forms, such as rectal, vaginal, urethral. Dosage forms are NOT interchangeable, so it is important that it is the right drug, administered in the right dosage form. It is also important to note when a drug dosage form has been changed by the prescriber (e.g., an injectable drug [IM] is changed to an oral dosage [po]). Every drug order should include the route of administration. If a question arises, proper dosage form should be confirmed before the drug is administered.

The right time

Time of drug administration (i.e., **dosage schedule** or frequency) is an important factor in pharmacotherapy. Drugs should be given at the time ordered allowing for an ordinary deviation of a half-hour, unless timing is critical. Diabetics should always receive their **hypoglycemic** drugs a half-hour before meals, unless otherwise specified. Patients on therapeutic drug monitoring are involved in pharmacokinetic laboratory studies. Dosage time is related to drug half-life and the time the phlebotomist will draw the blood for the serum analysis. Time of drug administration can be a critical factor in pharmacokinetic laboratory results. Time of a drug can be of great concern to the patient who is waiting. A patient who has been ordered an analgesic for the relief of pain to be given every 4 hours for the first 24 hours after the operation should receive this drug on time. Delays for this patient increase the pain and anxiety and slow the recovery process. Many drugs are now administered per parameters. An example is a cardiac medication to be administered if the heart rate and blood pressure are within a certain range and held if outside the range. Knowledge of when the physician wants the medication administered, any hospital-, unit-, or physician-specific per parameters policy applicable, and the actual monitoring required prior to administration are required. It is less confusing for the patient if, when possible, drug administration times in the hospital are kept close to when the patient would normally take them at home, especially being considerate of the patient's individual waking and sleeping times. This also facilitates an accurate assessment of therapeutic effect.

Oral Drug Administration

After the patient has been properly identified, the patient is either given the medication to swallow, to place under the tongue (sublingual), or to place between the cheek and the gum (buccal tablets) or the medication is appropriately injected, inserted, instilled, or inhaled in the case of respiratory drug therapy. If the patient is to self-administer an oral tablet, the nurse, pharmacist, or technician should remain with the patient until the drug has been swallowed. Drugs are never left at the patient's bedside without a doctor's order. Drugs left at the bedside may be forgotten, may be discarded, or may be hoarded for future use. The patient should be instructed to place a sublingual tablet (e.g., nitroglycerin) under the tongue and leave it there until it dissolves. A patient ordered a buccal tablet should be told to place the tablet between the gum and the cheek and allow it to dissolve. Throat and mouth troches or lozenges should not be swallowed or chewed but allowed to remain in the oral cavity until dissolved. In the case of a medicated mouthwash used for oral and throat infections, the patient should be told to swish the liquid around in the mouth and then either swallow or expectorate (spit out) according to the nature of the substance and the dosage directions.

Usually, the patient should be given an adequate amount of water (at least four ounces) to allow for easy swallowing, dissolution of the tablet or capsule, and prevention of esophageal erosion. Esophageal erosion can occur when an oral medication lodges and remains in the esophagus and does not move into the stomach. Particular care must be given to tablets with a corrosive potential, such as a compressed potassium chloride tablet.

The exceptions to the rule for administering sufficient water with an oral dosage form are in the cases of cough syrups intended to soothe and work in the throat area, medicated mouthwashes intended to be swallowed or expectorated, and after administering either a buccal or sublingual tablet. There are times when a liquid other than water may be indicated. If there is no contraindication, the patient may prefer to follow the drug with a drink of milk or a fruit juice. However, there are some definite contraindications. The person administering the drug should know the liquids that should not be administered with particular medications (e.g., fruit juices and sodas, such as cola beverages, should never be given with penicillin tablets; milk or milk products should not be given with the mycin-type antibiotics or certain laxatives, such as Dulcolax™).

Before leaving the patient, the person administering the drug should make sure the patient has taken the drug and has had no difficulty in swallowing the medication or following other instructions. If the patient asks questions about the drugs, an adequate answer should be given. If the person administering the drug is limited either on time or knowledge when the question is asked, a follow-up visit should be made. But such answers as "that is what the doctor orders" or "this is given to you to make you feel better" are not adequate answers. They are, in fact, dismissing the patient's questions and need for information. The patient is entitled to information regarding the drugs he or she is ordered. In most cases, the technician will refer these questions to the nurse or pharmacist responsible for the care of the patient who will further discuss the question. It is also important to document the medication administration immediately *after* the drug is taken. Documentation should never be done prior to administration because you could be called away from the bedside unexpectedly.

Topical Drug Administration

A **topical** drug is one applied to the skin or mucous membranes. Topical medications are intended to either produce local effect or provide a sustained release (e.g., transdermal patches). The person applying an ointment should wear disposable gloves and explain the procedure to the patient. The area should be cleaned and any remaining ointment removed. Ointments should be applied in thin layers using cotton swabs or a tongue depressor. Liquid medications such as lotions and suspensions should first be shaken well and then applied as directed with quick sprays. Both the patient and the drug administrator should be careful not to inhale the aerosol spray. In some cases, directions may require that the area be covered with sterile gauze after application. Special care should be given to burn-injured patients because they are most susceptible to infections. Generally, absorption of topically applied medications is less predictable than other routes.

Eyedrop and Eye Ointment Application

Always aseptically clean hands by scrubbing well or wearing disposable gloves before instilling eyedrops. To preserve the cleanliness of the delivery orifice, do not touch the tip of the dropper or container to the patient's eye or an external surface. Position the patient with head back. The lower lid can be gently pulled forward to create a well into which the drop or drops can be inserted. Be careful not to touch the eye or conjuctival sac with the medication dispenser.

Accurately apply the drop or number of drops as directed. Many eyedrops have systemic effects; therefore, additional drops should not be given. Before the drops are administered, check the label for name, strength and directions for use, including which eye, or if directed, both eyes should be treated. Check labels for expiration date. Never use any expired drug. If an ointment is used, discard the first bead as it is considered contaminated, instruct the patient to look up and then apply a thin line of ointment to the slightly retracted lower lid without allowing the tip of the tube to touch the eye. After instillation of either eyedrops or ointment, instruct the patient to close the eye for a few minutes to permit the dispersion of the drug through the eye. If a tear appears, wipe it away with sterile gauze. If there is any noticeable change in the eye (e.g., increased redness, discharge, signs of irritation), report it right away to the supervising nurse or pharmacist.

Administration of Ear and Nose Preparation

To instill eardrops, the patient should be sitting with the unaffected ear on the shoulder or lying down with the affected ear facing up. It will be more comfortable for the patient if the solution to be instilled is warmed slightly with your hand or by placing under warm water for a few minutes prior to instillation. For an adult or a child older than three, the ear should be gently pulled up and back, and for a child younger than three, the ear should be gently pulled down and back to make the ear canal more accessible. Drops are inserted directly into the canal without touching the tip of the dropper or nozzle to the ear. The patient should remain positioned for a few minutes to keep the drops from running out of the ear. If a cotton plug is ordered, it should be sterile and gently placed just at the opening of the canal. Administer only the prescribed number of drops after carefully reading the label.

Nose drops should be applied with the head resting on the back of the neck. The patient should be instructed to breathe through the mouth. Instill the required number of drops and instruct the patient to keep the head back a few minutes and not to blow the nose for a few minutes. Nose sprays are used with the patient's head in an upright position. The spray is applied by squeezing the applicator bottle quickly and firmly while it is placed in the tip of the nostril. Repeat the process with the other nostril. Use only as directed because active ingredients in the spray enter directly into the circulatory system and may have untoward systemic effects. Other drugs in nebulizer form come with specific instructions in the package insert. These should be carefully followed to properly administer the drugs.

Application of Transdermal Drugs

Transdermal drugs, often called drug patches, consist of an active drug ingredient inside a patch held in place by small adhesive tapes. The drug is applied externally for internal or **systemic action**. A drug such as nitroglycerin (for chest pain) is placed in a transdermal patch on the skin where it is picked up by the bloodstream for action over a sustained period of time. The area where the patch is applied should be clearly dry and free of hair (e.g., upper arm). The patch should not be applied to any area that is irritated, callused, or scarred. The location of the patch should be rotated when a new patch is applied. Do not place the patch below the knee or elbow. Care should be taken that the patch does not come off at night or during bathing. If the patch does fall off, check with the supervisor. The location of the patch needs to be documented.

Insertion of Suppositories

Prepare a treatment by checking the label on the box. Make sure the suppository feels firm. The cocoa butter base may begin to soften or melt at warm temperatures. If this occurs, briefly place the suppository, with foil wrapper intact, in cold water to increase firmness. Have a tube of lubricating ointment and a pair of disposable gloves on hand. Inform the patient concerning the drug administration procedure and position the patient as instructed. Drape the patient and provide for privacy. For rectal insertion, patient should be on one side (generally the left side unless contraindicated) with under leg extended and other leg flexed at knee. Don gloves, unwrap the suppository and lubricate the rounded end (or follow more specific manufacturer's instructions), and lubricate your gloved index finger. Instruct the patient to take slow, deep breaths. This will help them to relax. Insert the suppository into the rectum beyond the anal sphincter (approximately the length of your index finger for an adult, less for a child) and encourage the patient to retain it for at least 30–40 minutes. For vaginal insertion, encourage the patient to void then position her on her back with knees flexed and legs spread apart. The drug administrator should put on gloves and remove suppository foil wrapper. Rectal ointment and vaginal suppositories and ointments are inserted using an applicator that accompanies the suppository or cream. Further directions for use are found in the package insert.

Injectable Drug Administration

There are many techniques and various routes for the use of injectable medications. Injectable drugs can be given directly into a blood vessel (intravascular), into a vein (intravenous), into an artery (intra-arterial), into select muscles (intramuscular), under the skin (hypodermic or subcutaneous), into the skin (intradermal), into the spinal cord (intrathecal), or into the heart (intrapericardiac).

Many of these injection techniques require special manipulative skill. They are considered invasive procedures, frequently using very potent drugs. Information and competency development is beyond the scope of this manual.

Discontinuance of Drug Administration

Persons involved in drug administration need to be very alert to the times when drug discontinuance, interruption of dosage schedules, or modification of scheduled dosage patterns are prescribed or indicated.

Drug administration should be withheld if the patient gives evidence of experiencing an adverse drug reaction (e.g., hives; a rash occurring on the body, face, neck, arms or legs; difficulty in breathing; double vision or seeing various colors that are not objectively present). If the drug administrator observes any of these conditions or the patient speaks about them, the supervising nurse should be contacted before the next dose is given. In other clinical situations, there may be hospital policy or physician orders that direct stoppage of drug due to certain indicators (i.e., drugs by parameters). For example, do not give digoxin if apical pulse rate falls below sixty beats per minute.

Surgeons and anesthesiologists usually give specific orders for medication immediately before and after surgery. Many times, physicians or hospital policy will instruct that all or certain drugs be given with a sip of water prior to surgery even if the patient is npo (nothing by mouth). An example would be to continue the blood pressure medication even though the patient is npo for surgery to ensure the blood pressure remains within normal limits pre- and intraoperatively. Some physicians or hospital policies may discontinue all standing medication orders prior to the patient going to surgery. At that time, drugs needed prior to, during, and immediately after surgery are reordered. A drug administrator must carefully scrutinize the preoperative and postoperative drug orders for the surgical patient. Mistakes in this area could jeopardize the surgical outcome.

The patient may be scheduled for physical therapy, X-ray, or other activities that take the person off the floor during the times of medication administrations. If this occurs, the supervising nurse should be contacted as to the appropriate action to take regarding giving the medication when the patient returns.

Other interruptions of drug administration can occur when the patient's orders read "nothing by mouth" and the patient is on oral drug therapy. And in some situations, for various reasons, the patient may refuse to take the drug. In each case, the supervising nurse, the pharmacist, or the prescribing physician must be contacted to clarify the appropriate action to be taken regarding drug administration.

If a patient is in a program for therapeutic drug monitoring (TDM), the drug dosage schedule or laboratory phlebotomy schedule may have to be modified according to the half-life of the drug to obtain the accurate drug blood serum levels that are required for optimum drug therapy dosing. These patients may require an individualized drug dosage administration schedule to be planned by the physician, pharmacist, and medical technologist. Information regarding interrupted drug administration, refusal of the patient to take one drug, and modified drug schedules should always be charted in the medication records and reported to the supervising nurse.

Unit-Dose Drug Administration

A unit-dose drug comes individually packaged and labeled and requires no further packaging or labeling. This system cuts down on the problem of medication errors and preserves the integrity and safety of the product. In a unit-dose drug delivery system, a pharmacist checks every drug order prior to the administration of the drug. The unit-dose system provides each patient with a storage bin, usually in a medication cart, in which no more than a 24-hour supply of drugs is available for the individual patient. The package is opened at the patient's bedside and the name, label, strength, and patient are once again checked against the medication Cardex. Now unit-doses frequently include drug-specific barcodes to facilitate automation of the medication system.

Crushing Medications

Crushing medications to assist patients who have difficulty swallowing pills or capsules is recommended only after serious consideration and consultation between the physician and the pharmacist. Medications are designed in tablet or capsule form to ensure their absorption in the correct area of the gastrointestinal tract and to eliminate or minimize digestive problems. Crushing may seriously interfere with these safety measures. Crushing cannot be used for enteric-coated or sustained-action (e.g., Pronestyl-SR) medications. Notify the pharmacy about the need to crush specific medications and follow the pharmacist's advice regarding the safety of this action.

If crushing is necessary and approved by institution policy, each medication must be crushed individually, mixed with a palatable food (e.g., applesauce, Jell-O), and given to the patient separately. Attempt to give the patient as much of the drug in the first spoonful so that very little is wasted if the patient refuses the remainder. Never mix all the patient's medications in one cup.

Internal and External Medications

Any caregiver who has been in practice for an extended period of time can cite examples of inaccuracies that they read about, heard about, or were involved in. One that comes to mind was the elderly monk, admitted to the hospital for a severe scalp burn when someone attempting to dry up a wet lesion dropped a sunlamp on his head. The burn became infected and he was admitted to the hospital. His first morning in the hospital, his caregiver poured out and left at the bedside two ounces of mouthwash in a small waxed paper cup, the same as the one the patient had received a liquid medication in the previous evening. When the caregiver returned to assist him with oral hygiene, she asked what happened to the mouthwash. She got the simple answer, "I swallowed it." The aide reported it, the patient was carefully monitored, and outside of severe **diuresis** was fortunately discharged with no other apparent side effects. This story illustrates the fact that one cannot be too careful in providing medications for hospitalized persons.

Internal medications (to be swallowed, ingested, or injected) and external medications (to be applied to the outside of the body or an adjoining orifice) should always be kept separate. These drugs are labeled differently. External preparations require a red, external use label. Black or another color is used for internal medications. Drugs labeled for topical use are also external preparations and usually carry a red-lettered label.

Ancillary labels should be carefully read and followed (e.g., "Shake well before using," "Refrigerate," "Do not refrigerate," "For external use only").

Medication Teaching

Patients and families knowledgeable about their drug regimes can be an important link in ensuring safe medication administration, understanding the individual therapeutic medication effect, attaining the intended medication effect, and limiting untoward effects. It is key that as part of the medication team, you consistently involve them in the medication process and provide them as much information as appropriate. Active participation and an individualized approach based on patient needs are the standard. Remember that patients will be administering their own medications upon discharge. Listen carefully to your patients and families during medication administration. If they question a medication or a dose, you need to double-check it with your supervisor. Many errors have been prevented by an astute patient or family member and there is the potential for anyone to make a mistake. The provision of medication information to patients and their families takes some preparation and planning. The patient's physician, pharmacist, and nurse are responsible for establishing the teaching need and priorities, developing the teaching plan, and evaluating learning outcomes. Your role as a pharmacy technician is to participate in this process as requested and appropriate. As you administer medications, you will learn helpful information that will be important to communicate to the care team. You will also have a unique opportunity to participate in the teaching process. Information on the patient's readiness to learn, education level, best learning method (e.g., verbal, written, demonstration), and time available for teaching (i.e., expected discharge date) is needed to prepare to teach. It is always best to start with finding out what the patient knows and what the patient would like to know about the medications. There are many excellent sources of medication teaching materials and every hospital will have many resources available.

Readiness to Learn

With today's shorter lengths of stay, the best time for patient teaching may be a narrow window. Signs of readiness to learn include stable physical condition, pain control, patient alertness and the ability to concentrate for at least short periods of time, and patient interest in learning about medication. When the time frame available for teaching is particularly short, the teaching plan may include instruction done by others along the patient's "continuum of care," including long-term care facility staff, home care or visiting nurse, outpatient pharmacy, and family.

Age and Education Level

Age, developmental level, and educational level will all be considered as a teaching plan is formulated by the nurse or pharmacist. Age and years of schooling alone may not be the only guides to how to deliver information, but they do provide a starting point. When the patient's education has been of a basic level, it is best to address the teaching at an eighth-grade level. In many parts of the country, significant numbers of patients cannot read at all or have a very limited ability. Generally, patients will not share this type of information and do well covering up their limitations. It is a good rule of thumb to avoid the use of scientific or medical terminology and give examples to support and reinforce learning. Take clues from the patient; this is ultimately the best guide on patient understanding, application, and retention. Examples of teaching approaches based on developmental stages are as follows:

- ask adolescents if they want parents present during the teaching session
- provide the elderly patient with memory aids such as medication calendars or pill boxes
- let preschoolers handle and play with equipment before a procedure

Learning Method

How a person learns is a complex and individual process, but learning is facilitated when a number of methods and senses are involved. A good plan includes the methods of instruction. These may include a combination of the following: written materials, verbal instruction, demonstration, providing examples, video or audio tapes, and a question and answer session. Information is best absorbed when given over a period of time (e.g., give written material to the patient to read in the morning and return later in the day to discuss the information and answer questions). Many patients now have access to the Internet at home, and they can be given hospital or general Web sites that include patient educational materials on medication. Clear discharge instructions, medication information leaflets, and providing a number for the patient to call with questions after discharge are all standard ways to reinforce valuable information given to the patient under the stressful circumstances of illness, hospital discharge, or transfer to another facility.

Teaching Plan

The patient's nurse or pharmacist in collaboration with the physician will develop the teaching plan. Formation of a teaching plan focuses on the needs of the patient and the information to be taught. The plan will include learning objectives stated as outcome objectives (i.e., what the patient will learn by the completion of instruction). Objectives should be practical, achievable, and measurable. Include the patient's objectives in the plan when possible. Examples of teaching and learning objectives are as follows:

- The patient will be able to list three signs of digitalis toxicity that require physician notification.
- The patient will describe rotation of sites for insulin injection.
- The patient's son will demonstrate correct insulin injection technique.

Objectives provide a basis for evaluating the effectiveness for teaching. The ultimate objective is that the patient has the information and skill necessary for safe medication administration.

Teaching Process

When you participate in the teaching process, it is desirable to select the most suitable and comfortable location to provide instruction. A comfortable location with limited distractions will allow the patient to concentrate on the information and ask questions. Prior to initiating teaching, the teaching plan and the objectives should be reviewed. After, it is important to communicate what you covered with the patient to the other team members and ensure it is documented. At least two methods of instruction are recommended to improve understanding and retention.

When possible, provide the patient with written material from a patient teaching text, from a computerized program, or from the instructor. When a preprinted text is used, it needs to be reviewed for content, education level, size of type, and so forth prior to giving it to the patient. Teaching of complex information is generally done by the physician, nurse, or pharmacist and should be given in more than one session. The definition of "complex" information will vary according to the patient, but learning that requires cognitive and psychomotor capabilities is considered "complex." Examples of complex learning include self-injection, taking radial pulse prior to cardiac medication, and taking a child's temperature. In each of the situations, the patient or family members need to have information on the reason for the procedure, the skill or procedure, and what action they are to take based on the results, such as a radial pulse of 45 per minute or a temperature of 102°F. When participating in teaching complex information, a second or third teaching session should be scheduled to provide the patient an opportunity to absorb the information, formulate questions, and give a return demonstration as indicated.

Reinforcement

Provide patients with praise and encouragement during their learning process. Describe their progress in terms of readiness for discharge, self-independence, accomplishment of a skill, or being knowledgeable about their medication.

Evaluation of Learning

Since the ultimate goal of the teaching process is to effect learning and change behavior, the evaluation of learning is the final stage of the teaching/learning process. According to the nature of the information, the evaluation method may include a short written test, requesting the patient verbally state the information, or giving a return demonstration (e.g., taking a pulse).

Professional Responsibility for Drug Administration

Drug administration is the shared privilege and responsibility of different health disciplines, each one with carefully delineated functional activities. Medication administration is just one part of the medication process, which includes prescribing, dispensing, administering, monitoring, and systems and management control. Physician's delegates, such as physician assistants and nurse practitioners, have the responsibility to prescribe rational and selective drug therapy, dependent upon the patient's medical profile and the drug's therapeutic characteristics.

The pharmacists are responsible to screen these orders for rationality and appropriateness in particular, individualized cases. In some instances, the pharmacist is invited to participate in the multidisciplinary planning of a particular patient's drug regimen. The pharmacist evaluates the choice of drug for a particular pathology, and if doubt arises, the physician is contacted. Further consideration is given to the drug dose, the time intervals between cases, and the patient's past drug history regarding allergies, drug sensitivities, and past untoward drug reactions. The pharmacist further considers the drug benefit/risk ratio regarding the possibility of a drug-drug interaction, a drug-food interaction, or a drug-laboratory test interaction. If there is apparent serious drug risk involvement, the pharmacist further consults with the physician regarding appropriate drug administration. If the pharmacist evaluates the regimen to be within the bounds of sound therapy, the drug is dispensed, for an inpatient, through the nursing service in most situations. If the pharmacy completely controls the drug-usage process, a medication technician may then assume the final responsibility for proper drug administration. However, in most institutions, the nursing department in collaboration with the pharmacy department is responsible for the final step in the drug-usage process (i.e., administration of the drug and observation of the patient regarding the therapeutic outcome of the drug action). According to hospital policy, the task of actually giving the medication to a patient may be delegated to a technical assistant or trained medication technician. Yet the responsibility of the drug's outcome remains with the licensed health professionals involved. Basically, the right drug, for the right reason, must be given to the right patient at the right time in the right dosage strength and in the right drug dosage form.

This is the core responsibility of the drug administration process. Responsibility for the outcome is shared by the professionals of medicine, nursing, and pharmacy.

Legal Responsibilities in Drug Administration

Many states and many health care institutions have very specific policies and procedures that must be carried out exactly as written. Presently, many states require a registered nurse to administer all medications. At the same time, other states and health institutions, due to fiscal, technical, personnel, and patient loads, are changing or modifying existing regulations. Basic requirements do not change, even if the assigned or designated personnel change.

Every hospital is required to have a policy and procedural manual to ensure patient safety and patient care. It is necessary that these policies and procedures be known and observed by the persons involved in drug administration activities. When medication errors are made, they are usually related to the patient's five rights. To prove negligence, it must be established that drug administration policy was not followed, careless shortcuts were taken, or the medication order and administration procedure were not adequately checked by the responsible licensed professional.

For many years, health care has assumed a myth of infallibility. Errors have been underreported and covered up. Given the dramatic increase in prescription drugs, the toxicity of many medications, and the fact that health care professionals are human and do make mistakes, errors are a reality. Fortunately, most medication errors do not harm patients. The current thinking is that much will be gained in error reduction by refocusing from a culture of blame to one of systems improvement. The systems improvement approach recognizes that there are conditions and environments in which humans are more likely to err and that those conditions can be modified to reduce error. By having more errors and near misses reported, and by conducting studies to improve those environments, medication systems can be rewired for error prevention. Where do you fit in medication error prevention?

- Be aware of the risk and reality of medication errors. It is unrealistic to believe you will never be involved in an error.
- Report all errors and near misses consistently based on your hospital's policies and procedures.
- Utilize medication resources and attend inservices. Recognize it is no longer possible to be knowledgeable on every medication—there are just too many new drugs and too much new information constantly available.

- Know your patient's allergies.
- Be alert to high-risk medications, safe medication practices, and specific safety protocols.
- Recognize the role certain practices have in errors: illegible handwriting, trailing zeros, leading decimal points, abbreviations, use of the abbreviation "u" for units, etc.
- Practice meticulous medication administration practices such as identification of every patient every time, stating the drug-dose-reason for every drug every time, and always listening to patients and families.
- Provide information to patients and families and facilitate their active involvement in care.
- Participate in performance improvement activities, the implementation of computerized medication systems, and other medication safety improvements.

Adequate patient drug-use control, drug-use evaluation, and drug-use surveillance must be top priorities to ensure patient safety. Detected errors must be reported immediately to the licensed supervisor.

The goal of the performance improvement process is to identify individual and system problems which, if corrected, will help to avoid future errors.

Trends in Drug Administration

Drug administration methods are frequently called drug-delivery systems. Drug firms have made large investments in researching and developing new methods to target drug administration dosage forms to maximize effectiveness and to limit unwanted systemic effects. The future may see pharmacy technicians specializing in the maintenance, utilization, and monitoring of these new and often unique devices and drug administration delivery systems.

If contemporary trends, particularly the working definition for pharmaceutical care, continue to prevail, pharmacy technicians of the future may require the knowledge, judgment, techniques, and skills to participate in the health care team as competent pharmacy medication technicians.

Summary

The administration of medication is a serious responsibility, requiring the possession of clinical information and skills. It includes not only information about the drugs being given, but also the proper procedures for safe administration, communication with team members, and documentation. Skills in administration ensure that the patient receives medication in the safest and most therapeutic manner with the least chance of mistakes, untoward reactions, or spread of infection.

TEST YOUR KNOWLEDGE

Multiple Choice Questions

1. The drug administration process begins with
    a. the physician's prescription
    b. the pharmacist dispensing the drug
    c. the nurse evaluating the patient
    d. the technician's assignment
    e. the request for a drug

2. Medication orders include
    a. drugs ordered by the physician after medical rounds
    b. telephone drug orders in emergencies
    c. standing drug orders for particular patient categories
    d. STAT orders to be immediately administered
    e. all of the above

3. A prn drug is administered
    a. routinely
    b. at night before sleep
    c. before meals
    d. when the patient's condition requires it
    e. immediately

4. Patient rights include
    a. right drug
    b. right time
    c. right dosage strength
    d. right route/dosage form
    e. all of the above

5. Prior to administering a drug, the medication technician should
    a. check the patient's correct identification
    b. check the drug against the order three times
    c. leave the medication in the unit dose package
    d. tell the patient what drug is to be administered
    e. all of the above

6. A drug may be left at the patient's bedside if
    a. the patient requests that the drug be left
    b. the patient is asleep
    c. the patient is in X-ray
    d. the patient wants to discuss the drug with the pharmacist
    e. none of the above

7. At least four ounces of water should be given following the drug administration of
    a. a buccal tablet
    b. a medicated mouthwash
    c. an aspirin tablet
    d. cough syrup
    e. a sublingual tablet

8. Sufficient water given after administration of a solid oral dosage form
   a. assists the patient in swallowing
   b. prevents esophageal irritation
   c. aids drug solubility
   d. all of the above
   e. none of the above

9. After administration of eyedrops, the patient should be advised to
   a. not move the head
   b. not to sneeze
   c. close the eye(s) for a few minutes
   d. immediately wipe away any tears
   e. stay in a darkened room

10. Transdermal drug patches are placed
    a. on the upper arm or inside forearm
    b. below the knee
    c. directly above the wrists
    d. on the most accessible spot
    e. where directed by patient

11. Outcomes of the performance improvement process for medication errors include
    a. identifying problems in the medication administration process
    b. determining the need for staff education
    c. reducing the possibility of future errors
    d. all of the above
    e. none of the above

12. When administering an enteric-coated medication to a child or geriatric patient, the administrator may take the following action(s):
    a. give crushed in applesauce
    b. dissolve in water
    c. give with sufficient juice
    d. give sublingually
    e. none of the above

True/False Questions

13. _____ Drug administration requires a physician's or other authorized prescriber's drug order.

14. _____ If a person appears to be in serious distress, the medication technician selects a drug to bring relief.

15. _____ Any unusual or newly occurring physical or mental change observed by the medication technician should be reported promptly to the supervising nurse.

16. _____ Patient confidentiality regarding drugs, disease, and other personal and clinical matters is a responsibility of the medication technician.

17. _____ If a drug is not available as ordered as a capsule, the medication technician may substitute a tablet with the same active ingredient or strength.

18. _____   All drug discrepancies and errors must be immediately reported to the supervising nurse or pharmacist.

Matching Questions

19. _____   ointment   a.   internal drug

20. _____   topical preparation   b.   external drug

21. _____   tablet

22. _____   elixir

23. _____   intramuscular injection

References

Gourley, D. R., Wedemweyer, H. F., & Norvell, M. (1992). Administration of medications. In T. R. Brown & M. C. Smith (Eds.), *Handbook of institutional pharmacy practice* (3rd ed). Baltimore: Williams & Wilkins.

16 Drug Information Centers

COMPETENCIES

Upon completion of this chapter, the reader should be able to

1. Describe and perform the steps of the systematic approach to answering a drug information question.
2. Describe the characteristics of tertiary, secondary, and primary resources.
3. Differentiate between reputable and questionable Internet Web sites.
4. Identify useful tertiary resources and Internet Web sites.
5. List and describe the responsibilities of the pharmacy technician working in a drug information center.
6. Explain the qualities and skills that a pharmacy technician must have to contribute significantly to the functions of a drug information center.

Introduction

Pharmacy practice has evolved significantly over the centuries. Traditionally, pharmacy practice was focused primarily on compounding and dispensing medications. This changed in the 1850s when mass-manufacturers of drug products reduced the need for pharmacists to compound drugs. In the 1930s, 75% of prescriptions required compounding. This number dwindled down to every 1 in 100 prescriptions in the 1970s. Although the pharmacists' dispensing activities continued, pharmacy practice gradually changed to view the pharmacist as a source of reputable drug information and as an essential health care professional who assists in improving patient outcomes (i.e., pharmaceutical care). The need for pharmacists to provide drug information started the movement toward the concept of clinical pharmacy in the 1960s. Physicians and other health care professionals became so overwhelmed with high patient loads and by the rapidly increasing number of new drug products that they turned to pharmacists to provide them with sound, reliable, and unbiased drug information. Today the provision of drug information continues to be the most essential responsibility of all pharmacists. Pharmacy technicians, regardless of the setting in which they work, can assist the pharmacist in the provision of reliable drug information. This chapter will introduce the pharmacy technician to the area of drug information practice and will outline the pharmacy technician's role in this growing field. State laws and regulations describing the activities that can be delegated by the pharmacist to the pharmacy technician should always be reviewed and followed. The contents of this chapter may or may not be in compliance with all states' laws and regulations and, therefore, technicians are strongly encouraged to be knowledgeable of their state's laws and regulations.

Drug Information Specialists

Although all pharmacists are responsible for providing drug information, some pharmacists have chosen to undergo extensive training and specialization in the field of drug information practice. These pharmacists are referred to as drug information specialists. Drug information specialists have sophisticated knowledge of drug information resources, strong literature evaluation, problem solving, and analytical skills, advanced technical capabilities, and are effective communicators of verbal and written drug information. The responsibilities of a drug information specialist are outlined in the American Society of Health-System Pharmacists (ASHP) Guidelines in the "Provision of Medication Information by Pharmacists" section. The pharmacy technician should be familiar with these guidelines prior to working in a drug information center (DIC). One can find these guidelines for free on the ASHP's Web site (www.ashp.org).

Drug Information Centers

Drug information specialists usually work in drug information centers. The first drug information center was established in 1962 at the University of Kentucky Medical Center. Ever since then, the number of drug information centers has increased significantly across the United States. The purposes of a drug information center vary and depend on the practice setting in which the drug information center is located. A DIC is most commonly located in a hospital, academic institution, or pharmaceutical company. Since a pharmacy technician will most likely work in a hospital or academic setting, the information provided in this chapter will pertain predominantly to these settings.

A function common to all drug information centers is the handling of drug information requests. Requests can be received via the telephone, e-mail, regular mail, and in person. Requestors of information can be physicians, nurses, other pharmacists, and consumers or patients. The drug information specialist is required to obtain background information of a drug information request, extensively research the request, develop a response to the request, and communicate the response accurately. A systematic approach to answering drug information requests is used and described later in this chapter. The pharmacy technician working in a drug information center needs to be familiar with this systematic approach to assist the drug information specialist in performing daily operations of the center.

Other functions of a drug information center include, but are not limited to, the provision of education through lectures and newsletters, development of policies or guidelines for appropriate use of medications, provision of formulary management and quality assurance activities, and coordination of adverse drug reaction and medication error programs. Pharmacy technicians are instrumental in helping the drug information specialist perform all of the above activities.

Definition of Drug Information

The term *drug information* simply means information pertaining to drugs. This is an over-simplistic general definition and demonstrates how this term can mean just about anything. Drug information can be patient-specific in the process of providing pharmaceutical care or population-based. Patient-specific drug information most often involves the drug information specialist providing recommendations based on patient-specific information such as age, race, weight, height, past medical history, medication history, and lab values. Population-based drug information involves researching and evaluating drug information as it relates to patients in general. When providing population-based information, the drug information specialist focuses on the general use of a drug in a group of patients and not in an individual patient.

The Systematic Approach to Answering a Drug Information Question

The pharmacy technician working in a drug information center should have an understanding of the systematic approach to answering a drug information question originated by Watanabe and colleagues in 1975. The systematic approach was later modified to involve a total of seven steps:

1. determine the demographics of the requestor
2. obtain background information
3. determine and categorize the ultimate question
4. develop a search strategy and conduct search
5. evaluate, analyze, and summarize the information obtained
6. formulate and provide response, and
7. conduct follow-up and document the question from beginning to end.

Requestor Demographics

Usually requestors of information call and immediately provide you with an initial question. One should proceed by quickly writing down the initial question and then asking the requestor's full name (first names alone are not sufficient), profession, specialty, address, phone numbers, fax numbers, and any other contact information thought necessary. Understanding the requestor's profession or specialty is important in determining the depth and complexity of information needed. For example, a physician's question would most often require extensive research and a very detailed response while a consumer's inquiry could usually be answered rapidly without as much extensive research. In addition, when communicating with a consumer, it is necessary to use lay terms to ensure that the consumer understands the information provided. A pharmacy technician may perform the first step of documenting the information obtained on a drug information request documentation form (**Figure 16-1**) and should then arrange for the drug information specialist to perform the next step of obtaining background information, especially if the question appears to be of an urgent nature or of high complexity.

Background Information

Obtaining background information is the most important step in the systematic approach and requires effective communication and listening skills. To perform this

Date: _____ Time: _____ Received by: _____

Requestor's Demographics

Name: _____ Hospital Location: _____

Affiliation: _____

Address: _____
Street address

_____
City   State   Zip

Profession:
MD   RPh   PharmD   RN   PhD
Consumer/Patient

Specialty _____
Other _____

Phone Number: (   )   -   Fax Number: (   )   -

Pager Number: (   )   -   E-mail Address:

Background Information:

Patient Specific?   Yes   No   If yes, fill out below:
MR#_____ **Location:** _____ **Gender:** Female   Male **Age:**_____
Height: _____ **Weight:** _____ **Allergies:** _____
Relevant PMH / HPI / Diagnosis (including organ fxn):

Medications:

Initial Question:

Ultimate Question:

Classification of Request:

Product Availability   Compatibility/Stability   Reference Material
Pharmacokinetics   Dosage/Administration   Drug Interactions
Adverse Reactions/Toxicity   CAM/Dietary Supplements   Product Identification
Pregnancy/Lactation/Repro   Therapeutic Use   Compounding
Other _____

Urgency of Response: STAT   Other _____
Method of Request: Phone   In Person   E-mail   3rd Person   Other

FIGURE 16-1 Drug Information Request Documentation Form.

Actual Response Provided (attach continuation of response and support materials if necessary)**:**

All References Used (indicate whether information found or not)**:**

Response Information

Date: _____Time:_____   Verbal   Written

Answered by: _____ Approved by: _____

Response given via: Phone   Letter   In Person   Fax   E-mail   Other

Total time needed to complete request: _____

FIGURE 16-1   Drug Information Request Documentation Form (continued).

step well, an extensive knowledge base is needed of different medical conditions and medications. This step should be performed by the drug information specialist. If this step is not performed appropriately, serious consequences may occur in that inaccurate information may be provided and valuable time may be wasted. During this step, the drug information specialist will determine if the request is patient-specific or population-based and will proceed to ask important relevant questions to determine the ultimate question. Pharmacy technicians with extensive experience working in a drug information center may also perform this step if the question is deemed not urgent or is easily understood by the technician. An experienced technician will be able to use judgment to determine whether the question needs the attention of the drug information specialist. The experienced technician must demonstrate effective listening, communication, and interviewing skills to perform this step. The technician must also know what pertinent patient-specific information must be collected to allow for the drug information specialist to answer the request.

Determination and Categorization of the Ultimate Question

Determining the ultimate question is accomplished easily once sufficient background information is obtained. Often the initial question differs significantly from the ultimate or final question. Once the ultimate question is identified and clear, the pharmacy technician or the drug information specialist can then quickly categorize the request and the next step can begin. The question should be categorized by type. For example, the question can be categorized as a drug interaction question or a drug identification question. For a list of possible categories of drug information questions, see the drug information request documentation form in Figure 16-1. Categorization of the request is important in that it helps direct one to the resources that would best answer the question (e.g., a drug interaction textbook).

Search Strategy and Information Collection

The pharmacy technician can contribute significantly to the development of a search strategy and collection of pertinent information. The technician must first develop a search strategy starting with general resources (tertiary resources) and work towards more specific resources (primary resources) through use of indexing and abstracting services (secondary resources). These three different types of resources will be described later in this chapter. The experienced technician should be able to identify when a search through secondary and primary resources is needed for a given question (e.g., physician inquiry, detailed question) and when tertiary resources would be sufficient to answer the question (e.g., consumer or nurse inquiry, general question). The pharmacy technician must have good knowledge of all the resources available to answer drug information questions in the drug information center, in the affiliated medical library (if applicable), and on the Internet.

The technician must also be proficient in conducting literature searches, using computerized databases, and in the proper use of print resources. Once the necessary resources have been consulted and the information collected, the technician should then promptly provide this information to the drug information specialist for evaluation. The pharmacy technician must also remember to anticipate other questions that must be answered to provide a complete response. For example, if a requestor of information needs the drug of choice to treat a patient's community-acquired pneumonia, the drug name will most likely not be sufficient to completely answer the request. The drug dosing regimen, route of administration, duration of therapy, monitoring parameters, common side effects, and potential drug interactions would be additional information needed by the requestor, although the requestor did not specifically ask for it.

Evaluation, Analysis, and Synthesis of Information

This step requires strong literature evaluation skills and, therefore, should be left to the drug information specialist. Knowledge of study design, research, and statistical concepts is essential to be able to evaluate the medical literature and apply the information to clinical practice and patient-specific situations.

Formulate and Provide Response

After careful analysis and synthesis of information, the drug information specialist will formulate a response and then accurately convey the response back to the requestor of information. This requires strong verbal and written communication skills. If a written response is required, the pharmacy technician may assist in drafting and referencing the response. However, ultimately the drug information specialist must review the written response for accuracy and completeness.

Follow-up and Documentation

The pharmacy technician can assist in following up on all completed requests to determine whether the information provided was appropriate, recommendations provided were actually followed, and if the response was adequate to meet the requestor's needs. This process ensures and documents the quality of services provided by the drug information center. The pharmacy technician is also responsible for assisting in the appropriate documentation of all requests from beginning to end and should make sure all references used were properly documented on the drug information request documentation form.

Drug Information Resources

One of the technician's primary responsibilities in a drug information center is controlling the inventory of all resources in the drug information center. Resources should be stored in an organized fashion and kept up-to-date. The technician is also responsible for ordering references, keeping track of subscription expiration dates, and ensuring that ordered resources are actually received by the drug information center. The technician is also responsible for maintaining a filing system of important information for easy and rapid access by all drug information center personnel.

The pharmacy technician should also have knowledge of all the available resources in the drug information center, in nearby medical libraries (if applicable), and on the Internet. The technician must be proficient in the retrieval of drug information whether it be from the shelves of a library or from a computerized database. The technician will also assist in the printing and photocopying of necessary information.

The experienced technician should also be able to differentiate between reputable resources and those of questionable quality. There are three different types of drug information resources: (1) tertiary, (2) secondary, and (3) primary resources. Each type has advantages and disadvantages that the pharmacy technician should be able to describe and keep in mind when researching drug information requests.

Tertiary Resources

A list of tertiary resources (i.e., general resources) is provided in **Table 16-1**. Tertiary resources are textbooks, compendia, computer databases, and review articles. These resources are best if peer-reviewed, authored by an expert in the field the resource pertains to, and easy to navigate. Some compendia, such as the American Hospital Formulary Service and Drug Facts and Comparisons, are not peer-reviewed but are still considered very valuable and reputable resources of drug information. Tertiary resources can allow for rapid comprehensive access to information, are commonly consulted when initiating a search strategy, and are usually used to educate oneself on a medical condition or medication.

One of the significant disadvantages of tertiary resources is that they are usually somewhat out of date by the time they are published. This is due to the significant amount of time that elapses between when the resource is written and when it is actually published (i.e., long lag time). Therefore, one must always take into account the resource's date of publication when using it for drug information. Review articles published in journals and certain references published in updateable binder format (e.g., *Drug Facts and Comparisons*) do not have as significant a lag time. Also, one must keep in mind that the information provided in a tertiary resource is subject to the author's interpretation of the primary literature (i.e., original research) on the topic. Sometimes the author's opinion may not necessarily be accurate or complete. Since tertiary resources are general resources, they usually lack specific details, forcing the reader to conduct further research of the primary literature for more information.

Secondary Resources

Secondary resources are indexing and abstracting services such as MEDLINE (www.pubmed.gov), International Pharmaceutical Abstracts (IPA), Iowa Drug Information Service (IDIS), EMBASE (European Medline), and Journal Watch. Secondary resources are usually available electronically and quickly link the reader to the primary literature. The pharmacy technician must undergo training in properly searching secondary resources such as MEDLINE and IPA. This training will allow the technician to perform appropriate literature searches and identify useful information. The drug information specialist may either train the pharmacy technician on the proper use of secondary resources or inform the pharmacy technician of available educational programs. It is important to understand that each secondary resource indexes different journals and meeting abstracts; therefore, it is often necessary to search more than one secondary resource to perform a thorough literature search. Some secondary resources can be expensive to subscribe to (e.g., IPA, IDIS) while others are free (e.g., MEDLINE).

Primary Resources

Primary resources are the primary literature which includes original research articles published in journals such as the *Annals of Pharmacotherapy, American Journal of Hospital Pharmacy*, and the *Journal of the American Medical Association*. The primary literature also includes descriptive patient case reports, observational studies (i.e., cohort, case-control, cross-sectional studies), and experimental studies (i.e., clinical trials, crossover trials).

The primary literature is the most current source of information and provides a very detailed description of a study (i.e., objective, methods, statistics, results, and conclusion). This allows the reader to make his or her own evaluation and interpretation of the study, compare it to the results of other studies, and apply the

TABLE 16-1 Tertiary Resources Listed by Information Provided

Adverse Drug Reactions

Davies's *Textbook of Adverse Drug Reactions*

Meyler's *Side Effects of Drugs*

Compatibility and Stability Resources

King's *Guide to Parenteral Admixtures*

Trissel's *Handbook of Injectable Drugs*

Complementary and Alternative Medicine

AltMedDEX System published by Micromedex

The Complete German Commission E Monographs

Natural Medicine Comprehensive Database (www.naturaldatabase.com)

PDR for Herbal Medicines

The Review of Natural Products

Tyler's *Herbs of Choice*

Tyler's *Honest Herbal*

Compounding

Allen's *The Art, Science, and Technology of Pharmaceutical Compounding*

Allen's *Compounded Formulations: The Complete U.S. Pharmacist Collection*

Trissel's *Stability of Compounded Formulations*

Drug Availability

American Drug Index

Drug Facts and Comparisons

Drug Topics Red Book

Drug Identification

Ident-A-Drug Reference

IDENTIDEX System published by Micromedex

Drug Information and Literature Evaluation

Ascione's *Principles of Scientific Literature Evaluation: Critiquing Clinical Drug Trials*

De Muth's *Basic Statistics and Pharmaceutical Statistical Applications*

Malone's *Drug Information: A Guide for Pharmacists*

Riegelman's *Studying a Study and Testing a Test: How to Read the Medical Evidence*

Snow's *Drug Information: A Guide to Current Resources*

Drug Interaction Resources

Drug Interaction Facts

DRUG-REAX System by Micromedex

Hansten and Horn's *Drug Interaction Analysis and Management*

Foreign Drugs

European Drug Index

Index Nominum: International Drug Directory

Martindale: *The Complete Drug Reference*

USP Dictionary of United States Adopted Names (USAN) and International Drug Names

TABLE 16-1 Tertiary Resources Listed by Information Provided (continued)

General Drug Information References

American Hospital Formulary Service (AHFS) Drug Information

Drug Facts and Comparisons

Drug Information Handbook by Lexi-Comp Inc.

DRUGDEX System published by Micromedex

Mosby's GenRx

Physicians' Desk Reference (PDR)

Remington: *The Science and Practice of Pharmacy*

USP DI Volumes I (health care professional), II (patient), and III (legal requirements)

Geriatric Resources

Brocklehurst's *Textbook of Geriatric Medicine and Gerontology*

Geriatric Dosage Handbook by Lexi-Comp Inc.

The Merck Manual of Geriatrics

Immunology

Concepts in Immunology and Immunotherapeutics

ImmunoFacts

Infectious Disease

Mandell, Douglas, and Bennett's *Principles and Practice of Infectious Diseases*

Internal Medicine

Cecil's *Textbook of Medicine*

Conn's *Current Therapy*

Harrison's *Principles of Internal Medicine*

The Merck Manual of Diagnosis and Therapeutics

Laboratory Data Interpretation

Laboratory Test Handbook

Traub's *Basic Skills in Interpreting Laboratory Data*

Medical Dictionaries

Davies's Medical Abbreviations

Dorland's Illustrated Medical Dictionary

Stedman's Medical Dictionary

Nephrology

Drug Prescribing in Renal Failure: Dosing Guidelines for Adults

Nonprescription Products

Handbook of Nonprescription Drugs

PDR for Nonprescription Drugs and Dietary Supplements

Oncology/Hematology

DeVita's *Cancer: Principles and Practice of Oncology*

Dorr's *Cancer Chemotherapy Handbook*

Hoffman's *Hematology: Basic Principles and Practices*

Pediatric Resources

Nelson's *Textbook of Pediatrics*

Neofax

Pediatric Dosage Handbook by Lexi-Comp Inc.

Teddy Bear Book: Pediatric Injectable Drugs

Pharmaceutical Calculations

Stoklosa and Ansel's *Pharmaceutical Calculations*

Zatz's *Pharmaceutical Calculations*

Pharmacokinetics

Applied Pharmacokinetics: Principles of Therapeutic Drug Monitoring

Winter's *Basic Clinical Pharmacokinetics*

Pharmacology and Therapeutics

DiPiro's *Pharmacotherapy: A Pathophysiologic Approach*

Goodman and Gilman's *The Pharmacological Basis of Therapeutics*

Koda Kimble's *Applied Therapeutics: The Clinical Use of Drugs*

Melmon and Morrelli's *Clinical Pharmacology*

Pharmacy Law

Pharmacy Law Digest

Reproduction, Pregnancy, and Breastfeeding

Briggs's *Drugs in Pregnancy and Lactation*

Chemically Induced Birth Defects

REPRORISK System published by Micromedex

Shepard's *Catalog of Teratogenic Agents*

Toxicology

Casarett and Doull's *Toxicology: The Basic Science of Poisons*

Clinical Toxicology of Commercial Products

Ellenhorn's *Medical Toxicology: Diagnosis and Treatment of Human Poisoning*

Goldfrank's *Toxicologic Emergencies*

Material Safety Data Sheets (MSDS) from the USP

POISONDEX System published by Micromedex

TOMES System published by Micromedex

Veterinary Medicine

Merck Veterinary Manual

study results to patients encountered in practice. Excellent literature evaluation skills are necessary to critically evaluate each study and to be able to apply it to clinical practice. It often requires a significant amount of time to collect pertinent primary literature and evaluate all the primary literature on a particular topic.

The Internet

A discussion on drug information practice would not be complete without a discussion of the Internet and how it changed the provision of drug information. You may find tertiary (e.g., most Web sites), secondary (e.g., MEDLINE, Internet subscriptions to computerized databases), and primary literature (i.e., electronic full-text articles) on the Internet. Medication package inserts can be downloaded easily off the Internet (e.g., a package insert for metformin may be easily found at www.glucophage.com). The Internet allows for rapid and easy access to a wealth of information. It may help save space in the drug information center by allowing for electronic subscriptions. It also allows for rapid dissemination of important information to others through e-mail.

One must, however, be cautious when using the Internet for drug information. Anyone can create a Web site and many Web sites may provide false or misleading information. Each site providing drug or medical information must be carefully evaluated for reliability and accuracy. More reliable sites should provide balanced information (benefits and risks of medications), author's qualifications and expertise, protection of patient confidentiality, references, date information provided was last revised, and contact information for the site's creator. The funding sources of the site should be clearly stated so one can identify any possible conflicts of interest. In general, Web sites that sell products or advertise products are more likely to provide biased information. Even if a site provides all the above stated information, professional judgment and knowledge must always be used to determine whether information provided on the site is accurate and reliable. A list of reputable Web sites including governmental sites that are of good reputation and can be used for drug information with more confidence is provided in **Table 16-2.** Pharmacy technicians should always encourage patients to consult a health care professional prior to following any medical advice obtained from a Web site.

Necessary Skills for the Pharmacy Technician

In order to work in a drug information practice setting, the pharmacy technician must have effective communication and listening skills, should be able to properly pronounce medical and technical terms, and should be able to communicate on a level that is appropriate to the requestor. The technician must have a strong knowledge base of medical conditions, medications, resources, and strong research and technical capabilities. The technician must follow all ethical principles and behave in a courteous, professional, and caring manner.

The pharmacy technician is also expected to stay current with advances in pharmacy practice. The technician should participate in the drug information center's methods for staying current (e.g., journal clubs, educational conferences, continuing education, journal circulation).

TABLE 16-2

Useful Web Sites

Governmental Sites

Agency for Healthcare Research and Quality (*www.ahrq.gov*)

Centers for Disease Control and Prevention (*www.cdc.gov*)

Food and Drug Administration (*www.fda.gov*)

■ MedWatch Progam (*www.fda.gov/medwatch*)

National Guideline Clearinghouse (*www.guidelines.gov*)

National Institutes of Health (*www.nih.gov*)

■ ClinicalTrials.gov (*www.clinicaltrials.gov*)

■ National Center for Complementary and Alternative Medicine (*http://nccam.nih.gov*)

■ Office of Dietary Supplements (*http://ods.od.nih.gov*)

National Library of Medicine (*www.nlm.nih.gov*)

■ Directory of Health Organizations Online (*http://dirline.nlm.nih.gov*)

■ MEDLINEplus (*www.medlineplus.com*)

■ PubMed (*www.pubmed.gov*)

United States Pharmacopeia (*www.usp.org*)

Associations and Organizations

American Academy of Pediatrics (*www.aap.org*)

American Association of Colleges of Pharmacy (*www.aacp.org*)

American Association of Pharmacy Technicians (*www.pharmacytechnician.com*)

American Cancer Society (*www.cancer.org*)

American College of Clinical Pharmacy (*www.accp.com*)

American Council on Pharmaceutical Education (*www.acpe-accredit.org*)

American Diabetes Association (*www.diabetes.org*)

American Geriatrics Society (*www.americangeriatrics.org*)

American Heart Association (*www.americanheart.org*)

American Lung Association (*www.lungusa.com*)

American Medical Association (*www.ama-assn.org*)

American Pharmacists Association (*www.aphanet.org*)

American Society of Consultant Pharmacists (*www.ascp.com*)

American Society of Health-Systems Pharmacists (*www.ashp.org*)

American Society for Pharmacy Law (*www.aspl.org*)

Institute for Safe Medication Practices (*www.ismp.org*)

Joint Commission on Accreditation of Healthcare Organizations (*www.jcaho.org*)

National Association of Boards of Pharmacy (*www.nabp.net*)

National Association of Chain Drug Stores (*www.nacds.org*)

National Coordinating Council for Medication Error Reporting and Prevention (*www.nccmerp.org*)

Pharmacy Technician Certification Board (*www.ptcb.org*)

World Health Organization (*www.who.int*)

TABLE 16-2 Useful Web Sites (continued)

Other Miscellaneous Web Sites

CNN Health (*www.cnn.com/HEALTH*)

Doctor's Guide (*www.docguide.com*)

Health on the Net Foundation (*www.hon.ch*)

Medscape (*www.medscape.com*)

ReutersHealth (*www.reutershealth.com*)

RxList (*www.rxlist.com*)

WebMD (*www.webMD.com*)

Other Pharmacy Technician Responsibilities

In addition to the responsibilities already outlined in this chapter, the pharmacy technician is expected to assist in the supervision of pharmacy students or interns working at the center and collect statistics on the number of drug information requests received, the profession of the requestor using the drug information center, the type of questions asked, and the time spent answering questions on a monthly basis. The technician should maintain a filing system of old requests and a filing system of important information collected on medications or medical topics of interest to allow for rapid and easy access. In certain drug information centers where computerized databases are used to document and store drug information questions for subsequent easy retrieval, the technician can assist in maintaining and updating the database.

The pharmacy technician can help with compiling information to be published in a newsletter. A pharmacy technician with effective technological skills can help edit the newsletter to allow it to have a consistent appearance. The technician can also assist in the collection of data for research projects, adverse drug reactions, medication errors, quality assurance projects, and formulary management activities.

Summary

With the increasing complexity of information management and expanding responsibilities of the drug information specialist, pharmacy technicians are essential in assisting with the functions of a drug information center. In order for the pharmacy technician to assist in the daily operations of a drug information center, certain skills are required. The technician must become familiar with the many types of drug information resources available along with the reputability of such resources. Effective technical and communication skills are also necessary.

TEST YOUR KNOWLEDGE

Multiple Choice Questions

1. Place the following steps of the systematic approach to answering a drug information question in the order in which they should be performed.
   I.   Develop a search strategy and conduct search
   II.   Secure the demographics of the requestor
   III. Documentation and conduct follow-up
   IV.   Obtain background information
   V.   Formulate and provide a response
   VI.   Perform evaluation, analysis, and synthesis of information
   VII. Determine and categorize the ultimate question
   a. II, IV, VII, I, VI, V, III
   b. II, IV, VII, VI, I, V, III
   c. II, IV, VI, VII, V, I, III
   d. II, VII, IV, I, VI, V, III
   e. none of the above

2. Although all the steps of the systematic approach are important, which of the following steps is the most important?
   a. Secure the demographics of the requestor.
   b. Obtain background information.
   c. Formulate and provide a response.
   d. Perform evaluation, analysis, and synthesis of information.

3. Which of the following resources provides you with a general overview of a topic?
   a. tertiary resources
   b. secondary resources
   c. primary resources

4. Which of the following resources suffers the most from a long lag time (i.e., is somewhat outdated by the time it is published)?
   a. tertiary resources
   b. secondary resources
   c. primary resources

5. Which of the following statements regarding the use of the Internet for drug information are true?
   I.   Web sites that sell or advertise products are more likely to provide biased or misleading information.
   II.   Governmental Web sites are reputable and can be used for drug information with confidence.
   III. Patients should be encouraged to follow any medical advice obtained from a Web site without the need to consult with a health care professional.
   IV.   The Internet allows for rapid and easy access to a wealth of information and allows for rapid dissemination of information through e-mail.
   V.   You may find tertiary, secondary, and primary resources on the Internet.
   a. I, II, III, IV, V
   b. II, III
   c. I, II, IV, V
   d. III, V
   e. II, III, IV

6. More reputable Web sites should
   a. provide balanced information
   b. provide references
   c. provide the author's qualifications and expertise
   d. clearly state the Web site's funding source(s)
   e. all of the above

7. A useful tertiary resource to answer a drug information question on the safety of a certain medication during pregnancy is
   a. *American Drug Index*
   b. *Index Nominum*
   c. *Ident-A-Drug*
   d. *Brigg's Drugs in Pregnancy and Lactation*
   e. *Geriatric Dosage Handbook*

8. A useful tertiary resource to identify a medication is
   a. *American Drug Index*
   b. *Index Nominum*
   c. *Ident-A-Drug*
   d. *Brigg's Drugs in Pregnancy and Lactation*
   e. *Geriatric Dosage Handbook*

9. Which of the following is/are responsibilities of the pharmacy technician working at a drug information center?
   a. maintain a filing system
   b. maintain inventory of all informational resources held by the center
   c. perform literature searches
   d. retrieve drug information
   e. all of the above

10. Which of the following is/are necessary skills a pharmacy technician must possess to work effectively in a drug information center?
    a. effective verbal and written communication skills
    b. correct pronunciation of medical terms
    c. ethical and professional behavior
    d. strong knowledge base of medications and medical conditions
    e. all of the above

References

American Society of Health-System Pharmacists. (1996). ASHP guidelines on the provision of medication information by pharmacists. *American Journal of Hospital Pharmacy, 53,* 1843–1845.

Malone, P. M., Wilkinson Mosdell, K., Kier, K. L., & Stanovich, J. E. (2001). *Drug information: A guide for pharmacists* (2nd ed.). New York: McGraw-Hill.

Watanabe, A. S., & Conner, C. S. (1978). *Principles of drug information services: A syllabus of systematic concepts.* Hamilton, IL: Drug Intelligence Publications, Inc.

Watanabe, A. S., McGart, G., Shimomura, S., & Kayser, S. (1975). Systematic approach to drug information requests. *American Journal of Hospital Pharmacy 32*(12), 1282–1285.

17 Drug Distribution Systems

COMPETENCIES

Upon completion of this chapter, the reader should be able to

1. Outline the responsibility of the pharmacist and the role of the pharmacy technician in the various medication distribution functions.

2. Differentiate among the four major distribution systems.

3. Describe the purpose, functions, and advantages of the unit-dose drug distribution system.

4. Distinguish the main differences between a decentralized and a centralized drug distribution system.

5. Explain why the pharmacist must review a direct physician's order entry for a medication.

6. List the information that is included on a medication order.

7. Briefly explain the four methods by which a physician's original orders are directly transmitted to the pharmacy.

8. List the drug distribution activities that can be generated through computerization.

9. Describe various ways in which the pharmacy technician is directly involved in the computerization process.

10. List the checkpoints required by the pharmacist and by the pharmacy technicians when a physician's medication order is received in the pharmacy.

Introduction

Drug control, monitoring utilization, and assisting in the distribution of medications to patients are among the pharmacist's most important contributions to health care. With the advent of new regulations and the constantly changing health care system, methods of distributing and controlling drugs must undergo continuous re-evaluation and review. Only then can efficient systems that meet changing requirements be ensured. Advancing technology will permit the pharmacist to move from the traditional product-focused dispensing to that of a patient advocate and provider of clinical services. The pharmacist will assume a larger role in improved therapeutic outcomes in disease management. Greater efficiency and economy in disease therapy will be ensured.

The role of the technician in the area of dispensing and drug distribution is to assist the pharmacist. Technicians are an integral and important component of the health care team. However, the legal responsibility for dispensing still remains with the pharmacist.

After reviewing this chapter, the student should have a good understanding of drug distribution systems. The technician should be able to distinguish between the different types of distribution systems and clearly define the technician's role in each type of setting. This will allow the technician to actively participate in system planning and development.

Drug Distribution Systems

The Pharmacy and Therapeutics Committee is responsible for the development of broad policies and procedures that provide for the proper distribution of medications and pharmaceutical aids to patients. The drug distribution systems in use today are variations of four concepts: floor stock, patient prescription, combined floor stock and patient prescription, and unit-dose. Additional components of the drug distribution system are covered in other chapters of this manual and include intravenous admixtures, controlled drug distribution, and interdepartmental requisitions.

Floor Stock System

In the floor stock system of distribution, all medications are stocked on the nursing unit, with the possible exception of some rarely used or very expensive medications. Medications that require an expanded level of professional supervision and control, such as antineoplastic agents and antibiotics, may also be excluded from floor stock supplies. The nurse is totally responsible for all aspects of preparation and administration of medications. This is not the preferred drug distribution method for hospitals and long-term care facilities and should be strongly discouraged because of several inherent disadvantages:

- There is an increased potential for medication errors because a pharmacist does not review medication orders. Thus a nurse may select the wrong medication to administer from the vast array of drugs and dosage forms available.
- Economic loss may occur because of misappropriation or diversion by hospital personnel and lost medication charges. Expired, contaminated, and deteriorated drugs remaining on the unit may also mean loss and possible patient harm if administered from the floor stock supply.
- Increased drug inventory is necessary because of multiple inventories on each nursing unit. Thus drug inventory control is poor.
- Storage and control problems occur because of limited storage facilities on nursing units.

Individual Prescription System

In the individual prescription system, a multiple-day supply of each medication is dispensed for the patient upon receipt of prescriptions or orders. The nurse transcribes and prepares individual prescriptions or orders from the physician's original written order and forwards the request to the pharmacy for filling. Commonly, a three- to five-day supply is provided by the pharmacy. When the original supply is exhausted, the nurse prepares another request and the whole process is repeated. An enormous amount of time and manpower is required. Maintenance of drug containers by the nursing staff in an organized, easily accessible method is wasteful of nursing time. The pharmacy is usually responsible for charges and credits, which are individually entered into the patient's account or forwarded to the business office for processing. Altogether, much time is required of all participants. Although this system is an improvement over the floor stock system, it is not an efficient or practical method of drug distribution and is also not a preferred drug distribution method for hospitals or long-term care facilities.

Combined Floor Stock and Patient Prescription System

In the combined floor stock and patient prescription system of drug distribution, the primary method of dispensing is the individual prescription order supplemented with a limited number of floor stock items. This method possesses the benefits of both systems.

The floor stock items are generally over-the-counter medications (e.g., aspirin, acetaminophen, laxatives, vitamins) and selected controlled drug medications. Although this system is far superior to the previous two systems discussed, it also exhibits the disadvantages of both systems.

Unit-Dose Drug Distribution System

Unit-dose distribution represents a significant refinement of the individual prescription order system and is considered to be the safest, most economical method of distributing drugs in health care institutions. It is considered to be a hospital system, not simply a pharmacy system, because it involves many departments and disciplines in its planning, development, and operation.

The unit-dose has been preferred to the floor stock or individual system of drug distribution by federal government and non-federal regulatory agencies, including the Joint Commission on Accreditation of Healthcare Organizations (JCAHO), the Institute for Safe Medication Practices (ISMP), the Centers for Medicare and Medicaid Services (CMS), and state and local regulatory agencies. It has been proved to be the most effective drug distribution system available today. Following are the advantages of this type of system over the antiquated conventional approach:

- reduction in medication errors
- improved drug control
- decrease in the overall cost of medication distribution
- more precise medication billing
- reduction of medication credits
- reduced drug inventories throughout the institution

Numerous variations of unit-dose systems have been implemented throughout the world, but all share several common features. In all the systems, the nurse who administers the medication receives unit-dose packages of drugs from the pharmacy in a ready-to-administer form that requires no additional manipulation, measurement, or preparation.

A large- or small-volume injection may be considered a unit-dose, but it is not normally distributed in the same manner. Virtually all other medications can be dispensed as a unit-dose package, which is defined as containing the particular dose of the drug ordered for the patient. For example, a unit-dose liquid may contain from a fraction of a millimeter to 60 or more milliliters, but it is the exact amount ordered by the physician. A unit-dose of tablets or capsules may contain a fraction or one or more of a commercial dosage form, but it is the amount to be administered. A single-unit package contains one discrete form such as one tablet, 5 ml of liquid, or a prefilled syringe containing 25 mg in 1 ml. A single-unit package may be a unit-dose package if it contains the dose prescribed. In the event that dose prescribed and the dose sent vary, a *"Note Dosage Strength"* label may be helpful to alert the nursing staff of the difference.

Centralized Dispensing

In centralized dispensing systems, all activities required in the preparation and distribution of medications take place within the central pharmacy area.

Unit-dose medications are made available on the nursing floor one or more times daily, depending on the staff available and the logistics of moving supplies to and from the pharmacy and nursing locations. Patients' drugs are generally dispensed in amounts needed for the next 24 hours. In some institutions, nursing units are supplied twice or even three times daily. There may be many specific times during the day when drugs are scheduled to be administered to patients. In some cases, the pharmacy makes multiple drug deliveries each day to accommodate the need. Some drugs requiring special handling (e.g., antineoplastics, very expensive medications, items too large or unable to be safely sent in a pneumatic tube system) may be hand carried to the patient floor at the time of need.

The greatest number of technicians is usually involved in the unit-dose dispensing system. The technician assists in preparing all medication doses and fills the cabinets, carts, or cassettes. The technician utilizes the patient medication profile, which has been generated by either a manual or computerized system to prepare and deliver the medication to the patient care areas.

A pharmacist must check all medications before they are distributed to the patient care area. During this process, the pharmacist ensures that the correct drug and correct number of doses has been prepared. By visually inspecting the total drug supply for each patient, the pharmacist has another opportunity to confirm the absence of drug-drug interactions. The pharmacist is also able to assess the completeness of labeling, look for outdated supplies, and lastly, take full responsibility for the accuracy of the filling and distributing process.

Decentralized Dispensing

In a centralized system, all doses are prepared at a central location. In a decentralized system, the doses are prepared in a **satellite pharmacy** located in or near the nursing unit. The satellite may serve several nursing units or even one or more floors. Generally, the **centralized system** allows for somewhat greater management efficiency and control; the **decentralized system** allows closer pharmacist-physician-nurse-patient relationships. In addition, decentralization provides pharmacy services to the unit more quickly, accurately, and efficiently.

Physician's Original Order

Medications are dispensed only on the written order of a licensed physician or other licensed prescriber such as a physician's assistant, nurse practitioner, or dentist. The prescriber must also be certified by the institution as qualified to have privileges in the institution.

Basic Requirements of a Complete Medication Order

A medication order should be legible and include the following information:

■ patient's name, room number, and hospital number (the patient's age, weight, height, allergies, and gender should be included unless available in the patient's pharmacy profile)

■ name and strength of medication (the nonproprietary or generic name is preferred, although most physicians are inclined to utilize trade or brand names). Dosage strengths should always be written in the metric system (e.g., aspirin 325 mg, not aspirin 5 grains). Topical agents such as ointments, creams, ophthalmic solutions, and nasal solutions may have their strength expressed as a percentage.

■ intravenous solution orders, both large- and small-volume. Both should indicate the name and strength of each additive and the volume of the carrier or diluent with the flow rate or frequency (e.g., 125 ml/hr, q8h, over 24 hours).

■ route of administration (e.g., po, IM, IV, each eye, right ear)

■ frequency of administration (e.g., b.i.d., t.i.d., qhs, qam with meals)

It should be noted that when a prescriber verbally issues a medication order, only a pharmacist or a nurse can receive it; it cannot be received by a technician. The order should be immediately written on the medication order sheet (physician's order form) and should be noted as a telephone order (t.o.) or verbal order (v.o.). The physician is responsible for countersigning this order within 48 hours. It must be emphasized that only a pharmacist or a nurse is authorized to accept telephone or verbal orders.

Transmittal of Orders to Pharmacy

A multitude of methods are presently in use for obtaining the physician's order. The Joint Commission on Accreditation of Healthcare Organizations (JCAHO) and most state boards of pharmacy require that the pharmacy receive the physician's original prescription—or a copy of the original prescription—when filling medication orders. A direct copy of the order is most frequently utilized. This procedure eliminates transcription errors, which are a frequent source of medication errors. It is the pharmacist's responsibility to review, interpret, and evaluate the medication order.

Traditionally, the nurse was given the responsibility of transcribing the doctor's orders as written in the patient's chart onto a pharmacy order form. However, the more people involved in reviewing, evaluating, and transcribing an order, the greater the potential for error. By receiving a direct copy of the physician's original order, the pharmacist can review, clarify, and interpret the order, which is the pharmacist's legal and ethical responsibility. This process is now almost universally accomplished by the use of no-carbon-required (NCR) physician order forms. A direct copy of the original order is available and can easily be transmitted to the pharmacy for immediate processing. The orders may be hand-carried to the pharmacy or sent via a pneumatic tube system.

Electromechanical Systems

Several electronic methods are utilized to transmit orders from the nursing unit to the pharmacy. **Electrostatic copying machines** (photocopiers) and **facsimile transmitting equipment** (fax machines) can be used to copy or transmit orders. Evolution in technology has reduced paperwork by being able to transmit orders electronically from one computer to another. A physician is able to chart the patient's progress and order new medications, and then have them transmitted directly to the pharmacy for review and input, utilizing the patient's drug profile to note any problems. Like any mechanical equipment, provisions must be made for backup systems in the event of mechanical failure.

Computerization

One of the most important developments, which has significantly changed drug distribution systems, is the utilization of computers. A medical information system (MIS) based on computer technology has developed to varying degrees based on the diverse needs of pharmacy and other departments. There are, therefore, multitudes of pharmacy computer systems available today. Different hardware systems, software programs, and the need to interface with other hospital departments must be considered in the selection of a pharmacy support system.

Computerization offers the pharmacist a systematized method of order entry, patient profile development, label production, fill lists, and reports. It also provides clinical cross-checking mechanisms for allergy and sensitivity detection, dosage verification, drug interaction, and food-drug interactions.

Currently, a number of programs providing comprehensive drug information can be easily accessed during order entry. These allow the pharmacist to confirm the accuracy of drug use and dosage while checking for side effects, contraindications, laboratory test interferences, and so forth. This information may be printed immediately to assist in the education of the pharmacy staff, nurses, physicians, or other professionals within the institution.

An efficient computerized order entry system can generate **patient profiles** for a pharmacist, nurse, or physician to utilize. The profile includes all information necessary for adequately supervising appropriate drug usage within the institution. The information includes complete patient demographics, all scheduled and unscheduled (i.e., prn) drugs, and frequency and cautionary statements. The profile is used to generate the medical administration record (MAR) for the nurse. This tool allows the nurse to administer the drug at exactly the prescribed time for which it was intended. The MAR is essential for the accurate administration of medication to patients. A daily check of the MAR by nursing or pharmacy staff is essential and will help validate all changes on the patient's profile within the past 24 hours. It is essential to ensure that the MAR is up-to-date. The goal of a paperless, on-line MAR, along with an automated patient profile, is to have ready access for the review of a pharmacist, nurse, or physician.

Other applications which can be derived from the computerized profile include dispensing orders or fill lists from which the technician fills patient's cassettes or drug drawers for the next 24 hours or less. If the facility has automated dispensing cabinets, lists of drugs that are needed can be generated for the technician to fill the cabinet so that the appropriate drug and strength are available for the nurse to procure as needed.

The computerized profile should also be capable of transferring charges to the patient's account by a direct interface with the institution's financial system. Credits for drugs not used are also applied in the same manner.

Inventory control is managed by the computerized system by deleting items dispensed and their cost. Unused drugs returned to the pharmacy are credited to the inventory and to the patient simultaneously. Financial status is enhanced and the pharmacy administration is provided with valuable reports, which may be of importance to upper-level management.

The technician becomes directly involved in all aspects of computerization in most institutions. Order entry may be performed conditionally by the technician. The pharmacist validates the technician's entry before the order is activated. Other areas in which the technician's computer ability is utilized include floor stock entry, special patient charges and credits, labeling, report generation, and housekeeping or end-of-day functions. The areas of computerization and the technician's involvement are limitless.

Bar Code Applications

Presently, the use of bar code technology is used in the general retail industry. The retail applications, which have been widespread for many years, are mainly for pricing and inventory control. But bar codes are also used for customer identification and to collect demographic information. This information helps retailers address consumers needs. With refinements, these systems can be used to enhance health care.

The FDA proposed a rule change in 2003 that would require bar coded labels on all human drugs and biologicals. Even with the FDA mandate, there will probably be manufacturing issues and delays along with possible shifts in product availability that will likely slow down the process. Such delays should not preclude health systems from adopting bar code-enabled point-of-care systems to achieve gains in patient safety. Bar code technology is an enhancement from the traditional keyboard data entry by a technician. The information embedded in the bar code will help to promote an increased level of patient and medication safety. Verification of the right patient, right drug, right dose, right route, and right time will diminish mistakes. The health system must first establish a reliable process and procedure for identifying the correct patient and an identification of the caregiver. Every medication must have a unique bar code identifier to ensure the five rights of medication administration. When medications are not available from a manufacturer in a final product format, other means of applying an appropriate bar code must be utilized, including the use of unit-dose packaging equipment that produces a readable bar code. Overwrapping with a manual bar code and even outsourcing some medications to be bar coded in order to have every drug packaged with a readable and suitable bar code is an option that every facility that desires this technology must address prior to implementation. Policy and procedures and safety checks must be in place prior to use of bar coding. The future use of this point-of-care system with its reliable patient and caregiver identification and medication descriptions within a health care system can substantially increase the safe use of medications. This is our ultimate goal.

Physician's Order Entry Process

In recent studies, the value of a **physician order entry system** continues to be discussed and enhancements made to existing hospital information systems. Some of the beneficial effects of computerized physician order entry on the reduction of medical errors are as follows:

- complete and accurate information
- automatic dose calculation
- clinical decision support at the point of care

Applications may include

- formulary status of a drug
- cost considerations
- drug-drug interactions
- allergy checking
- standardized ordering, supported by evidence-based medicine

These processes and systems help ensure the equitable delivery of quality care, minimize human error, improve medication management, facilitate reporting and decision-making, and improve resource utilization. All these, while offering timely access to information and supporting compliance management and quality assurance initiatives, the final goal being that of enhanced positive patient care and associated positive outcomes of therapy.

Receiving the Medication Order

The functions of both the technician and the pharmacist have been previously described. The responsibilities are clearly defined for each individual in the dispensing system.

The Pharmacist's Role

It is the responsibility of the pharmacist to review and interpret every medication order prior to dispensing the medication. With the use of a computerized or manual patient profile, the pharmacist is able to evaluate the patient's complete medication regimen.

The patient profile

A patient profile is a complete listing of the patient's medications. For those institutions that do not utilize computers, the profile is designed to list all medications, strengths, directions, and patient data in addition to quantities and date dispensed. Depending on the institution, some profiles contain clinical data such as laboratory results, antimicrobial culture, and sensitivity reports. Previously used but discontinued drugs may also be visible.

When the unit-dose distribution system is used, a profile must be maintained so that the pharmacist may schedule, and the technician may prepare and distribute, individual medication doses according to the appropriate dosing schedule.

The drug profile system enables the pharmacist to identify potential drug interactions, dosage changes, drug duplications, overlapping therapy, and any drug that is contraindicated because of allergy or sensitivity. A complete patient profile should include, but not be limited to, the following information:

- patient's full name, location, age, weight, sex, hospital number, and admitting physician's name
- provisional diagnosis, secondary diagnosis, and confirmed diagnosis, if available
- allergies (e.g., food, drug, latex), sensitivities, and idiosyncrasies
- drug history from patient interview
- name of medication dispensed, strength, dosage, directions for use, quantity dispensed, date, and initials of pharmacist
- IV therapy (e.g., large- and small-volume intravenous solutions) with or without additives, hyperalimentation fluids, chemotherapy, etc
- laboratory data if known (e.g., electrolytes, creatinine, cultures, sensitivities)
- diet (e.g., low-sodium diet)
- selected diagnostic data related to coronary disease, diabetes, hypertension, etc.
- initials of dispensing technician and checking pharmacist

By receiving a copy of the complete physician's order, the pharmacist is able to seek information concerning laboratory test results, nursing procedures, and dietary intake, which might have been reordered. The pharmacist can then monitor possible drug-laboratory interactions, food-drug interactions, and other aspects of the patient's therapeutic program.

The pharmacist is also responsible for checking the technician's work in all aspects of the dispensing procedure.

- verification of the order entry on patient's profile to ensure that transcription or entry of doctor's medication order is correct
- verification of drug selection to be certain that the proper medication was set up for dispensing
- checking the drug label and contents to make certain that the finished product is complete, accurate, and ready for use
- checking unit-dose cassettes against the profile-generated fill list to verify that the drugs dispensed are correct and properly labeled. This process allows the pharmacist to conduct a final check of all unit-dose drugs that the patient will be administered.

The Technician's Role

It is the responsibility of the technician who receives the written prescription order to prepare the medication for dispensing. When the physician's order copy is received in the pharmacy, the technician must confirm that all necessary information pertaining to the patient's identification is available in the computer or on the profile (e.g., patient name, age, room number or location, hospital identification number, patient weight, allergies and sensitivities, the physician name). If a nurse has received a verbal or telephone order, the nurse's name should follow the name of the prescribing physician.

If all necessary information is present, the technician will enter the order into the computerized profile or transcribe it to a hand-generated profile, if that system is in use. It is the pharmacist's responsibility to review the order and the technician's order entry to validate its completeness and accuracy. The pharmacist will also take into consideration the patient's medication history, if available. (It is the policy in some hospitals to have a pharmacist interview patients upon admission to obtain a drug history to assist in evaluating the patient's drug therapy.) The use of technicians to enter medications into a patient's profile depends on the policies and procedures at that particular practice setting. If the facility allows technicians to perform these tasks, again, the final check and validation is the responsibility of the pharmacist.

Following order entry and validation, the technician prepares the drug for dispensing. The proper medication is selected from the appropriate storage site in either unit-dose or bulk form. For other than unit-dose drug distribution systems, the appropriate container must also be chosen. The technician prepares the label and counts or pours the designated quantity of the drug. Once the medication has been checked by the pharmacist, a positive, proactive practice would be to deliver the checked medication to the nurse taking care of that patient.

An important function of the technician is to answer the telephone. The technician functions in screening telephone calls and referring callers to the appropriate individuals. All questions of a clinical or drug-action nature should be directed to the supervising pharmacist for his/her professional judgment,

Compounding procedures

Qualified technicians may be allowed to conduct less critical compounding and manufacturing procedures under the pharmacist's direction and supervision.

If two or more drugs are compounded or mixed or prepackaged lyophilized powders are reconstituted for dispensing for a single dose, it may be considered "compounding."

If more than a single dose of a compounded product is prepared for future dispensing, it is known as "manufacturing" and requires the use of a manufacturing work sheet on which all components are identified by name, manufacturer, lot number, and quantitative amounts. Compounding directions are written or printed. A new lot number is assigned from a master control record. An expiration date is applied and should, where possible, be based on published stability information. Packaging information is also documented. The pharmacist must check all weights, measures, processes, and the completed product for uniformity and accuracy. The names of the technician and supervising pharmacist are recorded on the work sheet. After the procedure is completed and checked, the technician performs all necessary maintenance, housekeeping, and record-keeping duties.

Labeling and dispensing medications

The technician, in most cases, will be responsible for labeling medications. Labels may be computer generated, typed, or machine printed. Handwritten labels with pen, pencil, or marker are absolutely prohibited. One label should never be superimposed over another. The label should be clear, legible, and free from erasures and strikeovers. It should be firmly affixed to the container. The pharmacist confirms the original physician's order with the drug and label prior to dispensing.

Patients frequently judge the efficacy of a drug by the appearance of the label attached to the container. A neat label may signify to the patient that the drug is effective and will be of benefit. A sloppily printed label will indicate lack of concern by the pharmacy and its staff. The patient (and nursing and medical staffs) may interpret this indifference as a lack of effectiveness of the drug or lack of concern for the patient's well-being. Careful attention to the label indicates that careful attention has been given to preparing the medication as well.

With the exception of unit-dose or single-use products, the label should bear the name, address, and telephone number of the institution or pharmacy. Medications should never be relabeled by nursing personnel or anyone other than personnel supervised by a pharmacist.

Other points to consider in labeling are

- The metric system, rather than the apothecary system, should be utilized (e.g., 65 mg instead of 1 gr).
- When dispensing medications, the technician should be aware of any needed accessory labels, which should be attached to the container. These may include, but are not limited to the following:
  - "For the Eye"
  - "Keep in Refrigerator"
  - "Shake Well Before Use"
  - "Swallow Whole: Do Not Crush, Break, or Chew"
  - "For the Ear"
  - "Poison: Not For Internal Use"
  - "Take With A Full Glass of Water"
- There are a multitude of accessory labels available and every pharmacy should have a representative supply on hand to assist patients in understanding the appropriate use of the medication.
- When labeling a compounded prescription for inpatient use, the name and amount or percentage of each active ingredient should be indicated on the la-

bel. Prescription labels for outpatients should indicate the name of each therapeutically active ingredient.

■ In the event the medication being labeled requires further dilution or reconstitution, the label should provide appropriate directions. (**NOTE**: Effective unit-dose distribution systems do not require the nurse to conduct these operations; only in cases of extremely limited stability should this be allowed.)

■ Expiration dates should always appear on both unit-dose and prescription labels. There is little scientific information available to assist the pharmacist in determining how long the effectiveness of the medication can be ensured once it is removed from the manufacturer's original container. Many institutions will apply a 12-month expiration date unless the manufacturer's date arrives earlier. In no case should the expiration date exceed that of the original container. Special circumstances will require that a specific expiration date be assigned. For example, many antibiotics for oral suspension when reconstituted are stable for no longer than 7 to 14 days. Packaging materials, storage conditions, light conditions, and other factors must be considered in selecting an appropriate expiration date. The primary or secondary accessory label should indicate: "Expiration Date: _____" or "Use Before _____".

■ Parenteral medications may require special labeling in that the route of administration should be indicated (e.g., "For IM Use Only" or "Not for IV Use").

■ Labels for large- and small-volume intravenous solutions should be placed on the container so as to allow for visual inspection of the solution and should be readable in the hanging position of the container.

■ If the medication is an oncology or chemotherapeutic medication, an auxiliary label must be attached indicating "Special Handling—Chemo Hazard—Dispose of Properly". This should be applied to all forms of chemotherapeutic drugs whether they are oral, topical, or injectable.

■ Those containers that present difficulty in labeling, such as small tubes or bottles, must be labeled with a minimum of the patient's name and location. If possible, the drug name and strength should also be included. The small tube or bottle should be placed in a larger container bearing another label with all the necessary information.

Medication Delivery Systems

Transportation Courier

Some institutions have a centralized transportation courier system that delivers and transports medications, laboratory specimens, and supplies. In other hospitals and institutions, pharmacy technicians transport medications by providing order pickup and delivery. In a unit-dose exchange system, a technician uses a mobile cart to deliver medications in cassettes to the patient care area, exchanging full cassettes for those used during the previous 24-hour period and returning the used cassettes to the pharmacy for refilling.

Equipment

Various types of delivery equipment have been utilized to transport medications. The **pneumatic tube system** utilizes carrier cartridges that are sent from the pharmacy department directly to the terminal at the designated patient care area. All departments may be served depending on the number and location of terminals. In the event of mechanical problems, a backup system must be available to ensure rapid transfer of needed medications to the area or patient. Delays in drug delivery have been a major source of irritation for nurses and may result in medication errors when delivery time is excessive.

Dumbwaiters or elevators can also be used to transport medications. Unfortunately, these move in only a vertical direction. Personnel must then move the materials from the elevator's destination area to the patient care area. Elevators and dumbwaiters are also subject to mechanical failures and may impose the need for technicians to use stairways to deliver medications to their destinations.

Robotics are utilized in some institutions. These mobile, computerized, mechanical devices are programmed to move throughout the hospital and deliver medications. They are able to detect and move around obstacles and "speak" recorded messages. Other hospitals have found small, track-mounted carts that move to and from patient care areas delivering paper and supplies much like pneumatic tube systems to be useful. The big advantage to this type of transport is that it can handle bigger and heavier loads than the pneumatic tube system.

All mechanical systems are subject to failure and provisions must be made for alternate delivery methods when breakdowns occur. Drug security and control during transfer is a major concern that must always be considered in the selection and use of any transportation method. Pilferage, loss, and waste may create significant legal and financial problems.

Unit-Dose Picking Area

The area in the pharmacy where unit-dose carts are filled usually consists of slanted shelves on which plastic or cardboard bins are arranged to permit easy access by the technician's hands to select the doses needed. Bins are labeled in large letters showing the drug name, both generic and brand name, and strength. Circular shelves permitting one or two technicians to work with a minimum of movement are most efficient. Shelves should be within easy reach and should require minimal stooping or stretching. Adequate lighting is essential. Rubber mats on the floor reduce the strain of standing too long in one place.

One or more computer terminals and printers are located in the picking area to permit the technician to generate fill lists, post charges and issue credits, and review patient profiles. Sufficient space should be available outside the immediate picking area for storage of transfer carts where the pharmacist can also conduct the checking procedure. A telephone is essential and a small compounding and packaging area with a sink and running water should be immediately adjacent to the picking area.

The number and variety of drug bins in the picking area is never static. Change is constant and it is incumbent upon the technicians to ensure that the most frequently needed drugs are most readily retrievable. Infrequently used items should be relegated to the general stock area.

Return of stock to drug bins when patients are discharged or the drug is discontinued is a major source of error. Drugs in opened containers are never reissued. Unopened expired drugs are segregated for return to the manufacturer. Unit-dose packages may be dropped in the wrong bin and, if the technician becomes complacent and does not read and heed labels carefully, the wrong drug or dose may be issued in another cart-fill operation. The area should be kept free of clutter and trash. Maintenance of a clean and orderly picking area is absolutely necessary. Food or beverages should not be consumed in the picking area.

Medication Dispensing Units

Medication dispensing units or carts are available in many different configurations. They are designed to be wheeled from the nursing station to the patient's bedside, where the medication is administered directly to the patient.

Single-sided or double-sided carts may contain from a few to as many as 60 patient-identified drawers which hold those medications dispensed to each patient. The drawers may vary in length, width, and depth to accommodate the different needs of specific patient care areas.

Newer carts may also have computer terminals attached which enable the nurse to document the administration of each drug removed from the patient's drawer. This information may then be transmitted to the pharmacy computer system or the institution's mainframe for charging purposes, inventory control, and to update the patient's profile.

Individual patient bins or drawers are stored in portable cassettes. Each cassette may hold up to 30 drawers. The pharmacy technician uses a mobile cart to transport filled cassettes to the nursing station, unlocks the medication cart, and removes the cassette holding the empty drawers from the previous delivery period. The technician then inserts a filled cassette for the next 24-hour period and returns to the pharmacy with the empty drawers to repeat the filling process.

Proper maintenance of patient bins is an important responsibility of the technician. Each drawer or bin must be properly labeled with a computer-generated, typed, or machine-printed label showing the patient's name, room number, and physician's name. Sufficient dividers should be available to separate unit-dose packages and provide for efficient organization. In some institutions, drawer dividers serve to identify those drugs to be given at different dosing periods. For example, drugs prescribed to be taken early in the morning are located in the front of the drawer, those in the middle are to be given during the day, while those in the rear are scheduled for late evening or at bedtime. A final section might contain prn drugs. Dividers of different colors may also be used to further distinguish administration periods.

Carts and bins should be cleaned frequently. When possible, bins should be taken at regular intervals or when conditions indicate to a location where they can be thoroughly washed and sanitized.

Drug Distribution of the Future

With the advancements in technology and the increases in computerization, there will be monumental changes to the pharmacy profession. A pharmacist's clinical knowledge will be drawn upon to provide information to ensure the best clinical outcome for the patient. Technology will allow the pharmacist to move from labor-intensive medication distribution into a clinical resource for optimal patient care. Highly trained and motivated pharmacy technicians will be needed to handle the distribution of medications.

Also, with the advent of DRGs, patients will be receiving very intensive short-term care, with the pharmacist's role more firmly involved in therapeutic decision-making to ensure a rapid recovery with minimal adverse effects.

Automation has promised to decrease the number of pharmacists and technicians involved in the drug distribution process. In reality, those claims have not been realized. Automated systems require monitoring, preventative maintenance, upgrades, and database refinements besides the normal operation of restocking.

A definition of automated pharmacy systems has been adopted by the National Association of Boards of Pharmacy (NABP) and states that they "include, but are not limited to mechanical systems that perform operations or activities, other than compounding or administration, relative to the storage, packaging, dispensing, or distribution of medications, and which collect, control and maintain all transaction information."

Robotics

Many forms of robotic devices are currently available, with others being rapidly developed or improved, to mechanize the medication distribution process. Of primary concern with all products is medication safety and security. Mundane, repetitive tasks can be significantly reduced by the technology of these machines. The major advantage to automation is the increase in output with a notable decrease in medication errors. However, it must be remembered that restocking one of the machines with a wrong medication will cause multiple errors before it is detected and corrected. Undivided attention must be maintained when the restocking is being done. Checking and double-checking is a must to ensure that this type of error is not committed.

Pyxis, Omnicell, and HBOC/McKesson

These three companies are the industry leaders in decentralizing medication distribution. MedStation Rx System by Pyxis, Sure-Med by Omnicell, and AcuDose-Rx by HBOC/McKesson are similar in that medications are securely stored at remote sites throughout an institution. After the pharmacy has entered a physician's order on the patient's profile, the drug is available at the patient care unit for administration.

Authorized users, using a login password, have access via a color touch screen computer terminal. Once a patient has been identified, the profile is displayed, and the health care professional can choose the needed medication. A drawer opens and the drug can easily be removed. Updates to the patient's profile are done instantaneously via an interface with the main hospital computer software. Charges and credits are also issued automatically via another interface to the financial department.

Documentation of every aspect of the process is maintained and a variety of reports can be generated. The advantages of these systems are the elimination of end-of-shift counts for controlled substances, no need to have keys for medications that are locked in a cabinet, and missing doses becoming a thing of the past.

ATC Profile

In facilities that continue to have a cart exchange, the ATC Profile by AutoMed Technologies can be a substantial time saver. Over 200 of the most common oral drugs that are used in a facility are stored in individual canisters. The machine is interfaced to the main pharmacy computer system. The ATC Profile will unit-dose each medication on the patient's profile in the order in which the drugs will be administered. For example, drug A is to be given at 0800, 1400, and 2000; drug B is to be given at 1200; drug C is to be given at 0700 and 1900. The drugs are packaged in a strip with all the patient's information at the top. Drug C would be the first drug packaged, followed by drug A, drug B, another drug A, then drug C, and finally the last dose of drug A. The use of this machine assists the health care provider with the proper sequence for drug administration, virtually eliminates cart-fill errors, and unit-doses lower cost bulk medications so that unused doses may be credited and reissued. Charges are generated at the time of filling. Crediting for unused doses, however, must be done manually.

ROBOT-Rx

Automated Healthcare, Inc, a division of HBOC/McKesson, is one of the innovators in automated filling of carts. The difference between ROBOT-Rx and the ATC Profile is that the ROBOT-Rx can select items other than oral medications. A three-axis robot moves horizontally and vertically along rows of bar coded prepackaged solid oral meds or small-volume vials or ampules. The items are selected based on the patient's profile that is interfaced from the main pharmacy computer system to the robot's computer. Unlike the ATC Profile, the ROBOT-Rx is able to issue credits on unused doses and return them to stock for reissue.

The Future

In order to reduce medication errors, the demand for technology has been under an enormous strain to develop better, faster, and quicker ways to ensure patient safety. Direct physician order entry, bar coding at the patient's bedside, bar coding of medications, faster computers, and more efficient machinery are the current and future requirements that will provide a safe environment for a speedier recovery for a patient.

A Caveat

None of the current high-tech equipment briefly highlighted here, nor any future product, is going to be immune to hardware failure, power failure, and software failure. Humans still make mistakes when operating these systems, maintenance is sometimes delayed, or the equipment may be misused. All this can lead to medication mistakes. Backup systems must be provided for when and if these systems fail. The pharmacist and technician will have to return to a manual process to ensure that patients receive the right drug at the right time, in the right dose, and by the right route. A machine will never replace humans.

Summary

In this chapter, the technician's role in drug distribution has been generally described. The functions depicted are broad in nature and not all-inclusive. Only a small segment of duties have been outlined. Because each pharmacy is an entity of its own, it would be unrealistic or even undesirable to delineate a structured description of a technician's role. After a thorough orientation and training, the department's policy and procedure manual should be frequently consulted and followed throughout the technician's employment.

Because pharmacy is dynamic and not static, the roles of pharmacists and technicians are evolving from a product-oriented profession to a patient-oriented focus. The technician must be willing to continue the learning process, be open to innovative ideas, and be willing to assume newer responsibilities which may be required as the profession of pharmacy advances.

The time is coming for the use of technicians to fill some clinical roles. Experienced technicians will be trained to follow pain management therapy of patients. This will be of assistance to the pharmacist in evaluating drug therapy, while also spotting potential diversion of controlled substances. Identifying patients that are on IV therapy and able to switch to a more economical oral medication would be a major cost-containment process. Another function could be interviewing patients at time of admission to document their medication history. This would allow the pharmacist time to analyze what therapy may be appropriate during the hospital stay. As the procurement of medications becomes more challenging, analyzing drug usage and alternative therapies would assist the department's buyer and could reap monumental cost savings.

TEST YOUR KNOWLEDGE

True/False Questions

1. _____ Technicians are integral and important members of the health care team, in which they primarily assist the pharmacist. The legal responsibility for dispensing is with the technician.

2. _____ Unit-dose distribution represents a significant refinement of distribution systems and is considered to be the safest and most economical method of distribution.

3. _____ When a nurse or physician calls in an order to the pharmacy, it is referred to as a t.o. (telephone order).

4. _____ If a physician calls in the order, a pharmacist must take the call. If a nurse calls in, the technician can take the order.

5. _____ The use of NCR orders has eliminated the need for nurse transcription and thus reduces medication errors.

6. _____ Robots interfaced with computerized profiles are error-free and fail-safe.

7. _____ Automation is expected to replace the need for pharmacists and technicians as technology advances.

Matching Questions

8.	_____	ASHP	a. carrier cartridges
9.	_____	robotics	b. no carbon required
10.	_____	MAR	c. used by banks and hospitals for transportation
11.	_____	technician order entry	
12.	_____	pneumatic tube	d. national organization of pharmacists and technicians
13.	_____	JCAHO	e. Joint Commission on Accreditation of Healthcare Organizations
14.	_____	dumbwaiter	
15.	_____	NCR	f. computerized robot for cassette filling
16.	_____	scanner	g. medication administration record
17.	_____	facsimile equipment	h. must be validated by pharmacist
			i. elevator for transporting medications or orders
			j. fax

Completion Question

18. List five advantages of a unit-dose distribution system.

References

Barker, K. N., Felkey, B. G., Flynn, E. A., et al. (1998). White paper on automation in pharmacy. *Consulting Pharmacists, 46,* 2346.

Crawford, S. Y., Grussing, P. G., Clark, T. G., & Rice, J. A. (1998). Staff attitudes about the use of robots in pharmacy before implementation of a robotic dispensing system. *American Journal of Health-System Pharmacists, 55,* 1907–1914.

Garrelts, J. C., Koehn, L., Snyder, V., & Rich, D. S. (2001). Automated medication distribution systems and compliance with Joint Commission standards. *American Journal of Health-System Pharmacists, 58,* 2267–2272.

Klein, E. G., Santora, J. A., Pascale, P. M., & Kitrenos, J. G. (1994). Medication cart-filling time, accuracy, and cost with an automated dispensing system. *American Journal Hospital Pharmacist, 51,* 1193–1196.

Klink, L. (2003). Robots: Friend or foe? *The Pharmacist, 1,* 4–8, 10.

Lefkowitz, S., Cheiken, H., & Barnhart, M. R. (1991). A trial of the use of bar code technology to restructure a drug distribution and administration system. *Hospital Pharmacist, 26,* 239–242.

Marietti, C. (1997). Robots hooked on drugs. Robotic automation expands pharmacy services. *Healthcare Information, 14,* 37,38,40,42.

Neuenschwander, M., Cohen, M. R., Vaida, A. J., Patchett, J. A. Kelly, J., & Trohimovich, B. (2003). Practical guide to bar coding for patient medication safety. *American Journal of Health-System Pharmacists, 60,* 768–779.

Schwarz, H. O., & Brodowy, B. A. (1995). Implementation and evaluation of an automated dispensing system. *American Journal of Health-System Pharmacists, 52,* 823–828.

Manufacturers

Automed, 875 Woodlands Parkway, Vernon Hills, IL 60061, Phone: 888-537-3102. http://www.automedrx.com

McKesson Automation, 700 Waterfront Drive, Pittsburgh, PA 15222, Phone: (412) 209-1400, http://www.robot-rx.com

Omnicell, 1101 East Meadow Dr., Palo Alto, CA 94303, Phone: (800) 850-6664. http://www.omnicell.com

Pyxis Corporation, 3750 Torrey View Ct., San Diego, CA 92130, 858-480-6000 or 800-367-9947. http://www.pyxiscorp.com

18 Infection Control and Prevention in the Pharmacy

COMPETENCIES

Upon completion of this chapter, the reader should be able to

1. List four general causes of contamination of pharmaceuticals and sterile pharmacy products.
2. List three principal goals for infection control and prevention programs.
3. List three basic principles of asepsis.
4. Name the precautions used by health care workers to protect themselves and others from exposure to bloodborne and other pathogens.
5. Name three bloodborne pathogens of most concern to health care workers and for which OSHA exposure control plans are designed.
6. Recognize the routes of transmission of microorganisms.
7. List several components of the routine precautions used by health care workers to protect themselves and others from infections.
8. Describe what health care workers do when there is a possible occupational exposure to bloodborne pathogens.

Introduction

The infection control and prevention practices essential to ensure safe pharmaceuticals for patients are fundamentally rooted in good hygiene and sanitary practices. For example, handwashing is considered the single most important infection control measure practiced by health care workers. To prevent the spread of infection to themselves and to others, however, pharmacy workers need additional infection control education. Fortunately, the principles of infection control and prevention, once learned, are relevant to any health care setting. The information presented here is applicable to a freestanding pharmacy, acute-care hospital, skilled nursing facility, nursing home, home-care program, or any other setting where pharmacy personnel work.

Pharmacy personnel are responsible for ensuring that drugs and solutions are handled in a manner that prevents contamination and protects sterility when indicated. The pharmacy is responsible for the preparation and storage of most sterile medications and, in more and more instances, for managing intravenous therapy admixtures, including enteral nutrition products. The pharmacist and pharmacy staff need knowledge of infection control and prevention, first and foremost, because patient morbidity and mortality can result from contaminated pharmaceuticals. Meticulous attention is needed to prevent the introduction and transmission of germs.

Contamination of Pharmaceuticals

Contamination of pharmaceutical preparations has led to epidemics. Pharmacy personnel are required to know how to prevent contamination in the first place and must be prepared when contamination does occur to participate in curtailing disease. For example, the pharmacy staff may need to be involved in the identification of patients who have received specific products associated with an outbreak, and they may coordinate recalls of pharmaceutical preparations, such as occur in cases of manufacturer contamination.

Some of the general causes of contamination of pharmaceutical and sterile pharmacy products, and some recommendations for contamination prevention are listed here.

Preparation of intravenous products in areas outside of the pharmacy, in areas not providing a class 100 environment (no greater than 100 particles per square foot) may lead to contamination. Intravenous (IV) solution contamination rarely occurs, but when it does, bloodstream infections and diseases in the form of bacteremia, or fungemia, and septic shock are likely to result. Also, intravenous solution contamination has the potential to result in epidemics because of the likely wide distribution and use of the infected solutions. Solutions may be contaminated during production, which is known as intrinsic contamination. Intrinsic contamination of infusates during the manufacturing process has caused widespread epidemics of bloodstream infections. Extrinsic contamination, or contamination of IV fluids following manufacturing, is a constant threat during the admixture process or while the infusate is in use. The threat of extrinsic contamination is always possible when aseptic technique is not used and has resulted in bacteremia and septic shock. Recommendations for the prevention of contamination of intravenous infusions include the following:

- Compound admixtures in the pharmacy. The Centers for Disease Control and Prevention (CDC) and the Intravenous Nursing Society Standards of Practice both recommend that all parenteral fluids be prepared in the pharmacy using a laminar airflow hood.
- Prepare sterile products using facilities and equipment recommended by the American Society of Health-Systems Pharmacists (ASHP).
- The sterile product preparation area should have handwashing facilities with hot and cold running water. The ASHP recommends personnel preparing sterile products wear clothing covers or gowns that generate low numbers of particles, masks, and coverings for head and facial hair.
- All sterile products should be prepared in a class 100 environment with the use of a vertical or horizontal laminar airflow. The area should be separate from other areas with limited personnel traffic. Particle-generating items such as cardboard boxes should not be stored in the area surrounding the hood.

Improper aseptic technique may lead to contamination. To prevent contamination of pharmaceuticals, the use of proper aseptic techniques includes the following:

- Perform hand and forearm hygiene before preparing sterile products. Use an antimicrobial or detergent soap or use an alcohol skin hygiene product as directed by the latest guidelines.
- Eating, drinking, and smoking should not be allowed in the preparation area.
- The rubber stoppers of containers should be wiped or sprayed with 70% alcohol before entry.
- The ASHP recommends that the entire surface of ampules, vials, and container closures be disinfected appropriately before placement in the laminar airflow hood, including automated devices used for compounding sterile products that are to be placed in the laminar airflow hood.
- Personnel should avoid touch contamination of sterile supplies.

Contaminated multidose vials (MDVs) may lead to infections. Although contamination of in-use vials is rare according to several studies, epidemics have been traced to their use. In the past, most hospitals established policies to discard MDVs after a set period of time, but because there are no specific guidelines with respect to expiration of opened MDVs, recommendations no longer include dating to indicate when vials are first opened or to indicate when to discard vials. Recommendations for the prevention of contamination of MDVs include the following:

- When MDVs are used, CDC recommendations call for refrigerating the vials after opening if recommended by the manufacturer, cleaning the rubber diaphragm of the vial with alcohol before inserting a device into the vial, using a sterile device each time a vial is accessed, and avoiding touch contamination of the device before penetrating the rubber diaphragm. The MDV should be discarded when empty, when suspected or visible contamination occurs, or when the manufacturer's stated expiration date is reached.

Inadequate quality control practices may lead to contamination of pharmaceuticals. The pharmacy is responsible for the storage of all pharmaceuticals, for monitoring for expiration dates, and for monitoring the temperature of refrigerators and freezers used to store pharmaceuticals in all locations. Recommendations for the prevention of contamination include the following:

- Sterile products should be examined for leaks and cracks and for turbidity or particulate matter that could indicate contamination, although the growth of microorganisms, even in high numbers, may not be evident.
- Labeling all admixed parenterals according to ASHP recommendations provides for patient safety and the use of control or lot numbers for batch-prepared items should assist with recalls, if needed.
- Admixed parenterals may be stored in the refrigerator for up to one week providing that refrigeration begins immediately after preparation and is continuous unless stability of ingredients dictates a shorter storage time. According to the ASHP, some admixed parenterals may be stored longer depending on the sterile product preparation procedures used and the storage temperature.

Infection Control Fundamentals

The role of the pharmacy in infection control and prevention extends beyond assuring the integrity of pharmaceuticals. The dramatic increase in the last several decades of the loss of activity of standard antibiotics to common bacteria has led to an incredible challenge. There is a demand for a pharmacy leadership role in the selection, use, and control of antibiotics as hospitals and other health care facilities deal with infections caused by bacteria that are resistant to multiple antibiotics. Working in teams with physicians, microbiologists, and infection control professionals, pharmacists participate in programs that limit unnecessary antibiotic use and seek to prevent the spread of resistant microorganisms. These programs attempt to impact on practitioner antimicrobial prescribing practices and on the antibiotic habits of the public.

The Goals of Infection Control and Prevention Programs

The three principal goals for infection control and prevention programs are

1. protect the patient
2. protect the health care worker, visitors, and others in the health care environment
3. accomplish the previous two goals in a cost-effective manner, whenever possible

The Principles of Aseptic Techniques

To protect the patient and to prevent contamination, the basic principles of asepsis and the practices of aseptic techniques need to be understood.

- Microorganisms (germs) are capable of causing illness in humans.
- Microorganisms that are harmful to humans can be transmitted by direct or indirect contact.
- Interrupting the transmission of microorganisms from reservoirs to susceptible hosts can prevent illness.

Aseptic or clean techniques are practiced to reduce the numbers of microorganisms or to eliminate their transmission from one person, or environment, to another. The practices of aseptic technique include hand hygiene to reduce the numbers of skin microorganisms, the use of barriers such as gloves and gowns to avoid skin and clothing contact with contaminated surfaces, and environmental controls ranging from and including routine environmental cleaning and disinfection to the use of controlled airflow hoods.

Preventing Infections in Health Care Workers

Following the AIDS epidemic that began in the early 1980s, and in response to the threat of other serious on-the-job infections, federal and state legislatures have written into laws the requirement for institutional infection control and prevention programs and for health care worker infection control and prevention education. More recently, the health care industry was mandated to find ways to prevent health care worker injuries from contaminated needles and other sharp objects as part of programs designed to otherwise prevent health care worker exposures to sources of blood and other potentially infectious materials. These exposures primarily pose a potential threat of infection from the viruses of hepatitis B, hepatitis C, and AIDS (the human immunodeficiency virus [HIV]).

Health Care Worker Infection Control Education

All health care facilities are required to have infection control programs that establish infection control and prevention standards of care. Hospital staffs are required to review these infection control policies and procedures, some of which are specific to a department (such as the pharmacy), and others that relate to all members of the health care team.

Pharmacy personnel are not at high risk for occupational exposure to infectious diseases unless they are involved in direct patient care and have contact with body fluids. In some situations, the pharmacist might assist the medical team (e.g., during cardiac arrest response) and could possibly thereby have contact with body fluids. Other situations with less potential for pharmacy staff occupational exposure might nonetheless be harmful if basic infection control principles are not followed. For instance, during the delivery and distribution of pharmaceuticals to patient care areas, there could be an unexpected encounter with patients, patient linens, or with soiled patient care equipment. Health care worker duties that require contact with blood or body fluids, or with equipment that is contaminated with blood and other potentially infectious materials such as body fluids, create the most risk for exposure to serious infections.

To protect themselves and others from infection, all health care workers use **universal-standard precautions** whenever they are in a health care environment. The details of these precautions are mandated by the U.S. Occupational Safety & Health Administration (OSHA) and the Public Employee Safety & Health Administration (PESH) and are based on recommendations from the U.S. Public Health Services Centers for Disease Control and Prevention (CDC).

Through the Bloodborne Pathogen Standard (law), OSHA and PESH ordered that all health care facilities have in place **exposure control plans** to protect workers from exposure to infectious diseases. These plans must include infection control training for health care workers at risk for occupational exposure to blood and other potentially infectious material because these may contain **bloodborne pathogens**. Pathogens are microorganisms (germs) that cause infections. Additionally, control of tuberculosis is required to be reviewed because some health care workers may be at risk for exposure to this disease.

The bloodborne pathogens of most concern in health care include, but are not limited to, the **hepatitis B virus (HBV)** which causes hepatitis B, the **human immunodeficiency virus (HIV)** which causes acquired immunodeficiency syndrome (AIDS), and the **hepatitis C virus (HCV)** which causes hepatitis C. Other bloodborne pathogens include microorganisms that are considered to be less of a risk to health care workers from exposures, but can potentially cause diseases like syphilis, malaria, and viral hemorrhagic fever.

Not all tasks within the health care setting carry the same chance of contact with blood and potentially infectious body fluids. Tasks that carry a high risk of exposure require that the health care worker wear appropriate clothing, including cover gowns, gloves, masks and protective eyewear, known as personal protective equipment (PPE).

Infections

An infection cannot develop unless **pathogenic germs** are **transmitted** (or spread) from a **source**, such as an infected person, improperly decontaminated equipment, or contaminated food, **to a susceptible person**. Antibiotics, antifungal and antiviral medications are ordered by physicians to eliminate infectious agents causing disease. Environmental sanitation and the cleaning and disinfection or sterilization of hospital equipment and supplies is another way to eliminate germs. Health care workers use frequent handwashing or hand hygiene and various other precautions to prevent spreading pathogenic germs from infected persons or sources to themselves and to others. Knowing how to prevent transmission of germs is mandatory to prevent the spread of infections.

For an infection to occur, the three elements outlined in the triangle below must be present (**Figure 18-1**). An infection will be prevented if any one of the three parts is eliminated.

- a susceptible host
- a means for transmitting the pathogens to the host
- a reservoir or source of the infectious agent (pathogens)

Sources of Infectious Agents

Human sources of pathogens in health care may be patients, personnel, or, on occasion, visitors and may include persons with acute and obvious infectious diseases. But not all persons carrying infectious agents look sick. Those who are in the incubation period of a disease, for example, may not show symptoms of infection, and others who are **colonized**, or living with the infectious agents without being sick, may not show symptoms but still be capable of spreading pathogens. Some persons may be chronic carriers of an infectious agent. In particular circumstances, a person's own endogenous flora (i.e., the body's many normal indwelling microorganisms) that is mostly non-pathogenic can become pathogenic and be the source of infection. Other sources of infecting microorganisms may be inanimate environmental objects that have become contaminated, including equipment and medications.

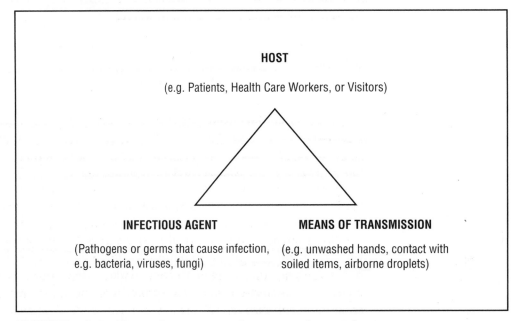

FIGURE 18-1   Three elements must be present for an infection to occur.

Host

Resistance and susceptibility among persons to pathogenic microorganisms varies greatly. Some persons may be immune to infection. Vaccines help the health care worker to be immune to some pathogens. For example, all hospital health care workers are offered the hepatitis B vaccine (unless they already have natural immunity from having had the disease hepatitis B).

Some people are naturally able to resist **colonization** by an infectious agent. Others exposed to the same germ may establish a balanced relationship with the infecting microorganism and become asymptomatic carriers (i.e., pathogens adapt to grow on the skin and mucous surfaces of the host, forming part of the normal flora without making the person sick). Still others may develop clinical disease.

Host factors may make persons more at risk for infection. For example, one's age affects one's ability to fight off infection. Children are known to be more susceptible and babies who are born prematurely are especially vulnerable. The elderly are also less able to fight off infections. Other conditions that disrupt the body's ability to fight infection include underlying diseases like diabetes and cancer and particular treatments including the use of antimicrobials, corticosteroid therapy, and other immunosuppressive agents, as well as radiation therapy.

Procedures performed for diagnosis and treatment of disease often place the patient at higher risk and can contribute to infection. For instance, the patient is at risk for infection when there are breaks in the skin or other natural body defenses as occurs during surgical operations, anesthesia, and when indwelling catheters are used.

Transmission

Microorganisms are spread five ways, or **routes**, and the same microorganism may be transmitted in more than one way.

Routes of transmission

Contact transmission, the most important and frequent mode of transmission of infections, is divided into two subgroups.

Direct-contact transmission involves direct body surface-to-body surface contact and physical transfer of microorganisms between a susceptible host and an infected or colonized person, such as occurs when nursing personnel bathe a patient or when physicians perform patient care activities that require direct personal contact. Direct-contact transmission can also occur between two patients, with one serving as the source of the infectious microorganisms and the other as a susceptible host.

Indirect-contact transmission involves contact of a susceptible host with a contaminated intermediate object, usually inanimate, such as contaminated instruments, needles, or dressings, or contaminated hands that are not washed and gloves that are not changed between patients.

Droplet transmission, theoretically, is a form of contact transmission. However, because the mechanism of transfer of the pathogen to the host is quite distinct from either direct- or indirect-contact transmission, the CDC considers droplet transmission a separate route of transmission. Droplets are generated from the source patient primarily during coughing, sneezing, and during certain procedures such as suctioning and bronchoscopy. Transmission occurs when droplets containing microorganisms generated from the infected person are propelled a short distance through the air and deposited on the host's conjunctivae (eye surface), nasal mucosa, or mouth. Because droplets do not remain suspended in the air, special air handling and ventilation are not required to prevent droplet transmission. Droplet transmission must not be confused with airborne transmission.

Airborne transmission occurs by dissemination of either **airborne droplet nuclei** (small-particle residue [five microns or smaller in size] of evaporated droplets containing microorganisms that remain suspended in the air for long periods of time) or dust particles containing the infectious agent. Microorganisms carried in this manner can be widely dispersed by air currents and may become inhaled by a susceptible host within the same room or over a longer distance from the source patient, depending on environmental factors. Therefore, special air handling and ventilation are required to prevent airborne transmission. Microorganisms transmitted by airborne transmission included *Mycobacterium tuberculosis* and the rubeola (measles) and varicella (chicken pox) viruses.

Common vehicle transmission applies to contaminated items such as food (salmonellosis), water (cholera, *E. coli*), medications, devices, and equipment.

Vector-borne transmission occurs when vectors such as mosquitoes (malaria, West Nile encephalitis), flies, rats, ticks (Lyme disease) or other vermin transmit microorganisms. This route of transmission is less significant in hospitals in the U.S. than in other regions of the world.

Control of Infections

Because host and agent factors are more difficult to control, interruption of the transfer of microorganisms in health care facilities is the primary aim of infection control and prevention programs. The greatest opportunity for health care workers to prevent infections comes from eliminating the transmission of germs.

Universal-Standard Precautions

For many years, the term and procedures for universal precautions, developed by OSHA, referred to infection control safety measures designed to protect health care workers from infections. The CDC, responsible for both health care workers and patients, expanded universal precautions to protect both health care workers and patients and used the term standard precautions. Today either term or a combination of the two may be used by a facility to name the infection control and prevention principle practices that need to be used for all exposures to blood and body fluids and to equipment that is potentially contaminated by blood and body fluid.

Since persons harboring infectious agents may not look sick, health care personnel must use precautions during the care of all patients, and for all contact with patients, clients, residents, and inmates regardless of the diagnosis or presumed infection status. Universal-standard precautions apply to any contact with

- blood
- all body fluids, secretions, and excretions except sweat, regardless of whether or not they contain visible blood
- non-intact skin (e.g., open cuts, wounds, surgical sites)
- mucous membranes (e.g., surface of the eye, inside of the nose and mouth)

Personal Protective Equipment (PPE)

Personal protective equipment (PPE) is made up of barriers used to prevent skin and mucous membrane exposure when contact with blood or other potentially infectious material is anticipated. PPE includes impermeable gowns or aprons, disposable non-sterile gloves, masks, masks with eye shields, goggles, resuscitation bags, mouthpieces, or other ventilation devices used for patient resuscitation, specimen transport bags, and red regulated medical waste garbage bags.

Health care workers use PPE when anticipating contact with blood, body fluids, secretions, and excretions, non-intact skin, and mucous membranes.

Health care workers must wear protective gloves when it can be reasonably anticipated that there may be hand contact with blood or body fluids, other potentially infectious material, mucous membranes, or non-intact skin and when handling or touching contaminated items or surfaces. For example, gloves must be worn during venipuncture or other vascular access procedures. Gloves must be changed after contact with each patient, client, resident, inmate, etc. Protective gloves are to be removed before touching non-contaminated items (e.g., telephones, doorknobs).

Health care workers must wear gowns or aprons for procedures that could involve splashing or spattering of blood or other body fluids and must wear face and eye protection when splashes, sprays, spatters, or droplets of blood or other potentially infective materials pose a hazard to the eye, nose, or mouth.

The following procedures must be observed with PPE :

- Wash hands immediately, or as soon as feasible, after removal of gloves or other PPE.
- Remove PPE after it becomes contaminated and before leaving the work area.
- Remove PPE either before leaving a contaminated area (e.g., a lab) or right after (e.g., a TB isolation room).
- Remove immediately, or as soon as feasible, any garment contaminated by blood or body fluids in such a way as to avoid contact with the outer surface.

Prevention of Needle-Stick and Other Sharps Injuries

Precautions must be taken to prevent injuries caused by needles, scalpels, and other sharp instruments or devices during and after use. To prevent needle-stick injuries, needles should NOT be recapped, purposely bent or broken by hand, removed from disposable syringes, or otherwise manipulated by hand. In the event a needle must be recapped, a "one-hand scoop" method must be employed. After use, disposable syringes and needles, and all other sharp items, both used and unused, should be discarded in appropriate puncture-proof sharps containers.

Handwashing

Hands and other skin surfaces must be washed immediately and thoroughly if contaminated with blood or other body fluids. Handwashing significantly reduces the transmission of pathogens in hospitals and is considered the most important infection control and prevention measure. Health care workers must wash hands frequently. Hands must be washed before putting on gloves and immediately after gloves are removed, between patient contacts, and when otherwise indicated to avoid transfer of microorganisms to other patients or environments.

To properly wash hands, wet hands with water and then add soap. Use friction to generate lather and wash hands. Use a vigorous 10- to 15-second rub to remove transient microorganisms (longer for more heavy contamination or after a possible exposure to bloodborne pathogens and other potentially infectious material). Follow with a thorough rinsing. In certain work areas, a counted scrub is used for hand washing (e.g., operating room, neonatal intensive care). Health care workers need to wash hands before beginning work, before and after giving treatments or handling used equipment, before eating, and before and after using the bathroom.

Waterless hand hygiene products containing alcohol are now available in most health care facilities for handwashing procedures. Health care workers like these products since they are easy to use and do not dry the skin because they contain emollients. Especially important when sinks are not available, dispensers can be located anywhere handwashing might be needed. In some instances, the health care worker may carry the hand hygiene product to use as needed. Soap and water must still be used when the hands are visibly soiled since the alcohol will not disinfect the hands through the soil. The waterless products are used for routine handwashing procedures, but do not replace counted or timed scrubs.

Cleaning and Decontamination of Surfaces and Spills

Environmental contamination is an effective method of disease transmission for microorganisms and particularly for the hepatitis B virus (HBV). The CDC states that HBV can survive for at least one week in dried blood on environmental surfaces used for contaminated needles and instruments. Cleaning of contaminated work surfaces after completion of procedures or after spills is required to ensure that employees are not unwittingly exposed to blood or other potentially infectious material remaining on a surface from previous procedures or from a spill. All cleaning should be done with infection control committee/institutional-approved disinfectants.

There are specific procedures used for spills of frank blood or other potentially infectious material. If you encounter a spill, call for help from the professional staff.

Biohazard symbols **(Figure 18-2)** or red bags are used to warn employees who may have contact with items of the potential hazard posed by their contents.

The storage of food, as well as eating, drinking, smoking, applying cosmetics or lip balm, and handling contact lenses is prohibited in patient care areas and in other work areas where there is the likelihood of occupational exposure.

Handle blood and other potentially infectious materials carefully, in order to minimize the potential for splashing and spraying.

Engineering and Work Place Controls

Engineering controls reduce the risk of employee exposures either by removing, eliminating, or isolating hazards.

Regulated medical waste (RMW) handling

Most hospital waste is not any more infective than residential waste. Consistent with most current state and local regulations, RMW is defined as sharps, culture/stocks, human pathological waste, animal research waste, and human blood or blood products. State regulations may vary and need to be checked on a state-to-state basis.

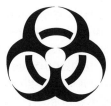

FIGURE 18-2 Biohazard symbol for universal precautions and standard precautions used to identify potential biologically infectious materials.

Bulk blood, suctioned fluids, excretions, and secretions may be carefully poured down a drain connected to a sanitary sewer or may be autoclaved. Only containers with free-flowing blood or blood products or discarded material saturated or dripping with blood (e.g., dressings, blood transfusion bags, or tubings) need be considered RMW. The determining factor for these materials to be RMW is that when compressed or squeezed they produce free-flowing fluid. All other hospital-related items are to be disposed of as regular waste.

RMW is placed in containers that are closable, constructed to contain all contents and prevent leakage, appropriately labeled as a biohazard or color coded, and closed prior to removal to prevent spillage or protrusion of contents during handling.

Sharps disposal containers

Leakproof, puncture resistant sharps disposal containers labeled with a biohazard label are located in all patient rooms, all patient care areas, and all other areas where contaminated sharps might be encountered. All sharps are to be discarded into such containers as soon as is feasible.

Safety devices and proper work practices

Needlestick-prevention devices with engineered safety features are part of the comprehensive program to reduce the risk of bloodborne pathogen exposures. Safer medical devices used to prevent percutaneous injuries before, during, or after use through safer design are becoming increasingly available on the market and are being evaluated throughout the United States in response to a recent OSHA rule. Examples of safer devices include shielded-needle devices, blunt needles, needleless IV connectors, and IV access devices.

Proper work practices, such as reducing hand-to-hand instrument passing in the operating room and no-hands procedures in handling contaminated sharps (including broken glassware picked up using mechanical means, such as a brush and dustpan), reduce the risk of bloodborne pathogen exposure. Examples of engineered devices that are used as part of proper work practices include mechanical pipetting devices, centrifuge safety cups, splashguards, and biological safety cabinets.

Hepatitis B Vaccination

Employees found to be nonimmune to hepatitis B must be encouraged to seek hepatitis B vaccination, which must be available at no charge to the employee. Nonimmune employees choosing to decline hepatitis B vaccination must sign a declination form. The employee may rescind a declination at any time.

Hospital Isolation Precautions

Isolation precautions are used in hospitals for patients known or suspected to be infected with highly transmissible microorganisms for which additional precautions beyond universal-standard precautions are needed to interrupt the transmission of disease. The particular isolation precautions used are based on the way infectious diseases or certain microorganisms are transmitted. These precautions might also be used in other parts of the health care system where the infectious disease is diagnosed prior to admission to the hospital.

Hospitals modify isolation systems to meet the needs of the patient population served and to meet federal, state, or local regulations. Each hospital isolation system, however, must preserve the principles of infection prevention and control and include precautions to interrupt the spread of infection by all routes that are likely to be encountered. Most hospitals today use a combination of standard precautions and transmission-based precautions.

Communicable diseases and conditions require different types of isolation. In most hospitals, a color-coded isolation sign (or card) is placed outside of the patient's room to alert health care workers and visitors to the procedures required to prevent infection from the disease or condition being isolated. The isolation sign lists the requirements of the isolation (e.g., whether masks or gowns are required). Before entering any hospital room, be sure to check for these signs.

Pharmacy personnel are not usually trained in transmission-based isolation precautions and, therefore, must not enter the room if there is a sign indicating "Isolation" or "Precautions." Those not trained in hospital isolation precautions are considered visitors and need to follow the instructions printed on the sign to "Report to the Nurses' Station before Entering the Room." The nurse instructs visitors on the precautions to take to prevent infection.

Transmission-Based Precautions

There are three types of transmission-based precautions: airborne precautions, droplet precautions, and contact precautions. They may be combined for diseases that have multiple routes of transmission. When used either singly or in combination, they are to be used in addition to standard precautions.

Airborne precautions

Airborne precautions require the use of a private room with a special air-handling system that creates negative air pressure and discharges room air to the outdoors or through a high-efficiency filter before the air is circulated to other areas in the hospital. National Institute of Occupational Safety and Health (NIOSH)-approved respirators are required to be worn by those entering the room except when the person is immune to the disease.

Airborne precautions are used for patients diagnosed with or suspected to have measles or varicella (chickenpox or disseminated *Herpes zoster*/shingles) and are used for patients diagnosed with or suspected to have tuberculosis.

The door to the room used for airborne precautions must remain closed to maintain negative air pressure in the room in relation to surrounding areas and to contain microorganisms that remain suspended in the air for long periods of time to prevent them from being widely dispersed by air currents.

Droplet precautions

Droplet precautions require the use of a private room or that the patient be placed in a room with a patient who has active infection or colonization with the same microorganism, but with no other infection (cohorting). Surgical masks with or without eye protection are used when entering the room or when within three feet of the patient.

Droplet precautions are used for patients diagnosed or suspected to have some types of meningitis, serious bacterial respiratory infections such as pertussis (whooping cough), Streptococcal pharyngitis, pneumonia or scarlet fever in infants and young children, and serious viral infections.

Transmission occurs when droplets are propelled a short distance through the air, but because droplets do not remain suspended in the air, special air handling and ventilation are not required to prevent droplet transmission. Droplet transmission must not be confused with airborne transmission.

Contact precautions

Contact precautions require the use of a private room or that the patient be placed in a room with a patient who has active infection or colonization with the same microorganism, but with no other infection (cohorting). Gloves are used when entering the room. Gowns are worn to enter the room if it is anticipated that clothing will have substantial contact with the patient, environmental surfaces, or items in the patient's room; if the patient is incontinent or has diarrhea; or if wound drainage is not contained by a dressing. When possible, patient care equipment (e.g., blood pressure machine, stethoscope) is dedicated to a single patient or cohort of patients or such equipment must be cleaned and disinfected before use on another patient.

Contact precautions are used for patients known or suspected to have illnesses easily transmitted by direct patient contact or by contact with items in the patient's environment including gastrointestinal, respiratory, skin or wound infections, or colonization with multi-drug resistant bacteria judged by the institution to be significant.

Occupational Exposures

Bloodborne Pathogen Exposures

Infectious body substances that carry a risk for bloodborne pathogen transmission include blood, bloody fluid, semen, vaginal secretions, synovial, pleural, peritoneal, pericardial, cerebrospinal, or amniotic fluid.

An exposure that may place a health care worker at risk for bloodborne pathogen infections is

- a percutaneous injury (e.g., a needlestick or cut with a sharp object)
- contact of mucous membrane, conjunctivae, or nonintact skin (e.g., when the exposed skin is chapped, abraded, or afflicted with dermatitis) with blood, tissue, or other body fluids
- contact with intact skin when the duration of contact is prolonged (i.e., several minutes or more) or involves an extensive area with blood, tissue, or other body fluids.

What to Do If Exposed

Clean affected area *immediately*. Wash with soap and water.

- For needlesticks, cuts, or skin contact, wash the area with soap and running water for several minutes. Do not vigorously disrupt the skin and do not use bleach or other strong chemicals since these can increase chances of infection through skin damage.
- For eye contact, flush the eyes with copious amounts of running water for several minutes.

Notify area supervisor *immediately*. Complete employee accident form. Report to the emergency department or to the employee health service as directed by the hospital *immediately*. Smaller hospitals and other institutions may make arrangements with area hospital emergency departments for their staff to be seen for occupational exposures.

Post-exposure prophylaxis (PEP) is recommended for individuals exposed to potentially infectious body substances within one to two hours of a reported event, ideally within one hour. Health care workers must not delay seeking evaluation and treatment. (CDC-specific antiretroviral recommendations may vary from state department of health recommendations.)

The risk of hepatitis B virus infection following a needlestick with infected blood appears to be approximately 6% to 30%. The risk of hepatitis C infection following a needlestick with infected blood appears to be approximately 3%. The risk of HIV infection following a needlestick with infected blood appears to be 0.3% to 0.5%.

Post-exposure services must be available to any employee who sustains an occupational exposure 24 hours a day, every day, in a designated center. All expenses for medical evaluations and procedures, vaccines, and post-exposure prophylaxis must be at no cost to the employee.

Post-Bloodborne Pathogen Exposure Evaluation and Follow-up

Health care workers need to be tested for hepatitis B, hepatitis C, and syphilis and referred for follow-up care. If the health care worker has never been infected with hepatitis B or has not been vaccinated against hepatitis B, the vaccine will be offered along with hyperimmune gamma globulin (HBIG).

Laws may vary by state, but usually the health care worker will be asked to consent to HIV testing. If consent is given, the source individual's blood will be tested as soon as feasible and after consent is obtained in accordance with state and local laws relating to this matter.

In some states, (e.g., New York) if already part of the health care team, the exposed employee may have access to the medical record and know the HIV status of the patient, as well as information about drug resistance. Alternatively, the patient may have signed an informed consent form authorizing disclosure of this information to the exposed worker or to undergo consented HIV testing with disclosure of the test results to the exposed worker. When neither of these situations applies, New York laws now authorize disclosure of existing HIV-related information to persons who have been exposed in the workplace when significant risk exposure has occurred.

Tuberculosis

All new employees in hospitals and other health care facilities must have a baseline evaluation for evidence of tuberculosis infection consisting of a two-stage **tuberculin skin test (TST)** unless they have a history of positive TST. Health care workers with negative TST must be retested at periodic intervals; annually in most cases; every six months, or more frequently for employees in work areas that are at high risk for tuberculosis. Health care workers with positive TST are evaluated to rule out active disease and must receive counseling regarding current recommended treatments and the symptoms of tuberculosis disease (including coughs and fevers that last two weeks or longer, night sweats, weight loss, blood in sputum). Persons with positive TST, but without active disease, have TB infection and may require treatment.

TB infection is not the same as TB disease. TB infection is a condition in which living tuberculosis germs are present in a person without causing continuing destruction of tissue. The healthy immune system usually keeps the infection in check, but prophylactic treatment with INH is needed to kill the *Mycobacterium tuberculosis*. If not treated and the immune system fails, TB disease may develop. TB disease is a condition in which living tuberculosis germs produce progressive destruction of tissue. TB disease is contagious. TB infection is not contagious.

Multi-drug resistant (MDR) TB

Some strains of TB have developed resistance to the drugs used to treat tuberculosis disease. The main reason that MDR strains of TB have developed is that TB patients have not followed their prescribed drug treatment. The drugs used to treat TB usually alleviate the symptoms within two to three weeks; however, they do not eliminate the underlying infection unless they are taken for at least six months. When patients do not adhere to their prescribed drug regimen, the bacteria can become resistant to the drugs being used. Symptoms can return and the patient can transmit these resistant organisms to others, including health care workers. Employees exposed to pulmonary tuberculosis in the workplace will be evaluated for evidence of infection as a result of the exposure through a post-exposure evaluation.

Health Care Worker Work Restrictions

Health care workers with infections can infect patients and other health care workers. Personnel with open draining lesions like abscesses or wounds must remain away from their jobs in the hospital and other health care settings and are to return only after cleared for work by the employee health service. Employees with herpetic lesions (herpes infections) should not care for patients in high-risk categories including nursery, oncology, and ICU until cleared by employee health. Health care workers should not work with rashes (especially if susceptible to varicella/chickenpox and after known exposure to chickenpox) or conjunctivitis until they have seen or spoken with their physician or employee health clinic.

Summary

The control of infection is a high priority in all health institutions. The pharmacy is an integral part of the health care system. The pharmacist and pharmacy technician are key players on the health care team. This chapter identifies areas of concern and methods to be employed to prevent and control the spread of infection in institutions where persons with infections are routinely treated.

An area of major concern that is addressed is preventing contamination of pharmaceuticals and ensuring sterility of all injectable medications.

TEST YOUR KNOWLEDGE

Multiple Choice Questions

1. Some of the general causes of contamination of IV fluids during preparation include
   a. not cleaning the rubber stopper of the medication vial with alcohol prior to entry with needle and syringe
   b. touching the sterile ports of IV fluids with sterile gloves.
   c. preparing parenteral nutrition solutions under the laminar airflow hood
   d. examining fluids for turbidity

2. Handwashing is
   a. used by pharmacy personnel mainly while handling sterile medications and solutions
   b. important in health care mostly when caring for patients in isolation rooms
   c. used by medical personnel primarily to protect themselves from infections
   d. considered the single most important infection control measure practiced by health care workers

3. The main goals of infection control and prevention programs are to
   a. protect the patient
   b. protect the health care worker
   c. use cost effective measures
   d. all of the above

4. The principles of asepsis include the idea that
   a. microorganisms can be completely eliminated from humans
   b. pathogens can be transmitted by direct or indirect contact
   c. pathogens do not cause infection in health care workers
   d. microorganisms cannot be spread in clean hospitals

5. Aseptic techniques
   a. are used to reduce or eliminate the transmission of germs
   b. are not used routinely by pharmacy personnel
   c. are needed only when working with items that are obviously soiled
   d. decrease the number of bloodborne pathogens in blood and body fluids

6. Pharmacy personnel
   a. as health care workers are at great risk for infection at work
   b. face no threat of infection on the job
   c. are not included in infection control education programs because they do not have direct contact with patients
   d. need to know how to protect themselves from contact with blood or body fluids or from equipment that is contaminated

7. OSHA mandates health care facilities have plans in place to protect health care workers from the following infectious diseases in particular:
   a. tuberculosis, influenza, measles, and mumps
   b. hepatitis A, hepatitis B, and hepatitis C
   c. hepatitis B, hepatitis C, HIV, and tuberculosis
   d. chickenpox, tuberculosis, and measles

8. For an infection to develop,
    a. germs have to be transmitted from people who have obvious infections
    b. microorganisms are transmitted from an infected or contaminated source
    c. the health care workers have to be very young or very old
    d. pathogens have to be contacted by hand

9. In hospitals, microorganisms are most frequently spread
    a. by mosquitoes and flies
    b. by contaminated food and water
    c. by contact with contaminated objects
    d. by droplets

10. Universal-standard precautions are used
    a. by doctors when shaking hands with patients and visitors
    b. by some health care workers in the laboratory
    c. by health care workers when they have contact with a patient's blood, body fluids, or wounds
    d. by health care workers when they have contact with a patient who is sweating profusely

11. Hospitalized patients are placed on isolation precautions
    a. to prevent the spread of microorganisms that are highly transmissible or resistant to multiple antibiotics
    b. to alert hospital staff to the special precautions required to prevent infection from the disease or condition being isolated
    c. to alert pharmacy personnel and other visitors there is a need to check with the nursing staff for special instructions before entering the room
    d. all of the above

12. An occupational exposure that might place a pharmacy worker at risk for hepatitis B infection includes
    a. a needle-stick from a needle that was used to inject medication into IV solution
    b. a needle-stick from a needle that was used to draw blood from a vein
    c. a needle-stick from an unused needle
    d. a finger skin cut from paper in the pharmacy

13. In the event of a possible or actual exposure to a patient's blood or body fluids,
    a. wash the area with bleach and call for help
    b. cover the area thoroughly with a dressing
    c. wash skin area immediately with soap and water or flush the eyes with copious amounts of running water for several minutes
    d. report to your supervisor during your next scheduled evaluation session

14. Tuberculosis
    a. might be spread to or from a pharmacy worker and, therefore, all pharmacy workers in hospitals must be screened
    b. does not exist in pharmacy personnel and, therefore, screening is not required
    c. is spread by persons with tuberculosis infection as evidenced only by a positive tuberculin skin test
    d. is a disease of third world countries and not a problem in the United States

15. Health care workers can infect others
   a. if they work while they have an open, draining wound or abscess
   b. have never had chickenpox and come to work with a rash
   c. if they have pink eye or conjunctivitis
   d. all of the above

References

American Society of Hospital Pharmacists. (1993). ASHP technical assistance bulletin on quality assurance for pharmacy-prepared sterile products. *American Journal of Hospital Pharmacy 50,* 2386–2398.

Bryan, D., & Marback, R. C. (1984). Laminar-airflow equipment certification: What the pharmacist needs to know. *American Journal of Hospital Pharmacy, 41,* 1343–1349.

Centers for Disease Control and Prevention. (1971). Epidemiologic notes and reports nosocomial bacteremias associated with intravenous fluid therapy. *Morbidity and Mortality Weekly Report, 20* (Suppl. 9), 81–82 (2, 3–5).

DeCastro, M. A. (2000). Aseptic technique. In *APIC Text of Infection Control and Epidemiology,* p. 27-1, Washington, DC: Association for Professionals in Infection Control and Epidemiology.

Department of Labor, Occupational Safety and Health Administration. Occupational exposure to bloodborne pathogens: Needlesticks and other sharps injuries. *Final Rule,* 29 C.F.R. §1910.1030 (b)(2001).

Felts, S. K., Schaffner, W., Melly, M. A., & Koenig, M. G. (1972). Sepsis caused by contaminated intravenous fluids. *Annals of Internal Medicine, 77,* 881–890.

Fernandez, C., Wilhelmi, I., & Andradas, E. (1996). Nosocomial outbreak of *Burkolderia picketti* infection due to a manufactured intravenous product used in three hospitals. *Clinical Infectious Diseases, 22,* 1092–1095.

Heller, W. M. (1980). Time limits on the use of opened multiple-dose vials. *American Journal of Hospital Pharmacists, 37,* 1610–1613.

Hospital Infection Control Practices Advisory Committee. (1996). Recommendations for isolation precautions in hospitals. *American Journal of Infection Control, 24,* 24–52.

Hospital Infection Control Practices Advisory Committee. (1996). Recommendations for the prevention of nosocomial intravascular device related infections. *American Journal of Infection Control, 24,* 262–293.

Hospital Infection Control Practices Advisory Committee. (1998). Guideline for infection control in health care personnel, 1988. *American Journal of Infection Control, 26,* 289–454.

Intravenous Nurses Society. (1998). Intravenous nursing standards of practice. *Journal of Intravenous Nursing, 21,* S1–S95.

Longfield, R., et al. (1984). Multidose medication vial sterility: An in-use study and a review of the literature. *Infection Control and Hospital Epidemiology, 5,* 165–169.

Maki, D. G., & Mermel, L. A. (1998). Infections due to infusion therapy. In J. V. Bennet & P. S. Brachman (Eds.), *Hospital infections* (4th ed). pp. 689–724. Boston: Little, Brown and Company.

Melnyk, P. S., et al. (1993). Contamination study of multiple dose vials. *The Annals of Pharmacotherapy, 27,* 274–278.

Montgomery, P. A., & Cornish, L. A. (2000). Pharmacy. In *APIC Text of Infection Control and Epidemiology,* p. 68. Washington, DC: Association for Professionals in Infection Control and Epidemiology.

Phillips, I., Eykyn, S., & Laker, M. (1972). Outbreak of hospital infection caused by contaminated autoclaved fluids. *Lancet, 1,* 1258–1260.

Scheckler, W. E., et al. (1998). Requirements for infrastructure and essential activities of infection control and epidemiology in hospitals: A Consensus Panel Report. *Infection Control and Epidemiology, 19,* 114–124.

PART

IV Clinical Aspects of Pharmacy Technology

Chapter 19: Introduction to Biopharmaceutics
Chapter 20: The Actions and Uses of Drugs
Chapter 21: Nonprescription Medications
Chapter 22: Natural Products

Introduction to Biopharmaceutics

COMPETENCIES

Upon completion of this chapter, the reader should be able to

1. Describe five key factors that can affect the absorption of a drug.
2. Define bioavailability and calculate it given the appropriate information.
3. Define the three parameters obtained from drug plasma concentration-time data to assess bioequivalence.
4. List factors that could decrease the bioavailability of a drug administered orally.
5. Describe the processes of drug distribution, metabolism, and elimination.

Introduction

Biopharmaceutics focuses on the interrelationship between the rate and extent of systemic drug absorption and the physiochemical properties of the drug molecule, the drug dosage form, and the route of administration of the dosage form. Bioavailability is the extent of drug absorption, and it is defined as the fraction of an administered dose that ultimately reaches the systemic or whole body circulation. The rate of drug absorption is evaluated by the magnitude or height of the maximum drug concentration and by how long it takes to reach that concentration.

Many factors can effect the rate and extent of drug absorption from a particular dosage form and, consequently, the therapeutic effect of the drug. These factors include the route of administration, formulation of the dosage form, the physiochemical properties of the drug, and various anatomical and physiological factors.

Routes of Administration

Drugs are given by many different routes of administration. These routes can be divided into two categories: (1) intravascular and (2) extravascular administration. Intravascular administration refers to the direct administration into the vasculature or bloodstream by an intravenous or intra-arterial route. Extravascular administration includes all routes of administration in which the drug is not delivered directly to the bloodstream. These routes include oral, sublingual, buccal, intramuscular, subcutaneous, transdermal or percutaneous, pulmonary or inhalation, rectal, and intranasal. Any drug administered extravascularly must first be absorbed from its site of administration to subsequently enter the bloodstream.

There are many factors to be considered when determining the best route of administration for a particular drug in a particular patient. These factors range from the physiochemical properties of the drug, anticipated patient compliance, severity of the disease state, concurrent disease states, and cost. There are numerous benefits of oral administration including ease of administration, patient acceptance, cost, and the ability to formulate modified release dosage forms. Therefore, the most common route of administration is oral, and a complete understanding of factors affecting absorption from oral dosage forms is very important.

Factors Affecting Drug Absorption

There are a number of barriers a drug administered by an extravascular route must overcome before it can reach the bloodstream. These barriers can affect both the amount of drug reaching the bloodstream and the rate at which the drug reaches the bloodstream. These barriers are drug release from the dosage form, dissolution of the drug in the surrounding fluid, and diffusion of the drug into the bloodstream. A simplified diagram of this process for an oral tablet is presented in **Figure 19-1**.

Drug Release From the Dosage Form

A solid drug product, such as a tablet, must disintegrate into smaller particles so the drug can be released from the formulation. Other dosage forms can release the drug without disintegrating. These include depot injections, implants, patches, creams, and ointments. The rate and extent that the drug is released from the dosage form directly influences the rate and extent of drug absorption into the bloodstream.

Dissolution

Unless the drug is already in solution when it is released from the dosage form, it must dissolve in the aqueous fluid surrounding it before diffusion can occur. The physiochemical properties of the drug determine its solubility in different biological fluids. The pH and composition of the fluid are also very important. The pH will affect the degree of ionization of the drug and, therefore, its solubility. The fluid may also contain substances that enhance the solubility of otherwise poorly soluble drugs. In general, compared to drugs with good solubility in the surrounding

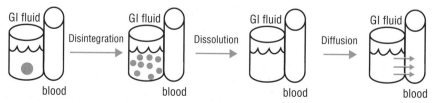

FIGURE 19-1 The process of a tablet disintegrating in gastrointestinal fluid (GI fluid), the drug particles going into solution, and finally the drug in solution diffusing across the gastrointestinal epithelium into the gastrointestinal capillaries.

biological fluid, a drug with poor solubility will be absorbed more slowly or incompletely.

Diffusion

Once the drug is in solution, it is able to diffuse across biological membranes. However, particular substances in gastrointestinal fluid, including some drugs, may then bind or adsorb the drug and prevent its diffusion. To prevent this type of interaction, the administration of certain combinations of drugs must be separated by several hours. For an oral dosage form, the drug must diffuse across the gastrointestinal epithelium. The lipid nature of biological membranes, including the gastrointestinal epithelium, results in their being more permeable to lipid-soluble substances.

Anatomic and Physiologic Considerations

Since orally administered drugs must diffuse across the epithelium of the gastrointestinal tract, the anatomic and physiologic features of the gastrointestinal tract are very important in determining how much of a drug diffuses. The amount of drug that will diffuse across the epithelium of the gastrointestinal tract is dependent on a variety of factors including the permeability of the epithelium, the surface area, the amount of time the drug is in the area of the epithelium, the blood supply, and the pH and nature of the gastrointestinal contents.

Stomach

The stomach has a relatively small surface area, so diffusion is usually very limited in the stomach. Parietal cells in the stomach secrete hydrochloric acid that yields a very acidic environment with a fasting pH of 2 to 6 and decreasing to 1 to 2 in the presence of food. Food, especially fatty food, inhibits the emptying of the gastric contents into the small intestine. Therefore, most drugs in which a rapid onset of action is desired should be taken on an empty stomach so they will reach the small intestine more quickly.

Small intestine

The small intestine consists of the duodenum, jejunum, and ileum. The total length of the small intestine is on average approximately 3 meters, and it extends from the pyloric sphincter to the ileocecal valve. The total surface area of the small intestine has been calculated to be approximately 200 m^2, or approximately the area of a singles tennis court. The permeability of the small intestine is greater than that of the stomach. It also has a large blood supply, with approximately one liter of blood passing through the intestinal capillaries each minute. The total transit time in the small intestine is approximately three to four hours in healthy individuals. All these factors contribute to the enormous absorptive capacity of the small intestine. Therefore, the principal site of absorption for most orally administered drugs is the small intestine.

Duodenum

The duodenum is the first section of the small intestine. Gastric contents are released into the duodenum through the pyloric sphincter. Bicarbonate from the pancreas buffers the contents coming from the stomach to a pH of 4 to 6. The anatomical structure of the duodenum includes villi and microvilli. These are small finger-like processes that project from the surface of the epithelium yielding a very large surface area. Due in part to this large surface area, the duodenum is the primary site of diffusion for many drugs into the blood. Bile salts from the liver and gall bladder and pancreatic enzymes are secreted into the duodenum via the hepatopancreatic ampulla. These secretions can increase the solubility of more lipophilic drugs in the luminal fluid and, therefore, enhance their ability to diffuse across the epithelium.

Jejunum

The jejunum is the center section of the small intestine. Although there is a gradual decrease in the diameter of small intestine and the number of villi and microvilli along its length, the jejunum still has a large surface area. The normal pH of the jejunum is in the range of 5 to 7. Due to these continuing favorable conditions, a significant amount of drug diffusion still occurs in the jejunum.

Ileum

The ileum is the terminal section of the small intestine. The diameter and number of villi and microvilli continue to decrease, but the ileum still has a relatively large surface area. The normal pH of ileum is in the range of 7 to 8. The blood supply to the ileum is much less than the blood supply to the duodenum and jejunum. Drug absorption continues to occur in the ileum, but not the extent that occurs in the duodenum and jejunum.

Large intestine

The large intestine is on average slightly over one meter in length and consists of the cecum, colon, and rectum. The contents of the small intestine are released into the cecum through the ileocecal valve. Due to a lack of villi and microvilli, the large intestine has a much smaller surface area than the small intestine. The contents of the large intestine are also more viscous and begin to take on a semisolid to solid form. These factors limit the capacity for the diffusion of drugs in the large intestine. However, certain drugs and peptides can be significantly absorbed in the large intestine due to the extended residence time of the contents in the colon (10–24 hours). These drugs are well suited for modified-release dosage forms. The pH of the large intestine can vary widely from 4 to 8. The rectum and anal canal are a straight, muscular tube that begins at the terminal colon and extend to the anus. Drug absorption by rectal administration can occur in the rectum via the hemorrhoidal veins.

First-Pass Metabolism in the Liver

Once an orally administered drug diffuses across the gastrointestinal epithelium into the blood of the hepatic portal vein, the drug is delivered directly to the liver before it can pass into the rest of the body (**Figure 19-2**). The liver then has the opportunity to metabolize the drug before it reaches the systemic or whole body circulation. This initial metabolism is known as first-pass metabolism or first-pass effect, because it occurs during the first pass of the drug through the liver. First-pass metabolism can significantly reduce the amount of an orally administered drug reaching the systemic circulation, even if the drug diffuses completely from the gastrointestinal tract into the blood. A drug with a very large first-pass effect cannot be administered orally because not enough of the drug will make it into the systemic circulation to achieve its desired therapeutic effect. The drug would have to be administered by routes not subject to first-pass effect (e.g., sublingually, transdermally, intravenously).

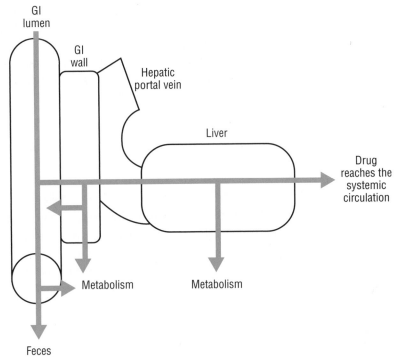

FIGURE 19-2   The barriers a drug in an oral dosage form must overcome to reach the systemic circulation include lack of diffusion through the gastrointestinal (GI) wall or epithelium, metabolism in the gut lumen, metabolism in the gut wall, drug being pumped back into the GI lumen, and first-pass metabolism in the liver.

Bioavailability

The amount of drug in the dosage form that ultimately clears all these barriers and reaches the systemic circulation unchanged is considered to be bioavailable. The bioavailability (F) of a dosage form can be defined by Equation 1.

Equation 1

$$\text{Bioavailability (F)} = \frac{\text{Amount of drug reaching the systemic circulation unchanged}}{\text{Amount of drug in the administered dosage form}}$$

Since intravenous doses are administered directly into systemic circulation, the bioavailability of an intravenous dose is always 100%. However, the bioavailability of any drug given by an extravascular route can range from 0% to 100% depending on the amount of the dose that reaches the systemic circulation unchanged.

Drug Distribution, Metabolism, and Elimination

Once a drug reaches the bloodstream, it must then move to the site(s) where it exerts its pharmacological action(s). This movement of drug from the bloodstream to other bodily tissues is called distribution. Several characteristics of the tissue

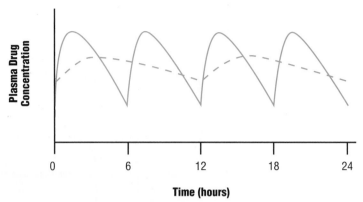

FIGURE 19-3   Plasma drug concentrations over time for both an immediate-release dosage form (solid line) and a modified-release formulation (dashed line) of the same drug. The immediate-release product must be given every 6 hours to maintain therapeutic concentrations. The modified-release product releases drug slowly, so it can be dosed every 12 hours and therapeutic concentrations are maintained with less peak-to-trough fluctuation in drug concentrations.

affect the distribution of a drug in and out of the tissue (e.g., regional pH, tissue composition and blood flow, lipid solubility of the drug, extent of drug bound to protein). For example, drugs with a high lipid solubility easily cross biological membranes and distribute extensively into adipose or fat tissue.

Drugs in the bloodstream are also subject to metabolism and elimination. The liver is the principal site of metabolism in the body, although drug-metabolizing enzymes do exist in other tissues. The typical purpose of drug metabolism is to convert the drug molecule to more water soluble and inactive metabolites. However, metabolism can also convert drugs to active or toxic metabolites. Finally, the drug or metabolites can be excreted by the kidneys into the urine and eliminated from the body. The amount of time it takes to eliminate one-half of the total amount of drug in the body is the elimination half-life. Drugs with short elimination half-lives must be dosed more frequently to maintain adequate amount of drug in the body to achieve the desired therapeutic effect. Alternatively, a modified-release formulation designed to slowly release the drug from the dosage form can be developed for drugs with short half-lives. The drug can then be given less frequently which increases the consistency and accuracy with which a patient follows the directions for taking the medication (**Figure 19-3**). Patient compliance with four-times-a-day regimens has been shown to average about 40%, whereas patients receiving once-daily and twice-daily regimens have average compliance rates of approximately 70%.

Methods to Assess Bioavailability

The bioavailability of dosage form can be determined by several methods depending on the objective of the study and the methods available to accurately measure the amount of the drug in biological fluids. The most commonly employed method is to measure consecutive blood or plasma drug concentrations after the administration of the same dose by non-intravenous and intravenous administration. Those data are used to create a concentration-time profile. The area under the drug

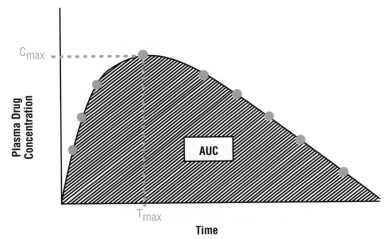

FIGURE 19-4   Plasma drug concentration-time profile in which each point (•) is a measured plasma concentration at a particular time after the dose was administered. The figure displays the C_{max} (maximum plasma concentration), T_{max} (time of maximum plasma concentration), AUC (area under the plasma concentration-time curve) in the shaded area and the elimination half-life.

concentration-time curve (AUC) can then be calculated (**Figure 19-4**). The bioavailability of the dosage form is determined by utilizing Equation 2, where the $AUC_{product}$ is the AUC of the non-intravenous dose being tested and AUC_{IV} is the AUC of the same drug dose given intravenously.

Equation 2

$$\text{Absolute bioavailability} = \frac{AUC_{product}}{AUC_{IV}}$$

Measurement of urinary drug excretion can also be used an indirect method to examine the bioavailability of a dosage form.

Bioavailability Studies

Bioavailability studies are generally conducted to determine both the rate and the extent (i.e., absolute bioavailability) to which a drug is absorbed from the dosage form into the systemic circulation. Information of the rate and extent of systemic absorption from a dosage form can be visualized graphically by the concentration-time profile (Figure 19-4).

During drug product development, bioavailability studies are routinely employed to compare different formulations of the same drug product. The formulation with the most desirable rate and extent of absorption can then be pursued. The desired rate and extent of absorption will depend on the therapeutic application of the drug in the dosage form. For example, it would be desirable for a dosage form of drug used to treat acute pain to provide a fast rate of release and absorption of the drug to quickly relieve the pain. In contrast, a drug needed to control a patient's blood pressure around-the-clock would be appropriate for manufacture as a controlled or slow-release product.

Bioequivalence studies are bioavailability studies specifically comparing two or more formulations of the same dose of the same drug in the same dosage form.

The purpose of bioequivalence studies is to determine if the concentration-time profiles produced by test formulations are similar to an innovator's product that is or soon will be off patent. If a test formulation is statistically found to be bioequivalent in terms of C_{max} (maximum plasma concentration achieved), T_{max} (time of the maximum plasma concentration), and AUC (area under the plasma concentration time curve) to the innovator's or reference formulation, then it is considered to be bioequivalent (Figure 19-4). Since the innovator product has already undergone extensive safety and efficacy testing to be approved by the Food and Drug Administration (FDA), it is assumed that the bioequivalent formulation will be unlikely to result in any clinically significant differences in therapeutic response or adverse events. Bioequivalence studies are one of the requirements for pharmaceutical companies trying to gain FDA-approved generic status for their formulation of off-patent products.

Summary

Biopharmaceutics focuses on the interrelationship between the rate and extent of systemic drug absorption, the physiochemical properties of the drug molecule, the properties of the dosage form, and the route of administration of the dosage form. There are many other complex factors, including anatomic and physiologic factors, that can affect the rate and extent of drug absorption that must also be taken into consideration.

Bioavailability studies are a commonly employed to assess the rate and extent of drug absorption from different dosage forms. Bioequivalence studies specifically examine the C_{max}, T_{max} and AUCs of different formulations of the same drug in the same dosage form to determine if the two formulations are similar in their release of the drug from the dosage form. If they are not found to be significantly different, then no differences in clinical outcome from them being substituted or administered interchangeably are expected.

TEST YOUR KNOWLEDGE

Multiple Choice Questions

1. Bioequivalence studies assess the similarity of plasma concentration-time profiles by comparing
   I. AUC
   II. C_{max}
   III. T_{max}
   a. I only
   b. III only
   c. I and II only
   d. II and III only
   e. I, II, and III

2. Drugs that are very lipid soluble tend to distribute extensively into
   a. skeletal muscle
   b. adipose tissue
   c. plasma
   d. bone

3. The bioavailability of drug administered intravenously is
   a. 0%
   b. 25%
   c. 50%
   d. 100%

4. The elimination half-life of a drug is
   a. the time required to completely eliminate the drug from the body
   b. the time required to eliminate one-half of the drug in the body
   c. the time required to absorb one-half of the drug from the dosage form
   d. the time required to completely absorb the drug from the dosage form

5. If 1000 mg of a drug is administered in an oral tablet and 400 mg of the drug is absorbed into the systemic circulation, then the absolute bioavailability (F) is
   a. 20%
   b. 40%
   c. 60%
   d. 80%

6. The bioavailability of an oral tablet could be decreased due to
   I. incomplete dissolution
   II. incomplete diffusion
   III. first-pass effect
   a. I only
   b. III only
   c. I and II only
   d. II and III only
   e. I, II, and III

7. Bioavailability is defined as
   a. the amount of an administered dose that reaches the systemic circulation
   b. the fraction of an administered dose that fails to reach the systemic circulation
   c. the amount of an administered dose that fails to reach the systemic circulation
   d. the fraction of an administered dose that reaches the systemic circulation

8. Which of the following is/are extravascular route(s) of administration?
   I. oral
   II. subcutaneous
   III. intravenous
   a. I only
   b. III only
   c. I and II only
   d. II and III only
   e. I, II, and III

9. Which one of the following represents the correct order of events an oral dosage form must go through for the drug to be reach the bloodstream?
   a. disintegration, dissolution, diffusion
   b. dissolution, disintegration, diffusion
   c. disintegration, diffusion, dissolution
   d. diffusion, dissolution, disintegration

10. The principal site of absorption for most orally administered drugs is the
   a. liver
   b. stomach
   c. small intestine
   d. large intestine

References

Ansel, H., Allen, L., & Popovich, N. (2000). *Pharmaceutical dosage forms and drug delivery systems* (7th ed.). Baltimore: Lippincott Williams & Wilkins.

Dipiro, J., Blouin, R., Pruemer, J., & Spruill, W. (2002). *Concepts in clinical pharmacokinetics: A self-instructional course* (3rd ed.). Bethesda, MD: ASHP.

Evans, W., Schentag, J., & Jusko, W. (1992). *Applied pharmacokinetics principles of therapeutic drug monitoring* (3rd ed.). Vancouver, WA: Applied Therapeutics.

Ganong, W. (2003). *Review of medical physiology* (21st ed.). San Francisco: Appleton & Lange.

Martin, A. (1993). *Physical pharmacy* (4th ed.). Baltimore, MD: Williams & Wilkins.

Rowland, M., & Tozer, T. (1995). *Clinical pharmacokinetics concepts and applications* (3rd ed.). Media, PA: Williams & Wilkins.

Seeley, R., Stephens, T., & Tate P. (2002). *Anatomy & physiology* (6th ed.). Boston: McGraw-Hill.

Shargel, L., & Yu, A. (1999). *Applied biopharmaceutics and pharmacokinetics* (4th ed.). Stamford, CT: Appleton & Lange.

CHAPTER
20

The Actions and Uses of Drugs

COMPETENCIES

Upon completion of this chapter, the reader should be able to

1. Describe the advantages and disadvantages of the various routes of drug administration.
2. Recognize and interpret the standard abbreviations for the various routes of administration.
3. Describe the major factors that affect variability in drug response.
4. Describe the role of drug therapy in some common disease states.
5. Know the therapeutic category for commonly prescribed drugs.
6. Match the generic and brand names of commonly prescribed medications.

Introduction

Drugs are prescribed to treat a wide variety of medical conditions and, therefore, the knowledge of the action and use of individual drugs is critical. This chapter describes the major therapeutic classes of drugs and categorizes drugs into these classes with both their trade and generic names. Once drug therapy is initiated in a patient, there are many factors that will affect the outcome of the drug therapy. All these factors combined can result in large patient variability, which is the difference in drug response from patient to patient.

The route of administration is one factor that can significantly affect drug response. Each route offers advantages and disadvantages that must be taken into consideration. There are also many patient-specific factors that affect drug response including patient compliance with administration directions, drug-food interactions, drug-drug interactions, drug-disease interactions, and the age, weight, and genetics of patients.

Factors That Affect Drug Response

Route of Administration

Drug dosage forms are given by many different routes of administration. These routes can be divided into two categories: (1) intravascular and (2) extravascular administration. Intravascular administration refers to the direct administration into the vasculature or bloodstream by intravenous or intra-arterial injection or infusion. Extravascular administration refers to all routes of administration in which the drug is not delivered directly into the bloodstream. These routes include oral, buccal, sublingual, translingual, intramuscular, subcutaneous, topical, transdermal, inhalation, rectal, vaginal, intranasal, ophthalmic, and otic. Several of these routes require the drug product to be sterile. Although the pharmacological effect of the same drug administered by different routes should be similar, the route can affect both the speed at which the desired effect is attained and the intensity of the effect.

Intravenous

The intravenous route of administration means directly injecting a sterile drug into a vein, and is abbreviated as "IV" on a prescription. Advantages to intravenous administration of drugs include a more rapid onset of drug action which can be very valuable in emergency situations and allowing the use of drugs that may not be suitable for extravascular administration due to poor absorption into the bloodstream or significant first-pass metabolism. Several disadvantages to intravenous administration include possible pain, irritation, and increased risk of infection at the injection site and in the bloodstream.

Intraarterial

Drugs are occasionally injected into arterial side of the bloodstream. This route is usually reserved for delivery of some anticancer drugs and diagnostic agents to a particular tissue or organ for localized effects. Otherwise, it offers the advantages and disadvantages of intravenous administration.

Oral

For oral administration, the drug dosage form is placed into the mouth and swallowed; it is abbreviated as "po" on a prescription. This route is the most common, convenient, and economical for many drugs. In addition, dosage forms can be designed to offer sustained or prolonged action of the drug, which decreases the frequency the drug must be taken. Disadvantages include limited absorption of some drugs, destructions of some drugs by digestive enzymes or the acidic pH of the stomach, and significant metabolism of some drugs during first-pass metabolism. When a drug is taken orally, it must pass through the liver before it can reach the systemic bloodstream. Therefore, the liver has the first chance to metabolize the drug before it reaches the rest of the body.

Buccal, sublingual, and translingual

Buccal, sublingual, and translingual routes represent the drug dosage form being placed into the mouth without swallowing it. For buccal administration, the dosage form is placed between the cheek and gum. For sublingual administration, the dosage form is placed under the tongue to dissolve and is abbreviated as "sl" on a prescription. For translingual administration, the drug is sprayed directly onto the tongue or mouth tissue. These routes of administration offer several advantages including rapid absorption and, therefore, rapid onset of drug action. The direct absorption into the bloodstream prevents the drug from the acidic environment of the stomach and first-pass metabolism. One disadvantage is that unless properly instructed, patients may swallow the medication before it is completely absorbed. Nitroglycerin preparations are often administered by these routes for rapid relief of anginal chest pain, but if the dosage form is swallowed, nitroglycerin will undergo a very large first-pass effect and be ineffective.

Intramuscular

Intramuscular administration means a sterile drug is directly injected into a skeletal muscle and is abbreviated as "IM" on a prescription. Common sites include the deltoid (shoulder) and gluteus maximus (buttocks). Absorption of the drug occurs as the drug diffuses from the site of injection into surrounding muscle fibers and into the blood vessels in those fibers. The rate of absorption into the bloodstream depends on the blood flow to the muscle. For example, the deltoid has a higher blood flow than the gluteus maximus and, therefore, absorption is normally quicker from the deltoid muscle. The rate of absorption is also dependent on the formulation of the injection. For example, aqueous or water-based injections are generally more rapidly absorbed than oil-based ones. Advantages include the potential for a sustained release while bypassing gastrointestinal absorption problems and first-pass metabolism. As with intravenous administration, disadvantages include pain, irritation, and risk of infection at the injection site.

Subcutaneous

Subcutaneous administration means the injection of a sterile drug just beneath the surface of the skin and is abbreviated as "subc," "subq," "SC," or "SQ" on a prescription. This route can only be used for drugs that are not irritating to the tissue and can be given in a small volume. The rate of absorption varies with blood flow to the area of the injection and formulation of the product. Advantages include the potential for a sustained release while bypassing gastrointestinal absorption problems and first-pass metabolism. Disadvantages may include pain and irritation at the injection site. Subcutaneous administration generally results in slower absorption into the bloodstream as compared to intramuscular injection of the same drug.

Topical and transdermal

Topical and transdermal administration involves applying a drug directly on the surface of the skin and is abbreviated as "top." on a prescription. Topical administration is used for local drug effects in the skin and is most commonly administered as a lotion, cream, or ointment. Transdermal administration is mainly used to deliver a drug into the bloodstream for systemic effects. However, transdermal patches can be used for local action (e.g., the Lidoderm patch). A transdermal patch is designed to control the release of drug and, therefore, provide a sustained absorption of the drug into the bloodstream. In addition to the potential for sustained effects, transdermal products bypass any problems with gastrointestinal absorption and first-pass metabolism.

Inhalation

Inhalation administration delivers a sterile drug directly into the lungs. This route is mostly used for local effects in the lungs, but is sometimes used for absorption of a drug into the bloodstream for systemic effects. The advantages of this route include a rapid onset of activity and avoidance of gastrointestinal absorption problems and first-pass metabolism. In addition, there are few to no systemic side effects when this route is used for local effects.

Rectal

Rectal administration means insertion of a drug suppository directly into the rectum and is abbreviated as "rect." or "PR" on a prescription. This route is used for either local effects in the rectum or for absorption of drug into the bloodstream for systemic effects. This route is an inexpensive alternative to the oral route for unconscious or vomiting patients when a systemic effect is desired. The administration of prochlorperazine (Compazine) suppositories for the management of nausea and vomiting is a good example of the effective use of the rectal route of administration. Advantages include a relatively low cost while bypassing gastrointestinal absorption problems and first-pass metabolism. The disadvantages of this route can include variable absorption and patients' dislike of inserting dosage forms into the rectum.

Vaginal

Vaginal administration involves the insertion of a drug directly into the vagina. This route is primarily used for local vaginal disorders, but some drugs can be absorbed into the bloodstream. Many vaginal preparations are antifungal agents in the form of creams, gels, ointments, and suppositories.

Intranasal

Intranasal administration means administering a drug directly into the nasal cavity. This route is used for either local effects in the nasal passages or for absorption of drugs into the bloodstream for systemic effects. The advantages of this route for systemic effects are the avoidance of gastrointestinal absorption problems and first-pass metabolism. When used for local effects, such as decongestant sprays, there are minimal systemic side effects.

Ophthalmic and otic

Ophthalmic and otic administration refers to giving a sterile drug directly into the eye or ear, respectively. Ophthalmic administration is designated by "o.u." or "o_2" for both eyes, "o.l." or "o.s." for the left eye only, and "o.d." for the right eye only. Otic administration is designated by "a.u." for both ears, "a.s." for the left ear only, and "a.d." for the right ear only. Both these routes are used for local drug effects which minimize or eliminate any systemic side effects.

Patient Variability

In addition to variability in drug response due to the route of administration, many patient-specific factors can affect an individual patient's response to drug therapy. The patient-specific factors include compliance, drug-food interactions, drug-drug interactions, drug-disease interactions, age, weight, or genetics.

Compliance

Compliance is the consistency or accuracy with which patients follow the prescribed directions for taking their medication. Compliance is a serious public health problem that has major health and economic implications. Studies report compliance rates in adults from about 8% to 93% depending on the medication and the frequency with which the medication should be taken. If not taken properly, the best possible therapeutic effect of the drug will not be achieved.

Drug-food interactions

Drug-food interactions occur when the presence of food results in altered absorption of orally administered drugs. Drug-food interactions can be a significant source of patient variability for certain drugs, and it can occur by several mechanisms. Some foods, particularly those high in fat, can significantly slow the rate of stomach emptying into the small intestine, thereby extending the drug's presence in the acidic pH of the stomach. The presence of food also influences the pH of the stomach. For these reasons, certain medications must be taken either with or without food according the instructions of the manufacturer.

Drug-drug interactions

Drug-drug interactions occur when a patient taking two or more drugs concurrently has an altered response to one or more of these drugs caused by the other drug(s). The effect of drug-drug interactions can be insignificant or it can decrease the therapeutic effect or increase the incidence and severity of side effects for one or more of the drugs the patient is taking. The interactions can be due to alterations in the absorption, distribution, metabolism, and elimination of one or more of the interacting drugs or a pharmacologic interaction (i.e., additive, synergistic, or antagonistic effects).

Absorption

Altered drug absorption due to the interaction of two or more drugs can occur by several mechanisms. The rate and extent of absorption of drugs depends on many factors that can be altered by the presence of other drugs. Drugs administered to elevate the pH in the stomach can affect the absorption of certain drugs. Absorption can also be altered by the binding of two or more drugs in the gastrointestinal tract, thereby preventing the drug's absorption. Finally, drugs that alter stomach emptying rate or gastrointestinal motility can affect the absorption of certain drugs by affecting the amount of time the drug takes to be absorbed.

Distribution

Altered drug distribution due to the interaction of two or more drugs normally occurs due to changes in plasma protein binding of drugs. Some drugs are highly bound to proteins in the blood. Interacting drugs that are also highly bound to these same proteins can competitively displace the other drug from its protein binding sites. This displacement leads to more unbound drug in the bloodstream which is free to diffuse out of the bloodstream into other tissue, which is the process of distribution. The net effect of this interaction is an increase in the distribution of the drug into tissues outside of the bloodstream. In addition, more unbound drug translates to more pharmacologic activity, which can lead to increased side effects.

Metabolism

Altered drug metabolism due to the interaction of two or more drugs can occur by two primary mechanisms: (1) enzyme induction and (2) inhibition. Most drugs are metabolized to some extent by various enzymes including the cytochrome P450 system in the liver and other parts of the body. These enzymes can have increased or decreased activity due to the presence of one or more drugs, as well as non-drug substances. These increases and decreases in metabolism due to other drugs are known as enzyme induction and enzyme inhibition, and the drugs causing these changes in activity are known as "inducers" and "inhibitors." Enzyme induction can lead to lower blood concentrations of drugs metabolized by that enzyme which can result in a decreased or lack of therapeutic effect. Enzyme inhibition can lead to higher blood concentrations of drugs metabolized by that enzyme which can result in an increased incidence of side effects.

Elimination

Altered drug elimination due to the interaction of two or more drugs can occur by several mechanisms. The kidney is the primary organ for drug elimination, and it is involved in both the elimination of the administered drug (i.e., parent drug) and its metabolites. Interacting drugs may increase or decrease the elimination of certain drugs by the kidneys. As with altered metabolism, these changes in elimination can lead to decreased drug concentrations in the blood and a corresponding decrease or lack of therapeutic effect or increased drug concentrations and a corresponding increased incidence of side effects.

Additive, Synergistic, and Antagonistic Interactions

Two or more drugs can combine to exert their individual pharmacological effects in an additive manner. Two or more drugs can also combine to exert their pharmacological effects in a manner that results in an overall effect that is more than what would result from a simple additive effect, analogous to "one plus one equals three." This type of interaction is known as a synergistic interaction. An antagonist interaction results when one or more drugs inhibit the pharmacological effect of another drug. These interactions can be beneficial and used in the treatment of a patient's medical condition. But these interactions can also decrease the effectiveness of the patient's drug therapy if they are not recognized.

Drug-disease interactions

Drug-disease interactions occur when a patient's disease state results in altered drug response. Therefore, the overall health of the patient can significantly affect the response to drug therapy. The liver is the primary location for drug metabolism, so diseases such as hepatitis and alcoholic liver disease can result in decreased drug metabolism. The kidney is the primary organ of drug elimination, so disease such as acute and chronic renal failure can result in decreased drug elimination. Both of these examples would lead to higher concentrations of drugs in the blood which can increase side effects and the drug's effectiveness.

Age and weight

Weight progressively increases from birth through adolescence, increases more slowly through adulthood, and then gradually declines in the elderly. Body water, muscle mass, and organ mass are all related to body weight. In addition, many bodily functions including organ blood flow and organ function are related to body weight. Some individuals may be considerably underweight or overweight compared to normal. All these factors can lead to the requirement of greatly different doses to achieve the desired therapeutic response depending on an individual patient's age and weight.

Genetics

Genetic variation can account for large variability in drug response. Genetic variation in drug-metabolizing enzymes usually results in severely decreased drug metabolism. These genetic variations are known as pharmacogenetic polymorphisms, and they have been identified in the cytochrome P450 system and other drug-metabolizing enzymes. The changes in drug metabolism due to pharmacogenetic polymorphisms can be very dramatic and can result in toxic concentrations of drugs when normal doses of the medications are taken. Pharmacogenetic polymorphisms can also result in lack of therapeutic effect if the administered drug is a prodrug, meaning it requires metabolic conversion in the body to an active compound. Codeine is a good example of a prodrug which requires conversion to morphine by cytochrome P450 2D6 to exert its analgesic activity. However, 8%–14% of Caucasians have pharmacogenetic polymorphisms of this particular enzyme and, therefore, cannot convert codeine to the active analgesic, morphine. Unmetabolized codeine results in a lack of pain relief and may cause nausea and vomiting.

Classification of Drugs

This section provides information on drugs and their therapeutic category. It is divided into bone and joint disorders, cardiovascular disorders, endocrinologic disorders, gastrointestinal disorders, gynecologic and obstetric disorders, infectious diseases, neurologic disorders, psychiatric disorders, and respiratory disorders. The list of medications is not all-inclusive, but attention has been placed on the most prescribed drugs in each category. Some prescription drugs are available without a prescription, but are usually in lower strengths as compared to their prescription counterparts. These over-the-counter (OTC) products will be marked with an asterisk (*).

Bone and Joint Disorders

Osteoporosis

Osteoporosis is a condition of diminished bone density. Many factors can contribute to osteoporosis, but the result is bone mass being lost faster than it is being formed. This decrease in bone density leads to an increased risk of fractures. Osteoporosis is most common in elderly women, but also occurs in men. Treatment and prevention of osteoporosis includes bisphosphonates, calcium supplements, estrogens, and vitamin D therapy. A list of drugs used to treat osteoporosis can be found in **Table 20-1**.

Osteoarthritis and pain

Almost 50% of individuals over age 65 are afflicted with osteoarthritis. Osteoarthritis is marked by a degeneration of cartilage, primarily in weight-bearing joints. The lack of cushioning between articulating bones results in inflammation, mild to moderate pain, and limited range of motion. Appropriate pain management is vital when treating osteoarthritis. It is best to begin therapy with an agent that will have the fewest side effects. These usually include aspirin, acetaminophen, and nonsteroidal anti-inflammatory drugs. Narcotic analgesics are rarely used in osteoarthritis, but are usually reserved for moderate to severe pain from other causes. Analgesics are often taken orally, while there are some available as transdermal and injectable products. Anesthetics can also be used in acute and chronic pain. These agents can be injected or applied topically and work by blocking

TABLE 20-1   **Drugs Used to Treat Osteoporosis**

Generic Name	Common Brand Name(s)
Bisphosphonates	
Alendronate	Fosamax
Risendronate	Actonel
Estrogens	
Conjugated estrogens	Premarin
Esterified estrogens	Estratab, Menest
Mircronized estradiol	Estrace
Transdermal estrogen	Climara, Estraderm, Vivelle
Miscellaneous Agents	
Calcitonin	Miacalcin
Calcium (*)	Tums, Viactiv, Oscal, Citracal
Raloxifene	Evista
Vitamin D (*)	Various

*Over-the-counter product

TABLE 20-2   Pain Medication

Generic Name	Common Brand Name(s)
Analgesics (Non-narcotic)	
acetaminophen (*)	Tylenol
acetylsalicylic acid (*)	Aspirin
celecoxib	Celebrex
diclofenac	Voltaren
ketoprofen (*)	Orudis KT
ibuprofen (*)	Motrin
indomethacin	Indocin
nambumetone	Relafen
naproxen (*)	Aleve, Anaprox, Naprosyn
rofecoxib	Vioxx
valdecoxib	Bextra
Analgesics (Narcotic)	
codeine (and combinations)	Tylenol w/Codeine #3, Various
fentanyl	Duragesic, Actiq
hydrocodone combinations	Lorcet, Lortab, Vicodin
hydromorphone	Dilaudid
meperidine	Demerol
methadone	Dolophine
morphine	MS Contin
oxycodone (and combinations)	OxyIR, OxyContin, Percocet, Tylox, Percodin
propoxyphene (and combinations)	Darvocet-N 100, Darvon
pentazocine	Talwin, Talwin NX
tramadol	Ultram
Anesthetics	
bupivacaine	Marcaine
dibucaine	Nupercaine
halothane	Fluothane
lidocaine	Xylocaine
procaine	Novocain
propofol	Diprivan
thiopental	Pentothal
tetracaine	Pontocaine

*Over-the-counter product

painful nerve impulses. Pain medications used in the treatment of osteoarthritis are found in **Table 20-2**.

Cardiovascular Disorders

Arrhythmias

An arrhythmia is a disruption in the heart's normal beating or rhythmic pattern. This abnormal electrical conduction can occur in different areas of the heart. Some common examples of arrhythmias are sinus bradycardia, sinus or ventricular tachycardia, atrial fibrillation, and ventricular fibrillation. Antiarrhythmic drugs are used to treat these arrhythmias (**Table 20-3**) and are classified into four types based on their electrophysiological properties.

Coronary artery disease

Coronary artery disease (CAD) develops as atherosclerotic plaques form on the inner walls of cardiac vessels. There are modifiable and nonmodifiable risk factors involved in the development of CAD. Angina pectoris is a common condition that is associated with coronary artery disease. When the vessels of the heart become blocked with plaque, or fatty material, the oxygen demand of the body may not be able to be met. Vasodilators, calcium channel blockers, and beta-adrenergic blockers are often used in the treatment of angina pectoris. A thrombus, or clot, can also form in vessels and block blood flow through those vessels. Antithrombotic agents can prevent platelet aggregation and reduce the likelihood of clot formation. Thrombolytic agents are used to dissolve previously formed clots. A list of agents used in the treatment of coronary artery disease can be found in **Table 20-4**.

TABLE 20-3

Classifications of Antiarrhythmic Drugs

Generic Name	Common Brand Name(s)
Type 1A	
disopyramide	Norpace
procainamide	Procanbid, Pronestyl
quinidine	Cardioquin, Quinaglute, Quinidex
Type 1B	
lidocaine	Xylocaine
mexiletine	Mexitil
tocainide	Tonocard
Type 1C	
flecainide	Tambocor
propafenone	Rythmol
Type 2	
beta-adrenergic blockers	
(see Table 20-6)	
Type 3	
amiodarone	Cordarone, Pacerone
bretylium	Bretylate
dofetilide	Tikosyn
sotalol	Betapace, Betapace AF
Type 4	
diltiazem	Cardizem, Dilacor XR, Tiazac
verapamil	Calan, Covera, Isoptin, Verelan
Miscellaneous Agents	
adenosine	Adenocard
digoxin	Lanoxin

TABLE 20-4   Agents Used in Coronary Artery Disease

Generic Name	Common Brand Name(s)
Antithrombotic Agents	
argatroban	Argatroban
dalteparin	Fragmin
enoxaparin	Lovenox
fondaparinux	Arixtra
heparin	Hep-Lock Liquaemin
warfarin	Coumadin
Thrombolytic Agents	
alteplase	Activase
streptokinase	Streptase
urokinase	Abbokinase
Beta-adrenergic Blockers (see Table 20-6)	
Calcium Channel Blockers	
amlodipine	Norvasc
diltiazem	Cardizem, Dilacor, Tiazac
felodipine	Plendil
nifedipine	Adalat CC, Procardia XL
verapamil	Calan, Covera, Isoptin, Verelan
Nitrates	
isosorbide dinitrate	Isordil
isosorbide mononitrate	Imdur
nitroglycerin	Nitrostat, Nitro-Bid, Minitran

Hyperlipidemia

Hyperlipidemia is an abnormally high concentration of lipids, or cholesterol, in the blood. Cholesterol is synthesized in the liver and is contained in many foods. The human body can use cholesterol as an energy source or store it. Cholesterol and triglycerides are two major lipids found in the body. A total cholesterol level of less than 200 mg/dl is desirable. Hyperlipidemia increases patients' chances of developing coronary artery disease (CAD) and peripheral vascular disease (PVD). Several classes of drug with different mechanisms of action are used to treat hyperlipidemia. Bile acid resins bind with bile acid to inhibit cholesterol absorption and storage. Fibrates cause an increase in enzymes which results in an increase in cholesterol metabolism. HMG-CoA reductase is an important enzyme that catalyzes in vivo cholesterol synthesis. HMG-CoA reductase inhibitors target this enzyme and inhibit its activity. Drugs used to lower cholesterol are listed in **Table 20-5**.

Hypertension

Hypertension, or high blood pressure, is a constant elevation in the systolic or diastolic blood pressure. Blood pressure is considered to be high when the systolic pressure is greater than 140 mmHg and the diastolic pressure is greater than

TABLE 20-5

Drugs Used to Treat Hyperlipidemia

Generic Name	Common Brand Name(s)
Bile Acid Resins	
colestipol	Colestid
colesevelam	Welchol
Fibrates	
clofibrate	Atromid-S
fenofibrate	Tricor
gemfibrozil	Lopid
HMG-CoA Reductase Inhibitors	
atorvastatin	Lipitor
lovastatin	Mevacor
pravastatin	Pravachol
rosuvastatin	Crestor
simvastatin	Zocor
Miscellaneous Agent	
ezetimibe	Zetia
niacin (*)	Niaspan

*Over-the-counter product

90 mmHg. There are numerous mechanisms that cause elevations in blood pressure. Drugs with different mechanisms of action can be utilized to reduce blood pressure effectively in individual patients. Alpha-adrenergic blockers hinder the nerve conduction to the heart and block nerve impulses that would make the heart beat faster. Angiotensin-converting enzyme inhibitors (ACE inhibitors) and angiotensin II receptor blockers (ARBs) work against the body's own mechanisms for raising blood pressure. Beta-adrenergic blockers regulate the heart rate. Calcium channel blockers weaken muscle contraction and decrease the workload placed on the heart. Diuretics lower blood pressure by lowering the volume of the vasculature, and vasodilators relax the walls of blood vessels. All of these agents are commonly used in treating hypertension (**Table 20-6**).

Endocrine Disorders

Diabetes mellitus

Diabetes mellitus is the body's inability to either produce or efficiently use insulin which results in high blood sugar, or hyperglycemia. Type I diabetes is characterized by the inability to produce insulin. Type II diabetes differs in that the body cannot efficiently utilize the insulin that it makes. Type I diabetics are usually diagnosed during adolescence while Type II diabetes usually manifests later in adulthood. The goal of therapy in diabetes mellitus is to maintain blood sugar levels within 80–120 mg/dl. Insulin is used more often by Type I diabetics as compared to Type II diabetics. However, both populations can utilize oral hypoglycemic agents to control blood glucose concentrations. Drugs used to treat diabetes are listed in **Table 20-7**.

Thyroid disorders

The thyroid gland plays a crucial role in growth, body development, and metabolism. Thyroid disorders involve either producing excess thyroid hormone or failing

TABLE 20-6   Drugs Used to Treat Hypertension

Generic Name	Common Brand Name(s)
Alpha-adrenergic Blockers	
doxazosin	Cardura
prazosin	Minipress
terazosin	Hytrin
Angiotensin-Converting Enzyme Inhibitors	
benazepril	Lotensin
captopril	Capoten
enalapril	Vasotec
fosinopril	Monopril
lisinopril	Prinivil, Zestril
quinapril	Accupril
ramipril	Altace
Angiotensin II Receptor Blockers	
candesartan	Atacand
irbesartan	Avapro
losartan	Cozaar
telmisartan	Micardis
valsartan	Diovan
Beta-adrenergic Blockers	
atenolol	Tenormin
bisoprolol	Ziac
carvedilol	Coreg
labetalol	Normodyne, Trandate
metoprolol	Lopressor, Toprol XL
nadolol	Corgard
propranolol	Inderal, Inderal LA
Calcium Channel Blockers	
amlodipine	Norvasc
diltiazem	Cardizem, Dilacor, Tiazac
felodipine	Plendil
nifedipine	Adalat CC, Procardia XL
verapamil	Calan, Covera, Isoptin, Verelan
Diuretics	
bumetanide	Bumex
furosemide	Lasix
hydrochlorothiazide	Esidrix, HydroDIURIL, Oretic
spironolactone	Aldactone
triamterene and hydrochlorothiazide	Dyazide, Maxzide

TABLE 20-6

Drugs Used to Treat Hypertension (continued)

Generic Name	Common Brand Name(s)
Vasodilators	
hydralazine	Apresoline
minoxidil	Loniten
sodium nitroprusside	Nitropress
Miscellaneous Agents	
clonidine	Catapres, Catapres-TTS
methyldopa	Aldomet
potassium chloride	K-Dur, Klor-Con, Micro-K, Slow-K

TABLE 20-7

Drugs Used to Treat Diabetes Mellitus

Generic Name	Common Brand Name(s)
Insulin Preparations	
intermediate-acting insulin	Humulin N, NPH-N, Novolin N
lente	Humulin L, Novolin L
long-acting insulin	Humulin U, Lantus
rapid-acting insulin	Humalog, NovoLog
NPH-regular combinations	Humulin 70/30, Novolin 70/30
short-acting insulin	Humulin R, Novolin R, Velosulin
Oral Hypoglycemic Agents	
acarbose	Precose
chlorpropamide	Diabinese
glimeperide	Amaryl
glipizide	Glucotrol
glyburide	DiaBeta, Glynase, Micronase
metformin	Glucophage
nateglinide	Starlix
pioglitazone	Actos
repaglinide	Prandin
rosiglitazone	Avandia

to produce an adequate amount. Hyperthyroidism is an increase in production of thyroid hormone. Hypothyroidism is a decrease in thyroid hormone production. Treatment consists of suppressing thyroid hormone production in hyperthyroidism, or supplying an exogenous source of thyroid hormone for hypothyroidism. Drugs used for this purpose are listed in **Table 20-8**.

TABLE 20-8   **Drugs Used to Treat Thyroid Disorders**

Generic Name	Common Brand Name(s)
Hyperthyroidism Agents	
methimazole	Tapazole
nadolol	Corgard
propylthiouracil	Propyl-Thyracil
Hypothyroidism Agents	
levothyroxine	Levothroid, Levoxyl, Synthroid
liothyronine	Cytomel
liotrix	Thyrolar
thyroid USP	Armour Thyroid

Gastrointestinal Disorders

Diarrhea and constipation

Diarrhea is an abnormally frequent occurrence of watery or semisolid stools. Diarrhea can be caused by disease, drugs, infection, and toxins. This increased frequency of watery defecation can lead to dehydration. Treatment consists of agents that can absorb the excess water or slow down the intestinal motility. Constipation is a decrease in stool frequency. This decreased frequency could be caused by certain medications. It is also often directly related to dietary fiber consumption. Common treatments of constipation are aimed at softening stools, increasing motility, and increasing bulk or volume of feces. Medications used to treat diarrhea and constipation are listed in **Table 20-9**.

Gastroesophageal reflux disease

Gastroesophageal reflux disease (GERD) is a condition where gastric acid and other stomach contents come back up into the esophagus causing pain and irritation. Common foods such as chocolate, coffee, and carbonated beverages can worsen GERD. Certain medications can also worsen gastroesophageal reflux disease. Treatment usually consists of over-the-counter antacids and histamine-receptor (H2) blockers, or prescription proton pump inhibitors (**Table 20-10**).

Gynecologic and Obstetric Disorders

Contraception and hormone replacement therapy

Contraception is simply the prevention of pregnancy or conception. There are various methods of contraception, but this section will focus on oral contraception. Oral contraception involves the manipulation of estrogen and its role in normal physiology. Most oral contraceptives contain a form of estrogen and a progestin component. Hormone replacement therapy usually begins during menopause to decrease associated symptoms. Drugs used as contraceptives and for hormone replacement are listed in **Table 20-11**.

TABLE 20-9

Drugs Used to Treat Diarrhea and Constipation

Generic Name	Common Brand Name(s)
Absorbing Agents	
attapulgite (*)	Kaopectate
polycarbophil (*)	Fiberall, Fibercon
Antimotility Agents	
diphenoxylate	Lomotil
loperamide (*)	Imodium
Laxative and Cathartic Agents	
bisacodyl (*)	Dulcolax
docusate (*)	Colace
gylcerin (*)	various
lactulose	Chronulac
mineral oil (*)	various
polyethylene glycol	GoLYTELY, MiraLax, NuLYTELY
psyllium (*)	Metamucil
saline (*)	various
senna (*)	Senokot

*Over-the-counter product

TABLE 20-10

Drugs Used to Treat GERD

Generic Name	Common Brand Name(s)
Antacids	
aluminum-containing (*)	AlternaGEL
calcium-containing (*)	Rolaids, Tums
magnesium/aluminum combinations (*)	Gaviscon, Maalox, Mylanta
sodium bicarbonate (*)	various
Histamine Receptor (H2) Blockers	
cimetidine (*)	Tagamet
famotidine (*)	Pepcid
nizatidine (*)	Axid
ranitidine (*)	Zantac
Proton Pump Inhibitors	
esomeprazole	Nexium
lansoprazole	Prevacid
omeprazole	Prilosec
pantoprazole	Protonix
rabeprazole	Aciphex
Miscellaneous Agents	
metoclopramide	Reglan
misoprostol	Cytotec
sucralfate	Carafate

*Over-the-counter product

TABLE 20-11   Drugs Used for Contraception and Hormone Replacement

Generic Name	Common Brand Name(s)
Estrogens	
conjugated estrogens	Premarin
esterified estrogens	Estratab, Menest
micronized estradiol	Estrace
transdermal estrogen	Climara, Estraderm, Vivelle
Progestins	
medroxyprogesterone	Provera
norethindrone	Aygestin, Micronor, Nor-QD
norgestrel	Ovrette
progesterone	Prometrium
Combined Oral Contraceptives	
ethinyl estradiol and desogestrel	Desogen, Mircette
ethinyl estradiol and norethindrone	Estrostep, Ortho-Novum, Ovcon
ethinyl estradiol and norgestimate	Ortho-Cyclen, Ortho Tri-Cyclen
ethinyl estradiol and norgestrel	Ovral, Lo/Ovral, Low-Ogestrel-28
conjugated estrogens and	
medroxyprogesterone	Premphase, Prempro

Infectious Diseases

Bacterial, fungal, and viral infections

Antibiotics used to treat bacterial infections are classified as either bacteriostatic or bacteriocidal. Bacteriostatic drugs inhibit the growth of an infecting organism, and bacteriocidal drugs kill the infecting organism. Antibiotics also work by various mechanisms of action. Penicillins and cephalosporins disrupt the cell wall of the organism. Aminoglycosides, fluoroquinolones, macrolides, and tetracyclines move into the cell to inhibit RNA and protein synthesis. Antifungal agents are used to treat both topical and systemic fungal infections. Antiviral agents are reserved for the treatment of viral infections. Antibiotics used to treat infections are found in **Table 20-12**.

Neurologic Disorders

Epilepsy

Epilepsy is a term that encompasses various symptoms that can range from some alteration in consciousness to uncontrollable convulsions or seizures that result from altered brain function. Decreasing the frequency of these attacks or seizures greatly increases the quality of life in epileptics. Drugs used to treat epilepsy are found in **Table 20-13**.

Psychiatric disorders

Psychiatric disorders range from depression, anxiety, and sleep disorders to more severe illnesses. Depression is an overwhelming feeling of sadness or guilt. There

TABLE 20-12

Drugs Used to Treat Infections

Generic Name	Common Brand Name(s)
Aminoglycosides	
amikacin	Amikin
gentamicin	Garamycin
neomycin	Mycifradin
streptomycin	various
tobramycin	Nebcin
Antifungal agents	
amphotericin B	Abelcet, Fungizone
clotrimazole (*)	Mycelex, Lotrimin
fluconazole	Diflucan
itraconazole	Sporanox
ketoconazole (*)	Nizoral
miconazole (*)	Monistat
nystatin	Mycostatin
voriconazole	Vfend
Antiviral agents	
acyclovir	Zovirax
amantadine	Symmetrel
didanosine	Videx
famciclovir	Famvir
ribavirin	Virazole
rimantadine	Flumadine
stavudine	Zerit
valacyclovir	Valtrex
zidovudine	Retrovir
Cephalosporins	
cefaclor	Ceclor
cefadroxil	Duricef
cefpodoxime	Vantin
cefprozil	Cefzil
ceftazidime	Fortaz
ceftriaxone	Rocephin
cephalexin	Keflex
Fluroquinolones	
ciprofloxacin	Cipro, Cipro XR
gatifloxacin	Tequin
moxifloxacin	Avelox
Macrolides	
azithromycin	Zithromax, Z-Pack
clarithromycin	Biaxin, Biaxin XL
erythromycin	E.E.S., Ery-Tab

*Over-the-counter product

TABLE 20-12 Drugs Used to Treat Infections (continued)

Generic Name	Common Brand Name(s)
Penicillins	
amoxicillin	Amoxil, Trimox
amoxicillin/clavulanate	Augmentin
ampicillin	Principen
ampicillin/sulbactam	Unasyn
penicillin G	various
piperacillin	Pipracil
piperacillin/tazobactam	Zosyn
ticarcillin	Ticar
Penicillin-related Agents	
aztreonam	Azactam
imipenem/cilastin	Primaxin
meropenen	Merrem IV
Tetracyclines	
doxycyline	Vibramycin
minocycline	Minocin
tetracycline	Sumycin
Miscellaneous Antibiotics	
isoniazid	INH
metronidazole	Flagyl, Flagyl ER
nitrofurantoin	Macrobid, Macrodantin
rifampin	Rifadin
sulfamethoxazole/trimethoprim	Bactrim, Septra

TABLE 20-13 Drugs Used to Treat Epilepsy

Generic Name	Common Brand Name(s)
Anticonvulsant Agents	
carbamazepine	Tegretol
clonazepam	Klonopin
fosphenytoin	Cerebyx
gabapentin	Neurontin
lamotrigine	Lamictal
phenobarbital	Luminal
phenytoin	Dilantin
valproic acid	Depakote
zonisamide	Zonegran

are numerous options for treating depression. Serotonin reuptake inhibitors are often used to treat depression. Anxiety disorders are characterized by abnormal restlessness and worry. Anxiety is commonly treated with benzodiazepines. With disruptions in mood, a lack of restful sleep often follows. Hypnotics are used to induce sleep in patients. Drugs used to treat psychiatric disorders can be found in **Table 20-14**.

Respiratory Disorders

Asthma and chronic obstructive pulmonary disease (COPD)
Asthma is a condition that is characterized by inflammation of the airways. Wheezing, chest tightness, and coughing occur frequently with asthma. Environmental factors, exercise, and certain drugs can all be triggers of asthmatic episodes.

TABLE 20-14

Drugs Used to Treat Psychiatric Disorders

Generic Name	Common Brand Name(s)
Antianxiety Agents	
alprazolam	Xanax
buspirone	BuSpar
clonazepam	Klonopin
diazepam	Valium
hydroxyzine	Atarax, Vistaril
imipramine	Tofranil
lorazepam	Ativan
oxazepam	Serax
velafaxine	Effexor XR
Antidepressants	
amitriptyline	Elavil
bupropion	Wellbutrin, Zyban
citalopram	Celexa
escitalopram	Lexapro
fluoxetine	Prozac
mirtazapine	Remeron
nortryptiline	Pamelor
paroxetine	Paxil, Paxil CR
sertraline	Zoloft
trazadone	Desyre 1
Hypnotic Agents	
flurazepam	Dalmane
midazolam	Versed
temazepam	Restoril
triazolam	Halcion
zaleplon	Sonata
zolpidem	Ambien

Chronic obstructive pulmonary disease (COPD) has two main causes: (1) chronic bronchitis and (2) emphysema. COPD has an inflammatory component along with airway obstruction. Treatments of asthma and COPD are similar. Bronchodilators are used to relax the bronchial smooth muscle and assist in breathing. Mast cell stabilizers and steroids are used to treat the inflammatory components of asthma and COPD. Drugs used to treat asthma and COPD are listed in **Table 20-15**.

Antihistamines and decongestants

Antihistamines block the activity of histamine that is released during colds, inflammation, and allergic reactions. Decongestants are often added to cold preparations to help alleviate a stuffy nose. Decongestants cause a constriction of blood vessels and allow for better breathing through the nose. It is important to note that individuals who have high blood pressure should contact their pharmacist or physician before using any products containing decongestants. Drugs used as antihistamines and decongestants are listed in **Table 20-16**.

TABLE 20-15 **Drugs Used to Treat Asthma and COPD**

Generic Name	Common Brand Name(s)
Anticholinergic Agent	
ipratropium	Atrovent
Beta-2 Adrenergic Agonists	
albuterol	Proventil, Ventolin
epinephrine (*)	Primatene Mist
levalbuterol	Xopenex
metaproterenol	Alupent
pirbuterol	Maxair
salmeterol	Serevent
terbutaline	Brethine
Mast Cell Stabilizing Agents	
cromolyn (*)	Intal, Nasalcrom
nedocromil	Tilade
Steroids	
beclomethasone	Beclovent, Beconase, Vancenase Vanceril
flunisolide	AeroBid
fluticasone	Flovent
prednisone	Deltasone, Orasone
triamcinalone	Azmacort

*Over-the-counter product

TABLE 20-16 Antihistamines and Decongestants

Generic Name	Common Brand Name(s)
Antihistamines	
brompheniramine (*)	Dimetapp
cetirizine	Zyrtec
chlorpheniramine (*)	Chlor-Trimeton
desloratadine	Clarinex
diphenhydramine	Benadryl
fexofenadine	Allegra
loratidine (*)	Alavert, Claritin
meclizine (*)	Antivert, Bonine
promethazine	Phenergan
Decongestants	
ephedrine (*)	Ephadron Nasal, Vatronol
phenylephrine (*)	Neosynephrine
pseudoephedrine (*)	Sudafed

*Over-the-counter product

Summary

This chapter first noted the advantages and disadvantages of the various extravascular and intravascular modes of drug administration. Drug action is also affected by patient characteristics such as compliance with directions for taking the drug, interactions of drugs with food and other drugs, and patient pathology, as well as age, weight, and genetic predispositions.

The second major part of the chapter dealt with the major therapeutic doses of drugs in use today and included both the generic and trade names of the drugs in each category.

Both the actions and the uses of drugs have been described and noted to provide the pharmacy technician with a sound basis for understanding the basics of drug therapy.

TEST YOUR KNOWLEDGE

Multiple Choice Questions

1. Which of the following route(s) of administration avoid first-pass metabolism?
    - I. oral
    - II. sublingual
    - III. intravenous
    - a. I only
    - b. III only
    - c. I and II only
    - d. II and III only
    - e. I, II, and III

2. Which one of the following routes of administration is best when a rapid on-set of systemic drug action is required in an emergency situation?
   a. transdermal
   b. rectal
   c. intravenous
   d. oral

3. Induction of drug-metabolizing enzymes is mostly likely to cause
   a. increased drug concentrations and increased side effects
   b. increased drug concentrations and decreased therapeutic effect
   c. decreased drug concentrations and increased side effects
   d. decreased drug concentrations and decreased therapeutic effect

4. Which drug listed below is a beta-adrenergic blocker?
   a. albuterol
   b. captopril
   c. propranolol
   d. fluconazole

5. Which of the following drugs is used to treat hyperlipidemia?
   a. diltiazem
   b. isoniazid
   c. minoxidil
   d. atorvastatin

6. Atrovent, Serevent and Flovent are common treatments for:
   a. coronary artery disease
   b. respiratory disorders
   c. hypertension
   d. bacterial infections

Matching Questions

Abbreviations   **Meaning**

7. _____ sl   a. intramuscular

8. _____ a.u.   b. subcutaneous

9. _____ IM   c. both ears

10. _____ o.d.   d. right eye

11. _____ SC   e. sublingual

Generic Name   **Brand Name**

12. _____ digoxin   a. Clarinex

13. _____ acetaminophen   b. Proventil

14. _____ warfarin   c. Dolophine

15. _____ salmeterol   d. Coumadin

16. _____ albuterol   e. Serevent

17. _____ desloratidine   f. Lanoxin

18. _____ methadone   g. Tylenol

True/False Questions

19. _____ Most patients are compliant with their prescribed medication directions.

20. _____ Decongestants are recommended for every patient with a stuffy nose.

References

DiPiro, J., Talbert, R., Yee, G. et al., (Eds.). (2002). *Pharmacotherapy: A pathophysiological approach* (5th ed.). New York: McGraw-Hill.

Hardman, J., & Limbird, L. (Eds.). (2001). *Goodman & Gilman's The pharmacological basis of therapeutics* (10th ed.). New York: McGraw-Hill.

Lacy, C., Armstrong, L., Goldman, M. et al. (Eds.). (2001). *Drug information handbook* (9th ed.) Hudson, OH: Lexi-Comp Inc.

Rowland, M., & Tozer, T. (1995). *Clinical pharmacokinetics concepts and applications* (3rd ed.). Media, PA: Williams & Wilkins.

Shargel, L., & Yu, A. (1999). *Applied biopharmaceutics and pharmacokinetics* (4th ed.). Stamford, CT: Appleton & Lange.

Nonprescription Medications

COMPETENCIES

Upon completion of this chapter, the reader should be able to

1. Define the term *over-the-counter agent* and be familiar with other common terms used to identify these agents.
2. Describe the various dosage formulations available as over-the-counter agents.
3. List the various therapeutic categories most commonly used for the purpose of self-care by patients.
4. Identify a specific nonprescription medication and recognize which therapeutic category it belongs to.
5. List common indications, adverse effects, and drug-disease interactions of select nonprescription medications.

Introduction

It is important for those practicing in a pharmacy environment to be familiar with agents that may be purchased by the consumer without a prescription from their health care provider. These medications are available for patients who are suffering from conditions that are considered self-treatable. An advantage is that they do not require patients to see their physician in order to gain access to them. This alleviates substantial burden on the health care community. It also allows the individual more control over his or her own personal health needs. The disadvantage is that without a physician's guidance, the patients may misdiagnose their condition and a far more serious condition may remain unrecognized. This can lead to inadequate treatment. In addition, over-the-counter agents (OTCs) have pharmacological activity, thus they have the potential to cause significant side effects and interact adversely with other medications that a patient may be taking. Certain nonprescription medications may not be safe for those patients with specific disease states, therefore, it is important for the pharmacist to be aware of the OTCs a patient is taking in order to effectively counsel a patient. For the above reasons, nonprescription medications are not benign and all considerations used by the pharmacist when evaluating prescription medications should be employed when a patient purchases an OTC. A technician can be of great assistance to the pharmacist in identifying patients who may require counseling or a visit to their physician. When patients come into the pharmacy to purchase a nonprescription medication or to fill a prescription, the technician may ask the patient about his nonprescription

tion medication use so that it can be placed in the patient's profile. Information that a pharmacy technician obtains during a casual conversation with the patient should be communicated to the pharmacist and will aid in identifying potential problems that may have otherwise gone unrecognized. In order to be able to do this effectively, a technician should be familiar with the numerous OTC products that are available. This chapter will highlight the most common therapeutic agents that are available for patients to purchase without a prescription.

Dosage Forms

OTCs are available in many different formulations, similar to prescription drugs. The most widely used agents are available as oral dosage forms and include capsules, tablets, suspensions, solutions, and effervescent tablets. It is important for patients to shake a suspension well, while solutions do not require this step. Effervescent tablets, such as Alka-Seltzer, need to be dissolved in water or another compatible liquid prior to ingesting. These agents also tend to have an increased amount of sodium, which becomes important in those patients who are on salt-restricted diets for disease states such as hypertension or heart failure. If an alternative dosage form is available, the pharmacist should make a recommendation that the patient take that rather than the effervescent tablet.

Topical agents are available as creams, ointments, and lotions. Other available forms include eardrops, eyedrops, suppositories, enemas, and shampoos. These dosage forms should never be taken by mouth since they are intended for external use only.

Pain

Analgesics are those agents that are used to treat a patient's pain. A patient may have pain for a variety of reasons and it may manifest as headaches, muscle pain, or bone or joint pain. Pain is often categorized as either acute or chronic. Acute pain is due to a recent, sudden occurrence such as an injury, medical procedure, or accident while chronic pain is usually the result of an underlying disease state such as cancer, rheumatoid arthritis, or multiple sclerosis. In general, nonprescription analgesics are most appropriately utilized in patients suffering from acute pain or as adjunctive agents in those with chronic pain. They are effective for mild to moderate pain. The pharmacist should direct the patient to see his or her physician for a complete evaluation if the pain has not resolved within ten days of taking an OTC analgesic. Analgesics are also commonly used as antipyretics to decrease a patient's fever. The pharmacist should direct the patient to see his or her physician for a complete fever workup if the fever has not subsided within three days of taking an OTC antipyretic.

Internal analgesics are those that can be taken by mouth (po) and include salicylates (e.g., aspirin), acetaminophen, and nonsteroidal anti-inflammatory drugs (NSAIDs). See **Table 21-1** for agents that are available without a prescription. OTC NSAIDs include ibuprofen, ketoprofen, and naproxen. The doses of OTC NSAIDs are considerably less than their prescription counterparts.

Common side effects of salicylates include bleeding and gastrointestinal irritation. These agents should be avoided in pregnant patients. Children and adolescents are at increased risk of developing Reye's syndrome, a fatal illness, especially

TABLE 21-1

Nonprescription Analgesic Agents

Therapeutic Category	Generic Name	Brand Name	Formulation
Salicylates	Aspirin	Anacin, Ascriptin, Bayer, Bufferin, Ecotrin	Tablets, caplets
	Magnesium salicylate	Doan's, Momentum	Caplets
	Choline salicylate	Arthropan	Liquid
Nonsteroidal anti-inflammatory drugs	Ibuprofen	Advil, Motrin, Nuprin	Tablets, chewtabs, caplets, capsules, geltabs, drops, suspension, liquid
	Ketoprofen	Actron, Orudis KT	Caplets, tablets
	Naproxen	Aleve	Caplets, tablets
Other	Acetaminophen	Tylenol, Tempra	Effervescent tablet, tablets, chewtabs, caplets, capsules, geltabs, drops, suspension, liquid
Counterirritants	Menthol	Absorbine Jr., BenGay, Flexall, Therapeutic Mineral Ice	Topical liquid, gel, cream
	Capsaicin	Capzasin, Zostrix	Topical lotion, gel, cream
	Trolamine salicylate	Aspercreme, Aspergel, Myoflex	Cream, lotion

if they have the flu or chicken pox. Therefore, salicylates are generally avoided in this population. An important drug interaction to consider with the salicylates is that they may cause increased risk of bleeding in those patients also taking warfarin. This interaction is also seen in patients taking NSAIDs and, to a lesser degree, acetaminophen.

Like salicylates, NSAIDs also cause significant stomach upset, dyspepsia, and heartburn. To help prevent stomach upset, the pharmacist should instruct patients to take these agents with food, milk, or antacids. The NSAIDs should be avoided in those patients who are allergic to aspirin or have asthma, ulcers, renal impairment, or heart failure.

Acetaminophen is also widely used for pain and is well tolerated, but may be damaging to the liver in higher doses, especially in those who are malnourished or drink heavily. Acetaminophen is available in several different dosage formulations and strengths for both the adult and pediatric populations. These include drops, syrup, suspension, suppositories, chewable tablets, caplets, tablets, and gelcaps.

Combination products are available for the consumer to purchase as well. The most common combination products include caffeine, which may increase the analgesic activity of the primary ingredient. They may also contain combinations of two of the agents discussed above.

Topical OTCs are available and are applied externally to the affected area of pain. External analgesics, including topical NSAIDs, are of questionable efficacy. They may decrease pain, itching, and burning. Counterirritants produce mild pain and inflammation at a site close to the affected area and decrease the severity of the pain that the patient is experiencing. This masks the pain that the patient has to make it more tolerable. Camphor, menthol, capsaicin, and trolamine salicylate are the most commonly used counterirritants. See Table 21-1 for available formulations. The pharmacist should warn users not to apply counterirritants to wounded skin or in the eyes. Bandages should not be placed over these products. Patients should be made aware that these agents might cause a burning sensation when applied and are never to be ingested.

Cold and Allergy

A **cold** is a self-limiting viral infection of the respiratory tract. The main goal in patients suffering from a cold is to alleviate their symptoms because a cold cannot be cured by the administration of antibiotics. Decongestants are used for patients' nasal stuffiness, analgesics for their fever and pain, and **antitussives** for their cough. **Antihistamines** can also be utilized to help control a runny nose and sneezing. Many combination products are available because many patients experience one or more cold symptoms. Multiple medications used separately can be quite confusing and cumbersome for the patient, and the likelihood of mistakes is much higher.

Allergies are characterized by sneezing, itchy and watery eyes, and an itchy, runny nose. The person with allergies may also experience increased fatigue, irritability, and worsening mood. These symptoms are triggered by an allergen, such as mold, pollen, cigarette smoke, dust, or pet dander. The symptoms of allergies are treated with antihistamines, intranasal cromolyn, and topical decongestants.

OTC decongestants are available as eyedrops, nasal sprays/drops/inhalers, and various oral formulations. Eyedrops contain naphazoline, oxymetazoline, phenylephrine, and tetrahydrozoline, and are utilized most often in those patients suffering from allergies. Intranasal formulations contain ephedrine, epinephrine, naphazoline, phenylephrine, tetrahydrozoline, xylometazoline, oxymetazoline, desoxyephedrine, and propylhexedrine. The oral form of pseudoephedrine is absorbed into the bloodstream and can result in cardiovascular and central nervous system stimulation. This results in increased blood pressure, palpitations, high heart rate, restlessness, tremors, anxiety, insomnia, and fear. The oral decongestants may worsen hypertension, hyperthyroidism, diabetes, coronary heart disease, ischemic heart disease, and benign prostatic hypertrophy. In general, patients with these conditions should avoid the oral decongestant agents.

Antitussives are those agents that are approved to suppress a patient's cough due to cold. The generic names of the nonprescription antitussives are codeine and dextromethorphan. Some states sell OTC codeine with certain restrictions, while others do not allow the sale of codeine as a nonprescription medication. Common side effects of codeine include nausea, vomiting, sedation, dizziness, and constipation. Codeine should not be used in those who have respiratory problems or a history of addiction. Dextromethorphan is well tolerated and does not cause sedation, respiratory depression, or have addictive properties. Guaifenesin is an expectorant that loosens thick secretions to make a cough more productive and, therefore, should only be used in those patients suffering from a productive cough. There is a popular nonprescription combination product that contains both guaifenesin and dextromethorphan. This product is irrational because it contains an agent that suppresses the cough and one that causes the cough to be more productive.

TABLE 21-2   Nonprescription Agents for Cold and Allergy

Therapeutic Category	Generic Name	Brand Name	Formulation
Topical decongestants	Oxymetazoline	Afrin 12-hour, Dristan 12-hour, Neosynephrine 12-hour, Vicks Sinex 12-hour	Nasal spray, pump, drops
	Phenylephrine	Afrin, Dristan, Little Noses, Neosynephrine, Vicks Sinex	Nasal spray, drops
	Xylometazoline	Otrivin	Nasal spray, drops
Oral decongestants	Pseudoephedrine	PediaCare, Sudafed, Triaminic	Liqui-Gels, drops, tablets, caplets, chewtabs
Antitussives	Dextromethorphan	Benylin, Robitussin, Sucrets, Vicks	Liquid, lozenges
Antihistamines	Diphenhydramine	Aler-Dryl, Benadryl	Caplets, tablets, liquid
	Chlorpheniramine	Chlor-Trimeton	Tablets
	Brompheniramine	Dimetapp, Dimetane	Tablets, elixir

Antihistamines are also used to control symptoms of the common cold and allergies. Some antihistamines that are available OTC can cause sedation, but some cause it to a greater degree than others. Brompheniramine and chlorpheniramine are the least sedating nonprescription antihistamines. Other antihistamines include diphenhydramine, doxylamine, and clemastine fumarate. Nonsedating antihistamines are available by prescription. OTC antihistamines can cause dry mouth, blurred vision, decreased urination, constipation, and an increased heart rate. They may also impair a patient's ability to perform tasks, such as those required for driving or working. The pharmacist should instruct patients with glaucoma or benign prostatic hypertrophy to avoid nonprescription antihistamines.

Cromolyn is used to treat the symptoms of allergies and is available as an intranasal spray. The pharmacist should inform the patient that it may take three to seven days to begin to take effect and up to a month for maximal benefit. The most common side effects include sneezing and nasal burning and stinging, primarily due to its administration. See **Table 21-2** for a list of commonly used nonprescription cold and allergy products.

Gastrointestinal Problems

Constipation

Constipation is defined as a decrease in the frequency of stool to below that of the patient's normal frequency. Constipated patients may experience abdominal discomfort, lower back pain, difficult passage of stool, bloating, and flatulence. Constipation is usually the result of inadequate exercise and the inadequate intake of water or fiber. Nonprescription treatment options that facilitate the elimination of stool include bulk laxatives, saline laxatives, hyperosmotic laxatives, stool softeners, mineral oil, and stimulant laxatives. See **Table 21-3** for common nonprescription agents within each class and their brand names.

Bulk-forming laxatives are fiber replacement therapy and are usually mixed with a liquid and taken by mouth. These include methylcellulose, polycarbophil, psyllium, and malt soup extract and are the safest of the laxatives. Bulk laxatives can be utilized for both prevention and treatment of constipation. These agents take as long as three days to work; therefore, patients who take these should not expect a bowel movement until then. The pharmacist must also instruct the patient to drink sufficient water with these agents to avoid blockage. They should also take the medications two hours prior to or two hours after taking other medications by mouth because they can interact with medications such as digoxin, warfarin, and salicylates.

Saline laxatives may be used to treat more severe constipation and should be used with caution in those who are dehydrated because these agents pull a significant amount of water into the intestine to soften the stool. There are magnesium- and sodium-containing saline laxatives available. The sodium-containing laxatives should be avoided in those patients on a low-salt diet, such as patient with hypertension or heart failure. Sodium-containing laxatives are most commonly used as enemas. Also, many sodium-containing laxatives contain phosphate; therefore, they should not be used in patients with kidney impairment. Patients with kidney impairment must also avoid magnesium-containing laxatives. The oral saline laxative will take effect in 30 minutes to three hours, while the enemas will take two to five minutes to work.

Hyperosmotic laxatives include glycerin and sorbitol. They can be given rectally in the form of suppositories and enemas, which may cause mild discomfort for the patient. The laxative usually takes effect within 15–60 minutes.

TABLE 21-3 **Nonprescription Agents for Constipation**

Therapeutic Category	Generic Name	Brand Name	Formulation
Bulk-forming laxatives	Polycarbophil	FiberCon, Mitrolan	Tablets
	Methylcellulose	Citrucel	Powder
	Psyllium	Konsyl, Metamucil, Perdiem	Powder, granules
	Malt soup extract	Maltsupex	Liquid
Saline laxatives	Magnesium citrate	Citroma	Liquid
	Sodium phosphate	Fleet	Enema
	Magnesium hydroxide	Milk of Magnesia	Suspension
Hyperosmotic laxatives	Glycerin	Fleet Babylax, Fleet suppositories	Liquid, suppositories
Stool softeners	Docusate sodium	Colace, Ex-Lax	Liquid, gelcaps, capsules
Lubricant laxative	Mineral oil	Fleet, Kondremul	Oil, enema
Stimulant laxatives	Bisacodyl	Correctol, Dulcolax, Fleet	Tablets, caplets, suppositories
	Senna	Ex-Lax, Correctol, Senokot	Tablets, herbal tea, syrup
	Castor oil	Neoloid, Purge	Oil

Stool softeners allow for easier and less painful passage of the stool by softening it. Docusate is the only available OTC softener. It is available as the sodium or calcium salt and takes 12–72 hours to take effect. Docusate is well tolerated and has minimal side effects.

Mineral oil is the only available lubricant laxative and is available as an enema or an oil that is taken by mouth. Mineral oil takes about six to eight hours to work. It should not be used as a first-line laxative because of its many adverse effects and interactions. Patients may aspirate the mineral oil; therefore, the pharmacist should warn the patient to remain upright when taking it and to take it at least 30 minutes prior to going to bed. Because mineral oil prevents the absorption of the fat-soluble vitamins, it should be taken two hours prior to or two hours after a meal.

Stimulant laxatives are available as liquids, tablets, granules, or suppositories. These laxatives force the bowel to expel its contents within six to twelve hours. Taking stimulants for an extended period of time may result in damage to the intestines. Senna, cascara, and, casanthranol are known as the anthraquinones. These agents turn urine a pink to red or brown to black color. It is important to warn the patient about this effect. Diphenylmethanes include bisacodyl which is the only bowel stimulant available as a suppository as well as a tablet. Castor oil is also a stimulant laxative. In most cases, the stimulant laxative should be combined with a stool softener. The stimulant alone may not soften the stool adequately, leading to pain and discomfort when the stool is passed.

Diarrhea

Diarrhea is characterized by an increased frequency of stool that is a loose and watery consistency. It can be the result of diet, infection, or medications. A pharmacist should always instruct parents or guardians of patients who are less than three years old and have had diarrhea for longer than two days or have a fever associated with their diarrhea to consult with a physician. Children under three years old are more prone to the effects of fluid losses and should consult with their pediatrician. Dehydration and electrolyte abnormalities can manifest from just two days of diarrhea depending upon the severity; therefore, these patients should see a physician. They may require the administration of intravenous fluids to correct the abnormalities. Patients with a fever may have an infectious cause of diarrhea and should be put on appropriate therapy, such as antibiotics rather than OTC products. Patients with infectious diarrhea should generally avoid OTC antidiarrheal agents because they inhibit the removal of the pathogen by slowing the gastrointestinal transit time, which could result in longer duration or increased severity of diarrhea. The nonprescription agents used to treat diarrhea include polycarbophil, attapulgite, bismuth subsalicylate, kaolin, loperamide, lactobacillus, activated charcoal, and oral rehydration solutions. Please see **Table 21-4** for a list of select agents and their brand names.

Calcium polycarbophil is a bulk laxative that was discussed earlier in the constipation section. It can be utilized for both constipation and diarrhea. It absorbs up to 60 times its weight in water to help "bulk up" the consistency of the stool. The pharmacist must inform patients that they should maintain adequate fluid intake and to chew the tablets before swallowing them. Patients who are on tetracycline should stagger their dose to minimize the effect of calcium binding to the tetracycline.

Adsorbents include attapulgite, kaolin, pectin, and bismuth subsalicylate. These agents work by binding to toxins, bacteria, and noxious materials that can cause diarrhea. Because these agents work by binding to substances which can result in decreased amount of drug available for activity, they should generally be given at least two hours prior to or two hours after other medications. Kaolin alone

TABLE 21-4   **Nonprescription Agents for Diarrhea**

Therapeutic Category	Generic Name	Brand Name	Formulation
Bulk laxative	Calcium polycarbophil	Equalactin, Mitrolan	Tablets
Adsorbents	Attapulgite	Donnagel, Kaopectate, Rheaban	Tablets, capsules, liquids, suspensions
	Bismuth subsalicylate	Pepto-Bismol	Tablets, capsules, liquids
Motility agent	Loperamide	Imodium AD	Caplets, liquid

may be effective, but has not been proven to be effective when given with pectin and was therefore removed from older products containing the combination. Older kaolin-pectin combination products were reformulated to contain attapulgite, which is effective in treating diarrhea. Bismuth subsalicylate is available as a suspension and contains salicylate. For this reason, caution should be used in the pediatric population, those who are allergic to aspirin, and in those who are taking other salicylates or anticoagulants such as warfarin. Bismuth subsalicylate may darken the tongue and stool.

Loperamide helps with the symptoms of diarrhea by slowing gastrointestinal motility and is available as caplets or a solution. Adverse effects are rare and include drowsiness, dizziness, and constipation.

Lactobacillus has not been proven effective, but may promote regrowth of normal flora in the bowel. This agent must be refrigerated and may cause flatulence. Activated charcoal is not proven to be effective and is not recommended for the treatment of diarrhea. Oral rehydration solutions may be helpful while a patient is waiting to see their physician.

Acid/Peptic Disorders

This section will emphasize the common gastrointestinal disorders that can be controlled with OTC medications. These include **gastroesophageal reflux disease (GERD)** and **peptic ulcer disease (PUD)**. PUD is ulceration of the stomach or duodenal lining. Patients must be seen by a physician and diagnosed with PUD before the pharmacist can aid in the selection of a nonprescription medication. Nonprescription medications used for patients with PUD are used as adjunctive agents in addition to prescription medications. Antacids can be used for pain relief and bismuth subsalicylate can be used as part of a regimen including prescription medications to treat *H. pylori,* an infectious cause of PUD. GERD, also called heartburn, is a process that causes a burning sensation in the chest area. This burning is the result of reflux of the acidic contents of the stomach up into the esophagus. The reflux causes irritation to the lining of the esophagus that can lead to discomfort and ulceration. Dietary and lifestyle modifications are key to the management of a patient suffering from heartburn. These measures include elevating the head of the bed, eating smaller meals, eating meals at least three hours before bedtime, and avoiding trigger foods such as mints, chocolates, citrus juices, spicy foods, foods with tomatoes, and coffee. It may also be helpful to lose weight, quit smoking, and avoid alcoholic beverages. Agents that are available without a prescription include antacids, alginic acid, and histamine$_2$ receptor antagonists. In general, these agents should not be used for longer than a two-week period unless the patient is being advised to do so by their physician.

Antacids neutralize the acid in the stomach to produce minimal irritation to the lining of the gastrointestinal tract. Calcium carbonate, sodium bicarbonate, aluminum hydroxide, aluminum phosphate, magnesium hydroxide, and magnesium chloride are the antacids available over the counter. Suspensions usually allow for quicker dissolution over tablet formulations; therefore, suspensions usually have a quicker onset of action. Calcium carbonate and aluminum hydroxide dissolve more slowly than sodium bicarbonate and magnesium hydroxide and take about 10–30 minutes to see an effect. Magnesium-containing antacids can cause diarrhea, while aluminum-containing antacids may cause constipation. For this reason, combination products are available to negate the effects of either agent. Magnesium can accumulate to cause central nervous system depression in patients with renal failure; therefore, the pharmacist should recommend an alternative antacid for these patients. Aluminum and sodium bicarbonate antacids should also be avoided in the patient with renal impairment due to accumulation. Alginic acid has been combined with sodium bicarbonate. This combination forms a viscous solution that floats on the acidic contents of the stomach and instead of acid refluxing into the esophagus, the viscous solution is refluxed which decreases irritation and symptoms. Antacids interact with many medications and the pharmacist should be aware of these in order to counsel the patient.

Histamine$_2$ receptor antagonists (H$_2$RAs) are available in prescription and nonprescription strength. The nonprescription strength is available in a lower dosage form. The H$_2$RAs that are available over the counter are cimetidine, famotidine, nizatidine, and ranitidine. These agents decrease gastric acid secretion which decreases damage done to the gastrointestinal mucosa. The nonprescription strength of these agents is not adequate to heal gastrointestinal ulcers due to GERD and PUD. The patient should be notified that these agents may not result in relief of symptoms for one to two hours; therefore, they should be taken one hour before a

TABLE 21-5 Nonprescription Agents for Acid/Peptic Disorders

Therapeutic Category	Generic Name	Brand Name	Formulation
Antacids	Magnesium hydroxide	Mag-Ox, Phillips' Milk of Magnesia, Uro-Mag	Tablets, suspension, capsules, chewtabs
	Aluminum hydroxide	ALternaGEL, Alu-Cap, Alu-Tab, Amphojel, Basaljel	Tablets, suspension, capsules, liquid
	Aluminum/magnesium hydroxide	Maalox, Riopan Mylanta, Tums	Suspension
	Calcium carbonate	Amitone, Chooz,	Chewtabs, liquid
	Calcium/magnesium	Rolaids, Mylanta	Chewtabs
	Aluminum/magnesium/ Alginate	Gaviscon	Tablets, suspension, chewtabs
H$_2$ receptor antagonists	Cimetidine	Tagamet	Tablets
	Famotidine	Pepcid	Tablets
	Nizatidine	Axid	Tablets
	Ranitidine	Zantac	Tablets

meal rather than at the time of symptoms. Common side effects from nonprescription doses of H_2RAs include headache, dizziness, constipation, nausea, and vomiting. Significant drug-drug interactions may occur with the H_2RAs. Cimetidine is associated with the most drug interactions of the drugs in this category. **Table 21-5** lists common agents for use in acid/peptic disorders.

Summary

It is imperative that those working in a pharmacy environment be familiar with agents that are sold over the counter to patients. These products have significant interactions and adverse effects and should be treated as prescription medications. The technician can aid the pharmacist in identifying those patients who need further counseling on nonprescription products. Knowledge of over-the-counter agents can help the technician do this effectively and with greater confidence. This chapter covers the most common problems that are self-treated with over-the-counter drugs.

TEST YOUR KNOWLEDGE

Multiple Choice Questions

1. All of the following are true statements regarding nonprescription medications except:
   a. OTCs are available for conditions that are considered to be self-treatable
   b. OTCs allow the patient more control over health care needs
   c. OTCs have pharmacological activity
   d. OTCs do not have the potential to cause adverse reactions

2. Which of the following products are options for the patient with hypertension?
   a. Alka-Seltzer
   b. Fibercon
   c. Sudafed
   d. Fleet's Enema

3. All of the following are examples of NSAIDs except:
   a. naproxen
   b. ketoprofen
   c. acetaminophen
   d. ibuprofen

4. Which of the following should be shaken well prior to administration?
   a. solution
   b. suspension
   c. elixir
   d. lotion

5. All of the following are topical dosage forms except:
   a. Doan's
   b. Capzasin
   c. Mineral Ice
   d. Icy Hot

6. Dextromethorphan belongs to which one of the following therapeutic categories?
   a. decongestant
   b. antitussive
   c. antihistamine
   d. expectorant

7. Which of the following antihistamines is not available OTC?
   a. diphenhydramine
   b. chlorpheniramine
   c. fexofenadine
   d. brompheniramine

8. In most cases, senna should be given with which of the following nonprescription agents to decrease pain and discomfort of constipation?
   a. Citroma
   b. Colace
   c. Maltsupex
   d. Milk of Magnesia

9. Which of the following can be used for the treatment of both constipation and diarrhea?
   a. polycarbophil
   b. docusate
   c. loperamide
   d. senna

10. Which of the following agents can be safely used in a patient with renal impairment?
    a. Alu-Tab
    b. Tums
    c. Milk of Magnesia
    d. Amphogel

References

Allen, L. V., Berardi, R. R., Desimone, E., et al. (Eds.) (2000). *Handbook of Nonprescription Drugs.* 12th ed. Washington, DC: American Pharmaceutical Association.

Mant, A., Whicker, S., & Kwok, Y. S. (1992). Over-the-counter self-medication. The issues. *Drugs Aging 2,* 257–261.

Pray, W. S. (1999). *Nonprescription product therapeutics* (1st ed.). Philadelphia: Lippincott Williams & Wilkins.

Smith, M. B., & Feldman, W. (1993). Over-the-counter cold medications. A critical review of clinical trials between 1950 and 1991. *Journal of the American Medical Association 269,* 2258–2263.

22 Natural Products

COMPETENCIES

Upon completion of this chapter, the reader should be able to

1. Describe what makes a product an herbal (or botanical) as opposed to a drug.
2. Describe how herbals are regulated by the Food and Drug Administration (FDA) in the USA.
3. List and briefly describe the plant natural product groups of secondary plant metabolites that are contained in the majority of herbals.
4. Explain the preparation and administration routes of most herbals.
5. Explain the potential for possibly dangerous interactions between herbals and standard drug therapy.
6. Be able to find current information on herbal safety and effectiveness.
7. List some common traditional uses of the major herbals.

Introduction

By definition, a **drug** is "any substance or mixture of substances intended for the cure, mitigation, diagnosis or prevention of disease." This definition comes, in large part, from the Pure Food Act of 1906 which formed the basis of what is now the Food and Drug Administration. Regulation of drugs in the United States is discussed in the next section.

An **herbal** substance is defined in the 1994 Dietary Supplement and Health Education Act (DSHEA) as a **dietary supplement**, not a drug. The DSHEA definition of a dietary supplement is any "product that contains a vitamin; mineral; amino acid; an herb or other botanical; a dietary substance for use by man to supplement the diet by increasing total daily intake; or a concentrate metabolite constituent, extract, or combinations of these ingredients."

Because they are not drugs, herbals and other dietary supplements cannot claim to cure, prevent, treat, or diagnose disease. They can claim to have a health action such as promoting healthy digestion. However, it is important to recognize that as a dietary supplement, herbal products are not evaluated by the FDA for either safety or effectiveness in the same manner that prescription drugs are evaluated. The reasons for this are discussed in the next section. In addition, the regulatory oversight that we have come to expect from the FDA with regard to drug manufacture is not necessarily followed for the production of herbal products. This lack of assurance as to safety, quality, and effectiveness often places the pharmacy in a difficult position when asked for recommendations about herbal products. One of the goals of this chapter is to provide some guidelines for the review of herbal preparations.

How Are Drugs and Herbals Regulated in the USA?

From colonial times until well into the 1900s, one of the primary roles of the pharmacy was the compounding or mixing of medicines. Pharmacists were not alone in this function. Unlike today, numerous physicians also compounded and dispensed medicines. Also unlike today, patients did not have to go to a physician to get a prescription to buy medicines. Indeed, as late as the 1920s, less than 25% of all medicines and drugs purchased in drugstores were bought using prescriptions.

Most of the early medicines compounded were based upon plant materials. One important example of such a medicine is digitalis, which was used to treat congestive heart failure. The active ingredients were usually harvested from the purple foxglove (*Digitalis purpurea*) or from the white foxglove (*Digitalis lanata*). In fact, the medicine derived its name from the genus name of the plants from which it was harvested. This medication was popularized by William Withering, a British physician, who published a monograph in 1785 on the use of extract of foxglove and the beneficial effects of digitalis on dropsy (the old name for congestive heart failure). Withering's treatise was one of the first published scientific studies of an herbal compound. Although crude digitalis extract is no longer used in the United States, digoxin and digitoxin (members of the cardiac glycoside drug class), which are the main components of the extract, are currently available.

To aid pharmacists in preparing compounds in a more a consistent manner, several national publications arose. The United States Pharmacopeia (USP) started in 1820 and the National Formulary (NF) started in 1888 by the American Pharmaceutical Association are two publications that have taken on the status of being official compendiums that set national standards. The USP describes standards for drug identity, strength, quality, purity, packaging, and labeling. The NF sets standards for excipients, botanicals, and other similar products. The NF was purchased by the USP in 1975, combining the two publications under one cover entitled the USP-NF.

Early on these publications had numerous monographs on the preparation of botanical products. At its peak, the USP published over 600 monographs on botanicals. By 1900, that number had decreased to about 169 monographs. Between 1900 to 1990, the increasing use of synthetic organic drugs resulted in a further reduction in attention to plant-derived medicines. Thus in recent decades the USP-NF had few monographs on botanicals.

Drug Regulation in the United States

At this point, a brief history of drug regulation in the United States is necessary. Prior to the early 1900s, there were few enforceable laws pertaining to medicines or what we would now call drugs. In 1906, the Pure Food Act was passed by Congress and signed into law. The legislation was enacted largely due to public concern over adulteration of foods as described by authors such as Upton Sinclair. Sinclair's book, *The Jungle,* described horrific practices at some meat packing plants and sparked public outrage demanding regulatory oversight over the production of food and medicines.

Although the title of the 1906 Pure Food Act suggests that it was about purity and food safety, in reality the law focused on making sure only that foods and drugs were truthfully and accurately labeled. The 1906 law had several important impacts on pharmacy. The law defined what constituted a drug and prohibited adulterated or misbranded drugs. However, it did not require that a drug be proven safe or effective. The 1906 law also converted the USP and NF from private publications into the official standards for the manufacture and compounding of drugs. And finally, the law essentially triggered creation of what has become the Food and Drug Administration (FDA).

To enforce the provisions of the 1906 legislation, the Department of Agriculture's Division of Chemistry headed by Harvey W. Wiley was enlarged and renamed the Bureau of Chemistry. The Bureau of Chemistry was charged with assaying and checking the accuracy of content labels. By 1927, the regulatory aspects of Bureau of Chemistry had become so large that they were moved to a new agency named the Food, Drug, and Insecticide Administration. In 1931, the name was shorted to the Food and Drug Administration (FDA).

As described above, the 1906 act was primarily concerned with truth in labeling. The Bureau of Chemistry could only act if a drug was misbranded or adulterated. There were no requirements that a drug be proven effective or even safe before being sold to the public. Then in 1937, the "elixir of sulfanilamide" tragedy occurred. A pharmaceutical company mixed sulfanilamide with diethylene glycol because it dissolved well and had a reasonable taste. Unfortunately, diethylene glycol, like ethylene glycol (the main component in automobile antifreeze), is poisonous to humans, causing potentially fatal central nervous system (CNS) and kidney (renal) damage. Over 100 of the patients who ingested the mixture died due to renal failure. Because there was no requirement that drugs be proven safe prior to sale, the FDA could only charge the pharmaceutical company with misbranding because the name of the drug used the term *elixir* in its name. Elixir is used to indicate an alcohol solution and there was no alcohol in the mixture. A fine of slightly more than $26,000 was levied on the company, but no other action could be taken.

Once again, public outrage led to enactment of new legislation. In 1938, the Federal Food, Drug, and Cosmetic Act was signed into law. This legislation focused on demonstration of drug safety. The law spelled out procedures for how applications for new drug approval had to occur. For the first time medical devices were included in FDA regulations. And perhaps most importantly, the regulations gave special treatment to prescriptions written by physicians, veterinary doctors, and dentists. They distinguished between prescription and over-the-counter (OTC) drugs, which led to the prescription-only method of drug acquisition common today. The 1938 Federal Food, Drug, and Cosmetic Act is the foundation of drug regulation as it exists in the United States.

However, the 1938 legislation still did not require a drug to be effective. This was corrected by the Drug Amendments of 1962 (often called the Kefauver-Harris Amendments) that required that all drugs marketed after 1962 in the United States be proven both safe and effective. Although already in committee in the Congress, enactment of this legislation was spurred by the thalidomide tragedy. Although never approved for sale in the United States, use of thalidomide in pregnant women often led to phocomelia, a birth defect in which the child is born missing one or more limbs. While nothing in the 1962 Drug Amendments would have specifically prevented clinical testing of thalidomide in the United States, it did encourage the mentality that the FDA should decide what drugs would be allowed on the market and then tightly regulate how they should be used.

To determine which drugs were effective, the FDA worked with the National Academy of Sciences' National Research Council to organize a drug efficacy study. This study examined the effectiveness of some 4,000 drugs that contained about

300 different chemicals. A final report was made in 1969. This report established much of how we think about prescription drugs in pharmacy today.

The drugs that could be purchased without a physician's prescription, the over-the-counter (OTC) drugs, were not examined (to any great extent) in the drug efficacy study. To deal with this lack, the FDA set up 17 panels in 1972 to evaluate the effectiveness of the active ingredients of OTC drugs. However, lack of sufficient data and resources to evaluate many of the OTCs led to a less than satisfactory result. The panels only examined ingredients if they were asked to do so and then only evaluated evidence presented to them. In 1990, when the final OTC study was released to the public, the safety and efficacy of many herbals was still in question. A few botanicals, such as senna leaves (which act as a laxative), were found to be safe and effective and classed as Category I (safe and effective). Almost 150 herbals were classed as Category II (unsafe or ineffective). However, over a hundred herbals were classed as Category III (insufficient evidence to evaluate). Note that a Category III designation does not mean that an herbal was not safe or effective. Category III means only that there was no decision because of lack of supporting evidence. For those looking for more direction on the use of herbals, this was a disappointing outcome.

Regulation of Herbals, Botanicals, and Dietary Supplements

A number of herbals are listed on the 1958 list of generally recognized as safe (GRAS) list of food additives. However, this list is directed primarily at food and flavoring agents and not at therapeutic actions. Finally, in 1994 the Dietary Supplement Health and Education Act (DSHEA) was signed into law. This law treats herbals as dietary supplements, not drugs, and allows them to make claims with regard to general health promotion but not disease claims (like drugs). Much like the 1906 Pure Food Act, DSHEA focuses on the labeling of herbals (as well as other dietary supplements) spelling out what constitutes a misbranded or adulterated botanical (herbal).

According to DSHEA, an herbal must (1) be labeled as a dietary supplement, (2) identify all ingredients by name, (3) list the quantity of each ingredient, (4) identify the plant and the plant part from which the ingredient is derived, (5) comply with any standards set by an official compendium (such as the USP and the NF), and (6) meet the quality, purity, and compositional specifications as established by validated assays. Failure to comply with these regulations means that an herbal is misbranded. The DSHEA also sets guidelines to prevent adulteration of dietary supplements. The DSHEA even states that a botanical or herbal must be "prepared, packed or held" under "good manufacturing practices" (GMP) protocols. Mandating GMP is meant to ensure quality at the manufacturing (or preparation) stage of herbal production. However, to follow GMP during manufacture or preparation requires standards that do not presently exist for many herbals. And the DSHEA regulations say that the FDA may not "impose standards for which there is no currently and generally available analytical methodology." For example, in the preparation of St. John's wort (an herbal often used for depression), which of the many components should be used by a company to standardize its manufacturing process? Two major components in St. John's wort are hypericin and hyperforin. Currently, many companies use hypericin levels as their assay standard for preparation of St. John's wort extract. However, there is no direct evidence that hypericin is the active ingredient in St. John's wort. Indeed, recent evidence suggests that if St. John's wort is effective in depression that the active ingredient may be hyperforin, not hypericin.

In summary, as the brief history of the regulation of herbals presented above indicates, herbals have a unique status in the United States. Manufacturers can only market them with health claims and may not make any claims as to their use in treating disease (i.e., disease claims). However, millions of consumers (and patients) are purchasing these preparations to treat disease. While health care professionals at many levels are concerned about the safety and effectiveness of these preparations, current limitations on the FDA make it unlikely that this agency will be able to address these concerns. This leaves the pharmacy in the difficult position of trying to counsel the consumer (patient) without adequate information. Certainly, the easiest, most conservative advice would be to not purchase or use herbals unless under the directions of a physician. However, without specific warnings (e.g., "Use of this preparation has caused liver failure in patients with your condition!"), the "Do not use" advice is likely to be ignored. Annual sales of dietary supplements are estimated to be in 10–15 billion dollar range. More and more people are turning to herbals as part of their health care. Thus the rest of this chapter is directed towards helping pharmacy understand and obtain up-to-date, useful information on herbals.

The Chemical Structure of Herbals: Secondary Plant Metabolites

Although the term *herbal* has been applied to any plant substance used for health purposes, most herbals are secondary plant metabolites. The name ***metabolite*** refers to a chemical synthesized within cells as part of a metabolic pathway. Primary plant metabolites are compounds that are essential for basic plant cell function and life. Primary metabolites fall into five general classes: proteins, nucleic acids, carbohydrates (sugars), simple organic acids, and lipids (fats). Secondary metabolites are derived from the primary metabolites, but have their own specialized pathways of synthesis. Secondary metabolites may be important for the success and health of the plant, but they are not as essential to cell survival as primary metabolites.

The functions of secondary metabolites in plants are quite varied. It is important to recognize that plants face many of the same environmental challenges that humans do, except they cannot change their location in response to these challenges. Thus some secondary metabolites evolved to help conserve moisture for the plant (e.g., the suberins and waxes), some evolved to help ward off herbaceous animals (predators) as a form of chemical self-defense (e.g., various plant toxins such as nicotine), and some evolved to fight fungal, bacterial, and viral infections in plants. It is this last group that is of particular interest to modern medicine and pharmacy because some of these compounds also fight infections in humans. A general scheme of the relationships of primary metabolites and secondary metabolites is shown in **Figure 22-1**.

For simplicity, secondary plant metabolites can be divided into three major groups or classes of compounds. Those three groups are (1) the terpenoids, (2) the alkaloids, and (3) the phenylpropanoids (including the flavonoids) and allied phenolics. Of these, the terpenoids are by far the most numerous in occurrence with more than 25,000 identified chemically. By comparison, there have been about

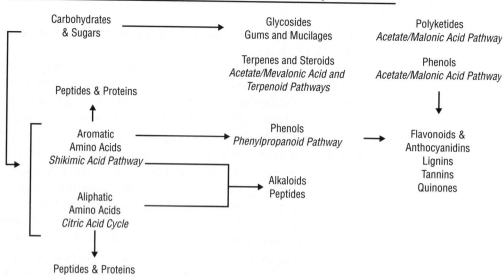

FIGURE 22-1 The relationship between primary and secondary metabolites.

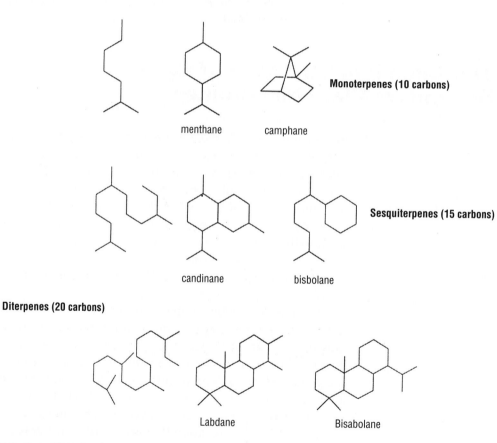

FIGURE 22-2 Structure of a terpenoid.

Nitrogen-Containing Ring Structures Common in Alkaloids

pyridine

piperidine

quinoline

isoquinoline

pyrrolidine

indole

imidazole

purine

tropane

Alkaloids

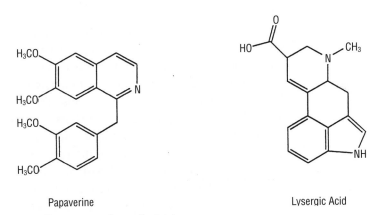

Papaverine

Lysergic Acid

FIGURE 22-3 Structure of an alkaloid.

12,000 alkaloids identified and approximately 8,000 plant phenolics characterized. Although these compounds have been characterized chemically, only a fraction of them have been tested for possible medicinal benefit.

Typical terpenoids (**Figure 22-2**), alkaloids (**Figure 22-3**), and flavonoids, which are phenylpropanoids (**Figure 22-4**), are shown below. Note that in the diagrams the standard organic chemistry graphics format has been used. Therefore, each "corner" or "bend" or end of a line represents a carbon atom. In many cases, the hydrogens and other atoms have been left out on purpose to better show the carbon "backbone" of a compound.

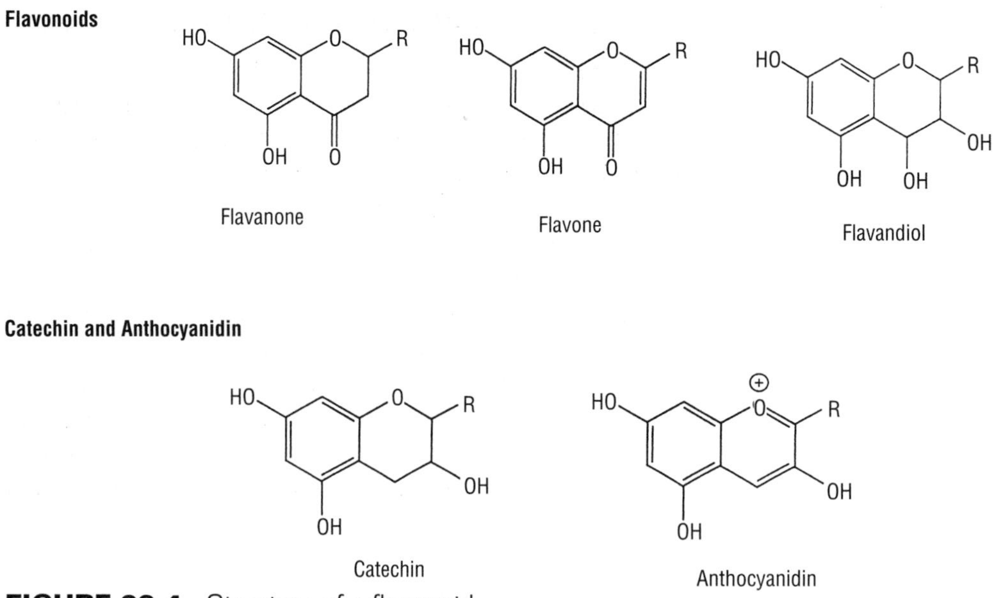

Flavonoids

Flavanone

Flavone

Flavandiol

Catechin and Anthocyanidin

Catechin

Anthocyanidin

FIGURE 22-4 Structure of a flavonoid.

Preparation and Routes of Administration of Herbals

Up until the mid-twentieth century, much of the work in the pharmacy was focused on preparation and compounding of plant material into herbal medicines. Today, however, most herbal preparations will enter the pharmacy already packaged. One reason for this is because few pharmacists are currently trained in pharmacognosy (i.e., the science of selecting and preparing plant materials for medical use). A second reason is economic; that is, it is cheaper to purchase the material ready to sell rather than to have to prepare and package it. This is certainly the case with many over-the-counter (OTC) preparations. There is also the matter of product safety which is more complicated for herbals (see below).

Many retail herbal preparations are supplied as tablets, capsules, lozenges, liquids, or tinctures to be taken orally (po). Some herbals are supplied in a dry form to be taken po as a powder or made into a tea or similar drink. A number of herbals are for external skin or topical use only and are supplied as a gel, cream, or ointment. For safety reasons, herbal products should not be given by injection, that is, by intravenous (IV), intramuscular (IM), or intra-arterial routes.

The Safety of Herbals

Advocates for herbals often state that they are more safe than modern drugs because they have been used by humans for a long time. In some instances, herbals have been used as a food or dietary supplement for generations. In general, most herbals are safe at low to moderate dosages. However, there are still a number of issues that must be considered by the pharmacy. The most important of these issues are (1) the potential of a hypersensitivity (i.e., allergic) response to an herbal, (2) that the product actually contains the herbal claimed, (3) potential contamination of the herbal product with toxic material, and (4) the potential for herbal-drug interaction.

Hypersensitivity (Allergic) Reactions

Just as with any newly administered drug or food, attention must be paid to the possibility of a hypersensitivity reaction to a component of the herbal product by the patient. A **hypersensitivity reaction** occurs when a patient has been exposed to a compound previously and has made antibodies against the compound. When the patient takes the compound again, a hyper or larger than normal immune response occurs and the patient's own antibodies begin to cause problems. An example of a hypersensitivity reaction is the pollen allergy. Hypersensitivity reactions can range from an immediate allergic reaction that can lead to anaphylactic shock and death to the skin rashes common in delayed hypersensitivity. Unfortunately, there is no easy way to predict which patients will have a hypersensitivity response to a particular food, compound, or drug. The patient should be counseled to be on the lookout for the signs and symptoms of hypersensitivity, to discontinue use of the product at once if they appear, and to seek appropriate medical treatment.

Content and Concentration of the Herbal Product

The concern that the product may not contain the herbal listed on the label or may have varying concentrations of the herbal is still a significant problem. Several analytical testing laboratories have examined herbal products from a number of manufacturers or producers and found a wide disparity in the contents of the product. An important next step in the herbal industry will have to be the standardization of various products. However, absolute nationally recognized standards do not exist at this time. Therefore, each retail outlet must investigate and decide upon an herbal supplier they trust to follow appropriate manufacturing (i.e., extraction) procedures. It is suggested that the pharmacy be involved in this process early on and the standards of good manufacturing practices (GMP) outlined by the FDA be applied.

Potential Contamination of the Herbal Product

This issue has taken on a heightened concern with the reported incidents of toxic contamination on the increase. In one case in Europe, an herbal product for weight reduction was found to be adulterated with the plant contaminant aristolochic acid. This compound has been reported to be nephrotoxic in laboratory animals. In an investigation reported in 2000, this compound was also associated with the development of urothelial carcinoma in a number of Belgian consumers of the weight-reduction herbal.

In another recent case, an herbal product was found to be contaminated with *Digitalis lanata* (white foxglove). The contamination was discovered when a consumer of the herbal was admitted to hospital with what was found to have been digitalis poisoning. After investigation by the FDA, the manufacturer voluntarily removed the product from the market. Although the manufacturer responded appropriately to protect the public safety, it should be noted that this contamination was only discovered after consumers had been exposed to the risk. Similar incidents have been reported with regard to heavy metal contamination such as lead, mercury, and cadmium of glucosamine products derived from mollusks. The only solution to such situations is extensive screening and testing for toxic contaminants by the manufacturer or producer of an herbal. Unfortunately, many manufacturers do not currently have the expertise or equipment for such screening. This issue is a major problem with the safe use of herbals.

Fortunately, in November 2001 the USP launched an initiative entitled the Dietary Supplement Verification Program (DSVP) in which manufacturers voluntarily submit their products to USP testing. Any product passing USP testing will be awarded the DSVP verification mark. The goals of the DSVP are to assure consumers and health care professionals that a dietary supplement product contains the ingredients listed on the label at the declared concentrations, the product meets requirements (as listed in the USP-NF) on potential contaminants, and that the product has been manufactured in compliance with GMPs proposed by the FDA and USP. Although voluntary at this time, this program sets a new standard for herbals in the United States and should be helpful to the pharmacy.

Potential Herbal-Drug Interactions

Just as with drug-drug interactions, the concomitant usage of herbal preparations with prescription drugs may lead to significant herbal-drug interactions with adverse outcomes. Herbals and orally administered drugs are absorbed across the GI tract, metabolized by the liver, and excreted by the kidneys. Therefore, it is not surprising that the presence of herbals may alter the absorption, metabolism, or excretion of drugs. For example, use of St. John's wort has been reported to decrease the absorption of digoxin and indinivar and to increase the metabolism of warfarin, cyclosporine, and oral contraceptives. Each of these interactions would decrease the amount of prescription drug concentrations in patients, potentially resulting in subtherapeutic doses. In short, the patient might be undertreated even though they were receiving the correct dosage of prescription drug. The difficulty of predicting such interactions with herbals is greatly complicated because they are not single compounds. There is no evidence, for example, that the above described effects of St. John's wort are due to a single constituent.

Where to Get More Information on Herbals

The concerns over safety and efficacy listed above clearly underscore the need for information on herbals that is updated in a timely manner and made rapidly available to the pharmacy. Until recently, it has been hard to obtain such information in the United States. Now, however, some very useful sources are available.

1. The United States Pharmacopeia has undertaken to develop and update at least 21 monographs on natural products (herbals) in the USP-NF. Included are the following herbals:

   Zingiber officinale Roscoe (Ginger)
   Valeriana officinalis Linné (Valerian)
   Allium sativum Linné (Garlic)
   Panax ginseng C.A. Meyer (Asian Ginseng)
   Ginkgo biloba Linné (Ginkgo)
   Tanacetum parthenium (Linné) Schultz-Bip. (Feverfew)
   Hypericum perforatum Linné (Hypericum or St. John's wort)
   Panax quinquefolius Linné (American Ginseng)
   Echinacea angustifolia DC (Echinacea)
   Chamomilla recutita (Linné) Rauschert (Matricaria Flower)
   Serenoa repens (Bartram) Small (Saw Palmetto fruit)
   Crataegus leavigata (Poir.) DC (Hawthorn)
   Hydrastis canadensis Linné (Golden Seal Root)

Silybum marianum (Linné) Gaertner (Milk Thistle)
Vaccinium macrocarpon Ait. or *Vaccinium oxycoccos* Linné (Cranberry)
Urtica dioica Linné (Nettle Root)
Ephedra sinica Stapf (Ephedra or Ma Huang)
Piper methisticum Linné (Kava Kava)
Eleutherococcus senticosus (Rupr. et Maxim) Harms (Siberian Ginseng)
Glycyrrhiza glabra Linné (Licorice)
Angelica archangelica Linné (Angelica)

Updates on the progress of these monographs can be found on the USP Web site at http://www.usp.org.

2. The USP recently launched Dietary Supplement Verification Program (DSVP), which sets a new standard for herbals in the United States. Manufacturers voluntarily submit their products to USP testing. Updates and details about the DSVP can be found at the USP Web site at http://www.usp.org. This program could be a major advance in addressing the safety issues concerning herbals. The pharmacy will know that an herbal product with the DSVP mark on the label actually contains the plant material at the declared concentration and that it is free of contaminants as specified in the USP-NF.

3. The NIH Office of Dietary Supplements Web site at http://ods.od.nih.gov. One of the provisions of the DSHEA of 1994 was the formation of an Office of Dietary Supplements at the National Institutes of Health (NIH). The mission of the ODS is to "strengthen knowledge and understanding of dietary supplements by evaluating scientific information, stimulating and supporting research, disseminating research results, and educating the public. . . .". ODS has created and maintains two large databases on herbals: IBIDS (the International Bibliographic Information on Dietary Supplements) and CARDS (Computer Access to Research on Dietary Supplements). CARDS covers all federally funded research projects such as those from the NIH from 1999 on. IBIDS covers all "published, international, scientific literature on dietary supplements" and includes almost 700,000 entries. Both databases can be accessed free of charge at the ODS Web site.

4. Another very useful Web site is the National Center for Complementary and Alternative Medicine at http://nccam.nih.gov/. This site contains information on current clinical trials and drug interactions between herbals and drugs.

5. Medwatch at http://www.fda.gov/medwatch/ contains information from the FDA Safety Information and Adverse Event Reporting Program. This site is not focused exclusively on herbals or dietary supplements, but adverse events, drug interactions, and important safety announcements are reported here. This is a very useful site for the pharmacy.

6. The publication in English of the German Commission E monographs on herbals provides an excellent reference based on the accepted medicinal uses of herbals in Europe. The text is entitled *Herbal Medicine: Expanded Commission E Monographs*. It is edited by M. Blumenthal, A. Goldberg, and J. Brinckman, published by Integrative Medicine Communications (2000), and is available in hardback (ISBN 0967077214) and as a CD-ROM.

The availability of these Web sites and CD-ROM-based expanded Commission E monographs greatly speed the pharmacy's access to necessary information for counseling patients on the safety and efficacy of an herbal. The availability of programs such as DSVP from the USP means that the pharmacy can begin to have confidence in the safety of compliant herbal products.

Some Traditional Uses of Herbals

Below are listed some common herbal products and their traditional or common uses. Please note that this section is not an endorsement of clinical efficacy of any particular herbal. Rather, these are merely examples of typical herbal products.

Common Name: Angelica
Botanical Name: *Angelica archangelica*
Typical Uses: To relieve symptoms of flatulence (i.e., GI gas), as a diuretic (i.e., to increase urine flow), and a diaphoretic (i.e., sweat producer). Also used as a flavoring agent in several liqueurs and in gin (along with juniper berries)

Common Name: Black Cohosh (black snakeroot)
Botanical Name: *Cimicifuga racemosa*
Typical Uses: To relieve symptoms of menopause and various menstrual problems

Common Name: Feverfew
Botanical Name: *Tanacetum parthenium*
Typical Uses: To relieve symptoms of migraine headaches, arthritis, and menstrual problems

Common Name: Garlic
Botanical Name: *Allium sativum*
Typical Uses: As a flavoring agent in salads, soups, and other foods; as a cholesterol-lowering agent

Common Name: Ginger
Botanical Name: *Zingiber officinale* Roscoe
Typical Uses: As a flavoring agent in foods; as a digestive aid; and as an antiemetic (i.e., to prevent vomiting)

Common Name: Ginkgo
Botanical Name: *Ginkgo biloba*
Typical Uses: As an antiasthmatic, bronchodilator, and to treat memory loss or headache

Common Name: Ginseng
Botanical Name: *Panax ginseng* (Asian ginseng) or *Panax quinquefolius* (American ginseng)
Typical Uses: As an "adaptogen" to increase resistence to environmental stress and to promote immune response

Common Name: Golden Seal
Botanical Name: *Hydrastis canadensis*
Typical Uses: As a bitter tonic for gastric and urogenital disorders

Common Name: Milk Thistle
Botanical Name: *Silybum marianum*
Typical Uses: As an anti-hepatotoxic agent (i.e., liver protectant) especially against poisoning from *Amanita* sp. mushrooms which contain compounds such as phallotoxins

Common Name: Purple Coneflower or Echinacea
Botanical Name: *Echinacea purpurea*
Typical Uses: As an anti-infective, antiseptic, and immunostimulant agent

Common Name: Saw Palmetto
Botanical Name: *Serenoa repens*
Typical Uses: To relieve the symptoms of benign prostatic hypertrophy (i.e., non-cancerous enlarged prostate gland)

Common Name: St. John's Wort
Botanical Name: *Hypericum calycinum*
Typical Uses: To relieve the symptoms of depression

Common Name: Valerian
Botanical Name: *Valeriana officinalis*
Typical Uses: To relieve the symptoms of restlessness, sleep disturbances, or nervousness

Summary

Historically, herbals, botanicals, and natural plant products have provided humans with a wealth of medicines. Herbals are currently regulated as dietary supplements and not as drugs under the 1994 Dietary Supplement Health and Education Act (DSHEA). According to DSHEA, herbals may not claim to cure, mitigate, diagnose, or prevent disease. However, herbals have been and continue to be used by many consumers to prevent or self-treat disease. While some herbal preparations may be useful, the effectiveness (efficacy) and safety of many herbals has never been proven. Fortunately, new regulatory initiatives and programs are beginning to address the safety and efficacy concerns over herbals. Moreover, reliable, professional health care information is becoming increasingly available on the Internet, allowing rapid access for the pharmacy. This chapter reviews the regulatory history of herbal products in the United States, the major classes of secondary plant metabolites that make up most herbals, and the sites where professional herbal information is freely available.

TEST YOUR KNOWLEDGE

Multiple Choice Questions

1. Which of the following is the best regulatory definition of an herbal?
   a. Plant material that smells nice
   b. Any substance or mixture of substances intended for the cure, mitigation, diagnosis, or prevention of disease
   c. A dietary supplement that contains an herb or other botanical for use to supplement the diet and to promote health
   d. All of the above

2. Which of the following prohibited misbranded or adulterated drugs, but did not require that a drug be safe or effective before being sold?
   a. 1906 Pure Food Act
   b. 1938 Federal Food, Drug, and Cosmetic Act
   c. 1962 Kefauver-Harris Drug Amendments
   d. 1994 Dietary Supplement Health and Education Act

3. Which of the following is the class of secondary natural plant metabolites that includes the flavonoids, which are potent antioxidant compounds associated with protection of the cardiovascular system?
   a. terpenoids
   b. phenylpropanoids
   c. alkaloids
   d. none of the above

4. To be compliant with DSHEA, an herbal must
   a. be labeled as a dietary supplement
   b. identify all ingredients by name and list the quantity of each ingredient
   c. identify the plant by genus and species and the plant part from which the ingredient is derived
   d. comply with any standards set forth by the USP-NF
   e. all of the above

5. Herbal remedies are never administered as
   a. tablet
   b. lozenge
   c. injection
   d. topical ointment
   e. tea

6. Which of the following is not an important safety concern with the use of herbal products?
   a. the potential of a hypersensitivity (allergic) response to the herbal
   b. the potential that the product does not contain the herbal declared on the label
   c. the potential that the herbal product is contaminated with toxic material
   d. The potential that the herbal product does not taste very good
   e. The potential for an herbal-drug interaction when taking other medication

7. Which of the following is the Web site for the Dietary Supplement Verification Program and the updates on the United States Pharmacopeia-National Formulary monographs on herbals?
   a. http://ods.od.nih.gov
   b. http://www.usp.org
   c. http://www.fda.gov/medwatch
   d. http://nccam.nih.gov
   e. none of the above

8. Which of the following is traditionally taken by individuals as an herbal treatment for depression?
   a. saw palmetto (*Serenoa repens*)
   b. milk thistle (*Silybum marianum*)
   c. St. John's wort (*Hypericum calycinum*)
   d. purple coneflower or echinacea (*Echinacea purpurea*)
   e. none of the above

9. Which of the following is traditionally taken by individuals to help prevent illness such as colds?
   a. saw palmetto (*Serenoa repens*)
   b. milk thistle (*Silybum marianum*)
   c. St. John's wort (*Hypericum calycinum*)
   d. purple coneflower or echinacea (*Echinacea purpurea*)
   e. none of the above

Matching Question

10. Match the following:

_____ cholesterol-lowering agent	a. ginger
_____ bronchodilator	b. ginsing
_____ anti-emetic	c. garlic
_____ stimulates immune system	d. valerian
_____ used for insomnia	e. ginkgo

References

Blumenthal, M., Goldberg, A., & Brinckman, J. (Eds.). (2000). *Herbal medicine: expanded commission E monographs*. Newton, MA: Integrative Medicine Communications.

Goldman, P. (2001). Herbal medicines today and the roots of modern pharmacology. *Annals of Internal Medicine, 135*, 594–600.

Harkey, M. R., Henderson, G. L., Gershwin, M. E., Stern, J. S., & Hackman, R. M. (2001). Variability in commercial ginseng products: An analysis of 25 preparations. *American Journal of Clinical Nutrition, 73*, 1101–1106.

Israelsen, L. D. (1998). Botanicals and DHSEA: A health professional's guide. *Quarterly Review of Natural Medicine, Fall*, 251–257.

Linde, K., Ramirez, G., Mulrow, C. D., Pauls, A., Weidenhammer, W., & Melchart, D. (1996). St. John's wort for depression—An overview and meta-analysis of randomized clinical trials. *British Medical Journal, 313*, 253–258.

Nortier, J. L., Martinez, M-C. M., Schmeiser, H. H., Arlt, V. M., Bieler, C. A., Petein, M., et al. (2000). Urothelial carcinoma associated with the use of a Chinese herb (*Aristolochia fanchi*). *New England Journal of Medicine, 342*, 1686–1692.

Slifman, N. R., Obermeyer, W. R., Aloi, B. K., Mussler, S. M., Correll, W. A., Cichowicz, S. M., et al. (1998). Contamination of botanical dietary supplements by *Digitalis lanata*. *New England Journal of Medicine, 339*, 806–811.

Srinivasan, V. S., & Kucera, P. (1998). Botanicals in the USP-NF. *Pharmacopeial Forum*, *24*, 6623–6626.

Temin, P. (1980). *Taking your medicine: Drug regulation in the United States.* Cambridge, MA: Harvard University Press.

Web Sites

http://www.usp.org/. The official Web site of the United States Pharmacopeia (USP-NF) and the dietary supplement verification program (DSVP).

http://ods.od.nih.gov/. The NIH Office of Dietary Supplements Web site with the IBIDS (International Bibliographic Information on Dietary Supplements) and CARDS (Computer Access to Research on Dietary Supplements) databases.

http://www.fda.gov/medwatch/. The Medwatch Web site with information from the FDA Safety Information and Adverse Event Reporting Program.

http://nccam.nih.gov/. The National Center for Complementary and Alternative Medicine Web site.

PART
V

Administrative Aspects of Pharmacy Technology

Chapter 23:   The Policy and Procedure Manual
Chapter 24:   Materials Management of Pharmaceuticals
Chapter 25:   The Pharmacy Formulary System
Chapter 26:   Computer Applications in Drug-Use Control
Chapter 27:   Preventing and Managing Medication Errors:
               The Technician's Role
Chapter 28:   Reimbursement for Pharmacy Services
Chapter 29:   Accreditation of Technician Training Programs
Chapter 30:   Pharmacy Technician Certification Board

23 The Policy and Procedure Manual

COMPETENCIES

Upon completion of this chapter, the reader should be able to

1. Define and differentiate a *policy* and a *procedure*.
2. Give five reasons to justify the need for a policy and procedure manual.
3. List the basic format requirements for such a manual.
4. Explain the steps involved in developing the manual.
5. List five topics that could be included in each of the following pharmacy areas: administration, distribution, and clinical.
6. Indicate three problems that may be encountered in the interpretation and implementation of departmental policies and procedures.

Introduction

In every organization rules or policies are developed to accomplish the objectives of the organization. There are also specific ways in which these policies are to be carried out. These ways of carrying out policies are called **procedures**. The formal definitions are as follows.

- A policy is a definite course or method of action; a high-level, overall plan embracing general goals and objectives of what is to be done.
- A procedure is a particular way of accomplishing the objectives set forth in the policy; a series of steps followed in a definite order; the established way of how things are to be done.

In summary, a policy is a decision by an organization or a department to do something; a procedure is a step-by-step method used to accomplish that policy.

Need for Policies and Procedures

When new employees begin work in a pharmacy, there are literally hundreds of things to learn. Not only must the newcomers learn the work, but they must also learn about lunch hours, benefits, hours of operation, the chain of command, what scope of services is provided by the department, and so on. By reading a manual in which policies and procedures are described, new employees should be able to learn a considerable amount about their respective jobs. So the first reason for having a policy and procedure manual is to use it in the training of new employees.

If written policies and procedures did not exist, employees would have to be trained and instructed verbally by other employees. Because not everyone is a good teacher or can explain things fully or clearly, having information in writing ensures it is presented in a clear and consistent manner. Therefore, the second reason to have a written policy and procedure manual is to prevent errors from verbal communication.

People handle different situations in different ways. In a pharmacy, however, it is important to ensure that the same accurate and consistent results occur and that people and situations are treated the same way every time. Thus a set way for doings things is established and set forth in a policy and procedure manual. Another reason for having a policy and procedure manual is consistency—to ensure that the same policy is followed in a particular situation all the time.

The pharmacy department uses a large number and variety of drugs and supplies. Although many drugs are expensive, labor and supplies used in compounding, packaging, and labeling in a pharmacy can also comprise a considerable component of the cost of bringing drugs to patients. If procedures are performed in an efficient and economical manner, waste can be minimized, thus reducing this cost. Thus a policy and procedure manual can minimize the waste of both materials and manpower, thus reducing the cost of providing services.

A good manager is responsible for seeing that the work is done and that employees are aware of how well they are performing in their jobs. One way in which this is accomplished is through periodic evaluations of personnel job performance (i.e., how well an employee is following procedures). Effective evaluations can be accomplished only if there are written policies and procedures against which job performance can be measured. Policy and procedure manuals are therefore used to evaluate job performance.

Because of potential harm to patients, pharmacy departments take considerable care to ensure that medications are purchased, stocked, packaged, compounded, labeled, dispensed, administered, and charted accurately. Despite this care, adverse outcomes do occur, resulting in lawsuits. Unfortunately, these are not uncommon and it is sometimes necessary to determine how a specific procedure was supposed to be performed. Policy and procedure manuals, therefore, often serve as legal documents in the event of a lawsuit to protect the individual and the institution.

Finally, it must be recognized that pharmacies and hospitals are highly regulated establishments. They are governed by laws, rules, regulations, standards, and guidelines that must be followed. Many of these federal, state, and local regulating agencies require written policies and procedures. During inspections, these written policies and procedures must be shown, and, therefore, it is necessary to ensure that they are accurate and current.

In summary, policy and procedure manuals exist for the following reasons:

- to train new employees or retrain existing employees
- to prevent errors that occur due to verbal communication
- to ensure consistency of policy and job performance
- to minimize the waste of human resources and materials
- to evaluate job performance
- to serve as legal documents in the event of a lawsuit
- to comply with regulatory and accreditation agencies' requirements

An example of an evaluation form for a technician is illustrated in **Figure 23-1**.

EVERBROOK UNIVERSITY HOSPITAL & MEDICAL CENTER

Performance Review

Review Form Name:	Technician
Employee Name:	Joe Technician
Address & Telephone No:	111 Main St._240-5991
Date of Hire:	8/1/20XX
Employee ID:	1234
Position Number:	99
Position Title:	Technician
Position Code:	1234
Division:	Pharmacy
Last Review Date:	8/1/20XX
Review Period Start:	8/2/20XX
Review Period End:	8/1/20XX
Next Review Date:	8/1/20XX
Next Review Due By:	Jane Chieftech
Reviewer Title:	Chief Technician

PERFORMANCE ELEMENTS

Personal Appearance   *Meets job requirements*

Joe dresses appropriately for the position and he presents a well-groomed appearance.

Initiative   *Meets job requirements*

Joe is quick to volunteer whenever others need help and he often seeks out additional responsibilities beyond the normal scope of his job. He takes independent actions and appropriate, calculated risks. Joe is resourceful at taking advantage of opportunities. He undertakes self-development activities on his own initiative and he usually indicates when he needs help.

Accountability   *Meets job requirements*

Joe responds promptly and reliably to requests for service and assistance. He follows instructions conscientiously and responds well to management directions. He is usually very punctual and he makes an effort to schedule time off in advance. In most situations, he assumes responsibility for his own actions and outcomes. He usually puts forth extra effort when asked and he generally keeps his commitments without delay or follow-up.

Interpersonal Skills   *Meets job requirements*

Joe regularly displays a positive outlook and pleasant manner. He usually establishes and maintains good working relationships. He exhibits tact and consideration in his relations with others. Joe assists and supports his coworkers. He works cooperatively in group situations and he takes responsibility to help resolve conflicts.

Technical Knowledge   *Meets job requirements*

Joe demonstrates competency in the skills and knowledge required. He learns and applies new skills within the expected time period. He is knowledgeable about current developments in his field and he works within the normal scope of supervision. Joe displays a good understanding of how his job relates to other jobs. He effectively uses the resources and tools available to him.

Accuracy   *Meets job requirements*

The work Joe produces is usually highly accurate and thorough. He displays a strong dedication and commitment to excellence. He looks for ways to improve quality. Joe applies the feedback he receives to improve his performance and he monitors his work to meet quality standards.

Productivity   *Exceeds job requirements*

Joe usually produces more work than expected and he often completes his work ahead of schedule. He demonstrates a strong commitment to increasing productivity and he works at a faster pace than normally expected for the position. Joe strives hard in the achievement of established goals.

Ability to Learn New Skills   *Meets job requirements*

Joe usually adapts well to changes in his job or his work environment. He normally is able to manage competing demands on his time and he generally accepts criticism and feedback well. Joe can adjust his approach or method to fit different situations.

Presentation Skills   *Meets job requirements*

Joe presents information and ideas clearly and persuasively. To better understand others, he listens well, displaying interest and asking questions. He responds well to questions and he has good presentation skills. Joe actively participates in meetings.

MANDATED IN-SERVICE ATTENDANCE & RETENTION

Has completed all mandated in-service education programs.

CONTINUING EDUCATION PARTICIPATION

Has participated in departmental educational programs designed for technicians.

FIGURE 23-1 Technician evaluation form.

POSITION-SPECIFIC RESPONSIBILITIES
Complies with position-specific responsibilities as outlined in policies and procedures.
SUMMARY
Meets all required criteria and job requirements.
PLANS FOR IMPROVEMENT
No recommendations at this time.
EMPLOYEE COMMENTS

Employee Acknowledgment
I have reviewed this document and discussed the contents with my manager. My signature means that I have been advised of my performance status and does not necessarily imply that I agree with the evaluation.

_____
Employee Signature/Date

REVIEWER COMMENTS

_____
Reviewer Signature/Date

FIGURE 23-1 Technician evaluation form (*continued*).

Composing a Policy and Procedure Manual

Let us now examine how the policy and procedure manuals are written and what information can be found in a pharmacy department's manual.

Format

To avoid confusion and for the sake of consistency, it is best if all policies and procedures follow a similar **format**. Some institutions use special preprinted forms on which to write their policies and procedures. Most institutions, however, follow some kind of standard format that sets forth the basic information required. Let us examine some of the items that should be part of every policy and procedure manual.

Title

First, every policy and procedure should have a title. This tells the reader what subject is covered in the policy and procedure. This title is also used in a **table of contents** or an index. Examples of policy and procedure titles include "Hours of Operation," "Drug Recalls," and "Labeling of Outpatient Prescriptions."

Date

Every policy and procedure should be dated. Initially, a date of implementation indicates when the policy and procedure went into effect. Often, however, it is necessary to change, update, expand, or modify an existing policy or procedure. Therefore, additional dates indicate when the policy or procedure was revised. Many institutions use just the original and latest revision dates. For example:

Approved and Implemented: 1-19-05
Revised: 10-25-05

Some departments use a code for a date composed of the year (two digits), the month (two digits), the day (two digits), and a letter (*A* for the first policy prepared that day, *B* for the second, etc.). For example, the second policy and procedure prepared on October 25, 1999, would be coded with the alphanumeric: 991025B.

Some hospitals use a classification number or letters on each policy so that the particular department, type of policy, and other facts can be determined from this information. Unless the system is easy to understand, however, it can often become confusing.

Signatures

Policies and procedures should also contain the signatures of the persons who wrote or approved the policy where the policy and procedure is most frequently carried out. These signature(s) are valuable because they indicate the person responsible for generating the policy and procedure and document the agreement of the administrative personnel on the highest level.

Many policies and procedures affect other departments as well. These policies and procedures should also bear the approving signature of an administrative person in that department to ensure agreement and cooperation. For example, pharmacy department policies and procedures on the requisitioning, distribution, control, and documentation of controlled substances should bear the signature of the director of nursing services. Similar policies regarding controlled substances to anesthesia personnel should bear the signature of the director of anesthesia. Policies and procedures that involve the monitoring of food-drug interactions should bear the endorsing signature of the director of the department of food and nutrition services. Such interdepartmental policies are often incorporated into the institution's policy and procedure manual.

Format

The body of the policy and procedure must contain the formal statement of policy, followed by the step-by-step, detailed procedure for carrying out that policy. Sometimes background material is included to explain why the policy exists. The body of a policy and procedure should designate the person who is responsible for carrying out the policy and procedure and the administrative staff titles of those responsible to ensure proper compliance. This section clearly delineates the chain of command and the responsibility for ensuring compliance. For example, policies and procedures carried out by staff personnel are supervised by a pharmacy supervisor or assistant director.

It has been suggested that a useful policy and procedure manual must answer the following questions regarding a specific activity.

- What must be done?
- Who should do it?
- How should it be done?
- When should it be done?

Figure 23-2 is an example of a format used in a large teaching hospital. This format has a place for all the elements described previously.

In summary, policies and procedures should follow a uniform appearance and format, have meaningful titles, possess dates of approval, implementation, and revision, be signed by the appropriate personnel, and be clear and logical.

**ADMINISTRATIVE PROCEDURES &
INFORMATION MANUAL
DEPARTMENT OF PHARMACY**

RE-REVIEW DATE:
(Assigned by Policy Review Committee)

SUBJECT: CLARIFICTION OF MEDICATION ORDERS

RESPONSIBLE DEPARTMENT, DIVISION OR COMMITTEE

EFFECTIVE DATE ORIGINAL POLICY: 8/29/xx	**EFFECTIVE DATE REVISED POLICY: 1/00** LAST REVIEW DATE: 3/05	**SUPERSEDES POLICY NUMBER: DATED:**

POLICY: No prescription or order is to be filled if there is any doubt in the mind of the pharmacist as to what is called for: the dose, how it is to be given, or whether it is appropriate.

PROCEDURE:

1. Orders being questioned are to be entered on the patient profile as a "pending" with documentation of the problem in the clinical notes and a statement in the Special Direction field "See Clinical Notes." The yellow copy of the order is to be placed in the "problem" box with a notation as to the problem. Orders with problems that could pose risk to the patient must contain the phrase "Do not dispense until clarified" on the yellow copy and in the Special Directions Field.
2. No medication is to be dispensed until the order is clarified.
3. It is the responsibility of the pharmacist to contact the <u>prescriber</u>.
4. In the event that the name of the prescriber cannot be determined from the signature or I.D. number, the nurse may be asked for the name of the prescriber.
5. The pharmacist will page the prescriber. If the prescriber is an intern and there is no response in 15 minutes, then page the resident. Repeat this procedure, if necessary. If still no response, contact the attending physician. This last step should be done when, in the pharmacist's professional judgment, the patient could be harmed by further delay.
6. If the matter has not been resolved by the end of the shift, the information must be communicated to a pharmacist on the next shift for follow-up and resolution.
7. Upon receipt of clarification, the pending order is cancelled and the corrected order is entered. Problem resolution is to be documented on the clinical notes.
8. If authorization to change an order has been obtained, a message is to be sent to the unit notifying the nurse of the change. (See "Change in Medication Order").
9. Documentation of a clarification/change will be made in the medical record by the authorized prescriber or the pharmacist.

J. Smith
Director of Pharmacy Services

FIGURE 23-2 Sample form from policy and procedure manual.

The Approval Process

In most hospitals, the Pharmacy and Therapeutics Committee serves as the liaison between the medical staff and the department of pharmacy services. The Joint Commission on Accreditation of Healthcare Organizations (JCAHO) requires that the Pharmacy and Therapeutics Committee annually review and approve the policies and procedures of the pharmacy department. Although some pharmacy departments indicate the approval of the Pharmacy and Therapeutics Committee on each policy and procedure itself, most pharmacy departments use a cover page at the beginning of the manual which indicates all approvals. Additional approvals

THE EVERBROOK UNIVERSITY HOSPITAL AND MEDICAL CENTER MULTIDISCIPLINARY POLICY & PROCEDURE			
SUBJECT:		**PAGE**	**OF**
ORIGINAL:	REVISED:	REVISED:	REVISED:
DEPARTMENT:			
CODE NAME:			
SECTION:			
POLICY: **PROCEDURE:**			

FIRST PAGE

THE EVERBROOK UNIVERSITY HOSPITAL AND MEDICAL CENTER MULTIDISCIPLINARY POLICY AND PROCEDURE	
SUBJECT:	**CODE:**
	PAGE: **OF**
DISTRIBUTION: **REFERENCE:** **INDEX:**	

LAST PAGE

FIGURE 23-3 Multidisciplinary policy and procedure format.

may also come from such individuals as the administrator responsible for the pharmacy department or the hospital's chief executive officer, as well as the chairman of the hospital's medical board or medical executive committee.

Many hospitals or other health care institutions have a subcommittee of the Pharmacy and Therapeutics Committee that deals specifically with medication procedures and may also serve as a pharmacy-nursing liaison committee. Many policies and procedures dealing with medication distribution, control, administration, and documentation are developed by the nursing and pharmacy department members of this committee jointly. The minutes of these meetings are then approved by the parent Pharmacy and Therapeutics Committee. Therefore, approval of the policies and procedures are accomplished before implementation.

Policies and procedures developed jointly with other departments should also have a uniform and consistent format. Different professional services may utilize drastically different formats for structuring and filing their policies and procedures. Because the recent trend by the JCAHO is to have patient-focused standards, they have shifted the emphasis from individual department standards to one that concentrates on the needs of the patient. Therefore, they are more concerned with the services provided to patients rather than which specific professional provides the care. This focus encourages a multidisciplinary approach to patient care and the development of policies and procedures that involve several disciplines.

Figure 23-3 is an example of a multidisciplinary policy and procedure format with space for three professional departments. Each department has a space for its code numbers in its specific system of filing. Every hospital department must be diligent in ensuring that all policies and procedures comply with governmental regulations and laws and that they are consistent with the requirements of all accrediting agencies as well as institutional policy.

Contents of a Policy and Procedure Manual

The format and contents of a policy and procedure manual will vary from hospital to hospital. In some institutions, there may be two manuals: policy and procedure manual (containing hospital-wide policies and procedures) and an **operational manual** (containing only those policies and procedures that affect the internal workings of the pharmacy department). Under such a system it is often confusing where a particular policy and procedure is to be found, although some departments elect to keep copies of institutional policies affecting their operations in their departmental manual as well.

The most common methods for organizing policy and procedure manuals fall into two main groups. The first has policies and procedures placed in a book in alphabetical order by title; for example, Abbreviations, Absenteeism, Administrative Services, Alcohol Dispensing and Control, Ambulatory Care, and Assay and Quality Control.

A second, more common method of organizing a manual is to group policies and procedures into categories and then divide the manual into separate sections for each category. Two examples of this format are outlined here.

The first example involves a format that is composed of five major categories.

- *Section I: Organization*—This section contains information on the hospital itself, organizational charts for both the hospital and the department, services offered, pharmacy department participation on hospital committees (e.g., Pharmacy and Therapeutics Committee, the Infection Control Committee), interdepartmental relationships, and so forth.

- *Section II: Personnel Policies*—This section may contain job descriptions; staffing information; policies on benefits, holidays, sick leave, disciplinary procedures, payroll periods, requesting vacations or other time off, medical and maternity leaves, educational benefits, and so forth.
- *Section III: Administrative Policies*—This section contains policies and procedures on the department's hours of operation; purchasing policies and procedures; inventory control; drug charging to patients, employees, and third parties; interdepartmental requisitions; alcohol and controlled drug record-keeping; administrative reports; annual reports; statistics gathered; and so forth.
- *Section IV: Professional Policies*—These policies and procedures involve the compounding, labeling, packaging, dispensing, and control of medications; patient profiles; drug therapy monitoring; pharmacokinetics consultation services; drug information services; investigational drugs; drug ordering; automatic stop orders; in-service education services; antineoplastic, parenteral nutrition, and intravenous admixture services; and so forth.
- *Section V: Facilities and Equipment*—These policies and procedures pertain to the use and maintenance of the department's physical facilities and equipment, their maintenance and repair, service contracts, requisitioning, and security.

This system requires a comprehensive table of contents or index so that any policy and procedure can be easily and readily located.

A second system that has been recently developed uses only three main sections for all policies and procedures: administrative, distributional, and clinical.

The **administrative section** contains those policies and procedures that pertain to the operation of the department, its personnel, and its place within the total organizational structure of the hospital. Policies and procedures that fall into this category include the following:

- job descriptions
- confidentiality of records
- hospital table of organization
- department table of organization
- formulary operation
- infection control
- incident reporting
- personnel policies
- continuing education
- personnel evaluations
- quality assurance
- orientation of personnel
- telephone operation
- others, depending on the institution or department

The **distributional section** contains those policies and procedures that deal with the acquisition, storage, ordering, dispensing, documentation, and disposition of drugs and supplies. Examples include the following:

- drug ordering
- unit-dose drug distribution
- pharmacy services to specialty areas
- dispensing to ambulatory patients
- sterile product preparation and dispensing
- compounding and manufacturing

- emergency boxes and crash carts
- investigational drugs
- interdepartmental requisitions

The **clinical section** contains those activities involved in patient-related monitoring and other activities of a clinical nature. Examples include the following:

- clinical monitoring of profiles
- discharge counseling
- interaction screening
- drug information services
- thrombolytic monitoring and control
- pharmacokinetic consultations

This system lends itself well to the use of electronic data processing. Traditional computer operating systems permit files to be saved using the 8-3 system, that is, eight letters (or select symbols), a period, and then three additional letters. Each policy and procedure is given a file name that ends in an appropriate three-letter designation that computer operating systems allow for file names. In the 8-3 system, the three last letters permit policies and procedures to use the following: "ADM" for administrative policies and procedures, "DIS" for distributional policies and procedures, and "CLN" for clinical policies and procedures. The use of such file names permits easy backup and the sorting of files by major categories. No matter which system a department uses to organize its policy and procedure manual, there is no one "right way." Some prefer not to include job descriptions in their manuals. Some have separate sections for inpatient and outpatient operations. The key factor of a good manual is that it meets the needs of the department and that it is a useful reference for the staff.

Distribution

A policy and procedure manual is a dynamic entity since it is constantly changing. Policies and procedures are being revised, added, or deleted on a continuing basis. Therefore, the more copies of a manual that are available, the more difficult it is to keep each issue current. A copy of the policy and procedure manual, however, should be readily available to every employee so that it may be used as a reference in handling both new and repeat situations. A copy should be available in every pharmacy area to ensure easy access. In addition, a number of copies should be available for the orientation of new employees.

In hospitals where pharmacy departments have computerized information systems, it is now possible to place the policy and procedure manual on the system's computer network. This permits access to the policy and procedure manual from any terminal and makes updating the policy and procedure manual quick and easy since the network file can be easily modified. Individuals can also generate a hard copy of any policy and procedure when necessary.

Updates to the policy and procedure manual should indicate if the new policy and procedure being distributed is a revision of an existing policy and procedure or a completely new policy and procedure. If it is a revision, it should indicate which policy and procedure it is replacing. Many hospitals put a cover sheet at the front of the manual on which revisions and updates are indicated. A space is provided for the signature of the person who placed the update in the manual.

In addition to this procedure, some hospital pharmacies post each new policy and procedure on a bulletin board with a signature sheet. Each employee is expected to review the posted policy and procedure and sign the posted sheet. The sheets are then filed. A permanent record is maintained showing that the employee has acknowledged reading the policy and procedure. If the institution has a good e-mail system, staff can be alerted to a new or revised policy and procedure in that manner.

Problems

In addition to the problem regarding distribution, policy and procedure manuals have other problems relating to their successful use. First, if policies and procedures have no method to ensure enforcement, they have no value. It is therefore necessary for all employees to understand the reason behind each policy and procedure. Supervisory personnel must ensure that policies and procedures are followed. If particular policies and procedures are not being followed, the supervisor must determine if they should be changed for some reason or if disciplinary action is warranted. At times, complying with certain policies and procedures becomes very difficult under certain circumstances. In this case, each employee has an obligation to bring this matter to the attention of supervisory personnel so that the procedure can be modified. Many times there are valid reasons for not following a particular procedure. Unforseen circumstances may require recourse to an alternative action. There are exceptions to every rule. Before you take it upon yourself to make such an exception, be sure to obtain your supervisor's approval.

Another major problem with policy and procedure manuals involves their update. In the past, modification on any one part of a long policy and procedure often meant that the entire policy and procedure had to be retyped, then photocopied and distributed. The advent of the relatively low-cost personal computer (PC) has changed this procedure significantly. Many pharmacy departments today maintain their policy and procedure manuals on computer disks or on the hard drive that is an integral part of the computer. Computer disks, also referred to as "floppy disks," can easily be duplicated so that copies can be transported and utilized in any other computer in which the common software program resides.

When policies and procedures are stored on a computer disk, they can be readily retrieved and modified in any way, and a revised copy can be printed out. Word-processing software programs permit easy changes, deletions, insertions, and other modifications of any policy and procedure. The newly revised policy and procedure are then stored on the computer disk in place of the old. Additional copies of the revised policy and procedure can be generated, if necessary, or can be photocopied and distributed. Making the policy and procedures available on a computer network simplifies any changes.

Computers use $3\frac{1}{2}''$ disks that can hold approximately 75 to 100 typewritten pages, more than enough for most policy and procedure manuals. Recently, disks and disk drives with two to ten times that capacity have become available. Internal hard drives can accommodate many thousands of typewritten pages.

The growth in PC use has led to a trend of placing the policy and procedure manual into the computer's memory where it can readily be accessed by any user, at any time. As a result, except for a master copy, there may be no written policy and procedure manual at all. In these cases, security must be considered. The ability to modify any policy and procedure on a personal computer or computer network must be limited to authorized personnel.

One additional problem that many pharmacy departments must address concerns "memos" versus "policies and procedures." When some new activity or service begins or if there is a modification of some long-standing activity or procedure, there is often a tendency to send out a memorandum instead of finding, updating, and distributing the appropriate policy and procedure. Memorandums are easy to generate, often take only a few minutes, and do not require the thought and effort needed to revise a policy and procedure. However, they are just as easily discarded, do not become part of the official departmental manual, and tend to make the appropriate policy and procedure obsolete and useless. Therefore, what may appear to be the easier way of handling a change should be avoided in favor of revising the policy and procedure in question or writing a new policy and procedure to cover the situation. A memo may be a good way to clarify an interpretation of a particular policy or to remind the staff that a particular policy exists.

Summary

Policy and procedure manuals that are comprehensive and current are necessary and useful tools in the proper management of any well-managed organization. They should be current and dynamic because the roles and responsibilities of the department change. They should be viewed as helpful guides in providing efficient and consistent service to the patients and staff whom the pharmacy department serves.

TEST YOUR KNOWLEDGE

Multiple Choice Questions

1. A policy is
   a. a series of steps to follow in a definite order
   b. a traditional way of doing things
   c. an organizational course of action
   d. a memorandum to accomplish a task
   e. all of the above

2. A procedure is
   a. a step-by-step method used to carry out a task
   b. a decision to do something
   c. a plan of general goals
   d. a verbal communication
   e. all of the above

3. New employees must become familiar with
   a. their job description
   b. the hours of work
   c. the policies and procedures
   d. the chain of command
   e. all of the above

4. Policy and procedure manuals are used to
   a. train and inform new employees
   b. prevent errors from verbal communications
   c. ensure that the same policy is followed in the same situation
   d. serve as legal documents in the event of a lawsuit
   e. all of the above

5. Which of the following is not true regarding policy and procedure manuals?
   a. Many regulating agencies require written policies and procedures.
   b. Any change requires approval of the chief operating officer of the institution.
   c. They minimize waste of manpower, time, and materials by providing direction in repetitive tasks.
   d. They provide a new employee with valuable information about his or her new job.
   e. They ensure accuracy and consistency in routine operational activities.

True/False Questions

6. _____ Policy and procedure manuals are used to evaluate job performance.

7. _____ Every policy and procedure should have a title.

8. _____ Policies and procedures should be signed by all persons affected by the policy.

9. _____ Every five years the members of the Pharmacy and Therapeutics Committee review and update the manual.

10. _____ Technicians should be familiar with policies and procedures that pertain to the administrative and technical aspects of the manual.

Matching Questions

11. _____ operational manual

12. _____ policy

13. _____ memo

14. _____ policy and procedure manual

15. _____ procedure

a. guidelines that contain goals and methods of carrying out the goals

b. a particular way of acting

c. a directive in message form

d. overall plan of general goals

e. internal workings of the pharmacy department

References

Aspen Reference Group. (1992). *Hospital pharmacy management: Forms, checklists & guidelines.* Frederick, MD: Aspen Publishers.

Brookdale University Hospital and Medical Center. (1998). *Policy and procedure manual of the Department of Pharmacy Services of the Brookdale University Hospital and Medical Center.* Brooklyn, NY: Author.

Brown, T. R. (Ed.). (1992). *Handbook of institutional pharmacy practice* (3rd ed.). Bethesda, MD: American Society of Health-System Pharmacists.

Hospital pharmacy policy and procedure manual. (1985). Tarzana, CA: AMI Pharmacy Management Services.

Trudeau, T. (Ed.). (annual). *Topics in hospital pharmacy management.* Frederick, MD: Aspen Publishers.

COMPETENCIES

Upon completion of this chapter, the reader should be able to

1. List the functions involved in the drug procurement process in the institutional pharmacy.

2. Explain the major methods used to distribute drugs in the hospital.

3. Describe the function of the Pharmacy and Therapeutics Committee in drug selection.

4. Distinguish between generic drugs and brand-name drugs.

5. Enumerate the seven basic principles that are essential for group purchasing.

6. List the records and reports required to be maintained in the materials management section.

7. State the information that must be included in a pharmacy purchase order.

8. Describe checkpoints to be observed when a drug order is received in the hospital.

9. List the environmental considerations required in the storage of drugs.

10. Define the following temperature requirements for drug storage: cold, cool, room temperature, warm, and excessive heat.

11. Name the drugs and pharmaceutical products that require special safety precautions.

12. Calculate an inventory turnover rate and state the desirable turnover level range.

13. Describe acquisition alternatives when manufacturer's back orders or distributor shortages impose a supply dilemma.

14. List the benefits associated with the use of a bar-coded medication system.

Introduction

This chapter will address the methods used to select, acquire, and organize a drug inventory for institutional use; describe the various systems of drug distribution and control; recognize the impact of cost-containment strategies used by pharmacy personnel; and describe the scope of activities that can be assumed by qualified pharmacy technicians.

Health care costs, at both the federal and state levels, have increased more rapidly than any other category of products or services used in our society. Private insurance companies and government agencies have been overwhelmed with requests for payment of expensive charges for state-of-the-art diagnostic procedures and sophisticated treatments and therapies. The costs associated with pharmaceuticals continue to increase at astronomical rates due to a constant flow of costly new **bioengineered therapies** resulting from advances in research and sophisticated marketing programs. As a result of increased costs for health care services and a decrease in resources to pay for them, it has become essential for pharmacy department managers to assess cost containment in all aspects of pharmacy service.

The objective of this chapter is to identify and describe the methods used by pharmacy personnel to deliver the appropriate drug to the right patient, at the right time, and at the most reasonable cost. Another way of stating this objective is "to identify pharmacy services that are both effective and affordable."

Controlling the costs associated with a complete pharmacy service includes not only the acquisition cost of drugs, but also the total cost of "managing" materials. An institutional pharmacy **materials management** program includes the following:

- *Procurement*—drug selection, source selection, cost analysis, group purchasing, **prime-vendor** relationships, purchasing procedures, record-keeping, receiving control
- *Drug storage and inventory control*—storage conditions, security requirements, proper rotation of inventory, computerized inventory control
- *Repackaging and labeling considerations*—unit-dose and extemporaneous packaging, labeling requirements
- *Distribution systems*—unit-dose, floor stock, compounded prescriptions, intravenous admixtures, emergency drugs
- *Recapture and disposal*—unused medication, returns and reuse, environmental considerations

In a hospital, the overall responsibility for the materials management of pharmaceuticals lies with the director of the pharmacy department. The Pharmacy and Therapeutics Committee selects drugs and therapeutic agents that are to be available in the institution. This committee is chaired by physicians who are appointed by the medical board, and the secretary is the director of the pharmacy services. The committee consists of representatives from the medical board, the pharmacy, nursing and dietary departments, quality assurance, and the hospital administration. It is essential to have the clinical and technical knowledge of pharmacists, physicians, and nurses available when making decisions regarding which drug products should be included in the formulary to ensure adequate and appropriate therapy.

The director of pharmacy delegates certain aspects of the pharmacy materials management program to trained pharmacy personnel to deliver effective and efficient pharmacy services. The official list of drugs available is known as the hospital formulary and is reviewed and modified on an ongoing basis as required.

Procurement

Drug Selection

The drug selection process may begin with a physician's request for a new drug. The pharmacist processes the request and prepares an objective review of the medication requested. If the drug required is similar to other drugs on the formulary, it is important to determine if the benefits justify admission to the formulary. Guidelines for the evaluation of drugs are provided by the ASHP Technical Assistance Bulletin on the Evaluation of Drugs for Formularies.

The pharmacy department's objective review includes cost analysis information—an important factor in this age of cost containment. The Pharmacy and Therapeutics Committee considers how much a drug costs per dose, per day, or even per treatment cycle. The decision regarding whether to add a new drug to the formulary is not based solely on whether it is a better therapeutic agent, but whether the perceived benefit is worth the additional cost (cost-benefit analysis). The pharmacy department's research and presentation can have a profound effect on whether a new drug is added to the hospital formulary.

The most cost-effective materials management programs are the result of combining the required expertise and specialty knowledge of a pharmacist with the materials management and systems expertise of a trained pharmacy technician. The pharmacist selects the brands or generic equivalents that are acceptable. The trained pharmacy technician may negotiate price, monitor inventory levels, input purchase order and receiving information into a computer system or manual record-keeping system, and organize inventory. Under supervision of the pharmacist, the technician will fill and deliver floor stock orders, repackage medication for unit-dose distribution, and may inspect medication storage areas for proper environmental conditions. The degree of supervision by a pharmacist will vary, depending on the ability of the technician and the policy of the pharmacy department. The pharmacist responsible for materials management supervises the entire process.

Source Selection

Another aspect of procurement deals with source selection. One aspect of source selection deals with the concept of **generic drugs** versus **brand-name drugs**. The pharmacist determines if the generic product is a **therapeutic equivalent** of the brand-name product and then makes the source selection.

The Food and Drug Administration regulates the manufacturing of generic drug products to make every effort to ensure therapeutic efficacy. To minimize therapeutic inadequacies, the pharmacist carefully considers the reputation of the generic drug manufacturer and reviews drug analysis data and information. Although cost savings associated with the use of generic drugs have proven to be of great value, selection is made on quality assurance of the product. Therapeutic equivalence is sometimes difficult to ascertain. However, the reputation of the generic manufacturer and an ongoing surveillance of the professional literature assist the pharmacist in determining if the amount of savings realized by purchasing a generic drug is cost-justified. Guidelines are provided by the ASHP Guidelines for Selecting Pharmaceutical Manufacturers and Suppliers.

Cost Analysis

Source selection also includes cost considerations. Drug product cost analysis is an essential step in assessing cost-containment strategies. Information regarding acquisition cost of the product is readily available and a price comparison of therapeutically equivalent drugs can be studied. Nonacquisition costs may include costs related to storage, time required to prepare products for patient use, and even packaging considerations. Nonacquisition costs include those related to getting the medication to the patient, not simply getting the drug to the pharmacy.

Group Purchasing and Prime Vendor Relationships

Group purchasing and prime vendor relationships are two important strategies utilized in an attempt to control the purchase price of drugs. In general, as a result of group purchasing, the unit cost of a drug is lowered as the projected quantity of the drug to be purchased is increased. Simply stated, group purchasing allows each participating hospital the benefit of quantity discounts as a result of pooling the projected quantities of each hospital and negotiating one contract that applies to all participating members. The seven basic principles that are essential for group purchasing to be effective are as follows.

1. Most hospitals should have generic formularies allowing across-the-board evaluation opportunities to all vendors.
2. All group members should be committed to buy from the awarded agreement.
3. The group should normally award each item to only one supplier.
4. A pharmacy committee should be established to ensure thorough product quality and vendor review. The pharmacy committee, when it addresses issues for the entire group, can direct the group to many years of successful agreements.
5. The management of individual hospitals should support group programs, especially pharmacy purchasing.
6. The group director should maintain open communication with vendors through newsletters, cooperation in dealing with compliance issues, and approval of regular visits.
7. The group should be willing and able to consider the addition of new products to the bid.

A prime-vendor relationship allows the pharmacy to reduce the size of inventory. This reduction frees dollars to pay other outstanding debts or to pay bills on time, which will minimize the amount of costly premiums associated with late payments. This is accomplished when the pharmacy department purchases as many products as possible from one single supply source, usually a drug wholesaler. A drug wholesaler can make same-day deliveries and acts as a local warehouse and distributor for various manufacturers. Some manufacturers maintain their own direct shipment service as well as a wholesaler distribution program, whereas others distribute exclusively through wholesalers thereby eliminating the need for their own distribution facilities.

Purchasing Procedures

Most wholesalers sell products at established contract prices plus an additional handling fee that can vary from 2% to 4% depending on the payment terms established with the hospital. The shorter the payment period, the lower the wholesaler markup. Prepayment schedules are usually necessary to realize discounts. If the hospital minimizes the markup charge by maintaining an efficient accounts payable schedule, the cost benefits realized from reducing the pharmacy inventory will far outweigh the additional cost associated with the wholesaler's fee. The following questions will assist the pharmacy technician to understand the intricacies of purchasing pharmaceuticals:

1. Is a single-brand purchasing policy in effect for the pharmacy department?
2. Has the Pharmacy and Therapeutics Committee approved a written generic substitution policy?
3. Has the Pharmacy and Therapeutics Committee approved a written therapeutic substitution policy?
4. Is competitive bidding used for high-cost items? For high-volume items?
5. Is either of these methods used to set prices: guarantee of bid prices or price ceiling set for the term of the contract?
6. Are the following considered when evaluating bids: prompt payment discount, terms of payment, nonperformance penalties, delivery time limitations, returned and damaged goods policy and services?
7. Are contracts negotiated when appropriate?
8. Are contracts renegotiated on a regular basis (e.g., annually)?
9. Is group purchasing used when advantageous?
10. If group purchasing is used, are prices guaranteed and is there a mechanism for determining that group prices are competitive?
11. Are primary wholesalers or wholesale contracts used for specific drugs when appropriate?
12. Are the wholesaler costs equal to or less than the costs of purchasing the same drugs directly? (Consider all factors such as increased investment revenues, decreased number of purchase orders, reduced inventory value, and receiving costs.)
13. Have inventories been adequately reduced?
14. Have ordering and receiving costs been adequately reduced?
15. Do outages that require payment of premium prices occur frequently?
16. Are there frequent outages?
17. Are volume discounts evaluated for net savings before purchase (i.e., gross savings minus increased carrying cost)?

Impact of Drug Shortages

The unavailability of drugs has increased in frequency and severity over the past few years for many reasons. One major factor is the overwhelming economic pressure that affects all aspects of the health care industry. Hospitals receive less reimbursement from insurers, and distributors and manufacturers compete for lower margin business affected by aggressive contracts from group purchasing organizations (GPOs). Unfortunately, there are strong indications that all parties in the supply chain are too aggressive in attempting to reduce costs and meet business objectives.

Drug shortages may cause treatment delays and a need for alternative therapeutic approaches sometimes resulting in less desirable treatment outcomes. There are many frustrations associated with drug shortages such as determining the cause of a drug shortage and the expected duration, locating an alternative source of the product or a generic substitution, selecting therapeutic alternatives, managing increased costs, and coping with strained relationships. Alternative agents may also increase the potential for medication errors leading to adverse reactions. Some of the contributing factors include poor communications throughout the supply chain, aggressive inventory practices, manufacturer issues, inaccurate product use projections, and the FDA's regulatory influence.

In an ideal world, providers of health care would be able to consistently anticipate and order the appropriate quantity of drugs in a timely manner so that manufacturers could produce sufficient quantities and distributors could deliver the drugs just prior to the time they are needed. The reason for a just-in-time (JIT) inventory strategy is to minimize tying up large sums of money for long periods of time and, in addition, to reduce the cost associated with inventory management. Hospitals, distributors, and manufacturers all implement a JIT strategy which leaves very little room for error. Using JIT strategies, manufacturers maintain approximately 30 days of raw material and product, distributors maintain approximately 43 days of product, and hospital pharmacies average between 10 and 16 inventory turns per year. A pharmacy technician working as an inventory manager or acting as a pharmacy buyer must consistently monitor the utilization trends of critical drugs and expensive products and communicate changes in utilization to the distributor every day. Distributors, in turn, need to frequently monitor the quantities being ordered and modify the quantities ordered from the manufacturer. Manufacturers should adjust production quantities as the demand for products change, but unfortunately, this is not always done.

There have been many factors that influence the production of drug products. Some of these factors include industry consolidation, complex manufacturing processes, raw material shortages, FDA certification problems, profitability, and obligation to shareholders. Sometimes production shortages occur when manufacturers underestimate the demand for product as a result of poor planning, shifts in clinical practice, new indication, and new treatment guidelines. Marketing strategies, unexpected withdrawals, contracting changes, or halting production when annual quotas are met can also cause drug shortages. An interesting phenomenon that is difficult to anticipate is when one drug shortage causes a rapid increase in the use of another product, which causes a secondary shortage.

The impact that drug shortages have on the hospital pharmacy can be devastating and may include increases in drug expenditures as a result of purchasing noncontracted drugs which may adversely affect bundled product contracts. There are sometimes costs associated with getting manufacturers to drop-ship emergency allocations of product that are no longer available from the distributors. There is also a tendency to overstock an item when it has been back ordered or difficult to obtain.

In order to be prepared, a hospital pharmacy buyer should take a proactive approach and establish contingency procedures. An excellent source of information on this topic can be found in the ASHP Guidelines on Managing Drug Product Shortages (2001).

Record-Keeping

The pharmacy department must also establish and maintain adequate records to meet government regulations, standards of practice requirements, accreditation standards, hospital policies, and management information requirements. These records include budget reports, productivity and workload documents, purchase orders, inventory, receiving and dispensing reports, and controlled substances and alcohol records. The pharmacy's materials manager should be intimately involved with the development and maintenance of many of these documents.

The purchase order
The purchase order document should be prepared at the time the order is placed by telephone, mail, computer, or fax. The information included on the purchase order includes the following:

- the name and address of the hospital
- the shipping address

- the date the order was placed
- the vendor's name and address
- the purchase order number
- the ordering department's name and location
- the expected date of delivery
- shipping terms (e.g., FOB, Net 30)
- the account number or billing designation
- a description of items ordered
- the quantity of items ordered
- the unit price
- the extended price
- the total price of the order
- the buyer's name and phone number

Receiving Control

Accepting the responsibility for receiving drugs for the pharmacy department is another important role that can be filled by the pharmacy technician. When receiving deliveries, the pharmacy technician should follow these basic rules.

- Check the shipping address to be sure the package received was intended for delivery to the pharmacy department.
- Check the outside of the package for visible signs of damage to the carton or the contents. Note any damage on the receiving document before you sign for the delivery.
- Look for any shipping documents attached to the outside of the package and determine if special handling is required (e.g., store in freezer, controlled substance).
- Carefully open the package and check each item for breakage.
- Check each item for expiration date and make note of any short-dated material for immediate use or return.
- Verify the order received against a copy of the purchase order. Make a notation of any variation. Refer to the shipping document or packing slip to determine if items are back ordered or out of stock.
- Refer any order discrepancies to the supervising pharmacist.

Complete accountability of drugs from receiving to patient administration requires a tightly controlled, coordinated effort on the part of all pharmacy and nursing personnel.

All drugs should be delivered directly to the pharmacy department or a secured pharmacy receiving area to prevent diversion of drug orders. Controlled substances and tax-free alcohol require special handling and must be closely supervised by a licensed pharmacist to minimize loss or adulteration. The pharmacist prepares purchase orders, receives and secures shipments, and monitors the inventory of controlled substances and tax-free alcohol. These practices are required by law in most states.

Drug Storage and Inventory Control

Storage

After drugs have been selected, ordered, and received, they must be properly stored. Appropriate storage requires environmental considerations, security issues, and safety requirements.

The inventory may be divided into an active drug inventory and a backup storeroom inventory for large, bulky items that require much space. The inventory may also be divided by how the drugs will be used. For example, parenteral medication for intravenous (IV) administration may be stored in the IV admixture room only.

Environmental consideration

Environmental considerations include proper temperature, ventilation, humidity, light, and sanitation. Standards have been developed and are referenced in various statutes as a basis for determining appropriate storage requirements since they affect strength, quality, purity, packaging, and labeling of drugs and related articles. These important standards are contained in a combined publication that is recognized as the official compendium, the *United States Pharmacopeia* (USP) and the *National Formulary* (NF).

For example, the USP defines *controlled room temperature* as the acceptable temperature when a variation is not specified. In addition, specific requirements are stated in some drug monographs where it is considered that storage at a lower or higher temperature may produce undesirable results. Specific storage conditions are required to be printed in product literature and on drug packaging and **drug labels** to ensure proper storage and product integrity. The conditions are defined by the following terms:

- *Cold*—any temperature not exceeding 8°C (45°F). A refrigerator is a cold place in which the temperature is maintained thermostatically between 2° and 8°C (36° and 46°F). A freezer is a cold place in which the temperature is maintained thermostatically between –20° and –10°C (–4° and 14°F).
  a. Protection from freezing—When freezing subjects an article to loss of strength or potency or to destructive alteration of its characteristics, the container label bears an appropriate instruction to prevent the article from freezing.
- *Cool*—any temperature between 8° and 15°C (46° and 59°F). An article for which storage in a cool place is directed may alternatively be stored in a refrigerator, unless otherwise specified in the individual monograph.
- *Room temperature*—the temperature prevailing in a working area. Controlled room temperature is a temperature maintained thermostatically between 15° and 30°C (59° and 86°F).
- *Warm*—any temperature between 30° and 40°C (86° and 104°F).
- *Excessive heat*—any temperature above 40°C (104°F).

When no specific storage directions or limitations are provided in the individual monograph, it is understood that the storage conditions include protection from moisture, freezing, and excessive heat.

Additional standards regarding the preservation, packaging, storage, and labeling of drugs are described in the "General Notices and Requirements" section of the USP/NF. Persons involved in any aspect of materials management of pharmaceuticals must be familiar with the official standards and definitions as they relate to the proper storage and handling of drugs. The pharmacy technician shares this obligation with all other members of the health care team involved in medication-related activities.

Security Requirements

Security requirements that restrict access to drugs to "authorized personnel only" are often the result of legal requirements, hospital policy, and established standards of practice. All medications must be maintained in restricted locations so that they are only accessible to professional staff who are authorized to receive, store, prepare, dispense, distribute, or administer such products.

Legend drugs (those that require a prescription) must be dispensed by a licensed pharmacist. However, a pharmacy technician under the direct supervision of a pharmacist can receive and fill floor stock orders and deliver the medication to a drug storage location. Medication storage areas located on nursing units must also be secured and restricted to authorized personnel only.

Controlled substances and tax-free alcohol require additional restrictions. Only a licensed pharmacist can order, receive, prepare, and dispense these drugs. However, a qualified pharmacy technician under the direct supervision of a pharmacist can assist in storing and delivering these products. Special security procedures, such as daily physical counts of pharmacy and nursing units inventories, are essential to ensure that there is no diversion or misuse of controlled substances. Tax-free alcohol, which is most often used only by the pathology department, is controlled by performing periodic record audits and physical inventories.

Safety precautions must also be carefully considered when handling materials that have a high potential for danger. For example, when storing volatile or flammable substances, it is important to have a cool location that is properly ventilated and has been specially designed to reduce fire and explosion potential. Another consideration would be to store caustic substances, such as acids, in a location that would reduce any potential for the container being dropped and broken (e.g., in a locked cabinet instead of an open shelf). Oncology drugs used to treat cancer are often cytotoxic themselves and, therefore, must be handled with extreme care. They should be received in a sealed protective outer bag that restricts the dissemination of the drug if the container leaks or is broken. These drugs should also be stored in a secure area that has limited access and a restricted traffic flow. When the potential exists for exposure to chemotherapy, all personnel involved must wear protective clothing and equipment while following a hazardous materials cleanup procedure. All exposed materials must be properly disposed of in chemo-hazardous waste containers.

Proper rotation of inventory

Segregating inventory by drug category also helps to prevent errors that could increase the potential for harm. For example, the standards of the Joint Commission on Accreditation of Healthcare Organizations (JCAHO) require that internal and external medications must be stored separately to reduce the potential for someone dispensing or administering an external product for internal use. Rotating inventory and checking expiration dates on products when drugs are received helps to reduce the potential for dispensing or administering expired drugs and also maximizes the utilization of inventory before drugs become outdated.

Computerized inventory control

Many of these functions can be better controlled with the use of computer programs dedicated to monitor the purchasing, receiving, and dispensing functions on an ongoing basis. Perpetual inventory systems are now being utilized to indicate when predetermined reorder points are reached. Most dedicated pharmacy systems can generate management reports that allow the materials manager to review drug use. For example, the monthly usage rate of each drug can be monitored, and utilization can be tracked to determine which clinical department or patient population is using specific drugs. Computers also enable the materials manager to closely monitor budget trends and year-to-date purchases by drug category. It is important for the pharmacy technician to remember that computer systems are only as effective as the users are accurate when inputting information. Therefore, the materials management technician must have a basic understanding of how the pharmacy computer works and must be properly trained to maximize the potential benefits of inventory control programs. More detail on pharmacy computerization is discussed in Chapter 26.

Turnover rate

Determining the pharmacy's inventory turnover rate is a good method of measuring the overall effectiveness of the purchasing and inventory control programs. The inventory turnover rate is calculated by dividing the total dollars spent to purchase drugs for one year by the actual value of the pharmacy inventory at any point in time. The number produced by this calculation offers an indication of how many times a year the inventory may have been used or replaced. The larger the number of inventory turnovers, the stronger the indication that the inventory control program is efficient.

In the 1980s, a turnover rate of 6% to 7% was considered to be acceptable. In the 1990s, turnover rates of 10% to 12% were easily achievable because of more efficient methods of purchasing, such as prime-vendor programs and computerized order-entry systems. Even higher turnover rates will be achieved in the twenty-first century due to new materials management techniques and business strategies such as consignment of inventory programs.

The following questions may further assist the pharmacy materials manager in his or her attempt to maintain adequate controls on a very large and complex inventory.

1. Has an inventory turnover rate been calculated for your hospital?
2. Is this rate optimal for the facility?
3. Is the storeroom checked at regular intervals to verify that appropriate purchasing and inventory methods are being followed?
   a. Are reorder points adjusted as needed?
   b. Is this rate optimal for the facility?
4. Are inventories controlled in dispensing areas?
   a. Are minimum and maximum inventories maintained?
   b. Is the space allotted for each product restricted?
   c. Is there a routine check for outdated drugs and excesses?
   d. Are exchange systems used when appropriate (e.g., carts, self-units, boxes)?
5. Are nursing-unit drug inventories controlled?
   a. Is an approved floor-stock list used for drug items?
   b. Are there maximum allowable quantities for each item?
   c. Are inventory dollar limits set for each nursing unit?
   d. Are units checked monthly for excesses and outdated drugs?
6. Are inventories controlled in the emergency, operating, and recovery rooms?

Repackaging and Labeling Considerations

In-house packaging and labeling are sometimes necessary when required dosage forms are not available commercially. The pharmacy technician is often directly involved in preparing unit-dose packaging that utilizes automated packaging equipment. The pharmacy technician must be adequately trained to ensure the stability of the product and appropriate labeling. Accordingly, the pharmacy technician must receive detailed training in this regard.

Depending on the product, the desired route of administration, and the method of dispensing, there are different container types from which to choose. For example, unit-dose packaging for solid oral forms (e.g., tray-fill blister packaging, cadet foil packaging) and oral liquids (e.g., Baxa cups, oral syringes). In addition, some of the new automated dispensing technologies require packaging unique to their dispensing design (e.g., APS Robot-ready cards, Envoy and SureMed dispensing cartridges).

Regardless of which type of packaging container is used, it should be clean and special precautions and cleaning procedures may be necessary to ensure that extraneous matter is not introduced into or onto the drugs being packaged. It is also essential to be sure that the container does not interact physically or chemically with the drug being placed in it so as to alter the strength, quality, or purity of the article beyond the official requirements.

Some drugs may have special packaging requirements as described in the manufacturer's literature and in official monographs published in the USP and NF. The following requirements for use of specified containers may apply when in-house packaging is required:

- *Light-resistant container*—protects the contents from the effects of light by virtue of the specific properties of the material of which it is composed, including any coating applied to it. Alternatively, a clear and colorless or a translucent container may be made light resistant by means of an opaque covering, in which case the label of the container bears a statement that the opaque covering is needed until the contents are to be used or administered. When it is directed to "protect from light" in an individual monograph, preservation in a light-resistant container is required.
- *Tamper-resistant packaging*—required for a sterile article intended for ophthalmic or otic use, except when extemporaneously compounded for immediate dispensing on prescription. The contents are sealed so that they cannot be opened without obvious destruction of the seal.
- *Tight container*—protects the contents from contamination by extraneous liquids, solids, or vapors, from loss of the article, and from efflorescence, deliquescence, or evaporation under the ordinary or customary conditions of handling, shipment, storage, and distribution, and is capable of tight reclosure.
- *Hermetic container*—is impervious to air or any other gas under the ordinary or customary conditions of handling, shipment, storage, and distribution.
- *Single-unit container*—is one that is designed to hold a quantity of drug product intended for administration as a single dose, or a single finished device intended for use promptly after the container is opened. Each single-unit container shall be labeled to indicate the identity, quantity, strength, name of manufacturer, lot number, and expiration date of the drug or article.
- *Single-dose container*—is a single-unit container for articles intended for parenteral administration only. Examples of single-dose containers include prefilled syringes, cartridges, fusion-sealed containers, and closure-sealed containers when so labeled.
- *Unit-dose container*—is a single-unit container for articles intended for administration by other than the parenteral route as a single dose, direct from the container.

Each label must at least include the following information:

- generic name of the product (brand name optional)
- strength in units (e.g., mg, ml, oz)

- drug form (e.g., tablet, capsule, suppository)
- lot number and manufacturer's name
- expiration date for repackaged drug

The expiration date used on repackaged drugs should be based on the prevailing community standard of practice or based on an evaluation of scientific information. In all cases, a maximum expiration date should be adhered to as identified in law and regulation. The seventeenth addition of the USP states, "In the absence of stability data to the contrary, such date should not exceed (1) 25% of the remaining time between the date of repackaging and the expiration date on the original manufacturer's bulk container, or (2) a 6-month period of time from the date the drug is repackaged, whichever is earlier."

All repackaged drugs must be carefully checked by a licensed pharmacist and approvals must be documented in writing before repackaged drugs are put into active inventory. Documentation of the repackaging process should include the following information:

- date of repackaging
- name and strength of drug
- quantity of drug repackaged
- manufacturer's name
- manufacturer's lot number
- manufacturer's expiration date
- in-house code number
- in-house expiration date
- initials of packaging technician
- initials of pharmacist

Benefits Associated with Bar Coding

In March 2003, the Food and Drug Administration (FDA) announced that it would require bar codes on all medication in an effort to reduce the high rate of medical errors. This is an important step in automating the medication use process and reducing the amount of human interpretation in the ordering, dispensing, and administration of drugs. During a study of more than 88 million doses from April 2002 to June 2003, it was estimated that only 36% of the dose level drugs had bar coding. The FDA estimates that it would cost pharmaceutical companies $50 million to add bar codes to all drugs manufactured and used in the U.S. and hospitals would spend over $7 billion on scanners and computer systems to support the initiative.

The Institute of the National Academy of Sciences has estimated that of the more than 98,000 people killed from medical errors each year, about 7,000 of those deaths were directly attributed to medication errors. According to Michael R. Cohen, president of the Institute for Safe Medication Practices, early studies indicate that bar coding should reduce the number of medications errors by over 50%.

There are early indications that some manufacturers will reduce the number of drugs presently available in individual dose packaging in order to avoid the increased cost associated with the new FDA requirement. This trend will result in an even greater need for providers to repackage and bar code drugs which will no longer be available in unit-dose packaging. This change will have a direct impact on the pharmacy technician's role and responsibilities. The pharmacy technician will need to become knowledgeable regarding the different types of packaging and scanning equipment available, the limitations and compatibility of bar-coding systems, and the associated changes in the medication use process. For example, bar-coded labels that are read by automated dispensing technology may not be compatible with a scanner used by a nurse at the patient's bedside. A bar-code label that is placed on a unit-dose product may or may not contain an expiration date which would be helpful for inventory management purposes. Due to the current lack of standardization related to bar coding in the health care industry today, pharmacy providers must carefully scrutinize the compatibility of the bar-coding systems and equipment in order to ensure that the outcomes desired are achieved.

The obvious goal of the government's initiative is to have all drugs bar coded to the dose level which, in turn, will make products available that can be used as part of an automated system that will reduce the incidence of medication errors. Additional benefits will be realized as a result of streamlining the entire medication use process. A physician can order medication for a patient online with less chance of a selection error or interpretation error occurring with a faster transmission time. A pharmacist can review the order as part of an electronic patient medication profile which is programmed to identify potential medication errors such as the wrong drug, wrong dose, or a drug that may not be compatible with other medication the patient is receiving. Patient profile systems can also identify drug-food allergies and possible allergic reactions as a result of known patient allergies. Drugs can also be dispensed using bar-coded labels or over-wrap containers compatible with automated dispensing technology either in the pharmacy or at the patient's point of care. A nurse can scan the patient' ID bracelet, her own ID badge, and the medication bar code as a final check to ensure the right medication and right dose is being administered to the right patient at the right time. If all of these checks are accepted, the medication administration documentation and the associated charge for the drug can be automatically processed as a post-administration step in the process.

The infrastructure required to accomplish these goals includes having medication with a bar-coded label, bar-coded patient ID bracelets, bar-coded nurse badges, a wireless network and point-of-care hardware (reader/scanner). Bar coding is the critical communication link, the common denominator used by automated systems to ensure that supply chain processes and the clinical checks and balances work in concert to support the best results. Bar coding uniquely identifies a specific product and a specific dose. The savings associated with automating the medication use process will eventually offset the cost of the technology and systems required to support a "closed loop" initiative, but the initial cost can only be justified as cost avoidance associated with reducing the incidence of medication errors and improving the quality of patient care. Pharmacy technicians will play a significant role in developing and supporting the Food and Drug Administration's bar-coding initiative.

Distribution Systems

Drug distribution systems have changed considerably in the last 10 years. In the past, it was acceptable to dispense large containers of drugs (bulk packaging) to be stored at the nursing unit for use whenever a nurse needed to administer a drug to a patient. This method, known as a floor stock system, does not allow the pharmacist to review drug therapy before it is administered to a patient. It is, therefore, potentially dangerous. Also, floor stock medication cannot be reused once it is removed from the original container because there is no way to guarantee product integrity. As a result, this method increases the potential for waste. Today the JCAHO and most state agencies require unit-dose dispensing and pharmacy-based intravenous additive programs. (The importance of these programs is discussed in Chapter 17).

Certain emergency drugs are still maintained as floor stock because they may be urgently needed. Emergency drugs may be stored in mobile units for quick transfer to a patient's bedside when resuscitation techniques are required. Emergency drugs are stored in a medication cabinet at the nursing unit for use when rapid blood levels are necessary in patients who cannot wait for drug orders to be processed and delivered by the pharmacy department. Determining when it is appropriate to circumvent a pharmacist review of drug therapy to have medication available for immediate administration is a difficult undertaking. It constantly challenges pharmacy and nursing relationships. The best way to minimize controversy regarding this consideration is to have comprehensive pharmacy services that meet the requirements of patient needs in a timely manner. Traditionally, emergency drugs are immediately available as circumstances require.

Recapture and Disposal

Returned Medications

Properly processing medication that is returned to the pharmacy department is an important role that can be fulfilled by a pharmacy technician. When unit-dose packaging is used, the pharmacy technician can check return medication for package integrity and proper dating before putting the drug back into stock. In case of a manufacturer's recall, each dose of medication can be located by lot number to ensure its removal. Records of all recall information should be maintained to ensure that a proper review of all potentially dangerous drugs has been completed.

Expiration Dates

All drug packages have expiration date notations that identify the date when the medication is no longer suitable for use. The expiration date will be designated in one of two ways: month and year (e.g., June 1999), which means that the packaged material, if properly stored, is good until the last day of the month; or more specifically as month, day, and year (e.g., June 15, 1999). Every hospital pharmacy must have a system whereby drugs are checked for expiration dates on a regular basis to guarantee that only properly dated drugs are available for use. Expired drugs must be segregated from active inventory to prevent a potentially dangerous dispensing error. Many pharmaceutical companies will give full credit for expired medication. It is essential for the pharmacy materials manager to determine the return policy for each company.

Environmental Considerations

When disposing of partially used drugs or expired drugs that cannot be returned for credit, it is important to consider the negative impact that certain drugs may have on the environment. For example, many oncology drugs used for the treatment of cancer are carcinogenic (i.e., they have the potential to cause cancer themselves). It is essential that strict precautions be taken and procedures followed to properly dispose of these items. Another concern is related to partially used injectable medication that may have come in contact with a patient who has a communicable disease. Once again the drug, needle, and syringe must be disposed of in a special puncture-resistant container that can be handled safely and then properly destroyed.

Materials management personnel must not only be concerned about the products they are obtaining, but they must also consider the type of packaging materials used by the manufacturers to ship their products. Many plastics and Styrofoam materials are not biodegradable and will have a detrimental effect on our environment for years to come.

Summary

It is important for the pharmacy technician to realize that the responsibilities of materials management are comprehensive and must be carried out in an organized and consistent manner to ensure patient safety and guarantee cost-effective pharmaceutical care.

TEST YOUR KNOWLEDGE

Multiple Choice Questions

1. An institutional pharmacy materials management program includes
   a. procurement
   b. drug storage
   c. inventory control
   d. drug distribution
   e. all of the above

2. In a hospital, overall responsibility for the materials management of pharmaceuticals lies with the
   a. chairman of the Pharmacy and Therapeutics Committee
   b. director of pharmacy services
   c. materials manager
   d. hospital administration
   e. chief pharmacy technician

3. Brand-name drugs are those drugs
   a. developed and marketed by the drug firm that did the original research and production
   b. that fall under a particular category of drugs
   c. developed by a drug firm after the original patent has expired
   d. b and c
   e. a, b, and c

4. A drug distribution system includes
   a. unit dose
   b. floor stock
   c. compounded prescriptions
   d. emergency drugs
   e. all of the above

5. Therapeutic equivalency indicates that the drugs
   a. are the same size, shape, and color
   b. have the same amount of active ingredient
   c. are equally effective in the same dose
   d. b and c
   e. a, b, and c

6. Environmental considerations in the storage of pharmaceuticals include
   a. proper temperature and ventilation
   b. proper humidity
   c. appropriate light
   d. proper sanitation
   e. all of the above

7. The pharmacy department is responsible for
   a. preparing purchase orders
   b. receiving and securing shipments of pharmaceuticals
   c. monitoring the inventory of controlled substances and tax-free alcohol
   d. coordinating the distribution of medical surgical supplies
   e. a, b, and c

8. Inventory control may include
   a. minimum and maximum reorder points maintained
   b. return of outdated stock
   c. restricted usage of pharmaceuticals
   d. drug usage report
   e. all of the above

9. It is estimated that the Food and Drug Administration's bar-coding rules will reduce the number of medication errors by more than _____%.
   a. 36
   b. 50
   c. 70
   d. 90

True/False Questions

10. _____ A legend drug is one that requires a prescription and must be dispensed by a licensed pharmacist.

11. _____ The calculation of the pharmacy turnover rate is a good indication of the effectiveness of a purchasing and inventory control program.

Matching I Questions

12. _____ cold temperature   a. −20° to −10°C (−4° to 14°F)

13. _____ freezer   b. 15° to 30°C (59° to 86°F)

14. _____ room temperature   c. not exceeding 8°C (46°F)

15. _____ refrigerator   d. 30° to 40°C (86° to 104°F)

16. _____ excessive heat   e. 2° to 8°C (36° to 46°F)

17. _____ warm   f. above 40°C (104°F)

Matching II Questions

18. _____ select the drug source

19. _____ prepare the drug order

20. _____ check the incoming
drug products

21. _____ maintain a proper drug
storage environment

22. _____ prepare formulary revision

a. pharmacist's
responsibility

b. technician's
responsibility

References

Abramowitz, P. W. (1984). Controlling financial variables—changing prescribing patterns. *American Journal of Health-System Pharmacy, 41,* 503–515.

ASHP guidelines on managing drug product shortages. (2001). *American Journal of Health-Systems Pharmacists, 58,* 1445–1450.

Joint Commission on Accreditation of Healthcare Organizations. Pharmacy services. (1996–1997). *Comprehensive accreditation manual for hospitals.* Oak Brook Terrace, IL: author.

Powers, J. R. (1987). Hospital pharmacy buying groups: The perspective of a contract sales manager. *Topics in Hospital Pharmacy Management, 7,* 12–13.

Rich, D. S. (1996). Expiration dating of pharmacy packaging. *Hospital Pharmacy, 31,* 1159–1160.

United States Pharmacopeial Convention (1995). General notices and requirements: Preservation, packaging, storage, and labeling. *The United States Pharmacopeia XXIII/The National Formulary XVIII,* 10–13.

25 The Pharmacy Formulary System

COMPETENCIES

Upon completion of this chapter, the reader should be able to

1. Outline the five core attributes of the formulary system.
2. List at least three strategies to gain the consensus of the medical community.
3. Explain why a formulary should be selective.
4. List three surveillance activities fostered by the formulary system.
5. Give an example of how the formulary system can define policy.
6. Illustrate why it is important to revise the formulary regularly.

Introduction

Throughout much of the history of pharmacy, the term *formulary* has referred basically to a listing of drugs. The spectrum of sophistication of a formulary can range from a simple list for use in a small institution to an elaborate compendium of detailed standards, which may, in fact, carry some official weight as a legally recognized standard. In some cases, an institution's formulary is actually a complete reference manual for the policies and procedures, guidelines for use, and criteria for evaluation of the medications approved for use at that particular institution. Formularies can be used for many purposes. Perhaps the most historically significant of the ancient formularies is the "Ebers Papyrus," a listing of complex prescriptions and cures from ancient Egypt. Formularies have documented the state-of-the-art therapeutic knowledge of the cultures that compiled them. Not all formularies are from the Old World. Some very complete ones, usually described as codices, are attributed to Central American native civilizations. In fact, some of the drugs, such as digitalis and cocaine, appeared in these formularies many years before they were "discovered" by Western or Oriental medicine. The most revered formulary in the United States is the *National Formulary.* Many pharmacists are familiar with the initials *"NF"* following drug names. The National Formulary has since been incorporated into the United States Pharmacopoeia (USP) as the official compendium of drug standards in the United States. Formularies, then, are a continuation of a worldwide, centuries-old pharmacy tradition.

In their modern form, formularies are usually associated with hospitals or other organized medical care settings, but increasingly larger organizations, such as pharmacy benefit managers (PBMs), managed care organizations (MCOs), and other payer-based entities have established their own formularies for their beneficiary or member populations. The utility and effectiveness of formularies, despite their ancient heritage and pervasiveness, are not without controversy. Some agencies and organizations seem to depend on them increasingly more. For example, the Veterans Affairs system has adopted a "national" formulary (not to be confused with the official compendium, *National Formulary*) and uses it to optimize therapy and as a tool to negotiate price savings due to its effect on standardization. Conversely, recent comments in various publications refer to the whole idea of formularies as archaic and ineffective. Formularies are tools, and like any tool, how one uses it determines the overall judgment of its value. As part of this tradition, certain attributes come to mind when using the term *formulary*. It is interesting that some ancient concepts embodied in formularies are now being used to expand the role of the pharmacy profession for its technician practitioners as well as for pharmacists.

The Formulary System

The formulary system is another concept associated with formularies. Essentially, the formulary system describes how formularies are derived and how the drug-use process can be guided, controlled, and accounted for when a particular formulary is in effect.

The core attributes of a formulary and formulary system include the following:

- The formulary system represents the consensus of the Pharmacy and Therapeutics Committee (P&T Committee) (Appendix B), which created it, regarding the most effective therapeutic agents to be used in the practice.
- Formularies represent a selective list of the drugs available from the pharmacy.
- Formularies should also contain additional information about the drugs and their use, such as dose regulations, tables comparing similar drugs within a related class, common drug interactions, suggestions for patient information, etc.
- The formulary system defines the policies and procedures established by the medical staff concerning drug use and defines the scope of the formulary.
- Formularies must be continuously revised.

Consensus is important for the formulary to be effective. Thus the members of the P&T Committee should be selected with this in mind. It would be frustrating if the committee failed to accurately reflect the feelings and expertise of the medical staff that it represents. In that case, the drugs listed in the formulary or the policies established by the committee would not accomplish what was intended, or their effectiveness might be significantly reduced over what might have been if the committee had been truly representative. The pharmacy department can play an important role in establishing consensus. Several strategies to gain consensus are provided next.

1. Additions to the formulary should be requested in a formal fashion through the use of a request form. This form can channel the thoughts of the requester by including some questions such as "Are there similar drugs on the formulary?" or "What are the advantages of this drug?"
2. Requests can be forwarded to the clinical chief of the department of the requester. Support of the chief eliminates a potential source of controversy.
3. The P&T Committee should prepare a "white paper" report on the advantages, disadvantages, therapeutic impact, and financial impact of the request. This task often falls to the drug information service. Subcommittees of the P&T Committee consisting of physicians and other professionals are often established, especially in large and complex institutions.

4. When the report of the committee indicates an unfavorable response to the request, it is advisable to share with the requester in writing the reasons why the drug will not be recommended for acceptance. Often the requester is asked to provide additional information in support of the request or is invited to attend the meeting at which the request will be presented.
5. The actions of the committee and the reasons for them should be published as soon as possible after the meeting. If actions were not to include a drug, it is particularly important to specify the reasons why.

It is important for formularies to be inclusive (i.e., they should be more than a list of drugs in a particular institution). Rather, the formulary should be selective and represent the best drugs available for the institution. The factors contributing to what the best drugs are for an institution can vary over a wide range; for example, cost, adverse events, factors affecting patient compliance, ease of administration, special storage or security requirements, and the inherent safety profile of the drug in a particular institution. There are many therapeutic reasons supporting a selective formulary—the elimination of unnecessary and potentially confusing duplications is one. A second reason deals with economics. It is now much more important for hospitals to watch carefully how the money is spent. The advent of high-tech drugs such as colony-stimulating factors, monoclonal antibodies, drugs produced by recombinant technology, and genetically engineered drugs can literally precipitate an economic crisis for the hospital if the potential economic impacts of these agents are treated in a cavalier fashion. The pharmacy budget as a percent of the total hospital budget has increased dramatically in the past few years. All indications are that this trend will continue indefinitely because of the many new, high-tech and innovative agents in the "pipeline." It is not unusual for the drug budget of a typical pharmacy to be 70% of the total pharmacy budget. You may read in other chapters about the challenges of the fiscal environment in hospitals today. The implications for the formulary are similar: there is less money to do more work at a higher cost. Selectivity, therefore, is becoming more important.

One method of viewing the economic impact of drug therapy is represented in the flow diagram shown in **Figure 25-1**. This figure represents a more global perception of pharmacoeconomic impact than merely considering the price of a drug or its impact on the pharmacy budget. Impact and possible decision alternatives are divided into three case scenarios.

Case 1 represents an uncomplicated situation when the proposed formulary change, in addition to being safe and effective, is cost neutral or represents a savings.

Case 2 becomes somewhat more complicated because the cost neutrality or potential savings of the choice involves another or several other departments. In this case, it is important to get a clear consensus from all parties to ensure that a cost burden in one area is actually offset by a savings in another. The economic analyses in these types of cases can be complex and usually involve financial experts and the clinical expertise of the P&T members.

Case 3 represents a truly global situation within the institution and requires sign-off at the highest administrative and clinical levels. These issues usually involve significant cost increases (often in the six- and seven-figure range), which clearly cannot be accommodated in either the pharmacy or the hospital budget. They require an approval at the strategic level of the organization. Although such cases were rare or nonexistent only a few years ago, they are rather common today.

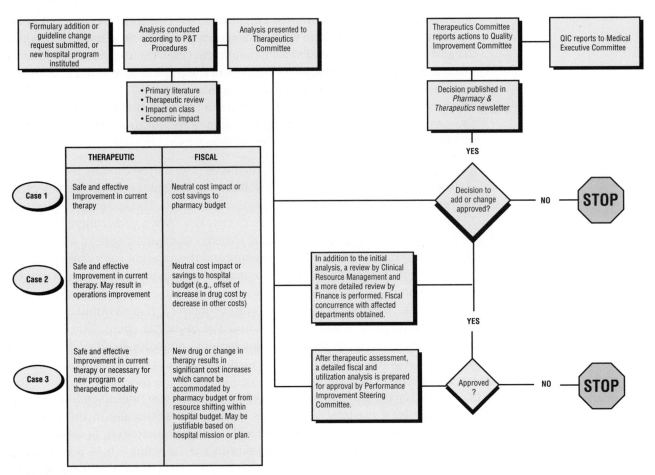

FIGURE 25-1 Flow diagram showing economic impact on drug therapy.

Complications can arise when trying to be selective and trying to reach a consensus at the same time. Little doubt remains that as pressure increases to become more selective, consensus will also become important and possibly more difficult to achieve.

The information a formulary contains, aside from the listing of the available drugs, can often be a decisive factor in determining its effectiveness and quality over another formulary. Pharmacy can be very effective when in consensus about how and which drugs are used. Reviewing formularies from similar institutions (e.g., university hospitals) would indicate a remarkable similarity in the drugs they contain. Although the additional information they convey is different, even in this aspect, uniformity seems to be more common. Additional information, for example, may list certain policies about drug use in a single place. Sample protocols for drug use can be listed. (Think of a protocol as a recipe for how to use a specific drug.) Often charts comparing the features or costs of an important drug class are included. Many large and small institutions have their formularies produced by outside vendors who prepare them from elaborate electronic databases. It is not surprising that many of these companies started in business producing cookbooks for various groups and organizations.

The formulary system defines the policies of drug use and can be effective in several aspects. For example, the system not only has the responsibility to select drugs and to foster rational drug therapy, but it can also function in an educational role as means of quality assurance. The educational role of the P&T Committee is carried out through the formulary system. Traditionally in the form of written communications, today's education involves more direct in-service programs sponsored or conducted by the P&T Committee.

Some surveillance activities fostered by the system have an educational and a quality assurance aspect. For example, monitoring nonformulary drug use can provide to the medical staff certain trends that would otherwise go unnoticed. Many monitoring activities, or drug utilization evaluations (DUEs), are discussed elsewhere that fall into this category. An exciting outgrowth of the formulary system linked to computer technology is the ability to track **adverse drug reactions (ADRs)**. Sophisticated database management programs often allow a more rapid identification of trends that might not otherwise be obvious and thus result in interventions to avoid such reactions. Recent literature has provided data that quantify the cost of ADRs—and the number is remarkable! For example, an overall average of the additional cost involved in ADRs is $2000 per incident, but the range may vary from $6700 per case for "bleeding" to $9000 for "induced fever" (Classen et al., 1997). These observations support the view that there is more to the relationship of formulary management, drug therapy, and cost than may be at first apparent.

The traditional application of the formulary system could be described as occurring in two dimensions: (1) mostly in writing and (2) often after the fact. However, the growing trend is to apply sophisticated computer techniques to how information is used. As a result, many of the formulary system's procedures and protocols can move away from the "scripture-like" status of written documents to a prospective and often interactive status. For example, in some computer applications, the program can alert the pharmacist to a drug's formulary status and to any restrictions that apply and document special criteria for use—all while the order is being entered. In a growing number of cases, physicians enter their own drug orders into the hospital information system. In these cases, certain checkpoints can be established that have to be answered before the order can proceed. You will no doubt hear more about the implications of such technology before too long, as more systems with these capabilities are installed. New ways to improve the medication use process are becoming the focus of medical safety efforts. Often referred to as computerized physician order entry (CPOE) or, more precisely, computer-assisted provider order entry (CAPOE), these systems are extremely complex, very expensive, and require major changes in the organizational culture affecting all aspects of the medication use process from drug selection through to administration and monitoring. While such technologies are promoted as the ultimate answer to medical safety, they are not an easy answer. The principles of the formulary system design discussed in this chapter will continue to play an important role in the success or failure of CAPOE system development and implementation.

We have included some examples of how the formulary system can define policy. Another aspect of the formulary system that should be discussed briefly is the relation of these concepts to the operation of the department of pharmacy. This relation involves some controversy and certainly much variation from hospital to hospital. In general, the P&T Committee must avoid trying to deal with operational pharmacy issues and stick to issues of broad therapeutic concern. In many institutions, the committee selects the drug entity to be included in the formulary, and the pharmacy determines the actual drug products to be procured.

Revision of the formulary is an important function because its effectiveness depends on how current it is. Keeping formularies current is a difficult task because they are created by the P&T Committee in hospitals, which meets several times a year or, in most cases, monthly. New drugs are also being introduced at a faster rate than in previous years. These factors combine to make formulary revision a constant activity.

Formularies are usually published once a year, even though they may be revised after each P&T Committee action. These changes that occur between official revisions can be communicated in several ways. Often the pharmacy department publishes them in a newsletter, or the P&T Committee releases a special publication when changes are made. The information contained in classic formularies is printed and published in book form. Formularies are revised continuously and the logistics of assuring that all previous copies are updated can be overwhelming. Typically, new editions of the formulary are published on a regular basis, and this too can get extremely expensive. More recently, a trend toward using modern electronic means to disseminate formularies and a vast array of drug information has revolutionized health care practice. Literally thousands of articles on the use of Web-based (Internet and Intranet) media and a bewildering variety of personal digital assistants (PDAs) or "pocket PCs" have been published and commercial information services are competing for attention in this dynamic market.

Summary

Formularies and the formulary system are ancient concepts that have been adapted to the dynamic environment of modern medical care. When sound therapeutic management principles are applied in a practical, scientific manner, they can also become very effective tools for clinical safety and quality of care.

TEST YOUR KNOWLEDGE

True/False Questions

1. The core attributes of the formulary system include
   a. _____ It represents the consensus of the P&T Committee.
   b. _____ It guarantees the best drugs at the lowest cost.
   c. _____ Formularies represent a selective list of drugs available in the pharmacy.
   d. _____ The formulary system defines the policies and procedures established by the medical staff concerning drug use and defines the scope of the formulary.
   e. _____ A properly established formulary needs little or no revision.

2. Three effective strategies to gain a consensus of the medical community include
   a. _____ The committee should hold a regular series of educational programs with free lunch.
   b. _____ The formulary process should be formal and encourage direct medical staff input.
   c. _____ When the evaluation process indicates an unfavorable response to a request, appropriate communications and additional participation should be solicited.
   d. _____ The actions of the committee and the reasons for them should be published as soon as possible.
   e. _____ Keep the important doctors happy at all times.

3. Appropriate surveillance activities of a formulary system might include which of the following:
   a. _____ a monitor of nonformulary drug use
   b. _____ a list of known "problem" salespeople who often interfere with the formulary
   c. _____ a system of drug utilization review (DUE) that is driven by criteria accepted by the medical staff
   d. _____ a report to administration of all physicians who prescribe expensive drugs
   e. _____ a system to tabulate and analyze adverse drug reactions (ADRs) and recommend steps to minimize them
   f. _____ incentive bonuses for physicians who use cheaper drugs

References

American Society of Health-System Pharmacists. (1996–1997). ASHP statement of the pharmacy and therapeutics committee. *Practice Standards of ASHP 1996–1997* (p. 4). Bethesda, MD: Author.

American Society of Health-System Pharmacists. (1996–1997). ASHP guidelines on formulary management. *Practice Standards of ASHP 1996–1997* (p. 60). Bethesda, MD: Author.

American Society of Health-System Pharmacists. (1996–1997). ASHP technical assistance bulletin on hospital drug distribution and control. *Practice Standards of ASHP 1996–1997* (p. 97). Bethesda, MD: Author.

American Society of Health-System Pharmacists. (1996–1997). ASHP technical assistance bulletin on drug formularies. *Practice Standards of ASHP 1996–1997* (p. 120). Bethesda, MD: Author.

American Society of Health-System Pharmacists. (1996–1997). ASHP technical assistance bulletin on the evaluation of drugs for formularies. *Practice Standards of ASHP 1996–1997* (p. 128). Bethesda, MD: Author.

American Society of Health-System Pharmacists. (1996–1997). ASHP technical assistance bulletin on assessing cost-containment strategies for pharmacies in organized health-care settings. *Practice Standards of ASHP 1996–1997* (p. 147). Bethesda, MD: Author.

Classen, D. C., Pestotnik, S. L., Evans, R. S., (1997, January). Adverse drug events in hospitalized patients: Excess length of stay, extra costs, and attributable mortality. *Journal of American Medical Association, 277*(4).

Joint Commission on the Accreditation of Health Care Organizations. *Accreditation manual for hospitals.* Oak Brook Terrace, IL: Author.

CHAPTER 26
Computer Applications in Drug-Use Control

COMPETENCIES

Upon completion of this chapter, the reader should be able to

1. List various pharmacy activities that automation and computerization have improved.
2. Describe how computer systems interact within the pharmacy and with other systems in the health care delivery process.
3. Describe how computerization within the health care system can better patient care.
4. Explain the concept of project management relating to the implementation of a computer system.
5. Describe the role of the pharmacist and the pharmacy technician in the management of a pharmacy information system.
6. Describe the general terms used in reference to information systems and automation.

Introduction

The management of medication administration plays a critical role in the patient care process. The data stored in the pharmacy information system is not only vital to the operation of the pharmacy, but it is also extremely important to other health care professionals in the management of the patient's care. Many extremely important decisions are made each day concerning drug therapy and the adjustment of drug therapy based upon the information that is retrieved from the pharmacy information system.

Pharmacy information systems have been used successfully in hospital and retail pharmacies for many years. In recent times, automation has become more and more prevalent in pharmacy practice. These automated systems not only improve productivity, but also help in reducing errors. Today it would be hard to find a pharmacy that does not have a pharmacy information system and some level of automation. As a matter of fact, without the use of a pharmacy information system, it would be nearly impossible to comply with all state, federal, and third-party insurance companies' demands.

As medical care becomes more and more complex, both clinically and administratively, pharmacy information systems have also become more and more complex. In the past, pharmacy information systems were nothing more than a system to retrieve prescription data in order to generate a label that was needed to fill either a prescription or drug order. Now pharmacy information systems screen for drug allergies and drug interactions, perform drug reviews, perform billing functions, automatically transmit information to insurance companies, allow the user to do sophisticated database searches or queries, interface with other information systems, such as laboratory computer systems, and link themselves to other devices in the pharmacy that are involved in automation.

It should also be noted that as more and more hospitals and pharmacies merge, the need for these information systems to communicate with each other (networking) becomes extremely important. Chain drugstores can now look up prescription data from any of the stores in their network or chain. The same holds true for hospitals. The sharing of information between hospitals not only helps with the efficiency of the member institutions, but it also helps disseminate vital information to members of the health care team.

In this chapter we will review the evolution of information systems within the hospital pharmacy and the role that pharmacists and technicians have played in their use. We will also review some of the basic terminology information technology specialists use when speaking of these integrated pharmacy information systems. Finally, we will attempt to look into our crystal balls and see what the future may hold for us.

Computer Terminology

Computer systems have a language all their own. Understanding of computer technologies hinges on understanding the language used. **Table 26-1** summarizes computer terminology.

Components of Computer Applications

There are four basic components of a pharmacy information system: (1) computer hardware, (2) application software, (3) system network, and (4) information server.

Computer Hardware

The computer hardware is the physical equipment that runs the application software. It is the part of the computer that can be physically handled. The function of these components is typically divided into three main categories: (1) input, (2) output, and (3) storage. Components in these categories connect to microprocessors, specifically, the computer's CPU.

Input hardware

Input hardware are external devices outside of the computer's CPU that provide information and instructions to the computer.

The keyboard and the mouse are examples of input hardware. The modem, which stands for modulator-demodulator, is also an example of input hardware. Modems transfer information from one computer to another. In order to do this, the modem takes the digital signals from the first computer, converts the digital signals

TABLE 26-1

Computer Terminology

abort	The abnormal termination of a program or process through user input or program failure
access speed	The average amount of time it takes for a storage device (floppy, hard or CD drive) to find a particular piece of data on a disk
ADT	Admission/discharge and transfer
agent	A type of software program that is instructed to perform a specific function.
algorithm	A detailed sequence of actions performed to accomplish a task of some kind.
alias	A name, usually short and easy to remember, that is translated into another name, usually long and difficult to remember.
alpha testing	Initial testing of software. Used to test software for problems (bugs) in the software.
application	Software that one uses to perform a specific task (e.g., word processors, spreadsheets, database programs).
backbone	A high-speed line or series of connections that forms a major pathway within a network.
backup	The action of copying important data to a second location to protect against data loss though equipment failure and unforeseen events.
beta	A version of an application or software made just prior to its accepted completion. Beta testing is carried out after alpha testing and involves ironing out any of the last few bugs or issues.
Boolean logic	A system used for searching and retrieving information using and combining terms such as AND, OR, and NOT.
booting	The act of starting up a computer and loading the system software into memory.
bus	An electronic pathway.
cache	A section of memory used to temporarily store files.
CD-ROM (compact disk, read-only memory)	A read-only optical storage technology that uses compact disks.
central processing unit (CPU)	The brain of the computer where most all information processing is carried out.
client	A computer that is able to access the resources of other computers on the network.
CPU	Central processing unit
crash	A sudden, unexpected system failure.
data	Any information stored in a electronic fashion.
DOS	Disk operating system
driver	A piece of software that tells the computer how to operate an external or added device, such as a printer or hard disk.
ethernet	A common method of networking computers in a LAN.
executable file	A file that is a program.

TABLE 26-1   Computer Terminology (continued)

file attributes	Markers assigned to files that describe properties of the file and limit access to the file. File attributes include archive, compress, hidden, read-only, and system.
file server	A computer that controls which other computers are allowed access to its storage media
file transfer	Transferring files electronically from one computer to another, whether the computer is in the same room or miles away
file transfer protocol (FTP)	Protocol used to move files between two computers linked via a network
firewall	A combination of hardware and software that acts as a gatekeeper. Firewalls restrict other computers from gaining access to data.
gigabyte	1,024 megabytes (MB) or 1,073,741,824 bytes
graphical user interface (GUI)	Allows users to click on buttons with a mouse, light pen, or touch screen instead of typing commands at the command line
hard drive	The main storage device in a computer.
hardware	Any physical device connected to a computer.
HIS	Hospital information system
kilobyte	1,024 bytes.
local area network (LAN)	A computer network limited to the immediate area, usually the same building or floor of a building.
megabyte	1,024 kilobytes or 1,048,576 bytes.
MIPS	Millions of instructions per second
motherboard	The main circuit board of a computer. The motherboard is the part of the computer where all other components are attached.
network	A group of computers set up to communicate with one another. A network can be as small as two computers linked together or millions of computers linked together.
operating system	The software on the computer that allows all other software to run. It is also the software that tells the computer how to run and execute commands.
peripheral	A piece of hardware that is located outside or external to the main computer. A printer or a monitor would be a peripheral.
post office protocol (POP)	The protocol used by e-mail clients to retrieve messages from a mail server.
print queue	A list of print jobs waiting to be sent to a printer.
print server	A software program that manages print jobs and print devices.
query	The process by which a user can ask for specific information from a database.
queue	A set of instructions waiting to be executed.
random access memory (RAM)	The physical memory installed in a computer.

TABLE 26-1

Computer Terminology (continued)

read-only memory (ROM)	Memory that can be read, but not erased
router	A network device that channels information from one computer to another across a network
T-1	A connection capable of carrying data at 1,544,000 bits per second.
token ring	A technology used to allow computers on a LAN to communicate.
uninterruptible power supply (UPS)	A device that has an internal power source (battery) that enables a computer to continue operations for a short period of time during a power outage.
upload	To send a file to another computer.
wide area network (WAN)	Any internet or network that covers an area larger than a single building or campus.
wildcard	A character (usually *) that can stand for one or more unknown characters during a search.
workstation	Any computer that is attached to a network.
WYSIWYG (what you see is what you get)	What you see on the screen will be pretty close to what you see in the finished product.

(modulation) to analog signals that can be transmitted over telephone lines, and sends these analog signals to the second computer. The modem on the second computer coverts the analog signals to digital signals (demodulation), which the second computer can understand.

Output hardware

Output hardware consists of external devices that transfer information from the computer's CPU to the computer user. A video display, the screen, printers, and speakers would be all examples of output devices.

Storage hardware

Storage hardware provides permanent or temporary storage of information and programs that can be retrieved and used by the computer. There are two main categories of these types of devices: (1) disk devices (e.g., hard drives, floppy disk drives, CD-ROM drives) and (2) memory. Memory on a computer usually refers to random access memory (RAM) chips.

The main difference between these two types of storage devices is that disk drives can store information and this information will only be erased if the user directs the computer to do so. All information stored on RAM chips will be lost when the computer is turned off or when it is rebooted.

The speed at which computers can access the information on disk drives and RAM memory differs greatly. It takes the computer much longer to access information on disk drives than it does to access information on RAM. So what typically happens when you run a particular program is that some of the information needed to run the program is copied to the RAM chips inside the computer. The computer now runs the program from the RAM and not the disk drives. This speeds up processing of information. When you are finished working on a particular program and intermittently at specified times determined by the application, information is transferred back to the disk drive for safety. Remember that if at any time power is lost to the RAM chips, all information on these chips will be lost.

Some devices serve more than one purpose. For example, floppy disks may also be used as input devices if they contain information to be used and processed by the computer user. In addition, they can be used as output devices if the user wants to store information for archival purposes.

Application Software

Application software is nothing more than the programs one uses. Application software is the software that is running on your computer system that you use. Application software could be the pharmacy software package that you use to enter physician orders and prescriptions into the computer. It could be the software used by the laboratory department or software used by the payroll department to pay the employees within the company or institution. Application software used in pharmacies is usually leased from companies that supply the same software to many different pharmacies or hospitals. Usually, the organization will pay an initial fee for the installation of the software in the pharmacy or on the hospital's network and then pay monthly maintenance fees to the software company which ensures that the software is kept current. These monthly maintenance fees also pay for any technical support that the end user might need.

System Network

The system network, simplistically, is a collection of wiring, hardware, and software that allows all computers that are linked to the network the ability to share information. Network management (i.e., client-server technology) controls the security of the network as well as the transfer of all data crossing over on the network. Client-server technology determines what information is passed back and forth from computer to computer. It also determines where information will be processed and on what machine the data will be stored. An example of this would be the calculation of a drug dosage. A pharmacist using a local computer in the pharmacy would obtain age, weight, height, sex and all other information needed to calculate the correct dosage from demographic information that most likely is stored on the hospital's main information server. Once all the necessary information or data is obtained, the process of calculating the dosage can be done on the local pharmacy computer. The results of this calculation can then either be stored on the server or on the pharmacy system depending on the way the network is set up. Normally, information is stored locally only when that information is specific for that one department.

The important thing to remember here is that, in most cases, specific data is never stored in more than one place. It would be foolish to store everything about every patient on every computer in the network. Modern networking applications allow the local computer to run local applications which obtain specific data only when needed. Storing data on multiple computers or storage devices could lead to individual users having different data sets. Storing the data on one computer or storage device ensures that everyone in the network has access to the exact same data.

Until recently, all computers on a network were physically linked together by high-capacity copper or fiber cable. More recently, wireless networks are beginning to appear. There are many advantages to wireless networks. Probably the biggest one is that buildings no longer would have to be "wired." One must remember that wiring a large building with high-speed networking cable can be very expensive and adding new computers to the network after the building is already wired is always an ongoing and expensive chore. With a wireless network, any new computer can very easily be added to the network. These wireless networks are, at the present time, in their infancy, but one can easily predict that within the near future copper or fiber networks will be a thing of the past.

Information Server

The information server is usually a larger capacity computer that aims to serve as an online repository of information resources. Demographic information such as name, address, phone number, age, and sex are all kinds of information that would be stored on the information server. Other computers on the network access this information according to the software running on the computer and the privileges that the operator of the computer has.

System Management

Computer systems throughout most hospitals are administered or controlled by the institution's information technology (IT) department. The IT department is broken down into many divisions, but typically most IT departments will have people assigned to

- *Integration*—The role of this department is to make sure that the applications you are running integrate with the other applications on the network.
- *Help desk*—This is a support group that helps the client use his applications. It is analogous to a technical support number that you might call with software or hardware questions at home.
- *Medical informatics*—This is a group of people that make sure state-of-the-art clinical information is present for your use. This could include anything from drug information applications to video conferencing between other hospitals.
- *Networking services*—This group of people maintains the institution's network.
- *Patient information services*—These are the people who ensure proper patient information (e.g., demographic information, previous admission information, drug history information) is available to all end users.
- *Technical services*—These are support personnel that maintain the information system.

Individual departments might have someone designated as the liaison between his or her department and the IT department. This person could be anyone in the department that has more than the usual computer skills. This person works with the IT department to make sure his system is running correctly and also makes sure training is available to all staff members who use applications on the system. The liaison would also be involved in the decision-making process if and when new hardware or software is deemed necessary.

Changing primary system applications or, for that matter, making major hardware revisions usually involves a team effort and is not an easy undertaking. Data on the old system must be able to be integrated into the new application and any new hardware must be able to perform its given tasks.

Because of the complexity of such changes, a team effort is usually needed to make these major changes in operation run smoothly. The team participates in the tasks necessary to implement the system project in accordance with a well-defined work plan. The implementation of the system follows a well-defined project management methodology. A systems administrator will handle the ongoing management of the system once it is put into production.

When large revisions in hardware or system applications are necessary, it is the end users responsibility for justifying and obtaining funding for the procurement and ongoing enhancements for his particular system. This individual also defends departmental initiatives for the system.

Generally, when these types of large projects are initiated, someone within the department is named the project manager. The project manager is the field boss during the implementation or upgrade of the computer system. In the pharmacy, a pharmacist or pharmacy technician best fills this job. That person should have an intimate knowledge of the operation to be automated and must understand the goals and objectives of the project. In addition, this individual should possess sufficient skills to manage the pharmacy staff, participating staff from other departments, vendors, and assigned technical personnel. The project manager develops the work plan and uses it to manage the project team through to its completion.

One job of the project manager is to manage the expectations of all who are involved in the project. The project manager must manage the expectations of the department, the members of the project team, and the other members of the hospital community who will be relying on the system when it goes into production. The work plan developed by the project manager must be realistic. Project milestones and other deliverables should take into consideration all steps necessary to complete the assigned tasks in a professional manner.

The project manager becomes the principal architect in designing how the system will be used in the pharmacy and how it will interact with other systems and departments throughout the hospital. The project manager also will coordinate how the work flow of the area(s) being automated will interact with the system.

A computer system can serve as a change agent to facilitate improvements of the processes being automated. If a system project automates a manual process without materially improving that process, the benefits of the system investment may be subject to question. Through the work-flow design process and the development of policies, procedures, and forms, the project team has a real opportunity to effect positive change.

A well-managed system project is supported by a team working under the direction of the project manager. The project team should consist of people containing the right mix of skills, experience, and knowledge to build the desired system. The team should consist of representatives of the areas being automated. They should be intimately familiar with the work flow in their areas of responsibility and all relevant policies and procedures of the area. Subject to the components of the system being implemented, the project team should include information systems staff with hardware, network, or programming expertise. Additional participants should be considered from areas with which the pharmacy interfaces on a regular basis (e.g., nursing, admitting, medical staff). These additional team members can assist in designing into the system those features and functions that will promote increased customer satisfaction through the use of the system.

To begin the discussion about pharmacy computer applications, we must first understand how this application fits within the framework of the hospital's other critical applications.

Hospital Information System Application Relationships

Patient Flow Cycle

The basic hospital information system (HIS) manages the processes of patient admission, charge capture, and billing. Although this is an oversimplification, it is in essence the set of features and functions performed within the HIS.

The admission process is, of course, a more complex process, which is often referred to as the admission/discharge and transfer system (ADT). The ADT is the system that first acknowledges a patient's existence in the hospital to every other system. The pharmacy system depends on the ADT system to know that a patient is a current patient of the hospital. It also distinguishes whether or not the patient is and outpatient or an inpatient. The ADT provides the pharmacy system with basic demographics on each patient (e.g., name, address, telephone numbers of the patient and next of kin, medical record number, bill/account number, date of birth, sex). The ADT keeps the pharmacy system informed as to each patient's location in the hospital. It also constantly updates the pharmacy system when patients are transferred or discharged. With this information, the pharmacy will know the room and bed location of each patient, where to send medication orders, where to send reports concerning patients, and if the patient has been discharged and is no longer entitled to filled orders.

In addition, the ADT provides other systems with critical information necessary to manage other processes within the hospital. Insurance information is collected here to facilitate the billing process. The ADT can also be used to help the hospital collect other valuable information such as whether the patient has a living will or durable power of attorney, who referred the patient to the hospital, and the name of the patient's physician.

The next component of the patient flow cycle is the charge capture system. A modern HIS system is referred to as the order entry system. Every time an order is entered on a patient, a charge is being captured for billing purposes, and a statistic is being captured for management monitoring purposes. Depending on the nature of an order, some charges are not computed until a test is resulted or the order is completed. In the case of physical therapy, an order for such a service typically is not finalized until after the physical therapist can assess the patient's condition and determine the amount of therapy required.

Medical records owns a piece of the patient flow cycle. At discharge, the medical records department codes the chart with procedure and diagnostic information. This information is required for regulatory and billing purposes. A link between this coded information, charge information, and admitting information forms the basis of the billing and accounting functions performed relative to the services rendered to each patient.

The patient accounting component forms the last piece of the patient flow cycle, which is the final piece into which all previously collected information flows, and allows the hospital to bill and collect for its services. Components of this system include charge capture, accounts receivable, collection system, and cash receipts system. This system, and its relationship to the other components of the patient flow cycle, forms the basis for compliance with regulatory reporting standards of state, federal, and other accrediting organizations.

Ancillary Systems

The pharmacy system is one of many ancillary departmental systems. Other departments have specialized systems that support their operations such as radiology, clinical pathology, surgical pathology, food and nutritional services, the operating room, and other procedure areas and specialty labs. These systems relate to the patient flow cycle systems in the same manner as the pharmacy system.

The relationships of systems in many hospitals allow ancillary systems to communicate with one another to support patient care needs. For example, if a lab result indicates the need for an adjustment of a patient's medication, then such a result can be triggered to automatically place a notification in the pharmacy system for a pharmacist to review. Because a dietitian may have a similar need to manage patients' nutritional intake, certain lab values can also be automatically sent to the food and nutritional services system.

Services provided by the ancillary department are captured within the ancillary system. Each order entered is processed to interact with the inventory that the department manages. Issuing an item results in a reduction of the inventory on hand. The item that has been ordered and issued to the patient, with the patient's identifying information, is communicated back to the hospital's billing system so that the hospital can bill correctly for the item. To the extent that test results would accompany this communication from the ancillary system (in the case of radiology or laboratory systems), the result would be placed in a portion of the hospital's information system where it can be retrieved by caregivers who have a need to access such information.

Many HIS environments support order entry via the HIS. These orders can be transmitted directly to each ancillary system via an automated interface. Order entry interfaces and their implications in the pharmacy will be addressed later in this chapter.

Business Systems

Several other systems support the day-to-day activities of a hospital. For the purposes of this chapter, they are classified as business systems.

The finance department requires a number of systems to support its operations: payroll systems, accounts payable systems, general ledger and budgeting systems, and cost-accounting systems. For the most part, the functions performed by these systems are self-evident by their names. It is also important to understand that the pharmacy interacts with each of these systems on paper or in an automated sense as it relates to the business processes of the pharmacy.

The hospital's payroll system is the vehicle that will pay the employees of the pharmacy as well as other employees within the institution. Hours have to be collected for input at the end of each pay period. Adjustments in vacation time, sick time, and staffing shift differential pay (for evening and night shift staff) need to be collected and submitted by the pharmacy's management in a timely manner so that payroll can pay all employees.

The accounts payable system processes the pharmacy's bills for payment, as it does for every other department of the hospital. This system requires that the pharmacy verify all purchases of supplies, products, or services on invoices prior to processing payment. Accounts payable systems are often linked to materials management systems to facilitate the link between purchasing and receiving and accounting for the payment of purchases.

The general ledger and budget systems allow the pharmacy to submit its budget for the coming year and track its actual expenditures against the approved budget.

Although only one system may reside in the pharmacy, it must interact with the vast majority of other computer systems in the hospital to conduct its day-to-day business.

The Hospital Pharmacy Application

Pharmacy information systems are designed to support the specific needs of pharmacy operations. These systems support activities that fall into several broad categories: inventory management, purchasing, distribution/production, and clinical support.

Inventory Management

A good place to start is the maintenance of the pharmacy's inventory. The level or quantity of an item in inventory triggers the need to order more product. What this means is that when the quantity on hand of a particular item reaches a certain predefined level or quantity (sometimes called the par level), some sort of notification must be sent out so that the materials management people or the purchasing component of the system knows that the item needs to be reordered.

When shipments are received, they must be checked against the purchasing documentation and then logged into inventory. Many pharmacy systems employ bar code scanners, which speed up the process of item identification and input into the system. When an order received is incomplete, the pharmacy system will track open order or back order situations. When the inventory level dips to a critical low, it will notify the purchasing component of the system and the key system user that follow-up is necessary.

As patient medication orders are filled, stock levels are automatically reduced in the inventory system. As stock items are taken to create new products (e.g., IV admixtures), the inventory system also reduces the inventory by the quantity of the item used.

The term *perpetual inventory* is best understood as the quantity count of items in stock, based on the computer's calculations of purchases, less medications dispensed plus the inventory item count at the last physical inventory. Its accuracy is dependent on several variables, including compatibility of the unit of issue with the unit of purchase, the accurate reporting of inventory shrinkage (e.g., items removed from stock due to expiration), and the accuracy of reporting of every item added to and removed from stock. It is up to the pharmacist or pharmacy technician to maintain the definitions in the inventory system in a manner so that the system can correctly perform the necessary calculations. Periodic physical counts of the inventory in stock must be performed and the results compared with the system inventory. This procedure will ensure the integrity of the information in the system and will alert the pharmacy as to any shrinkage of inventory that requires follow-up.

Purchasing/Receiving

When drugs, supplies, or other items in inventory require restocking, or new items must be purchased, the purchasing system is the vehicle that serves to facilitate the process. The purchasing system enables the management of orders placed, tracks open orders and back orders, and possesses the capability to electronically communicate new purchases to suppliers.

Whether the order for restocking is computed electronically (i.e., calculated by the system) or an item is entered for purchasing, most modern systems will be able to create a purchase requisition. Subject to the nature of the item(s) to be purchased, the system provides analysis tools to assist in analyzing supplier pricing. Once the supplier for each item is identified, requisitions are converted into purchase orders. Each purchase order contains those items to be acquired from one supplier and contains all agreed terms and conditions of the purchase.

When a purchase order is generated by the system and signed by an authorized signatory, it becomes a legally binding agreement when accepted by the supplier. Most suppliers will ship an order based only on receiving a purchase order number. Pharmacy computer systems are usually capable of generating purchase orders and transmitting them to suppliers electronically. In these instances, both the pharmacy (hospital) and the supplier are usually bound by certain terms and conditions as if a purchase order was duly signed by the purchaser and accepted by the supplier.

An electronically transmitted purchase order employs a technology referred to as electronic data interchange (EDI). EDI technology is commonly used for ordering merchandise, transferring funds (e.g., electronic payroll deposits), and billing.

Upon receipt of merchandise ordered, pharmacy personnel must count the items received and compare them with the items, quantities, and pricing ordered. Although the process can occur directly online on a computer terminal, it typically is more expeditious to check the order against the vendor's packing list, and then check the packing list against the order and the invoice. If there is any discrepancy in the shipment against the order, the system will facilitate correcting the error. It is important to understand that the system will not correct the error, but merely provide the pharmacist or technician sufficient information to follow up on the discrepancy. When ordered merchandise is acknowledged to the system as received, the inventory on hand is updated.

Clinical Support

The production side of pharmacy operation relates to the receipt of medication orders for patient care, the processing of the orders, and the tracking of patients' medication history. The features and functions of pharmacy information systems and the relationship they bear to a hospital's order entry system vary widely.

Most physicians generate medication orders in their own handwriting. The issues surrounding physicians entering orders directly into a system are complex and will be discussed briefly later in this chapter. In most hospitals today, physician orders are keyed into systems in the pharmacy. Fax machines, pneumatic tubes, and couriers or transporters are all being used to transmit orders from nursing units to the pharmacy. In some instances, physicians are entering orders directly into the HIS, which is interfaced to the pharmacy system or order entry.

Upon entry of the medication order, some systems will immediately identify existing medication orders, laboratory test results, or allergies that may be incompatible with the order just placed. Other systems have functionality which will suggest to the user that certain laboratory tests should be ordered with the medication order and other open orders should be discontinued based on the current literature. Still other features include suggesting more cost-effective medications than the one ordered. In such instances, the system is not designed to terminate the order, but merely to suggest to the pharmacist that the physician who wrote the order should be contacted to verify that the order is as intended.

The pharmacy system will generally receive relevant information on every patient from the HIS to facilitate the processing of appropriate doses. Date of birth, sex, height, weight, medical record number, and admitting (or billing) number are critical pieces of information. These data, coupled with the history of medications already ordered and dispensed to the patient, laboratory results, vital signs, diet orders and restrictions, and knowledge of procedures which have been ordered or scheduled, provide the system and the pharmacist with critical information to assist in managing the patient toward a speedy recovery.

When orders are entered, the system queues up the orders for a regular production cycle. Pharmacists and technicians prepare medication doses in accordance with schedules prepared by the system. The system also generates the appropriate labels for the medication to be administered. When robotics is being utilized, pharmacy information systems can electronically pass the order to the robot.

As the orders are packaged for shipping to the patient units, the inventory system is automatically adjusted to reflect a reduction in stock. In addition, each patient's medication administration record is updated to reflect the order and the medications dispensed. Medication lot numbers are also tracked so as to facilitate patient identification in the event of a manufacturer's recall.

Orders issued are communicated to such other systems as the hospital patient-accounting (or billing) system, cost-accounting system, utilization review system, or other systems which have authorized access.

For a pharmacist to fill a medication order for a patient, the pharmacist must determine that the order was written by a physician and that the medication, dosage, and frequency of its administration is in accordance with the physician's order. The two accepted mechanisms to accomplish this process are (1) the pharmacist visually inspects the physician's written order and then enters it into the system, or (2) the physician enters the order directly into the system and uses a secret password that only he or she would know. Medication orders that are transcribed by a unit secretary or other personnel may result in many errors and should not be considered reliable. Most of the HIS implementations to date have not been successful in inducing the medical staff to enter medication or other orders directly into the computer without transcription.

Over the years, a number of information system vendors have designed order entry systems which have attempted to induce physicians to enter orders directly into the system. Some of the newer systems have simplified the number of steps necessary to input an order. Some vendors have linked the order entry process with other patient information and current literature concerning the medication order. As of this writing, very few hospitals have successfully implemented systems in which medication orders are entered directly by the medical staff.

Most clinical pharmacy information that is available comes from third-party vendors that link their products with pharmacy software. The vendors' core business is the maintenance of current information concerning medications, general pharmacology, drug-drug and drug-food interactions, and other related health care information in the form of numerous computerized database products.

The Future of Pharmacy Information Systems

The future of pharmacy information systems appears to be heading in two distinct directions. The first is the integration of the data- and information-driven systems with robotics for drug dispensing. The second is the improvement of voice recognition technology to attract more physicians to enter their own orders directly into a system.

In a truly integrated environment, the management of patient medications is closely tied with laboratory results and diet. Abnormal laboratory test results can trigger alerts to clinical decision makers, which can result in a change to the patient's medications or diet. As physician order entry occurs, integrated systems can provide educational reminders or a series of cost-effective options for physicians and other clinical decision makers to consider. When orders are about to be entered that are inconsistent with the patient's treatment plan, the system can also alert the system user to the potential problem.

An order system that is linked to a robotics system can then complete the automation loop by processing and filling the orders without human involvement from the moment the order is entered. Pharmacy personnel must manage these robotic systems. Inventory levels within the robot must be periodically checked. The restocking of the robot's inventory levels also must be manually supervised.

True integration allows the hospital to operate as a whole. Information concerning all services provided to a patient can interact against a common data repository, which will form the true source for all patient information. These repositories will not only hold patient data, but also diagnostic images such as X-rays and lab slides.

Clinical data repositories will form the basis of online, computerized patient records. This record will contain information concerning the most recent patient encounter and all information concerning a patient's medical history throughout a patient's life.

Voice recognition is the vehicle that holds a lot of promise for bringing more physicians into the world of automated order entry. Consider the fact that the effort required to write an order is much easier than the effort involved in signing onto a system, flipping through order entry screens, identifying medications from the formulary, and validating the entry. Many physicians are reluctant to undertake this responsibility. Once perfected, voice recognition will provide a vehicle that will require little training and actually ease the effort for physicians.

Although the technologies described in this section do exist today, they are not widely used or are in early stages of development or release. By looking at what they are being designed to accomplish, they create a clear vision of what the near future will look like.

Summary

Early forms of automation dealt with speeding the processing of information so that productivity gains could be reached. As computers and technology have become more sophisticated, speeding the ability to access information has allowed decision makers to make more intelligent decisions. This is true for the pharmacy, as well.

This chapter was written with the goal of letting the reader understand that the role of the pharmacist and pharmacy technician is a critical one in the implementation and management of systems in a hospital pharmacy operation. A systems consultant can certainly play a role in managing a system, but ultimately leaves the project when it is completed. The pharmacists and pharmacy technicians are the individuals who will be responsible for the care and feeding of the system after the consultants leave. The pharmacists and pharmacy technicians are the people who are responsible for linking the features and functions of a system with the operational needs of the workplace. And lastly, it will be the pharmacists and the pharmacy technicians who will play a major role in the evolution of these systems.

Society has grown to be more dependent on automation over the years. Successful pharmacy professionals will be those who understand what automation can contribute, are able to harness its power, and are able to align its power with the tactical and strategic requirements of the business of pharmacy and hospital management.

TEST YOUR KNOWLEDGE

Multiple Choice Questions

1. The software that provides the desirable features and functions is the
   a. operating system software
   b. files
   c. application software
   d. data

2. Under a software lease, a user
   a. pays an installation fee
   b. pays a monthly maintenance fee
   c. receives technical support
   d. all of the above

3. A benefit of using a server for file storage is *not*
   a. to facilitate sharing common files
   b. to store computer programs
   c. to facilitate communications between different computer systems
   d. to provide improved access security

Matching Questions

4. _____ ADT
5. _____ BUS
6. _____ CPU
7. _____ DOS
8. _____ firewall
9. _____ HIS
10. _____ MIPS
11. _____ query
12. _____ RAM
13. _____ UPS

a. disk operating system

b. hospital information system

c. a combination of hardware and software that acts as a gatekeeper that restricts other computers from gaining access to data

d. millions of instructions per second

e. an electronic pathway

f. the process by which a user can ask for specific information from a database

g. admission/discharge and transfer

h. the physical memory installed in a computer

i. a device that has an internal power source (battery) that enables a computer to continue operations for a short period of time during a power outage

j. central processing unit

References

Austin, C. J., & Boxerman, S. B. (2003). *Information systems for healthcare management* (6th ed.). Ann Arbor MI: Health Administration Press.

Campbell-Kelly, M., & Aspray, W. (1997). *Computer: A history of the information machine.* New York: Basic Books.

Drazen, E. L., Ritter, J. L., Schneider, M. K., & Metzger, J. (1995). *Patient care information systems: Successful design and implementation (computers in health care).* New York: Springer Verlag.

Dudeck, J., Blobel, B., Lordieck, W., & Burkle, T. (Eds.). (2000). *Studies in health technology and informatics* (Vol 45). Amsterdam: IOS Press.

Englander, I. (2002). *The architecture of computer hardware and systems software: An information technology approach.* New York: John Wiley.

Haux, R. (Ed.). (2003). *Strategic information management in hospitals: An introduction to hospital information systems (health informatics).* New York: Springer Verlag.

Kreider, N. A., & Haselton, B. J. (1997). *The systems challenge: Getting the clinical information support you need to improve patient care.* San Francisco: Jossey-Bass.

Long, L., & Long, N. (2003). *Computers: Information technology in perspective* (11th ed.). Upper Saddle River, NJ: Prentice-Hall.

Reis, R. A. (1986). *Understanding electronic and computer technology.* Chico, CA: Technical Education Press.

Turban, E., Kelly Rainer, R., & Potter, R. E. (2002). *Introduction to information technology.* New York: John Wiley.

27 Preventing and Managing Medication Errors: The Technician's Role

COMPETENCIES

Upon completion of this chapter, the reader should be able to

1. Discuss the role of the pharmacy technician in preventing medication errors.
2. Determine the cause of system breakdowns that result in medication errors.
3. Define the types of medication errors that occur during the ordering and dispensing process.
4. State the 11 steps necessary for proper dispensing of medications.
5. List some commonly used drugs that result in medication error-related deaths.
6. Define confirmation bias.
7. List the steps that should be taken to minimize errors when taking verbal orders.

Introduction

With increasing attention to medical and medication errors by the lay media, concern has intensified in both the public and health care sectors. Health professionals acknowledge that medication errors are a growing concern because of the increased numbers of critically ill patients, the development of more potent and potentially dangerous drugs and methods of administration, and more emphasis on fiscal constraints that affect hospital staffing and workloads in all sectors. Protecting patients from inappropriate administration of medications has become an important focus for pharmacists and technicians, including those in community and institutional settings.

Technicians play a major role in modern pharmacy practice. Based on a summary of several studies in hospitals and long-term care facilities, Allan and Barker estimated that medication errors occur at a rate of about one per patient per day. While most of these errors probably have minimal clinical relevance and do not adversely affect patients, many experts believe that the medication error rate in less controlled environments—such as in the ambulatory setting where a patient purchases nonprescription medications or picks up prescription medicines from a community pharmacy—is probably higher.

In this chapter, we will focus on system enhancements and the checks and balances needed to provide the maximum degree of safety as pharmacists and technicians prepare, dispense, and control medications in both community and institutional pharmacy settings.

Background

When a medication error occurs, it is the result of deficits in one of two areas: knowledge or performance. Because no individual knows everything and because everyone has occasional lapses in performance, all people occasionally make errors. To minimize the errors associated with medications, society has devised a system whereby one practitioner—usually a physician, but increasingly nonphysician primary care providers—order medications via prescriptions and another professional, the pharmacist, is responsible for interpreting prescriptions, filling them accurately, and providing important information to patients. This system filters out errors and prevents them from reaching patients.

Health care professionals must apply the five "rights" of medication prescribing, dispensing, and administration for medications to be both safe and effective. The *right* medication in the *right* dose has to be administered by the *right* route at the *right* time to the *right* patient. When all five of these "rights" are assured, medication errors are impossible.

Ordering Medications

Physicians or their designees (i.e., pharmacists, nurses, nurse practitioners, physician assistants) initiate the drug-dispensing and administration process through the medication order or prescribing process. Because prescribers are people, errors occur because of a lack of knowledge or because of poor performance. Computerized order entry systems are being developed and implemented and will likely become commonplace in a few short years. These systems may help reduce certain types of errors, such as illegible handwriting errors (although they will introduce new types of errors as prescribers make other types of mistakes). But for now, most pharmacists dispense from handwritten medication orders. When illegible, ambiguous, or incomplete, handwritten prescriptions or medication orders can contribute to many errors made by nurses, pharmacists, pharmacy technicians, and other health care workers.

Illegible Handwriting

To minimize the chance of misinterpretation, physicians with poor handwriting should print prescriptions and medication orders in block letters. In the institutional setting, physicians can review orders with the nursing staff before leaving the patient care area. In addition, including the purpose of the medication as part of the prescription or medication order can help readers distinguish the drug names when legibility of handwriting is less than ideal. Many medications have similar names, but very few name pairs that are spelled similarly are used for similar purposes. Preprinted orders, dictation, and direct order entry into the computer by physicians are other solutions for poor handwriting and improper orders.

Because even skilled individuals can misread good handwriting, a system of order/prescription transcription should be in place in which several individuals interpret and transcribe an order. In many hospitals, each order is read by a unit secretary and reviewed by a nurse. At the same time, an exact copy of the order is sent to the pharmacy either directly or by facsimile. In the pharmacy, pharmacists and technicians have a number of opportunities to check the order, including a double check against labels, printouts, and the drug containers. A technician often screens the order and sometimes enters it into the computer. After data entry, a label is printed and a pharmacist interprets the original order/prescription and verifies the technician's computer entry by comparing it to the label. Later, the order and label again will be read by technicians and pharmacists as doses are prepared and dispensed. In the outpatient setting, this system should include a final check when providing counseling to the patient. In no case should pharmacy technicians interpret orders on their own since this process does not offer enough checks in the event an error is made. In addition, orders must not be filled only from computer-generated labels; rather, the original order should accompany the label to serve as another check.

Look-Alike Drug Names

Medications with names that are spelled similarly can easily be misread for one another. Technicians must be alert to this problem and should never guess about the prescriber's intent (see Appendix D).

Study the handwriting in **Figures 27-1** through **27-7**. Would you have had difficulty reading these medication orders correctly? These are actual examples of handwritten orders in both the inpatient and outpatient setting, and each led to medication errors. The problem was not uncertainty. On the contrary, each order was misread from the start; no consideration was ever given to the alternative drug, because in each case the pharmacy staff members thought they were reading the order correctly.

When pharmacists and technicians interpret prescriptions and medication orders, new drugs are a particular problem. Staff members are not as familiar with names of newly marketed drugs, and they tend to misinterpret them as older drugs. This is a good reason for health care facilities to establish policies that prohibit oral requests for medication without the pharmacy reviewing of a copy of the order. Facsimile machines on each nursing unit and in the pharmacy make the process of having a pharmacist review the order easier. In the community, physicians can write both the generic and trade names legibly on the prescription, and they can add the intended purpose of the medication to further alert pharmacy staff to the correct medication name.

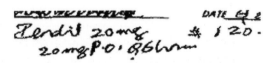

FIGURE 27-1 Prescription order for Isordil 20 mg misread as Plendil 20 mg.

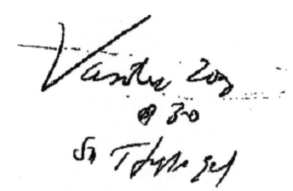

FIGURE 27-2 Order for Vantin 200 mg misread as Vasotec 20 mg.

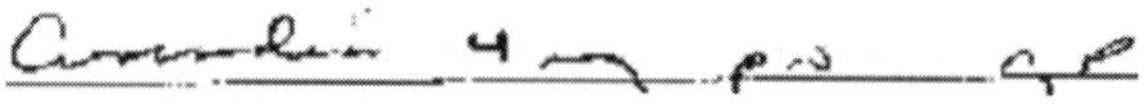

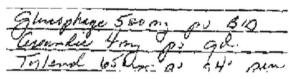

FIGURE 27-3 Order for Avandia 4 mg misread as Coumadin 4 mg.

FIGURE 27-4 Order for Avandia 4 mg misread as Coumadin 4 mg (second order).

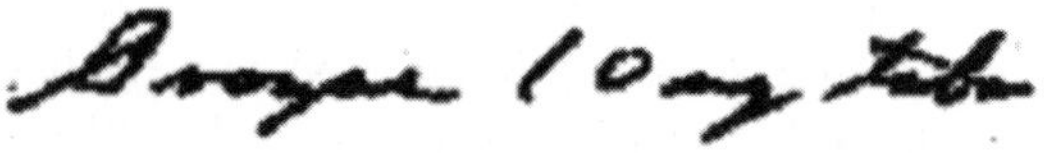

FIGURE 27-5 Order for BuSpar 10 mg misread as Prozac 10 mg.

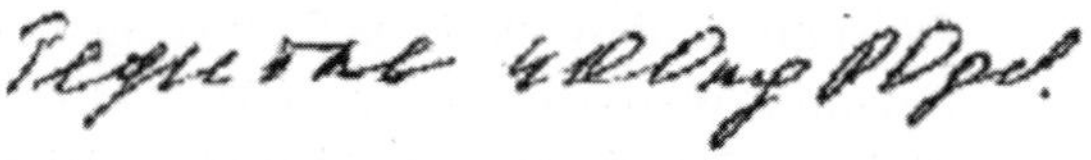

FIGURE 27-6 Order for Tequin 400 mg (misspelled with an "e") misread as Tegretol 400 mg.

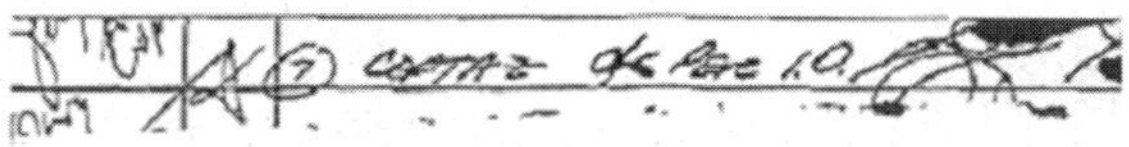

FIGURE 27-7 Ceftazidime "OK" per I.D. misread as ceftazidime "d/c" per I.D.

Sound-Alike Drug Names

Drug orders communicated orally often are misheard, misunderstood, misinterpreted, or transcribed incorrectly. Celebrex and Cerebyx sound alike, as do Celexa and Zyprexa, Sarafem and Serophene, Lopid and Slo-bid, and thousands of other name pairs. All of these have been confused at one time or another, resulting in patients receiving incorrect medications. In many cases, serious injuries have occurred because of misinterpreted verbal orders. Sound-alike drug names present many of the same problems as look-alikes. Obviously, when uncertainties exist, the pharmacist must contact the prescriber for clarification.

To decrease the opportunity for misunderstanding, health care facilities and community pharmacies should seriously discourage verbal orders. Greater use of facsimile machines among hospital areas, medical offices, pharmacies, and nursing units will help.

When verbal communication is unavoidable, strict adherence to these procedures for verbal orders can minimize errors.

- Verbal orders should be taken only by authorized personnel.
- If possible, a second person should listen while the prescription is being given.
- The order should be transcribed and read back, repeating exactly what has been understood, sometimes spelling the drug name for verification and the strength.
- The prescribed agent must make sense for the patient's clinical situation.

To prevent sound-alike and look-alike errors, physicians must be encouraged to include complete directions, strengths, route of administration, and indication (purpose) for use. All of these elements can serve as identifiers. It cannot be stressed enough that even if such information is lacking on orders, by knowing a drug's purpose as well as the patient's problems, skilled health care professionals can judge whether the drug ordered makes sense for the patient in the context in which the order is written. For example, knowing that the patient has a diagnosis of diabetes would be an important clue in determining that Avandia is intended by the orders in Figures 27-3 and 27-4. Diagnostic procedures along with orders also could provide important information. This is why it is important for pharmacists to verify all orders processed by technicians. Never guess on an order. When in doubt, check with the pharmacist, who can call the physician for clarification if the intent is not completely clear. A list of sound-alike drug names can be found in Appendix D.

Ambiguous Orders

Errors can result when ambiguous orders are interpreted in a manner other than what the prescriber intended. Proper expression of doses is vital in a drug order. Technicians should be able to recognize improper expressions of doses—and the potential for error—when they see them, and they should bring them to the pharmacist's attention. When the prescriber's clarification is needed, the pharmacist must contact the prescriber. Pharmacists and technicians should avoid using improper expressions of doses as they process orders, type labels, and communicate with others. Several improperly expressed orders are analyzed and corrected in the following examples.

- *Decreased doses*—A patient with diabetes had been receiving 80 mg of prednisone daily for several months. After an office visit, the physician decided to decrease the daily dose by 5 mg, from 80 mg to 75 mg, and wrote the order, "Decrease prednisone—75 mg." The order was misinterpreted as meaning 80 mg *minus* 75 mg and was transcribed as, "Prednisone 5 mg po daily." As a result, a 5-mg dose was given, and the unintentional, sudden, large decrease in dosage caused the patient to collapse. "Decrease prednisone by 5 mg daily" would have been clearer, but the safest way would have been "Decrease prednisone by 5 mg daily. New dose is 75 mg daily."

■ *Tablet strengths*—Orders specifying both strength and number of tablets are confusing when more than one tablet strength exists. For example, "Atenolol ½ tablet 50 mg qd" appears clear enough; however, when you realize this product is available in both 50 mg and 100 mg tablets, it becomes clear that this order is ambiguous. What is the intended dose, 50 mg or 25 mg? Orders are clearer if the dose is specified regardless of the strengths available: "Atenolol 50 mg qd." For doses that require several tablets or capsules, the pharmacy label should note the exact number of dosage units needed. For example, the label on a 80-mg dose of furosemide, which is available in 40-mg tablets, should read "2 × 40 mg tablets = 80 mg." For a 2.5 mg dose of prednisone, which is available in 5 mg tablets, the label should read "½ × 5 mg tablet = 2.5 mg." If your pharmacy prepares a computer-generated medication administration record (MAR) for the nurses, this same type of notation should be used.

■ *Liquid dosage forms*—Expressing the dose only in milliliters (or teaspoonfuls) for liquid dosage forms is confusing. For example, acetaminophen elixir is available in many strengths including 80 mg per 5 mL, 120 mg per 5 mL, and 160 mg per 5 mL. If the prescriber wrote "5 mL," the intended number of milligrams would be unclear, but "80 mg" is clear. The amount of drug by metric weight as well as the volume always should be included on the pharmacy label: "Acetaminophen elixir 80 mg/5 mL." Further, the patient dose should also be included; for a 320 mg dose the label should read, "320 mg = 20 mL." The same holds true for unit-dose labels and bulk labels.

■ *Injectable medications*—For injectable drugs, the same rule applies. List the metric weight or the metric weight and volume—never the volume alone—because solution concentrations are variable. An error occurred from this problem at a hospital where hepatitis B vaccines were being administered. A preprinted doctor's order form was used to prescribe the vaccine, listing only the volume to be given. When the clinic switched to another brand of vaccine, containing a different concentration of vaccine, the same preprinted forms continued to be used, underdosing hundreds of children until the error was discovered. This could have been avoided had the amount of vaccine been prescribed in micrograms, rather than just the volume in milliliters.

■ *Variable amounts*—A drug dose should never be ordered solely by number of tablets, capsules, ampules, or vials because the amounts contained in these dosage forms are variable. Drug doses should be ordered with proper unit expression; for example, 20 mEq of magnesium sulfate. A patient whose doctor orders "an amp" of magnesium sulfate might get 8 mEq, 40 mEq, or 60 mEq. Under certain circumstances, the higher doses could be lethal.

■ *Zeros and decimal points*—When listing drug doses on labels or in other communications, never follow a whole number with a decimal plus a zero. For example, "Coumadin 1.0 mg" is a very dangerous way to express this dose. If the decimal point were not seen, the dose would be misinterpreted as "10 mg" and a 10-fold overdose would result. The same could happen if "Dilaudid 1.0 mg" is written. The proper way to express these orders would be "Coumadin 1 mg" and "Dilaudid 1 mg," respectively. On the other hand, always place a zero *before* a decimal point when the dose is smaller than 1. For example, "Synthroid .1 mg" may be seen as "Synthroid 1 mg," especially when a poor impression of the decimal is written, such as on faxes or carbon or no-carbon-required copies. Avoid using decimal expressions at all where recognizable alternatives exist because whole numbers are easier to work with. In the above example, "Synthroid 0.1 mg" would be good, but "Synthroid 100 mcg" would be better. Use "Digoxin 125 mcg" rather than "Digoxin 0.125 mg." Use "500 mg" instead of "0.5 grams."

- *Spacing*—When typing labels, always place a space after the drug name, the dose, and the unit of measurement. It is difficult to read labels when everything runs together. Do not type "Tegretol300mg," because this can be misinterpreted as "Tegreol 1300 mg." Instead, type "Tegretol 300 mg."
- *Apothecary system*—Use the metric system exclusively. Although you have learned about the apothecary systems and its grains, drams, minims, and ounces, it is very inaccurate. For example, symbols for dram have been misread as "3" and minim misread as "55." Orders for phenobarbital 0.5 gr. (30 mg) have been mistaken for 0.5 grams (500 mg). The use of the apothecary system is no longer officially recognized by the *United States Pharmacopeia.*

Abbreviations to Avoid

Certain abbreviations are easily misinterpreted. Controlling dangerous abbreviations can reduce communication errors. Although many health care facilities have lists of abbreviations that are approved for use by the professional staff, it would be far safer if each hospital also developed a list of abbreviations that should *never* be used. In fact, such a negative list is easier to maintain and enforce. In addition, the Joint Commission on the Accreditation of Healthcare Organizations (JCAHO), a national accrediting agency for health care organizations, has recommended that accredited organizations standardize abbreviations, acronyms, and symbols used throughout an organization, including a list of abbreviations, acronyms, and symbols not to use.

Table 27-1 contains several easily misinterpreted abbreviations. These should never be used in medication orders, on pharmacy labels, in newsletters or other communications that originate in the pharmacy, or in pharmacy computer systems because they may find their way to medication orders, labels, and reports.

Consider some of the abbreviations shown in Table 27-1. The abbreviation "U" for units is an example of what can go wrong; it should be on every organization's list of unacceptable abbreviations. Errors have occurred when the letter "U" was mistaken for the numerals 0, 4, 6, and 7, and even "cc," resulting in disastrous drug overdoses with insulin, heparin, penicillin, and other medications whose doses are sometimes expressed in units. For example, orders written as, "6U Regular Insulin," have been misinterpreted as "60 Regular Insulin," with patients receiving 60 units rather than the intended 6 units.

D/C is another example of an abbreviation that should not be used. It has been written to mean either discontinue or discharge, sometimes resulting in premature stoppage of patient's medications. In Figure 27-7, the "d/c" order was incorrectly interpreted as discontinuation of an antibiotic that the patient had never even received. In reality, the "d/c" is really "OK," meaning that the drug was approved for use by the infectious disease physician.

Do not abbreviate drug names. For example, "MTX" means "methotrexate" to some health professionals, but others understand it as "mitoxantrone." "AZT" has been misunderstood as "azathioprine" (Imuran) when "zidovudine" (Retrovir) was intended. In one case, this misinterpretation led to patient with AIDS receiving azathioprine, an immunosuppressant, instead of the intended antiretroviral agent. The patient's immune system worsened, and he developed an overwhelming infection. In another example, an order for "HCTZ 50 mg" (hydrochlorothiazide) was mistaken for an order for "HCT 250 mg" (hydrocortisone).

TABLE 27-1   **Misinterpretation of Abbreviations and Associated Errors**

Abbreviation/ Dose Expression	Intended Meaning	Misinterpretation	Correction
℥	dram	Misunderstood or misread as "3."	Use the metric system.
m	minim	Misunderstood or misread as "mL."	Use the metric system.
AU	aurio uterque (each ear)	Mistaken for OU (oculo uterque—each eye).	Do not use this abbreviation.
D/C	discharge discontinue	Premature discontinuation of medications when D/C (intended to mean "discharge") has been misinterpreted as "discontinued" when followed by a list of drugs.	Spell out "discharge" and "discontinue."
μg	microgram	Mistaken for "mg" when handwritten.	Use "mcg."
o.d. or OD	once daily	Misinterpreted as "right eye" (OD—oculus dexter) and administration of oral medications in the eye.	Use "daily."
TIW or tiw	three times a week	Mistaken as "three times a day."	Do not use this abbreviation.
per os	orally	The "os" can be mistaken for "left eye."	Use "po," "by mouth," or "orally."
Drug names			
ARA-A	vidarabine	cytarabine (ARA-C)	Use the complete spelling for drug names.
AZT	zidovudine	azathioprine	
CPZ	Compazine (prochlorperazine)	chlorpromazine	
HCl	hydrochloride salt	potassium chloride (The "H" was misinterpreted as "K")	
HCT	hydrocortisone	hydrochlorothiazide	
HCTZ 50	hydrochlorothiazide 50 mg	hydrocortisone (seen as HCT250 mg)	
$MgSO_4$	magnesium sulfate	morphine sulfate	
MSO_4	morphine sulfate	magnesium sulfate	
MTX	methotrexate	mitoxantrone	
TAC	triamcinolone	tetracaine, adrenalin, cocaine	
$ZnSO_4$	zinc sulfate	morphine sulfate	
Stemmed names			
Nitro drip	nitroglycerin infusion	sodium nitroprusside infusion	Use the complete spelling for drug names.
Norflox	norfloxacin	Norflex (orphenadrine)	

TABLE 27-1   **Misinterpretation of Abbreviations and Associated Errors (continued)**

Abbreviation/ Dose Expression	Intended Meaning	Misinterpretation	Correction
q.d. or QD	every day	Mistaken as q.i.d., especially if the period after the "q" or the tail of the "q" is misunderstood as an "i."	Use "daily" or "every day."
qn	nightly or at bedtime	Misinterpreted as "qh" (every hour).	Use "nightly."
qhs	nightly at bedtime	Misread as every hour.	Use "nightly."
q6PM, etc.	every evening at 6 PM	Misread as every six hours.	Use 6 PM "nightly."
q.o.d. or QOD	every other day	Misinterpreted as "q.d." (daily) or "q.i.d." (four times daily) if the "o" is poorly written.	Use "every other day."
sub q	subcutaneous	The "q" has been mistaken for "every" (e.g., one heparin dose ordered "sub q 2 hours before surgery" misunderstood as every 2 hours before surgery).	Use "subcut." or write "subcutaneous."
SC	subcutaneous	Mistaken for SL (sublingual).	Use "subcut." or write "subcutaneous."
U or u	unit	Read as a zero or a four, causing a 10-fold overdose or greater (4U seen as "40" or 4u seen as "44").	"Unit" has no acceptable abbreviation. Use "unit."
IU	international unit	Misread as IV (intravenous).	Use "units."
cc	cubic centimeters	Misread as "U" (units).	Use "mL."
×3d	for three days	Mistaken for "three doses."	Use "for three days."
BT	bedtime	Mistaken as "BID" (twice daily).	Use "hs."
ss	sliding scale (insulin) or 1/2 $\overline{ss}$	Mistaken for "55."	Spell out "sliding scale." Use "one-half" or use "1/2 $\overline{ss}$"
> and <	greater than and less than	Mistakenly used or interpreted as the opposite symbol.	Spell out "greater than" or "less than."
/ (slash mark)	separates two doses or indicates "per"	Misunderstood as the number 1 ("25 unit/10 units" read as "110" units.	Do not use a slash mark to separate doses. Spell out "per" when that is intended.

Abbreviation/ Dose Expression	Intended Meaning	Misinterpretation	Correction
Name letters and dose numbers run together (e.g., Inderal 40 mg)	Inderal 40 mg	Misread as Inderal 140 mg.	Always use space between drug name, dose, and unit of measure.
Zero after decimal point (1.0)	1 mg	Misread as 10 mg if the decimal point is not seen.	Do not use terminal zeros for doses expressed in whole numbers.
No zero before decimal dose (.5 mg)	0.5 mg	Misread as 5 mg.	Always use zero before a decimal when the dose is less than 1.

Preparing and Dispensing Medications

An important safety enhancement for preventing dispensing errors is the development of a system of redundant checks from the time a prescription order is first written in the physician's office or on the nursing unit, to receipt in the pharmacy, through dispensing and administration. Such a system is suggested in this section. Obviously, the more "looks" an order receives (while efficient work flow is maintained), the better. Health professionals can review orders at several checkpoints and thereby maximize the chances of errors being discovered. Pharmacies with computerized drug distribution systems have an advantage because labels and reports can be printed so that at various steps order interpretation and order entry can be verified.

Steps in Prescription-Filling

Even pharmacies without computer systems should incorporate most of this suggested work flow since many of the options are available in a manual system.

1. The physician sees the patient; performs an assessment; determines appropriate medication, dose, and frequency; and writes the order. In the institutional setting, unusual orders or orders for new drugs not yet on the hospital formulary also are communicated verbally to nursing personnel.
2. In the institution, a unit secretary reads and transcribes the order onto the medication administration record (MAR). This step is unnecessary in hospitals where computers generate the MAR or where physicians can enter orders by computer, although the nurse and the pharmacist still must verify the order.
3. In the institution, a nurse checks the unit secretary's transcription for accuracy.
4. In both community and institutional settings, a direct copy of the order is carried or faxed to the pharmacy or the physician's computer entry reaches the pharmacy. The pharmacy technician reads the order and enters it in the phar-

macy computer system. If the technician finds a duplicate order, incorrect dose, an allergy, or the like, it is documented and called to the attention of the pharmacist during the clinical screening in step 5.

5. A pharmacist reviews the technician's computer entry, compares it with the original prescription (handwritten or electronic), and performs a clinical screening of the prescription with respect to the need for the drug, allergies or other contraindications, proper dose, and proper route of administration.

6. A label or a medication profile is printed. A copy of the original prescription or medication order continues to accompany the label or medication profile while the order is filled. No orders are filled solely on the basis of what appears on the label or medication profile because the computer entry may have been in error.

7. To choose an item for dispensing, a technician reviews both the label and the medication order for possible discrepancies.

8. A pharmacist checks the technician's work, reviewing the label against the medication order copy and the dose that has been prepared. The drug is dispensed. In the community setting, the pharmacist uses the patient counseling session to further assess that the correct medication is being dispensed and that the patient has a condition treatable with the product being provided.

9. In the community, ambulatory patients should ask the pharmacist any questions they have about the medication. For refills and medications patients have taken in the past, they should ask the pharmacist about any changes in appearance of the product. In the institution, the nurse receives the drug and compares the medication and pharmacy label against the copy of the physician's order as well as the handwritten transcription made earlier in the MAR.

10. Patients in the community should know the common adverse effects of medications they are taking, and they should understood what clinical signs to watch for and report to health professionals. In the institution, the nurse administers the dose, explaining the drug's purpose and potential adverse effects, and answers questions and concerns raised by the patient.

11. The final step in the process is the assurance of adherence to medication therapy. When ambulatory patients return to the pharmacy for refills, they should be asked if they are early or late in picking up the medications. If the patient is taking too much medication or is not taking the drug as frequently as prescribed, the pharmacist should counsel the patient to determine the reasons for and address the variation. In addition, patients should be asked about common adverse effects and about signs of serious drug toxicities. In the institution, pharmacy personnel check unit-dose bins and MARs to make sure that nursing staff is administering the medication on the proper schedule.

Selecting Medications

The importance of reading the product label while selecting medications and filling prescriptions cannot be overemphasized. Too often the wrong drug or wrong strength is dispensed, and such errors usually stem from failure to read the label.

During drug preparation and dispensing, the label should be read three times: when the product is selected, when the medication is prepared, and when either the partially used medication is disposed of (or restored to stock) or product preparation is complete.

Selecting the correct item from the shelf, drawer, or bin can be complicated by many factors. Similar labeling and packaging as well as look-alike names are a common trap that leads to medication errors. Restocking errors are quite common and can lead to repeated medication errors before being detected.

Automated dispensing machines have become more common on the nursing units of many hospitals. The nurse must punch in a security code and a password into the dispensing device, along with the name of the patient and the name of the medication, before the machine will allow access to remove the medication. This system allows more control of items kept on the nursing unit and serves as a check for the nurse who retrieves the medication, more so than for regularly stocked floor stock items. In some cases, online communication with the hospital computer information system or pharmacy system allows a pharmacist to review medication orders before nursing access to the medication is allowed.

Automated dispensing devices create several situations that can easily result in errors. The machines are restocked daily and the incorrect restocking of items (i.e., placing the wrong drug into the wrong bin) can occur. Devices that have multiple medications in each drawer and that do not require pharmacist review of orders before access have drawbacks that are identical to flaws in the old floor stock systems.

- the nurse can retrieve either the wrong item or additional items to use for other patients
- lack of pharmacist double-checking and screening of orders allows prescribing errors, wrong dosages, incorrect routes of administration, and other clinical errors to occur

When errors occur in selection of medication by either pharmacy or nursing staff, the term *confirmation bias* is used to describe the phenomenon. When choosing an item, people see what they are looking for, and once they think they have found it, they stop looking any further. Often the health professional chooses a medication container based on a mental picture of the item. Staff members may be looking for some characteristic of the drug label, the shape and size or color of the container, or the location of the item on a shelf, in a drawer, or in a storage bin instead of reading the name of the drug itself. Consequently, they may fail to realize that they have the wrong item in hand.

A number of approaches can be used to minimize the possibility of such errors in the pharmacy and in automated dispensing machines. Physically separating drugs with look-alike labels and packaging reduces the potential for error. Some pharmacy technicians also separate drugs with similar names and overlapping strengths, especially those labeled and packaged by the same manufacturer. For example, chlorpromazine 100 mg tablets and chlorpropamide 100 mg tablets, both from the same unit-dose packager, might pose a problem. So might hydroxyzine 50 mg and hydralazine 50 mg. Another strategy would be to change the appearance of look-alike product names on computer screens, pharmacy shelf labels and bins, and pharmacy product labels by highlighting, through boldface, color, or by the use of "tall man" letters, the parts of the names that are different (e.g., hydrOXYzine, hydrALAzine). In fact, the FDA Office of Generic Drugs requested manufacturers of 16 look-alike name pairs to voluntarily revise the appearance of their established names in order to minimize medication errors resulting from look-alike confusion. Manufacturers were encouraged to visually differentiate their established names with the use of "tall man" letters. Examples of established names involved include chlorpro**MAZINE** and chlorpro**PAMIDE**, vin**BLAS**tine and vin**CRIS**tine, and ni**CAR**dipine and **NIFE**dipine.

Pharmaceutical companies are aware of labeling and packaging problems, and many have responded to suggestions made by technicians and pharmacists. Health professionals can alert manufacturers about errors caused by commercial packaging and labeling problems by using the USP-ISMP (Institute for Safe Medication Practices) Medication Error Reporting Program (MERP). Reports are forwarded to the individual pharmaceutical company and the U.S. Food and

Drug Administration (FDA), and ISMP provides follow-up when appropriate. Call 1-800-23-ERROR, or complete a USP-ISMP MERP report (**Figure 27-8**). All reports are confidential.

In institutional settings and community pharmacies with several staff members, everyone should have input in deciding how and where drugs are available, how doses are prepared, who is responsible for preparing them, the appearance of the storage containers, and how they are labeled. Procedures to ensure safe medication use must be written, and the importance of adhering to the guidelines must be shared by all involved pharmacy, medical, and nursing staff members.

FIGURE 27-8 Form used to report medication errors or problems to the USP/ISMP Medication Error Reporting Program. (Reprinted with permission of the United States Pharmacopeia. All rights reserved. © 2002.)

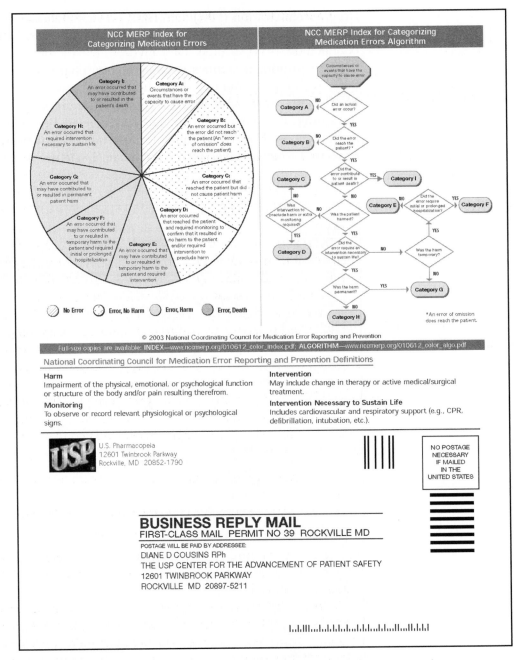

FIGURE 27-8 Form used to report medication errors or problems to the USP/ISMP Medication Error Reporting Program. (Reprinted with permission of the United States Pharmacopeia. All rights reserved. © 2002.) (*continued*).

Selecting Auxiliary Labels

To help prevent errors, pharmacists and technicians should apply auxiliary labels in certain circumstances, especially in the community setting. For example, amoxicillin oral suspension is available in dropper bottles for pediatric use. When the suspension is used for an ear infection, some parents have been known to place the suspension in the child's ear rather than give it properly, that is, orally. An auxiliary label, "For Oral Use Only," would help prevent this error. Other such labels are "For the Ear," "For the Eye," and "For External Use Only."

Similar labels are sometimes used in institutions, especially nursing homes and other types of long-term care facilities, where bulk containers of ear and eye drops may be dispensed for administration over several days.

Sterile Admixture Preparation

In preparing fluids for injectable administration, the potential for grave error is increased for several reasons. First, patients often are sicker when they need intravenous drugs, so the medications used have more dramatic effects on the body's function and physiology. Further, most injectable solutions are simply clear, colorless, water-based fluids, so they all look alike, regardless of what drug and how much of it is actually in the fluid.

Thus in the sterile admixture preparation setting, the chance of dosage miscalculation or measurement error must be minimized by systems designed with procedures that require independent double checks by two staff members. The independent double check in some pharmacies might be required for all calculations or measurements, while others require it only for calculations falling into special categories, such as dosage calculations for admixture compounding for any child under 12, critical-care drug infusions requiring a dose in micrograms per kilogram per minute, insulin infusions, chemotherapy, and patient-controlled analgesia. Calculators and computer programs may improve accuracy, but they do not eliminate the need for a second person to review the calculations and solution concentrations used.

Another important way to minimize calculation errors is to avoid the need for calculations. This can be accomplished by using the unit-dose system exclusively through the following:

- using commercially available unit-dose systems such as premixed critical care parenterals products
- standardizing doses and concentrations, especially of critical-care drugs such as heparin, dobutamine, dopamine, or morphine

Similar steps can be taken in community pharmacies that provide sterile admixtures to physician's offices, home care programs and patients, long-term care facilities, and other clients.

The use of standard dosage charts on the floors and standard formulations in the pharmacy minimizes the possibility of error and makes calculations much easier for everyone. For example, in critical care units, physicians need order only the amount of drug they want infused and list any titration parameters. No one has to perform any calculations because dosage charts can be readily available for choosing appropriate flow rates by patient weight and dose ordered.

Standard concentrations for frequently prepared formulations should be recorded and be readily accessible for reference in the admixture preparation area in the pharmacy. Of course, all calculations must be double-checked and documented by the pharmacist. Diluents as well as active drugs must be checked. The stock container of each additive with its accompanying syringe should be lined up in the order it appears on the container label to facilitate the checking procedure. The final edge of the plunger piston should be aligned with the calibration marks on the syringe barrel indicating the amount used.

In many hospitals, automated compounders are being used for admixing both large- and small-volume parenterals. Automated equipment has been known to fail occasionally. Also, some accidents have occurred in which solutions were placed on the wrong additive channel. In either case, the result could be a serious medication error. Therefore, it is important that the pharmacy have an ongoing quality assurance program for the use of automated compounding equipment. This program should include double checks and documentation of solution placement within the compounder, final weighing or refractometer testing of the solution to assure that proper concentrations have been compounded, and ongoing sampling of electrolyte concentrations. Pharmacists that prepare special parenteral solutions in batches (e.g., total parenteral nutrition base solutions, cardioplegic solutions) should have additional quality assurance procedures in place, including sterility testing and quarantine until confirmation.

Effective Medication Error Prevention and Monitoring Systems

All drug-dispensing procedures should be examined regularly, and the cause of system breakdowns must be discovered so that prevention measures can be designed. Pharmacy technicians need to communicate clearly to their pharmacist-supervisors what it takes to do the job correctly in terms of personnel, training programs, facilities design, equipment, drug procedures and supplies, computer systems, and quality assurance programs.

Multidisciplinary educational programs should be developed for health care personnel about medication error prevention. Because many errors happen when procedures are not followed, this is one area on which to focus through newsletters and in-service training. It also is important for pharmacy staff to focus not just on their own internal errors, but to look at other pharmacies' errors and methods of prevention and to learn from these. ISMP provides ongoing features to facilitate these reviews in publications such as *Pharmacy Today, U.S. Pharmacist, Hospital Pharmacy*, and *Pharmacy & Therapeutics*. ISMP also publishes its own biweekly *ISMP Medication Safety Alert!* for hospitals and a monthly newsletter for community/ambulatory care practices that reports on current medication safety issues and offers recommendations for changes.

Summary

In institutions, the pharmacy department is responsible for the drug-use process throughout the facility. Pharmacists and other members of the pharmacy department should lead a multidisciplinary effort in examining where errors arise in this process. Pharmacists and pharmacy technicians should work together in designing quality assurance programs to obtain information that helps establish priorities and make changes. For example, joint reviews of the accuracy of unit-dose cart fills are of great help in detecting reasons for missing or inaccurate doses and changing the drug-dispensing system accordingly. Programs can be established to monitor the accuracy of order entry into computers in the pharmacy. Quality assurance efforts that include a review of medication error reports help to develop a better understanding of the kinds of system or behavioral defects being experienced so that necessary corrections can be identified. The medication error problem will never be completely eliminated, but pharmacists and pharmacy technicians, working together, can use their expertise to address issues of safety and thus ensure the safest environment possible.

TEST YOUR KNOWLEDGE

Multiple Choice Questions

1. Medication errors are a growing concern in hospitals because of
   a. increased numbers of critically ill patients
   b. development of more potent medications
   c. increased media awareness
   d. all of the above

2. According to Allan and Barker, medication errors are estimated to occur at a rate of
   a. one per patient per day
   b. one per hospital per day
   c. one per health care personnel per day
   d. one per nursing unit per day

3. The five "rights" of medication prescribing, dispensing, and administration for medications include all but
   a. patient
   b. route
   c. dose
   d. prescriber

4. Which of the following changes in process could minimize the chance of mis-interpretation of handwritten orders?
   a. prescribers printing prescriptions and medication orders in block letters
   b. physicians can review orders with the nursing staff before leaving the patient care area
   c. including the purpose of the medication as part of the prescription
   d. all of the above

5. An order for a drug whose strength is a whole number should never be followed by a zero (e.g., 10.0 mg) because
   a. the patient could be underdosed 10-fold
   b. the patient could be overdosed 10-fold
   c. the patient could be underdosed 100-fold
   d. the patient could be overdosed 100-fold

6. Which order below is most clearly written and least ambiguous?
   a. "Synthroid 100mcg daily"
   b. "Synthroid 1 tablet daily"
   c. "Synthroid 0.1 mg daily"
   d. "Synthroid 100 mcg daily"

7. Which order below is most clearly written and least ambiguous?
   a. "Phenobarbital elixir 15 mg/5 mL: Give 15 mg = 5 mL at bedtime."
   b. "Phenobarbital elixir: Give 5 mL at bedtime."
   c. "Phenobarbital elixir 15 mg/5 mL: Give 5.0 mL at bedtime."
   d. "Phenobarbital elixir: Give one teaspoonful at bedtime."

8. When you see an order for "AZT" written, it could stand for
   a. Azidothymidine
   b. Azathioprine
   c. Aztreonam
   d. all of the above—better check with prescriber before filling

9. Computerized order entry enhances routine drug dispensing activities by
   a. serving as a double check of the patient's medication for physicians, nurses, and pharmacists
   b. eliminating the pharmacist from having to check technician's bin filling
   c. eliminating the technician from having to restock floor stock items
   d. none of the above

10. Confirmation bias occurs when
    a. a physician orders medication for the wrong patient
    b. an item is chosen once you confirm what you think you are looking for on the label
    c. a nurse confirms the identity of a patient before administering medication
    d. a pharmacist does a clinical screening of a patient's medication profile

11. Medication errors can be reported to the USP-ISMP MERP by:
    a. pharmacists
    b. pharmacy technicians
    c. the public
    d. all of the above

True/False Question

12. _____ When a pharmacy technician is very experienced, he can review and interpret the orders himself without a double check by the pharmacist.

References

Allan, E. L., & Barker, K. N. (1990). Fundamentals of medication error research. *American Journal of Hospital Pharmacy, 47,* 555–571.

Cohen, M. R. (Ed.) (1999). *Medication errors.* Washington, DC: American Pharmaceutical Association.

Davis, N. M., Cohen, M. R., & Teplitsky, B. S. (1992). Look-alike and sound-alike drug names: The problem and the solution. *Hospital Pharmacy, 27,* 95–110.

Flynn, E. A., Pearson, R. E., & Barker, K. N. (1997). Observational study of accuracy in compounding IV admixtures at five hospitals. *American Journal of Health-System Pharmacy, 54,* 904–912.

Lambert, B. (1997). Predicting look-alike and sound-alike medication errors. *American Journal of Health-System Pharmacy, 54,* 1161–1171.

Lesar, T. S., Briceland, L., & Stein, D. S. (1997). Factors related to errors in medication prescribing. *Journal of the American Medical Association, 277,* 312–317.

Reimbursement for Pharmacy Services

COMPETENCIES

Upon completion of this chapter, the reader should be able to

1. Describe the factors that affect product and service reimbursement for the drug product in hospitals, skilled nursing facilities, and community practice.
2. List factors that affect prescription coverage and reimbursement in community pharmacy practice.
3. Differentiate between the criteria in reimbursement issues in acute care and long-term care.
4. Explain existing and possible avenues for reimbursement for cognitive services.
5. Describe the role of the pharmacy technician in increasing reimbursement for a health care provider.

Introduction

Reimbursement and insurance coverage for pharmacy services is a subject that is discussed widely by patients and their families. This issue now receives widespread coverage in the media because of the discussions of the impending federal drug coverage legislation. Although it is a relatively small part of total health care expenditure, it is a highly visible one. While drug marketers present drugs as a small component of overall health care expenditure, we must remember that for a large segment of the population, it is the least reimbursed health care component and, therefore, the most costly portion of health care. The average Medicare beneficiary with hypertension and minor coronary disease may spend $8.00 on a monthly physician visit and $100.00 on medication each month. Therefore, opportunities for reimbursement must be carefully considered.

Ambulatory Care (Community Pharmacy) Reimbursement

In most instances, there is little variance regarding reimbursement for medication products between Medicaid, indemnity insurance companies, and managed care coverage. In general, the cost of medication is reimbursed plus a fee for dispensing, monitoring, and record-keeping. The parameters for cost reimbursement and the dispensing fee vary from carrier to carrier. Some agreements utilize **average wholesale price (AWP)**, others **maximum allowable cost (MAC)**, and others utilize **wholesaler acquisition cost**. The latter may take into account contracts negotiated between the provider and the pharmaceutical industry. Most carrier contracts utilize a **closed formulary**, where there is a list of medications that will be reimbursed. In some cases, if the prescriber demonstrates evidence for individual patient need, medications outside the formulary will be reimbursed. This process is generally done according to a prior approval protocol. Clinical pharmacists who work for third-party payers usually review cases of non-formulary prescribing and grant approval to the member pharmacy to release non-formulary prescriptions. The evidence to grant prior approval for non-formulary drugs usually must indicate

- patient intolerance of existing drug choices
- treatment failures
- diagnoses without any listed treatments on the formulary
- new drug modalities

There are large segments of the population without ambulatory pharmacy prescription coverage. The largest group is Medicare fee-for-service patients without supplemental coverage. Since most of these patients are elderly, they use more medications and, therefore, have the greatest out-of-pocket expense. Another group is employed individuals who have health insurance, but no prescription coverage. Employed patients without the health insurance benefit is a group that has no prescription coverage, but probably is not eligible for Medicaid because of income higher than Medicaid maximums. Another group is the unemployed, who have no coverage, which includes those who are Medicaid eligible, who are awaiting coverage, or who have not applied for coverage. These groups all have one thing in common: their out-of-pocket expense for drugs represents a higher percentage of their total health care outlay than one would anticipate by examination of the overall cost of health care.

It must be kept in mind that for these patients, maintenance at a higher level of health care costs them less out of pocket for medications. This is true because Medicare pays a rate that includes medications in acute care and long-term care. Patients without prescription coverage cared for in acute care, long-term care, or in an emergency department will also receive their medication without expense directly attributable to drug cost. These higher levels of care are obviously more costly to the health care system, but patients have the incentive to seek higher levels of care to avoid out-of-pocket expense. A challenge for pharmaceutical care providers is to demonstrate the value of ambulatory pharmacy services in keeping patients at a lower level of care and to convince carriers to reimburse for this service to reduce risk of admission to a higher level of care.

Reimbursement for Ambulatory Care Parenteral Therapy

Significant opportunities exist for revenue generation through ambulatory care parenteral therapy. Payers have long understood that it is less expensive to treat patients in the ambulatory setting than to admit them for such treatments as chemotherapy and hemodialysis. Therefore, significant reimbursement for these services is available even in the Medicare population. The Centers for Medicare and Medicaid Services (CMS) has created a list of health insurance continuation programs (HICPs) codes for drugs utilized in this setting. Reimbursable costs are also included in this listing, which provide for revenue generation between acquisition cost and reimbursable costs. This is in addition to the professional fee component and the facility fee. With this "fee-cost spread" facilities and freestanding practices are able to underwrite treatment of patients covered by other payers where the reimbursement is not so favorable. Formulary choices are detailed by manufacturers based upon "cost-reimbursement spread" rather than improvement in clinical outcomes. It is necessary for pharmacy to uncover and present outcomes evidence to ensure that the most safe and effective drug modality is utilized. Over time, patient outcome evidence must be presented because in addition to better patient care, evidence will demonstrate overall cost savings by maintaining patients at a lower level of care.

Reimbursement for Long-Term Care

Unlike ambulatory care, reimbursement for long-term care is often done at a constant rate. A percentage of the daily rate paid by the resident or the resident payer is based upon medication cost. The per diem rate is calculated by factoring in previous medication cost incurred by the facility Therefore, changes in medication utilization because of patient acuity (i.e., how "sick" a patient is), new diagnoses, or new treatments do not occur until far into the future. Patient acuity is related to the degree of severity of illness or combination of illnesses and is utilized to attempt to predict how intensive care will need to be. At this level of care, it is incumbent upon those who are involved in drug administration decision-making to evaluate choices. This includes formulary control and examination of epidemiological, microbacteriological, and outcomes evidence. It is necessary for caregivers to utilize an ordered process to evaluate modalities to choose low-cost, safe, and effective modalities. The safety issue cannot be overemphasized. This is why the regulatory agencies developed a list of unnecessary drugs which were determined to have excessive risk of adverse reactions. Although these medications are inexpensive, it is clear from the evidence that these medications had higher adverse event rates and poorer outcomes when compared to more expensive, newer drug modalities. The greater risk and poorer outcomes are more expensive to the facility in the long run and less contributory to good patient care as well.

Unfortunately, long-term care **per-diem reimbursement** (i.e., reimbursement on a preset daily rate) is adversely affected by the new treatments that have become available. Oral medication for long-term care patients was previously obtainable as a five-drug regimen for about $2.50 per day. Now many oral solids can cost from $3–$10. We can see even at a low patient acuity, medication costs can quickly rise way above 10 times what they were five years ago. Therefore, the case mix index, a description of patient acuity utilized to provide evidence for higher costs and, therefore, higher reimbursement, is not sufficient to recover these increased medication costs. Specific treatment areas where oral solid medication costs have skyrocketed include antimicrobials, antifungals, pain management, psychotropics, antidepressants, cardiovascular medications, antilipidemics, antidiabetics, and antihypertensives. Patients at all acuity levels receive these medications routinely. Because there has been such a great increase in oral solid medication costs, it is no longer just high level of care patients, such as rehabilitation or ventilator therapy or sub-acute care patients, who receive high-cost medications. It has become important for pharmaceutical care to address these reimbursement shortfalls. Medicaid does allow "carve-out" reimbursement for a small number of medications. Carve-outs are the ability to charge for medication above the pre-established daily rate. This includes colony-stimulating factors such as erythropoietin, immune system mediators like GM-CSF, and the newer major tranquilizers. However, this list is not comprehensive and some large classifications of high-use, high-cost modalities are omitted. Therefore, efficient pharmaceutical care will still conserve resources for new drug treatment modalities.

Reimbursement for Acute Care

Reimbursement for acute care pharmacy services has evolved over time and, for the most part, does not allow pharmacy services to generate profit. Often, pharmacy-related costs are calculated into the per diem hospital charge. Therefore, high medication usage is often not reimbursable and causes funds to have to be allocated from other cost centers. This presents challenges for acute care pharmacists in terms of management and distributive and clinical services. The value of pharmaceutical care in the acute care setting must be examined for its efficacy and its effect on direct and indirect costs. Examples of this are as follows.

- labor costs to procure, store, and distribute medications efficiently
- labor costs to assess medication use and monitor its effect
- assessment of value of treatments to determine efficient outcomes and to demonstrate that medication is cost effective even if it is expensive
- assessment of risk of adverse events that can be caused by an individual drug or drug combination leading to drug-associated morbidity—inexpensive medication can really be more expensive in the long run
- labor costs to monitor formulary adherence and conformity with clinical guidelines
- labor costs to research the practice of patient care at a facility and to examine and evaluate clinical evidence in the literature to determine if the treatments utilized have the best probability of successful and efficient outcomes
- labor costs to assess and recommend treatments for individual patients
- labor costs to plan pharmaceutical care post-discharge and convey self-care instructions to patients to ensure that they can benefit from a lower, less costly level of care for as long as possible

All of these services require labor costs that are not directly reimbursable, but need to be provided by a pharmacy service committed to involvement in the assessment and treatment of patients. The most efficient manner of provision of these services is to conserve labor costs from the procurement and distribution side. This process will allow existing pharmacists to monitor and assess the effect and modify treatments. Some of the methods for improving distributive efficiencies include

- assigning the pharmacy technician responsibilities in the dose preparation and distribution functions
- partnering with distributors to facilitate procurement and inventory maintenance
- utilizing of current technology to distribute medication to the point of care

- computerizing inventory and billing functions at the point of care
- utilizing computer physician order entry to eliminate error risk and allow interactive prescribing with "rules engines" to provide executable orders at the time of prescribing to prevent discussion with prescribers long after the orders are written. Rules engines are protocols placed in the automated order entry system that prompt prescribers to modify orders when prescribing errors are present before the orders are sent to the individual providing direct patient care.
- initiating interactive medication administration recording with automated medication administrative records, which provide patient identification, proper administration times, prevention of dose duplication, prevention of administration of discontinued orders, and rules for medication administration as indicated

Although these functions are not reimbursable at present, their efficiencies at the point of care eliminate duplicate paper entries, minimize risk, and lead to better outcomes which positively impact the bottom line of a health care system. Utilization of these patient-care systems also provides data that the facility can use to demonstrate the value of pharmaceutical care. This information can be presented to payers, such as managed care organizations. These organizations will recognize that utilization of a specific treatment may appear costly at first, but may lead to superior outcomes such as decreased length of stay, decreased need for monitoring of adverse effects, and maintenance at a lower level of care. Tangible results of this recognition include carve-outs (i.e., reimbursement for drug charges in addition to the pre-established daily rate), such as reimbursing a facility for the cost of an expensive medication outside of the typical per diem cost. This additional reimbursement conserves funds to pay for unreimbursed new technologies, enhanced pharmaceutical care, and capital investment in new drug-order and delivery systems outlined above. It is necessary for pharmacy departments to continue to outline the value of medication to contribute to a care plan that benefits the health care system, the patient, and the payer. This will foster a climate where new drug technologies will be reimbursable once they develop a track record both in clinical trials and experiential use.

Reimbursement for Cognitive Services

Reimbursement in this area covers a wide variety of services across all levels of care.

- prescriptive authority by the pharmacist
- administration of medications by the pharmacist
- patient assessment and treatment
- pharmacist intervention with prescribers and other health care providers
- patient education
- patient reassessment and monitoring of the progress of medication use

The benefits of all of these services have to be presented in a way that demonstrates value and indicate that provision of these services will maintain a patient at a lower level of care. Reimbursement levels to the pharmacist pale in comparison to the costs incurred at the higher level of care. Examples of this include shorter inpatient length of stay to free an acute care bed for another patient. Another example is a switch of a patient to oral medication so the patient can be transferred to a skilled nursing facility. Maintenance of a patient's anticoagulation status to diminish the risk of a gastrointestinal bleed readmission also falls into this category. The more outcomes data presented that express this value, the more payers will be inclined to encourage these services with reimbursement.

An obstacle for reimbursement for acute care pharmacy costs is in the retrospective-payer system. This means that costs are calculated from retrospective (i.e., total costs from previous years) data. This causes delays in inclusion of reimbursement for new treatment modalities. If these treatments are more expensive than old ones, reimbursement will not go up for at least two years. In addition, costs do not include unfunded mandates (i.e., rules that health care systems have to follow without being paid for the resources needed to adhere to them). It costs money to pay individuals to perform these tasks. Sometimes additional equipment, such as computer programs, has to be purchased as well. Examples of these requirements include rules promulgated by regulatory agencies such as the Joint Commission of Accreditation of Healthcare Organizations, peer review organizations, the Occupational Health and Safety Administration, and many others. Funds for new cognitive services must be derived at the expense of other cost centers or must be conserved from reduction of existing costs.

Evidence that priority has been placed on reimbursement for cognitive services can be seen at the national pharmacy organizational level. The National Community Pharmacists Association, through its National Institute for Pharmacist Care Outcomes, provides training for pharmacists that includes patient assessment, disease state management, and methodologies for capturing reimbursement for cognitive pharmacist outpatient services that culminate in the Pharmacist Care Diplomate certification.

The Role of Pharmacy Technicians in Increased Reimbursement

The role of pharmacy technicians in efforts to enhance reimbursement cannot be overestimated. The aging of the population and the increased complexity of drug regimens require increased utilization of support personnel. In addition, experienced, trained support staff can uncover circumstances that can increase patient risk. Examples of this include risk of medication error, duplicate therapy, overdosage, unnoticed drug allergy, and polypharmacy. Teamwork of the pharmacy technician with the pharmacist will lead to avoidance of many of these pitfalls.

Utilization of automation as well as increased technician utilization can free pharmacists from distributive services and allow greater participation in cognitive services. Excellence in technical support will allow organizations to provide cognitive clinical services and as their value is proven, resources will follow. Technicians fill medication orders, compound intravenous solutions, provide point-of-service distribution, bill for medications and cognitive services, triage telephone calls, and assist in procurement, inventory, and distribution. As with all job categories, performance varies from organization to organization and from individual to individual. Good technical support must be fostered and must be retained and compensated for in an organization. Compensation, vacation priority, regular performance review, and advancement must be incorporated. Performance review must include technical support to enhance pharmaceutical care development and reimbursement.

Summary

Reimbursement for pharmaceutical care requires a proactive approach that demonstrates the inherent value of these services to provide evidence for provision of resources. Development of efficiencies in the provision of this care is necessary to preserve scant resources available to seed reimbursement for pharmaceutical care. Utilization of pharmacy technicians is proven to both extend resources and release pharmacists to provide pharmaceutical care and provide evidence of its benefits. A stable, efficient, and reliable pharmacy technician staff is inherent in any successful, financially solvent pharmaceutical care program anywhere in the continuum of care.

TEST YOUR KNOWLEDGE

Multiple Choice Questions

1. Which of the following statements is true regarding ambulatory medication costs?
   a. They are a major component of a typical Medicare patient's cash outlay.
   b. Is not an important issue to senior citizens.
   c. Reimbursement is often duplicated by employee prescription benefits.
   d. None of the above.

2. Which of the following is true regarding pharmacy reimbursement in ambulatory care?
   a. Payers usually reimburse costs plus a dispensing fee.
   b. Pharmacists are routinely reimbursed for non-dispensing related interventions.

3. Reimbursement for acute care pharmacy costs has which of the following pitfalls?
   a. Costs are calculated from retrospective data, causing delays in inclusion of new treatment modalities that may be more costly than previous treatments.
   b. Costs do not include unfunded mandates such as rules promulgated by regulatory agencies.
   c. Funds for new cognitive services must be derived at the expense of other cost centers.
   d. All of the above.

4. Evidence required for prior approval for non-formulary drugs usually must include
   a. patient intolerance of existing choices
   b. treatment failures
   c. diagnoses without any representative treatments on the formulary
   d. all of the above

5. Which of the following improve efficient utilization of labor resources?
   a. dose preparation and distribution involving pharmacy technicians
   b. utilization of current technology to distribute medication
   c. computerization of inventory and billing at the point of care
   d. all of the above

6. Use of computerized recording of medication administration can assist with
   a. patient identification
   b. prevention of dose duplication
   c. prevention of administration of discontinued orders
   d. all of the above

7. Unfunded mandates are
   a. physician requirements
   b. regulatory requirements placed on health care systems without allowing an increase in reimbursement
   c. not applicable to acute care facilities
   d. are not an issue in the eastern U.S.

8. Regular performance review is useful in a pharmacy technician utilization program because
   a. it can demonstrate how well technician support allows pharmacists to provide cognitive services.
   b. it can link compensation to retention of excellent technicians
   c. it can establish and measure goals for increased technician task load
   d. all of the above

True/False Questions

9. _____ Long-term care providers are generally reimbursed for all medications administered at cost

10. _____ It is possible for a patient to have less out-of-pocket expense in acute care than in ambulatory care.

References

Cortese Annecchini, L. M., & Letendre, D. E. (1998). Funding of pharmacy residency programs—(1996) *American Journal of Health-System Pharmacy 55,* 1618–1619.

Miller, D. E., & Woller, T. W. (1998). Understanding reimbursement for pharmacy residents. *American Journal of Health-System Pharmacy, 55,* 1620.

The Expanding Role of the Pharmacist and Reimbursement ASHP Government Affairs Division ASHP Web site 2003.

Transforming Pharmacy Reimbursement: A Roadmap For Success. ASHP 2003 Summer Meeting, June 4th, 2003.

Accreditation of Technician Training Programs

COMPETENCIES

Upon completion of this chapter, the reader should be able to

1. State four objectives of the accreditation process for pharmacy technician training programs.
2. Articulate the primary reason for a differentiated workforce in the pharmacy profession.
3. Explain ASHP's involvement in accrediting pharmacy technician training programs rather than in evaluating competency achievement of individual pharmacy technicians.
4. List the eight areas that comprise the Accreditation Standard for Pharmacy Technician Training Programs.
5. Outline the objectives that form the basis for pharmacy technician training programs.
6. List the organizations that have endorsed the Model Curriculum for Pharmacy Technician Training.

Introduction

The objectives of the **accreditation** process for pharmacy technician **training programs** are to (1) upgrade and standardize the formal training that pharmacy technicians receive, (2) guide, assist, and recognize those health care facilities and academic institutions that wish to support the profession by operating such programs, (3) provide criteria for the prospective technician trainee in the selection of a program by identifying those institutions conducting accredited pharmacy technician training programs, and (4) provide prospective employees a basis for determining the level of competency of pharmacy technicians by identifying those technicians who have successfully completed accredited technician training programs.

The Need for a Differentiated Workforce

During the past decade, many of ASHP's initiatives have centered on pharmacy's movement toward becoming a full-fledged clinical profession. ASHP has long recognized that as we continue to move in this **clinical** direction, other health care professions and the public will increasingly look to pharmacy for answers to complex questions in drug therapy. With pharmacists' continuing efforts to enhance the degree to which they better utilize their knowledge and skills by providing direct patient care services, it becomes more evident that many, if not all, of the technical tasks routinely done by pharmacists must be delegated (with appropriate guidance and supervision) to nonprofessional personnel.

Development of a differentiated workforce will provide a core of well-trained pharmacy technicians who can assist the pharmacist in the delivery of pharmaceutical care by performing routine tasks that were formerly part of the traditional role of the pharmacist.

ASHP Initiatives

For over two decades, ASHP, in response to an obvious void, has promulgated documents that specifically address **outcome competencies** for pharmacy technicians. However, to date these have not been uniformly recognized and accepted throughout pharmacy. While these documents are gaining a greater degree of acceptance among pharmacists, it remains clear that the job category of technician continues to be interpreted differently because no two technicians are necessarily measured by the same yardstick.

ASHP has remained steadfast in its belief that an absolute prerequisite for the orderly development of pharmacy support personnel is uniform recognition and acceptance of a competency or performance standard. Moreover, it has agreed that such a standard provides the basic **objective** for supportive personnel training programs.

Early on, ASHP recognized that a competency standard alone could not suffice for development of pharmacy technician training programs. In fact, ASHP considered as part of its early deliberations about such programs whether competency-based training would be acceptable. Key to these deliberations was the realization that the structure and process of these training programs would be of secondary importance; competency outcomes would be the primary concern. Further, it was agreed that the feasibility of developing competency-based training programs, which depend largely on the ability to evaluate competency achievement, would not be difficult. Despite these considerations and due in large measure to the advice of its members, ASHP expressed uneasiness about promoting establishment of competency-based technician training programs. As a consequence, ASHP decided to follow the more traditional pattern of evaluating each training program through the process of accreditation. It is easy to understand how ASHP chose this avenue since it already had a well-established accreditation process for postgraduate pharmacy residency training programs in place since 1963.

Accreditation is defined as the process by which an agency or organization evaluates and recognizes a program of study or an institution as meeting certain predetermined qualifications or standards. It applies only to institutions and their programs of study or their services.

Obviously, to establish an accreditation program, ASHP knew firsthand that it was necessary to develop an accreditation standard that would delineate specific facilities and process requirements in addition to competency outcome criteria. Therefore, in November 1980 the ASHP Board of Directors requested that an accreditation standard for technician training programs be developed. They also authorized implementation of an accreditation process for such programs at the earliest possible time.

An accreditation standard for pharmacy technician training programs was approved by the ASHP board in April 1982. The first program was accredited in September 1983.

Accreditation Program

As noted in the ASHP regulations on accreditation of pharmacy technician training programs, the accreditation service is conducted by authority of the ASHP Board of Directors under the direction of the **Commission on Credentialing**. The commission reviews and evaluates applications and survey reports and, as delegated by the board, takes final action on all applications set forth in the regulations.

All pharmacy technician training programs applying for accreditation by ASHP are evaluated by **site survey** against the ASHP Accreditation Standard for Pharmacy Technician Training Programs. The standard outlines specific requirements for administrative responsibility for the training program, qualifications of the training site, qualification of the **pharmacy service** that is used to provide trainees with practical experience, qualifications of the pharmacy director and preceptors, qualifications and selection of the applicant, the overall structure of the pharmacy technician training program, experimentation and innovative approaches to training, and issuance of the certificate of completion.

With respect to the competency-based objectives that must be developed as a fundamental component of any ASHP-accredited technician training program, individuals are encouraged to use the Model Curriculum for Pharmacy Technician Training, Second Edition. This is the updated version of the manual that was developed as a nationwide project to provide technician educators with a prototype for training technicians in all practice settings and geographic locations. Specifically, it provides a guide for structuring the curriculum of a technician-training program, a checklist of quality components of existing training programs, suggestions for strengthening technicians' skills in specific areas, a list of job responsibilities and tasks that technicians can assume to allow pharmacists time to provide direct patient care, and a descriptive list of tasks to assist technicians when writing job descriptions. A user's guide is included with the curriculum to help pare down the training menu to suit individual training needs. The curriculum consists of four components including (1) goal statements, objectives, and instructional objectives, (2) a curriculum map with suggested sequencing of the modules for instruction, (3) descriptors for each of the instruction modules, and (4) a tracking document that identifies where each objective and instructional objective are taught. Introduction of the technician's role in enhancing safe medication use, tech-check-tech, and assisting in immunizations are included in the curriculum. The Model Curriculum was a collaborative project undertaken by the American Association of Pharmacy Technicians, American Pharmaceutical Association, American Society of Health-System Pharmacists, National Association of Chain Drug Stores, and Pharmacy Technician Educators Council. The project was under the leadership of the American Society of Health-System Pharmacists. A free copy can be obtained by going to www.ashp.org, under the technician section.

The ASHP accreditation standards accommodate training programs offered by hospital and health-system pharmacy departments, managed care facilities, community colleges, vocational/technical institutes, proprietary agencies, and military facilities. Currently, there are approximately 85 ASHP-accredited programs that are conducted in each of these types of training facilities. A directory of these programs is located at www.ashp.org, under the technician section.

Additional information about the ASHP program for accreditation of pharmacy technician training programs can be obtained at www.ashp.org, under the technician section, or by contacting the Accreditation Services Division, American Society of Health-System Pharmacists, 7272 Wisconsin Avenue, Bethesda, MD 20814, (301) 657-3000, ext. 1251.

TEST YOUR KNOWLEDGE

Multiple Choice Questions

1. ASHP has accredited pharmacy technician training programs in
   a. colleges of pharmacy
   b. vocational/technical schools
   c. military institutions
   d. hospital pharmacy departments
   e. all of the above
   f. none of the above

2. Continuing accreditation of a pharmacy technician training program is dependent upon
   a. a site visit
   b. adherence to accreditation standards
   c. increased number of graduates over previous years
   d. at least one graduating class every two years
   e. all of the above
   f. none of the above

3. A pharmacy technician may engage in the following activities:
   a. packaging and labeling medication doses
   b. maintaining patient records
   c. preparing intravenous admixtures
   d. inventory of drug supplies
   e. all of the above

4. A differentiated workforce is needed in pharmacy because
   a. pharmacists provide direct patient care services
   b. technicians answer complex questions in drug therapy
   c. pharmacists must perform many technical functions
   d. personnel best suited for the role perform specialized functions

References

American Society of Health-System Pharmacists (2001). *Model curriculum for pharmacy technician training* (2nd ed.). Bethesda, MD: Author.

ASHP accreditation standard for pharmacy technician training programs. *American Society of Health-System Pharmacists, Practice Standards of ASHP 1998–1999.* Bethesda, MD: American Society of Health-System Pharmacists.

American Society of Health-System Pharmacists (1980, September). ASHP position on long-range pharmacy manpower needs and residency training. *American Society of Hospital Pharmacists, 37,* 1220.

ASHP regulations on accreditation of pharmacy technician training programs. *American Society of Health-System Pharmacists, Practice Standards of ASHP 1998–1999.* Bethesda, MD: American Society of Health-System Pharmacists.

COMPETENCIES

Upon completion of this chapter, the reader should be able to

1. Identify the organizations for the Pharmacy Technician Certification Board (PTCB).
2. Provide an overview of the PTCB, including management and exam structure.
3. Define the process of certification.
4. Describe the eligibility requirements to sit for the PTCB examination.
5. List the major stakeholders of the PTCB.
6. Describe ways to become more involved with PTCB.

Introduction

The Pharmacy Technician Certification Board (PTCB) develops, maintains, promotes, and administers a certification and recertification program for pharmacy technicians. The PTCB provides programs and services that offer technicians an opportunity to demonstrate that they have mastered knowledge and skills across practice settings. Through the PTCB program, pharmacy technicians are able to work more effectively with pharmacists to offer safe and effective patient care and service. Pharmacy technicians must sit for and pass the National Pharmacy Technician Certification Examination (PTCE) to use the designation Certified Pharmacy Technician (CPhT). To continue to hold certification, a CPhT must successfully complete the recertification process, including obtaining 20 hours of continuing education within two years of original certification or previous recertification. PTCB offers a reinstatement program that allows technicians whose certification has lapsed to once again become actively certified.

Since its first exam in 1995, the PTCB has certified over 95,000 pharmacy technicians through the examination and transfer process.

Background

The PTCB, a 501(c)6 organization, was established in January 1995 by the American Pharmaceutical Association (APhA), the American Society of Health-System Pharmacists (ASHP), the Illinois Council of Health-System Pharmacists (ICHP), and the Michigan Pharmacists Association (MPA). Together the four organizations created one consolidated national certification program for pharmacy technicians. In 2002, the National Association of Boards of Pharmacy (NABP) joined the PTCB. The PTCB is responsible for the development and implementation of policies related to the national certification of pharmacy technicians.

The goal of the PTCB's certification program is to enable pharmacy technicians to work more effectively with pharmacists to offer greater patient care and service. Certification is the process by which a nongovernmental association or agency grants recognition to an individual who has met certain predetermined qualifications specified by that association or agency.

Structure

A Board of Governors, consisting of the chief executive officer from each of the five organizations (APhA, ASHP, ICHP, MPA, and NABP) and the PTCB Chief Executive Officer and Executive Director, provides strategic direction to the PTCB, focusing on policy and fiscal matters. The Board of Governors appoints a broadly constituted Certification Council which is comprised of pharmacists, certified pharmacy technicians, subject matter experts, and educators drawn from various practice settings, geographical areas, and diverse backgrounds to administer the certification program by establishing the rules and regulations that govern the program. Certification Council members serve a three-year term.

The Certification Council sets requirements for candidacy, recertification, examination content and administration, and issuing certificates. The Certification Council develops recommendations for eligibility, builds each examination form, sets the minimum passing point for the examination, and makes decisions on candidate challenges regarding the content of the examination. It also maintains a registry of those certified and manages the appeals process.

Current Examination Practices

The methods used to develop and administer the Pharmacy Technician Certification Examination are designed to promote the validity, measurement precision, and integrity of the examination program. These methods follow testing procedures relevant to certification examinations recommended in the Standards for Educational and Psychological Tests and guidelines published by the National Organization for Competency Assurance (NOCA), and the Council on Licensure, Enforcement, and Regulation (CLEAR).

The national Pharmacy Technician Certification Examination samples pharmacy technicians' knowledge and skill base for activities performed in the work of pharmacy technicians. To ensure that the examination is psychometrically sound and legally defensible, the content framework of the entire examination is supported by a nationwide study of the work pharmacy technicians perform in diverse settings, including community and institutional.

The PTCB administers its national certification examination three times annually, in March, July, and November, at 120 locations per test administration. The PTCB selects test sites with input from the PTCB's state marketing partners, national pharmacy associations, and other stakeholders. The examination currently is in paper-and-pencil format. To be eligible to take the PTCE, the candidate must have a high school diploma or GED and have never been convicted of a felony. A felony conviction is not an absolute bar to apply for certification. Each case will be evaluated individually. If this applies to you, please enclose a signed letter of explanation and a copy of all pertinent court documents or arrest reports related to the conviction by the application receipt deadline. (Those convicted of drug or pharmacy-related felonies are not eligible to sit for the PTCE). The application fee for the PTCE is $120.

Technology

PTCB established a Web site, www.ptcb.org, to provide information to potential candidates and serve as an important resource on pharmacy technician issues. The Web site is recording over 1 million hits per month! Candidates use the online process to register for the examination and to complete the recertification process. The Web site also serves as an interactive web forum and information bank for CPhTs, pharmacy technicians, pharmacists, and employers.

Get Involved with PTCB

Item Writers

Each fall, the Pharmacy Technician Certification Board recruits volunteers to participate as item writers for the national Pharmacy Technician Certification Examination. The examination items are prepared by these volunteers, who are pharmacists, certified pharmacy technicians, or pharmacy technician educators who serve as subject matter experts. Over 100 subject matter experts prepare items for the Pharmacy Technician Certification Examination. The volunteers for this group have practice experience and have demonstrated the ability to logically define and categorize the array of tasks technicians perform in various practice environments and have the familiarity with pharmacy association work.

A select number of item writers are invited to participate in an item writing workshop normally held every summer in Washington, D.C. to review, refine, and edit items for the examination.

Stakeholder Policy Council

In 2002, the PTCB created the PTCB Stakeholder Policy Council (the Council). The Council is comprised of 12 involved, knowledgeable, experienced, and committed stakeholders. They bring expanded perspectives, experience, and special skills to PTCB. The Council provides input on current issues and trends including marketplace expectations and changes, communications, target marketing, and the future of the PTCB program. The purpose of the Council is to develop policy and make recommendations to the Board of Governors regarding the PTCB's direction.

Information gathered from the Council is analyzed along with the PTCB's extensive information about stakeholders gathered from candidate and employer survey data, the PTCB meetings and presentations, and the PTCB Web site (www.ptcb.org). This information will be developed into a needs analysis that will determine critical needs of stakeholder groups, which include employers, certified and noncertified technicians, regulators, trainers and educators, state affiliates, national pharmacy organizations, etc.

Communication Vehicles

The PTCB uses several vehicles to communicate with candidates. In addition to issuing application instructions that are carefully designed to provide information about the program and to facilitate the application process, PTCB collaborates with state pharmacy organizations to market the national certification program for pharmacy technicians. In 1995, PTCB extended an offer to the pharmacy association and society of hospital pharmacists in each state to participate in the certification program. PTCB state marketing partners build awareness and encourage participation in the program. All fifty states are represented as PTCB state marketing partners. Specific roles for PTCB state marketing partners are in marketing the examination to technicians and in nominating pharmacists and technicians for PTCB committee assignments.

The PTCB recognizes the value in communicating with stakeholders. These stakeholders include pharmacists, pharmacy technicians, technician educators, major employers of pharmacy technicians, state marketing partners, and other national pharmacy organizations. PTCB has initiated several outreach efforts including a fax network with state marketing partners, presentations and an exhibit at national and state pharmacy meetings, public relations including media briefings and news releases, and information on the Internet. The PTCB also established communication vehicles with the American Association of Pharmacy Technicians and the Pharmacy Technician Educators Council. The PTCB also established a data collection process to document the value of PTCB certification for pharmacy technicians and gather demographic information to create a national certified pharmacy technician databank. The PTCB surveys for examination candidates, transfer candidates, and those recertifying CPhTs were developed to collect demographic data and demonstrate the positive impact of the use of certified pharmacy technicians.

Regulation of Pharmacy Technicians

State rules and regulations as well as job-center policies and procedures may specifically define functions and responsibilities of pharmacy technicians. The pharmacy technician is accountable to the supervising pharmacist, who is legally responsible by virtue of state licensure for the care and safety of patients served by the pharmacy.

Over the past five years, a majority of states have revised their pharmacy practice acts in areas related to pharmacy technicians. Some states have made PTCB certification a requirement for registration. Other states have revised pharmacist-technician ratios, responsibilities, supervision, or other requirements on the basis of a technician's certification status. Finally, with the addition of NABP to the PTCB Board of Governors, NABP is working with state boards to encourage the acceptance of the PTCB certification program as the recognized assessment tool for pharmacy technicians. The use of the PTCB certification program has been incorporated into NABP's Model State Pharmacy Practice Act and Model Rules.

Future for Pharmacy Technicians

Since its inception in 1995, PTCB has committed its resources to the recognition of certified pharmacy technicians in all sectors of practice who have demonstrated their mastery to work more effectively with pharmacists to offer safe and effective patient care and service. This mission will serve to benefit all aspects of the pharmacy profession as the health care industry continues to evolve through the next century.

Summary

The PTCB program offers technicians opportunities for recognition and greater job flexibility and satisfaction. Certification for pharmacy technicians encourages technicians to look beyond their present job and may also increase their likelihood of getting a better job. Certification may enhance the opportunities for promotion or merit increases. Through national surveys, PTCB has learned that the reasons for undertaking the certification process is the personal satisfaction that is derived from the effort, the pride of mastering a unique body of knowledge, and the skills and joy of applying them to something meaningful and worthwhile.

The PTCB has been able to change the lives of thousands of pharmacy technicians across the United States. The successful launch of the certification program has not gone unnoticed in the credentialing and association management fields. In fact, PTCB has been selected for several awards since its inception. PTCB also has established strong external relationships with the National Organization of Competency Assurance and the Washington, D.C. Certification Networking Group. With over 100,000 certified pharmacy technicians since 1995, PTCB has proven that pharmacy technicians are an integral part of the pharmacy team.

TEST YOUR KNOWLEDGE

Multiple Choice Questions

1. The organizations for the Pharmacy Technician Certification Board are
   a. The American Pharmaceutical Association
   b. The American Society of Health-System Pharmacists
   c. The Illinois Council of Health-System Pharmacists
   d. The Michigan Pharmacists Association
   e. all of the above

2. In recent years, pharmacists have increased their use of pharmacy technicians due in part to which of the following?
   a. trends in pharmacy practice
   b. new pharmacy schools
   c. third-party reimbursement
   d. both a and b
   e. both a and c

3. What are some benefits for employers who use certified pharmacy technicians?
    a. Better able to manage risk
    b. reduced technician training times and lower training costs
    c. increased employee satisfaction
    d. employees encouraged to improve performance
    e. all of the above

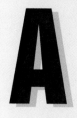

APPENDIX A

Long-Term Care

A-1: Examples of Guidelines for Automatic Stop-Order Policy in a Skilled Nursing Facility (Unless Otherwise Specified by Physician)

Drug Type

Analgesics . . . . .30 days
   Darvon, Darvocet

Antianemia drugs . . . . .30 days
   iron

Antibiotics . . . . .7 days
   Keflex, tetracycline

Antiemetics . . . . .4 days
   Compazine, Tigan

Anticoagulants . . . . .30 days
   Coumadin

Antihistamines . . . . .7 days
   Chlor-Trimeton, Seldane, Sudafed

Antineoplastics . . . . .30 days
   Nolvadex, Hydrea

Barbiturates . . . . .30 days
   phenobarbital

Cardiovascular . . . . .30 days
   digoxin, Vasotec, quinidine

Cathartics . . . . .30 days
   Pericolace, Colace, Senokot

Cold preparations . . . . .5 days
   Phenergan Expectorant, Robitussin

Dermatologicals . . . . .30 days
   Lidex, hydrocortisone, Synalar

Diuretics . . . . .30 days
   HCTZ, Dyazide, Aldactazide, Lasix

A-2: Medication Order Entry Flow Chart

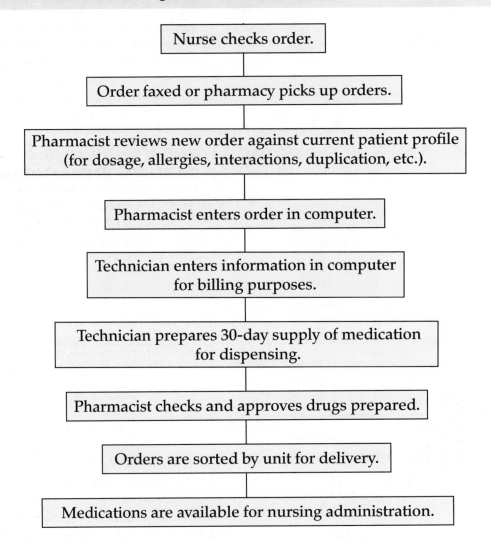

Nurse checks order.

Order faxed or pharmacy picks up orders.

Pharmacist reviews new order against current patient profile (for dosage, allergies, interactions, duplication, etc.).

Pharmacist enters order in computer.

Technician enters information in computer for billing purposes.

Technician prepares 30-day supply of medication for dispensing.

Pharmacist checks and approves drugs prepared.

Orders are sorted by unit for delivery.

Medications are available for nursing administration.

APPENDIX

B The Hospital Formulary System

B-1: The Pharmacy and Therapeutics Committee

The Pharmacy and Therapeutics Committee is a standing committee of the medical staff and is responsible to the Quality Improvement Committee. This committee shall be so selected as to represent different medical departments or divisions. A chief medical resident, a member of the nursing staff, and the director of Drug Information Services or his/her pharmacist designee, shall serve as members. A representative of the administration who has administrative responsibility for the department of pharmacy services shall also serve as a member.

The committee's duty shall be to review periodically the therapeutic agents and devices used in the hospital and clinics to ensure that their quality meets specifications of the *United States Pharmacopeia (U.S.P.), Good Manufacturing Practices,* other pertinent publications, and applicable hospital committees. This will in part be accomplished through a continually revised hospital formulary.

The committee shall function in both an advisory and an educational capacity.

1. It shall deal with contemporary problems in therapeutics.
2. It shall select for routine use within the institution and its ambulatory services and clinics, therapeutic agents that represent the best available for the prophylaxis or management of disease.
3. It shall recommend the deletion of drugs from the formulary that no longer meet the needs of the hospital patients.

The department of pharmacy services shall recommend to the committee quality control specifications, methods of distribution and control, and drug-utilization reviews.

Function

1. To serve as an advisory group to the medical staff, to the hospital administration, and to the department of pharmacy services on matters pertaining to drug utilization, drug-use control, and standards of practice concerning the use of drugs.
2. To recommend the adoption group to the medical staff, to the hospital administration, and to the department of pharmacy services on matters pertaining to drug, utilization, drug-use control, and standards of practice concerning the use of drugs.
3. To assist in the formulation and implementation of programs designed to meet the needs of the professional staff of physicians, nurses, pharmacists, and others for complete and current knowledge on matters related to drug practice.
4. To serve in an advisory capacity to the medical staff in the selection or choice of drugs that meet the most effective therapeutic quality standards and to evaluate objectively clinical and scientific data regarding new drugs or agents proposed for use in the hospital.
5. To differentiate between similar therapeutic agents and to recommend the best agent for use in the hospital.
6. To develop a formulary of accepted drugs for use in the hospital and to provide for its constant revision. This formulary shall reflect the modern teachings of pharmacotherapeutics and will present a listing of selected therapeutically effective drugs that should be the optimum in drug therapy.
7. To recommend policies regarding the surveillance of investigational drugs.
8. To study problems relating to the administration of medications and make recommendations where applicable.
9. To serve as a focal point for collecting data obtained from drug utilization reviews throughout the hospital.
10. To review and, if necessary, take action on observations made.

473

B-2: Definitions and Categories of Drugs to Be Stocked in the Pharmacy

Formulary Drug

A formulary drug is a therapeutic agent whose place in therapy is well established. It is selected by the Pharmacy and Therapeutics Committee as essential for the best patient care. Such a drug shall be listed in the formulary and stocked in the pharmacy.

Clinical Evaluation Drug

A clinical evaluation drug is a commercially available, nonformulary agent that is temporarily made available to a particular physician or physicians for the purpose of evaluation for formulary inclusion. Any attending physician, with the approval of the chief of service, may request to evaluate a nonformulary drug. It is the responsibility of the Pharmacy and Therapeutics Committee to review these requests. If approved by the chief of service, the requesting physician shall complete a Clinical Evaluation Drug Request Form and submit it to the secretary of the Pharmacy and Therapeutics Committee. The request for the evaluation may be approved by the chair of the Pharmacy and Therapeutics Committee.

The request form will seek the following information:

- objectives of the clinical evaluation
- criteria for selection of patients who will receive the drug
- parameters to be assessed
- estimated number of patients to be studied
- duration of study

The requesting physician shall submit the results of the evaluation after an interim period of time (usually 6 months) to the Pharmacy and Therapeutics Committee.

The final report shall contain conclusions of the requesting physician and a recommendation to the Pharmacy and Therapeutics Committee concerning the drug's role relative to formulary alternatives. If admitted to the formulary, the investigating physician will be expected to assist the Drug Information Service in developing criteria for the appropriate use of the agent.

During the evaluation, the investigating physician(s) need not complete a Nonformulary Drug Request Form for each patient. The department of pharmacy services will be responsible for monitoring the usage of the evaluation drug.

Restricted Drug

A restricted drug is a therapeutic agent, admitted to the formulary, the use of which is authorized by a specific group of physicians designated by the committee (see Administrative Guidelines). The following procedures will apply:

- Drugs in the category will be dispensed only if prescribed by a full-time faculty member of the designated group of physicians.
- Other members of the medical staff may prescribe the drug for an individual patient if they have the drug order authorized by one of the designated physicians.

Investigational Drug

An investigational drug is a therapeutic agent undergoing clinical investigation. It is not approved for general use by the Food and Drug Administration. Or it has been approved by the FDA only for a cause different from that being investigated.

The medical executive committee, through the Pharmacy and Therapeutics Committee, has charged the department of pharmacy services with the administrative control of experimental therapeutic agents. This administrative control includes storage, disposition, and record keeping. In addition the pharmacy is charged with the responsibility for providing drug information relative to these agents.

In order to implement the change, physicians are asked to comply with the following procedures:

- Obtain approval for any study of investigational agents from the Institutional Review Board.
- Complete the Investigational Drug Data Form and return it to the pharmacy.
- Provide the pharmacy with a copy of the signed consent form.
- Instruct the manufacturer to supply the pharmacy with all available pharmacologic and stability data.
- Make arrangements for transfer of the drug to the pharmacy if it is to be received directly by the chief investigator.
- Arrange with the pharmacy for a minimum inventory level and indicate if the pharmacy is to reorder.

Nonformulary Drug

A nonformulary drug is any drug other than one classified as a formulary drug, evaluation drug, restricted drug, or investigational drug. Nonformulary medications may only be prescribed by chiefs of service or attending physicians. These medications will not be dispensed without the prior submission of a Nonformulary Drug Request Form.

Upon receipt of a medication order, the pharmacist will notify the prescriber if the prescribed medication is nonformulary. The pharmacist will suggest to the prescriber alternative medications in the same therapeutic class. If the prescriber still wishes to use the nonformulary medication, a Nonformulary Drug Request Form shall be submitted for each individual patient. The pharmacist will inform the prescriber that there might be a delay in obtaining the requested medication due to possible problems.

B-3: Additions to the Formulary

Requests for the addition of drugs to the formulary may be initiated by an attending physician of the medical staff. A Request for Formulary Addition Form must be completed and signed by the requesting physician, cosigned by the chief of service, and submitted to the secretary of the Pharmacy and Therapeutics Committee. Incomplete forms will be returned to the requesting physician for completion.

The Drug Information Service shall be responsible for preparing all drug evaluation reports. These reports will review the pertinent literature concerning the requested drug and will make recommendations to the committee on the appropriate formulary status of the drug.

The recommendations of the Drug Information Service will be discussed with the requesting physician. The requesters may address the committee when the drug is discussed.

The committee may admit a drug monograph to the formulary without restriction or may restrict the drug's use to the following categories:

1. Restricted to previously established criteria for use. The use of drugs in this category is regularly audited by the drug-use evaluation program of the department of pharmacy services. The audit criteria are based on the established explicit criteria.
2. Restricted to use by full-time faculty within designated departments, divisions, or services.
3. Restricted to prior approval by full-time faculty within designated departments, divisions, or services.

The formulary status of a particular drug may be reviewed and evaluated by the committee after a specific period of time, usually 6 months.

A drug that is reviewed by the committee for formulary addition becomes official on the first day of the month following the meeting upon publication in the formulary update.

B-4: Deletions from the Formulary

Drugs may be deleted from the formulary as a result of the addition of more efficacious or safer agents, or at the request of a committee member of the Drug Information Service. Drugs may also be deleted upon review of the annual Low Volume of Use report.

Proposed deletions from the formulary will be published in the formulary update so that the medical staff may comment before final action is taken. If no objections to the deletion are heard, the drug will be removed from the formulary.

Body Surface Area Nomogram

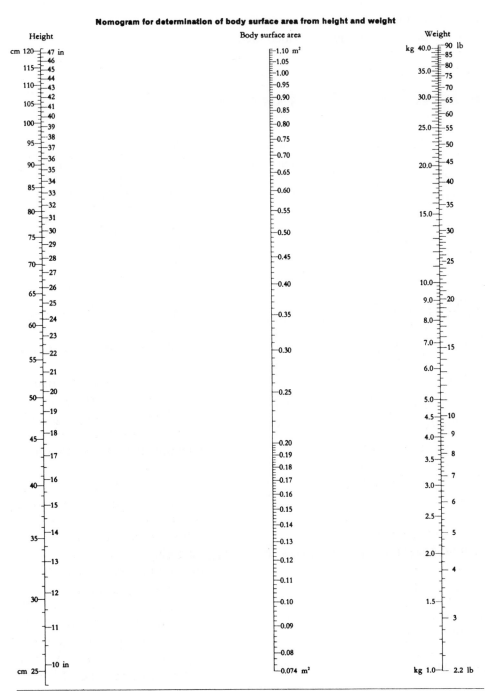

Nomogram for determination of body surface area from height and weight

Height	Body surface area	Weight

From the formula of Du Bois and Du Bois, *Arch. intern. Med.*, 17, 863 (1916): $S = W^{0.425} \times H^{0.725} \times 71.84$, or
$\log S = \log W \times 0.425 + \log H \times 0.725 + 1.8564$ (S = body surface in cm², W = weight in kg, H = height in cm)

D Common Sound-Alike Drug Names

The following is a list of common sound-alike drug names; trade names are capitalized. In parentheses next to each drug name is the pharmacological classification/use for the drug. (Reprinted from *PDR Nurse's Drug Handbook* by G. R. Spratto and A. L. Woods. Clifton Park, NY: Thomson Delmar Learning, 2004.)

Accupril (ACE inhibitor)	Accutane (antiacne drug)
acetazolamide (antiglaucoma drug)	acetohexamide (oral antidiabetic drug)
Aciphex (proton pump inhibitor)	Accupril (ACE inhibitor)
Aciphex (proton pump inhibitor)	Aricept (anti-Alzheimer's drug)
Actos (oral hypoglycemic)	Actonel (diphosphonate—bone growth regulator)
Adriamycin (antineoplastic)	Aredia (bone growth regulator)
albuterol (sympathomimetic)	atenolol (beta-blocker)
Aldomet (antihypertensive)	Aldoril (antihypertensive)
Alkeran (antineoplastic)	Leukeran (antineoplastic)
Alkeran (antineoplastic)	Myleran (antineoplastic)
allopurinol (antigout drug)	Apresoline (antihypertensive)
alprazolam (anti-anxiety agent)	lorazepam (anti-anxiety agent)
Amaryl (oral hypoglycemic)	Reminyl (anti-Alzheimer's drug)
Ambien (sedative-hypnotic)	Amen (progestin)
amiloride (diuretic)	amlodipine (calcium channel blocker)
amiodarone (antiarrhythmic)	amrinone (inotropic agent)
amitriptyline (antidepressant)	nortriptyline (antidepressant)
Apresazide (antihypertensive)	Apresoline (antihypertensive)
Aripiprazole (antipsychotic)	Lansoprazole (proton pump inhibitor)
Arlidin (peripheral vasodilator)	Aralen (antimalarial)
Artane (cholinergic blocking agent)	Altace (ACE inhibitor)
Asacol (anti-inflammatory drug)	Avelox (fluoroquinolone antibiotic)
asparaginase (antineoplastic agent)	pegaspargase (antineoplastic agent)
Atarax (antianxiety agent)	Ativan (antianxiety agent)
atenolol (beta-blocker)	timolol (beta-blocker)
Atrovent (cholinergic blocking agent)	Alupent (sympathomimetic)
Avandia (oral hypoglycemic)	Coumadin (anticoagulant)
Avandia (oral hypoglycemic)	Prandin (oral hypoglycemic)
Bacitracin (antibacterial)	Bactroban (anti-infective, topical)
Benylin (expectorant)	Ventolin (sympathomimetic)
Brevital (barbiturate)	Brevibloc (beta-adrenergic blocker)
Bumex (diuretic)	Buprenex (narcotic analgesic)
bupropion (antidepressant; smoking deterrent)	buspirone (anti-anxiety agent)
Cafergot (analgesic)	Carafate (antiulcer drug)
calciferol (vitamin D)	calcitriol (vitamin D)
carboplatin (antineoplastic agent)	cisplatin (antineoplastic agent)
Cardene (calcium channel blocker)	Cardizem (calcium channel blocker)

Cardura (antihypertensive)	Ridaura (gold-containing anti-inflammatory)
Cataflam (NSAID)	Catapres (antihypertensive)
Catapres (antihypertensive)	Combipres (antihypertensive)
cefotaxime (cephalosporin)	cefoxitin (cephalosporin)
cefuroxime (cephalosporin)	deferoxamine (iron chelator)
Celebrex (NSAID)	Cerebyx (anticonvulsant)
Celebrex (NSAID)	Celera (antidepressant)
Cerebyx (anticonvulsant)	Celera (antidepressant)
chlorpromazine (antipsychotic)	chlorpropamide (oral antidiabetic)
chlorpromazine (antipsychotic)	prochlorperazine (antipsychotic)
chlorpromazine (antipsychotic)	promethazine (antihistamine)
Clinoril (NSAID)	Clozaril (antipsychotic)
clomipramine (antidepressant)	clomiphene (ovarian stimulant)
clonidine (antihypertensive)	Klonopin (anticonvulsant)
Combivir (AIDS drug combination)	Combivent (combination for COPD)
Cozaar (antihypertensive)	Zocor (antihyperlipidemic)
cyclobenzaprine (skeletal muscle relaxant)	cyproheptadine (antihistamine)
cyclophosphamide (antineoplastic)	cyclosporine (immunosuppressant)
cyclosporine (immunosuppressant)	cycloserine (antineoplastic)
Cytovene (antiviral drug)	Cytosar (antineoplastic)
Cytoxan (antineoplastic)	Cytotec (prostaglandin derivative)
Cytoxan (antineoplastic)	Cytosar (antineoplastic)
Dantrium (skeletal muscle relaxant)	danazol (gonadotropin inhibitor)
Darvocet-N (analgesic)	Darvon-N (analgesic)
daunorubicin (antineoplastic)	doxorubicin (antineoplastic)
desipramine (antidepressant)	diphenhydramine (antihistamine)
DiaBeta (oral hypoglycemic)	Zebeta (beta-adrenergic blocker)
digitoxin (cardiac glycoside)	digoxin (cardiac glycoside)
diphenhydramine (antihistamine)	dimenhydrinate (antihistamine)
dopamine (sympathomimetic)	dobutamine (sympathomimetic)
Edecrin (diuretic)	Eulexin (antineoplastic)
enalapril (ACE inhibitor)	Anafranil (antidepressant)
enalapril (ACE inhibitor)	Eldepryl (antiparkinson agent)
Eryc (erythromycin base)	Ery-Tab (erythromycin base)
etidronate (bone growth regulator)	etretinate (antipsoriatic)
etomidate (general anesthetic)	etidronate (bone growth regulator)
E-Vista (antihistamine)	Evista (estrogen receptor modulator)
Femara (antineoplastic)	Femhrt (estrogen-progestin combination)
Fioricet (analgesic)	Fiorinal (analgesic)
Flomax (alpha-adrenergic blocker)	Volmax (sympathomimetic)
flurbiprofen (NSAID)	fenoprofen (NSAID)
folinic acid (leucovorin calcium)	folic acid (vitamin B complex)
Gantrisin (sulfonamide)	Gantanol (sulfonamide)
glipizide (oral hypoglycemic)	glyburide (oral hypoglycemic)
glyburide (oral hypoglycemic)	Glucotrol (oral hypoglycemic)
Hycodan (cough preparation)	Hycomine (cough preparation)
hydralazine (antihypertensive)	hydroxyzine (antianxiety agent)
hydrocodone (narcotic analgesic)	hydrocortisone (corticosteroid)
Hydrogesic (analgesic combination)	hydroxyzine (antihistamine)
hydromorphone (narcotic analgesic)	morphine (narcotic analgesic)
Hydropres (antihypertensive)	Diupres (antihypertensive)
Hytone (topical corticosteroid)	Vytone (topical corticosteroid)
imipramine (antidepressant)	Norpramin (antidepressant)

Inderal (beta-adrenergic blocker)	Inderide (antihypertensive)
Inderal (beta-adrenergic blocker)	Isordil (coronary vasodilator)
Indocin (NSAID)	Minocin (antibiotic)
K-Phos Neutral (phosphorus-potassium replenishment)	Neutra-Phos-K (phosphorus-potassium replenishment)
Lamictal (anticonvulsant)	Lamisil (antifungal)
Lamictal (anticonvulsant)	Ludiomil (alpha- and beta-adrenergic blocker)
Lamisil (antiviral)	Ludiomil (alpha- and beta-adrenergic blocker)
Lanoxin (cardiac glycoside)	Lasix (diuretic)
Lantus (insulin glargine)	Lente insulin (insulin zinc suspension)
Lioresal (muscle relaxant)	lisinopril (ACE inhibitor)
Lithostat (lithium carbonate)	Lithobid (lithium carbonate)
Lithotabs (lithium carbonate)	Lithobid (lithium carbonate)
Lodine (NSAID)	codeine (narcotic analgesic)
Lopid (antihyperlipidemic)	Lorabid (beta-lactam antibiotic)
lovastatin (antihyperlipidemic)	Lotensin (ACE inhibitor)
Ludiomil (alpha- and beta-adrenergic blocker)	Lomotil (antidiarrheal)
Medrol (corticosteroid)	Haldol (antipsychotic)
metolazone (thiazide diuretic)	methotrexate (antineoplastic)
metolazone (thiazide diuretic)	metoclopramide (GI stimulant)
metoprolol tartrate (beta-adrenergic blocker)	metoclopramide hydrochloride (GI stimulant)
metoprolol (beta-adrenergic blocker)	misoprostol (prostaglandin derivative)
Monopril (ACE inhibitor)	minoxidil (antihypertensive)
nelfinavir (antiviral)	nevirapine (antiviral)
nicardipine (calcium channel blocker)	nifedipine (calcium channel blocker)
Norlutate (progestin)	Norlutin (progestin)
Noroxin (fluoroquinolone antibiotic)	Neurontin (anticonvulsant)
Norvasc (calcium channel blocker)	Navane (antipsychotic)
Norvir (antiviral)	Retrovir (antiviral)
Ocufen (NSAID)	Ocuflox (fluoroquinolone antibiotic)
Orinase (oral hypoglycemic)	Ornade (upper respiratory product)
Percocet (narcotic analgesic)	Percodan (narcotic analgesic)
paroxetine (antidepressant)	paclitaxel (antineoplastic)
Paxil (antidepressant)	paclitaxel (antineoplastic)
Paxil (antidepressant)	Taxol (antineoplastic)
penicillamine (heavy metal antagonist)	penicillin (antibiotic)
pindolol (beta-adrenergic blocker)	Parlodel (inhibitor of prolactin secretion)
Platinol (antineoplastic)	Paraplatin (antineoplastic)
Pletal (antiplatelet drug)	Plavix (antiplatelet drug)
Pravachol (antihyperlipidemic)	Prevacid (GI drug)
Pravachol (antihyperlipidemic)	propranolol (beta-adrenergic blocker)
prednisolone (corticosteroid)	prednisone (corticosteroid)
Prilosec (inhibitor of gastric acid secretion)	Prozac (antidepressant)
Prinivil (ACE inhibitor)	Prilosec (GI drug)
Prinivil (ACE inhibitor)	Proventil (sympathomimetic)
Procanbid (antiarrhythmic)	Procan SR (antiarrhythmic)
propranolol (beta-adrenergic blocker)	Propulsid (GI drug)
Provera (progestin)	Premarin (estrogen)
Prozac (antidepressant)	Proscar (androgen hormone inhibitor)
quinidine (antiarrhythmic)	clonidine (antihypertensive)
quinidine (antiarrhythmic)	Quinamm (antimalarial)
quinine (antimalarial)	quinidine (antiarrhythmic)
Regroton (antihypertensive)	Hygroton (diuretic)

Reminyl (anti-Alzheimer's drug)	Robinul (muscle relaxant)
Retrovir (antiviral)	Ritonavir (antiviral)
Rifamate (antituberculous drug)	rifampin (antituberculous drug)
rimantadine (antiviral)	flutamide (antineoplastic)
Roxicodone (oxycodone alone—analgesic)	Roxicet (oxycodone/acetaminophen analgesic)
Sarafem (for PMS)	Serophene (ovulation stimulator)
Seroquel (antipsychotic)	Serzone (antidepressant)
Serzone (antidepressant)	Seroquel (antipsychotic)
Soriatane (antipsoriasis)	Loxitane (antipsychotic)
Stadol (narcotic analgesic)	Haldol (antipsychotic)
sulfadiazine (sulfonamide)	sulfasalazine (sulfonamide)
Tegretol (anticonvulsant)	Tequin (antibacterial)
terazosin hydrochloride (anti-hypertensive)	temazepam (sedative-hypnotic)
terbinafine (antifungal agent)	terfenadine (antihistamine)
terbutaline (sympathomimetic)	tolbutamide (oral hypoglycemic)
Ticlid (antiplatelet drug)	Tequin (fluoroquinolone antibiotic)
tolazamide (oral hypoglycemic)	tolbutamide (oral hypoglycemic)
torsemide (loop diuretic)	furosemide (loop diuretic)
trifluoperazine (antipsychotic)	trihexyphenidyl (antiparkinson drug)
Trimox (amoxicillin product)	Diamox (carbonic anhydrase inhibitor)
Ultram (analgesic)	Ultrase (pancreatic enzymes)
Vancenase (corticosteroid)	Vanceril (corticosteroid)
Vasosulf (sulfonamide/decongestant)	Velosef (cephalosporin)
Versed (benzodiazepine sedative)	Vistaril (antianxiety agent)
Versed (benzodiazepine sedative)	VePesid (antineoplastic)
Xanax (antianxiety agent)	Zantac (H2 histamine blocker)
Xenical (antiobesity)	Xeloda (antineoplastic)
Xydis	(see note)
Zantac (H2 histamine blocker)	Zyrtec (H1 antihistamine)
Zebeta (beta-blocker)	DiaBeta (oral hypoglycemic)
Zinacef (cephalosporin)	Zithromax (macrolide antibiotic)
Zocor (antihyperlipidemic)	Zoloft (antidepressant)
Zofran (antiemetic)	Zantac (H2 histamine blocker)
Zosyn (penicillin antibiotic)	Zofran (antiemetic)
Zovirax (antiviral)	Zyvox (antibiotic)
Zyrtec (antihistamine)	Zyprexa (antipsychotic)
Zyvox (antibiotic)	Vioxx (COX-2 inhibitor)

Note: Xydis is a technology consisting of a freeze-dried wafer that dissolves almost instantly on the tongue or contact with saliva. The name of the technology has been confused because it is written on prescriptions as if it were a drug name.

Glossary

accelerated care unit (ACU)—separate unit in the hospital where patients are prepared to better care for themselves and their condition after being discharged from the hospital

accreditation—the process by which an agency or organization evaluates and recognizes a program of study or an institution as meeting predetermined qualifications

achlorhydria—absence of hydrochloric acid in the stomach

acidosis—acid/base imbalance causing the blood and body tissues to become excessively acidic

action plan—a concise, written document listing the objectives an employee will accomplish in a specific period of time, such as one year. The objectives are mutually agreed upon by the employee and the supervisor and should be clear, measurable, and obtainable

active transport—movement of drug molecules against a concentration gradient (i.e., from an area of low concentration to an area of higher concentration)

acute—a severe condition, rising rapidly to a peak and then subsiding

acute illness—an illness with severe symptoms and of short duration

additive (parenteral)—an addition of an active ingredient to a solution that is intended for intravenous administration or irrigation

administer—give a patient medication, once it is checked for accuracy

administration (or route of administration)—refers to how a drug or therapy is introduced into the body. Systemic administration means that the drug goes throughout the body (usually carried in the bloodstream), and includes oral administration (by mouth) and intravenous administration (injection into the vein). Local administration means that the drug is applied or introduced into a specific area affected by disease (e.g., application directly onto the affected skin surface, called topical administration). The effects of most therapies depend upon the ability of the drug to reach the affected area, thus the route of administration and consequent distribution of a drug in the body is an important determinant of its effectiveness.

administrative section—that part of the manual containing the policies and procedures that pertain to the operation of the department

admixture—term used to denote one or more active ingredients in a large-volume parenteral solution

ADT—computer program for admission/discharge and transfer which provides significant demographic and clinical information for each patient

adverse drug reaction—any unexpected obvious change in a patient's condition that the physician suspects may be due to a drug

aerosol—finely nebulized medication for inhalation therapy

AIDS—acquired immune deficiency syndrome

airborne transmission—infection by contact with airborne particles that contain infectious organisms

alkaloid—a nitrogenous basic substance found in plants or synthetic substances with structures similar to plant structures (e.g., atropine, caffeine, morphine)

alkalosis—acid/base imbalance causing the blood and body tissues to become excessively alkaline (basic)

allergen—an agent that provokes the symptoms of an allergy

allergy—a disorder in which the body becomes hypersensitive to a particular antigen (called an *allergen*)

allopathy—a method of treating a disease by administering an agent that has the opposite characteristics of the disease

allopathy—treatment of diseases with drugs that cause the opposite effect (e.g., antipyretics to reduce fever)

almshouse—a home for the poor and indigent

ambulatory care—care provided to persons who do not require either an acute care (hospital) or chronic care (skilled nursing facility) setting

ambulatory care—patients come in for treatment and go home the same day; they are not hospitalized

ambulatory patient—a patient who is able to walk and is not restricted to bed

American Council on Pharmaceutical Education—the accrediting body for colleges of pharmacy by which high educational standards are established and monitored

American Druggist Blue Book—provides prices and other miscellaneous information about prescription drugs, over-the-counter products, cosmetics, toiletries, and other items sold in pharmacy stores

American Society of Health-System Pharmacists (ASHP)—a national organization established in 1942 and presently includes pharmacists in various institutional health care settings; presently contains a section for pharmacy technicians

amphetamine—a stimulant drug; also known as uppers, bam, bennies, browns, bumblebee, butterflies

anabolic agent—a substance that builds up tissue protein

anabolism—the body process during which proteins are synthesized and tissues are formed

analgesic—an agent that relieves pain without causing loss of consciousness (e.g., codeine)

anaphylaxis—a hypersensitivity reaction that is immediate, shocklike, and possibly fatal; severe allergenic reaction caused by a drug or biological

anesthetic—a drug used to decrease sensation

aneurysm—a dilation or bulging out of a blood vessel wall

angiotensin-converting enzyme (ACE)—helps inhibit the renal mechanism for blood elevation

anhydrous—containing no water

anionic—carrying a negative charge

antacids—an agent that neutralizes gastric acid

antagonist—a drug that opposes the action of another drug or a natural body chemical

antepartum—before the onset of childbirth

antianginal—drug used to relieve chest pain

antiarrhythmic—agent that restores normal heart rhythm

antibiotic—medication that is derived from living cells or synthetic compounds and is antagonistic to other forms of life, especially bacteria; a soluble substance derived from a mold or bacterium that inhibits the growth of other organisms and is used to combat disease and infection

anticholinergic—a drug that blocks the passage of impulses through parasympathetic nerve fibers

anticoagulant—a drug that prevents or delays coagulation or clotting of blood; a "blood thinner"

antidote—a remedy for counteracting a poison

antiemetic—controls nausea and vomiting

antiflatulent—a drug that facilitates expulsion of gas from the GI tract

antigen—an agent that stimulates antibody formation

antihistamine—reduces runny nose and sneezing

antihypertensive—an agent that reduces blood pressure

antineoplastic—a substance that prevents the development or spread of tumor cells

antineoplastic agent—chemotherapy agent or cancer drug

antipruritic—a drug that relieves itch

antipyretic—a drug that reduces fever

antiseptic—an agent that inhibits the growth of microorganisms but does not necessarily kill them

antitoxin—a specific agent neutralizing a poison or toxin

antitussive—a drug used for the relief of cough

apothecary—early American or European term for a pharmacist

apparent volume of distribution—the apparent volume of plasma that would be required to account for all the drug in the body; rarely corresponds to a real volume space in the body

application software—referred to as programs, accepting data from the user; it calculates, stores user-specific data, and presents information according to the prescribed instructions

arrhythmia—an abnormal, irregular heartbeat

arteriosclerosis—disorder characterized by thickening, loss of elasticity, and calcification of the walls of the arteries

arteriosclerosis—hardening of the arteries

arthritis—inflammation of joints

ascites—accumulation of fluid within the abdominal cavity

aseptic—a condition in which there are no living microorganisms; free from infection

aseptic technique—a method of preparation that will prevent contamination of a site (e.g., wound) or product (e.g., IV admixture)

asylum—an institution for the relief or care of the destitute or afflicted and especially the insane

atherosclerosis—lipid (fat) deposits in large and medium size arteries

atonic—weak tone or absence of tone

automated pharmacy systems—mechanical systems that perform operations and activities, other than compounding and drug administration, relative to storage, packaging, dispensing, and distribution of medications and that collect, control, and maintain transaction information

average wholesale price (AWP)—cost of drugs and pharmaceuticals purchased from a drug wholesaler

B.S. degree—bachelor of science degree; an initial entry degree originally required for admission to a state board examination to obtain a license to practice as a pharmacist

backup systems—alternate procedures in the event the computer system should fail

bactericide—an agent capable of killing bacterias

bacteriostat—an agent that inhibits the growth of bacteria

bar coding—a series of vertical bars and spaces of varying thicknesses and heights to represent information

benign—not malignant or invasive

beta blocker—a drug that selectively blocks beta receptors in the autonomic nervous system

bile—a fluid secreted by the liver

bile salts—naturally occurring surface-active agents secreted by the gall bladder into the small intestine

bioavailability—term used to indicate the rate and relative amount of administered drug that reaches the circulatory system intact

biodegradable—can be broken down by living organisms

bioengineered therapies—the process used in the manufacture of therapeutic agents through recombinant DNA (deoxyribonucleic acid) technology

biological equivalents—those chemical equivalents that, when administered in the same amounts, will provide the same biological or physiological availability

biological fluids—includes blood, serum, plasma, lymph, etc.

biologicals—medicinal preparations made from living organisms or their products; include serums, vaccines, antigens, and antitoxins

biopharmaceutics—the branch of pharmaceutics that concerns itself with the relationship between physicochemical properties of a drug in a dosage form, and the pharmacologic, toxicologic, or clinical responses observed after drug administration

biopsy—excision of a small piece of tissue for diagnostic purposes

biotech drugs—genetically engineered therapeutic agents

biotechnology—the application of biological systems and organisms to technical and industrial processes

black plague—a worldwide epidemic of the fourteenth century in which some 60 million persons are said to have died; descriptions indicate that it was pneumonic plague, also called *black death* or *the plague*

blending—mixing

blister packages—cardboard and plastic material that is heat-sealed to individually package medication

blood urea nitrogen (BUN)—an indication of kidney function

bloodborne pathogens—microorganisms that are transmitted through exposure to contaminated blood products

board of trustees/directors—body responsible for governing the hospital in the community's best interest

bolus—an injection directly from the syringe barrel into a vein, also called *IV push*

botany—the science of plants, including structure, functions of parts, and classification

bradycardia—slow heart rate

brand-name drugs—drugs that are research-developed, patented, manufactured, and distributed by a drug firm

buccal—between the gum and cheek

budget—the projected costs allocated on a yearly basis for personnel, supplies, construction, and operating expenses

buffer—offers a resistance to pH change

calibrate—standardization of the graduations of a quantitative measuring device

calibration—a method of standardizing a measuring device

candida—a yeast organism that normally lives in the intestines, but can flourish in other parts of the body at times of immune suppression

caplet—tablet shaped like a capsule

capsule—soluble container enclosing medicine

carcinogen—any substance that causes cancer

cardiotonic—an agent that has the effect of producing or restoring normal heart activity

carminative—a medicine that relieves stomach/intestinal gas

catabolism—the breakdown of body proteins

cataract—loss of transparency of the lens of the eye

cathartic—an agent that causes bowel evacuation

catheter—a tubular device used for the drainage or injection of fluids through a body passage; made of silicone, rubber, plastic, or other materials

cationic—carrying a positive charge

central processing unit (CPU)—the unit of the computer that accomplishes the processing or execution of given calculations or instructions

central service—an area in the hospital where general sterilization procedures are performed; serves as a storage facility for various types of equipment

centralized system—a system of distribution in which all functions, processing, preparation, and distribution occur in a main area (e.g., the main pharmacy)

chain pharmacy—a retail pharmacy owned by a corporation that consists of many stores in a particular region or nationally

chelating—making a complex formation

chemical equivalents—those multiple-source drug products that contain identical amounts of the identical active ingredient in identical dosage forms

chemotherapy—the treatment of an illness with medication; commonly refers to the treatment of malignancy with agents that are cytotoxic (i.e., the medication kills cells); more specifically, use of chemicals to treat cancer

cholinergic—a drug that is stimulated, activated, or transmitted by acetylcholine

chronic—of long duration or frequent recurrence

chronic illness—a disturbance in health that persists for a long time, usually showing little change or slow progression over time

Class 100 environment—a room or hood designed for the preparation of sterile products which indicates the environment has less than 100 particles of dust and particulates per cubic centimeter of air

Class A prescription balance—a sensitive balance scale with a range of 6 mg to 650 mg

clean room—a specially filtered room to create a sterile environment

clinical—involving direct observation of the patient

clinical pharmacokinetics—that branch of pharmaceutics that deals with the application of pharmacokinetics to the safe and effective therapeutic management of the individual patient

clinical pharmacy—patient-oriented pharmacy practice that is concerned with health care through rational drug use

clinical pharmacy practice—the application of knowledge about drugs and drug therapy to the care and treatment of patients

clinical section—that section of a policy and procedure manual describing patient-related monitoring activities

closed formulary—a list of reimburseable medications

coagulation—blood-clotting process

cocaine—a topical anesthetic, also known as coke, crack, snow, blow, white horse, 8-ball

collaborative drug therapy agreement—an agreement between a physician and a pharmacist that allows the pharmacist expanded prescription authorization regarding managing drug therapy

colonized—a group of microorganisms that have grown from a single infectious microorganism within a particular part of the body causing an infection

colostomy—creation of an opening into the colon through the abdominal wall

Commission on Credentialing—the body appointed to formulate and recommend standards and administer programs for accreditation of pharmacy personnel training programs

common vehicle transmission—infection through contact with contaminated food or water

community pharmacy—pharmacy service provided in pharmacy health care; sometimes called the "family drugstore" in which ambulatory individuals are provided prescription and nonprescription drugs and other health-related supplies

community relations and fund development—a department that communicates with and markets hospital programs to the local community

compliance—act of adhering to prescribed directions

compliance rate—an indicator of how many times out of a hundred (expressed as a percent) that a quality event occurs or fails to occur

compounding—preparation of a pharmaceutical that contains more than one ingredient according to a prescription or formula

Comprehensive Drug Abuse and Prevention Control Act—a federal statute through which the DEA (Drug Enforcement Agency) promulgates and enforces rules and regulations that control narcotic use

computer—a programmable electronic device used to store, process, or communicate information

computer application—a series of computer programs written for a particular function (e.g., inventory management)

computer file—collection of like elements of information stored under a common name (e.g., Hospital Formulary)

computer network—the technology that supports the connection of multiple computers including application, processors, printers, and microcomputers

computer server—a computer that collects and stores information for use by other computers

computer system—a combination of hardware and software working together to perform specific functions

computer terminal—a device that contains a keyboard and screen; functions as both the inpatient and outpatient device

congestive heart failure (CHF)—failure or diminished ability of the heart to pump an adequate blood supply to the rest of the body

constipation—difficult, incomplete, or infrequent bowel evacuation

consultant pharmacist—responsible for monitoring drug usage and drug therapy of residents in nursing homes

contaminated—unclean; microorganisms introduced into an area where they had not previously been present

continuous infusion—administration of an intravenous drug at a constant rate over a prolonged time period

contraindicate—to indicate against; to indicate the inappropriateness of a form of treatment or a drug for a specific disease

control—any method used to eliminate or reduce the potential harm of the distributed medication

control documents—forms, such as records, sheets, logs, or checklists, that track conformance with standards that have been established to reduce the likelihood of an error or negative outcome

controlled substances—drugs, controlled by the federal or state Drug Enforcement Administration, that can produce dependence or be abused (e.g., narcotics, select psychotropics, steroids)

Controlled Substances Act—federal law regulating the manufacture, distribution, and sale of drugs that have the potential for abuse

coring—a needle rips a piece of the vial stopper at the site where the needle was inserted into the vial

counter balance—a double-pan balance capable of weighing relatively large quantities

counterirritant—an agent, such as mustard plaster, that is applied locally to produce an inflammatory reaction for the purpose of affecting some other part, usually adjacent to or underlying the surface irritated

covered entities—entities which HIPAA regulations apply to, namely health plans that provide or pay the costs of medical care, health care clearinghouses that facilitate the processing of health information from another entity, to health care providers of medical or health services

CPU—central processing unit of computer hardware; the brain of the computer

crack—an illicit, pure form of cocaine, usually smoked in a pipe

cream—water-based, semisolid external dosage form

creatinine clearance—a measure of renal function

credentialling—a process in which a formal, organized agency recognizes and documents the competencies and abilities performed by an individual or an organization

criteria—a set of statements that define quality

cyber—cultural revolution; computerization and telecommunication that transport information through fiber optics, CD-ROM, satellites, and the Internet

cytotoxic—a substance that causes cellular deterioration

data entry—the input function that involves recording, coding, or converting data to a form that the computer can recognize

decentralized system—a system of distribution in which all functions (processing, preparation, and distribution) occur on or near the nursing unit (e.g., satellite pharmacy)

decongestant—a drug used to open the air passages of the nose and lungs

decubitus ulcer—a bedsore

dedicated—limited to processing information for one area

defenses—legal arguments that are raised by defendants in support of their case

deinstitutionalization—discharge of persons with a history of long-term mental health care in a hospital back to the community

Delphi Study—a futuristic study employed to gain insight into desirable courses of action to achieve the mission of the group

density—weight per unit volume

deoxyribonucleic acid (DNA)—a double-stranded structure that is the molecular basis of heredity

departmental manual—lists only those policies and procedures that affect the internal working of the pharmacy department

deposition—out-of-court, sworn testimony made in response to questioning by an attorney and recorded by a court reporter

diabetes mellitus—a metabolic disorder in which faulty pancreatic activity decreases the oxidation of carbohydrates

diagnosis—the determination of the nature of a disease or symptom through physical examination and clinical tests

diagnosis-related group (DRG))—utilized by Medicare, Medicaid, and other third-party payers to reimburse hospitals a predetermined fee for each patient based on the patient's diagnosis, irrespective of the quantity or cost of the care. Costs over this predetermined fee are not reimbursed by the government but are allocated to the hospital. The intent of implementing the DRG system was to regulate and control Medicare's health care expenditure. *See also* **prospective payment system (PPS)**.

diagnostic equipment—articles or implements used to detect physical conditions that may be related to disease or biological changes; usually used at home by one patient

diarrhea—increased frequency of stool that is loose and watery

diastolic pressure—the force exerted by the blood on the blood vessels when the ventricles of the heart are in a state of rest before systole

didactic instruction—formalized, structured, lecture-type education program

dietary supplement—any product containing a vitamin, mineral, amino acid, or herb that is intended to supplement the diet by increasing overall intake of a particular substance

Dietary Supplement Verification Program (DSVP)—program developed by the USP to establish standards for herbal and vitamin supplements

differentiated manpower—the distinction of responsibilities among available personnel to achieve the overall purpose of the entire group

diluent—an agent that dilutes or reconstitutes a solution or mixture

direct contact transmission—infection through body surface to body surface contact with an infected person

discharge planning—a program developed to ensure continued appropriate care after the patient leaves the hospital

discovery—the formal pretrial process by which evidence is obtained by one party from another party to a litigation

disease state management—a continuous, coordinated, and on-going process that manages and improves the health status of defined patient populations over the course of an entire disease

disinfectant—a substance used to destroy pathogens; generally used on objects rather than on humans

dispensatory—a treatise on the quality and composition of medicine

dispensing—the process of selecting, preparing, checking, and delivering prescribed medication and associated information; must be under the supervision of a pharmacist

dissolution—the act of dissolving

distributional section—the part of a policy and procedure manual that presents those policies and procedures that deal with the appropriate storage, ordering, dispensing, documentation, and disposition of drugs and supplies

diuresis—increased excretion of urine

diuretic—an agent that causes an increase in the excretion of urine

dosage—the determination and regulation of the size, frequency, and number of doses

dosage forms—the various pharmaceutical forms whereby drugs are made available (e.g., capsules, patches, injections)

dosage schedule—the frequency, interval, and length of time a medicine is to be given

dosage strength—the quantity of a drug in a given dosage form

dose—a quantity of a drug or radiation to be given at one time

DRG—*see* **diagnostic-related group**

droplet transmission—infection through contact with microscopic liquid particles coming from an infected person

drug—any substance intended to cure, prevent, or diagnose a disease or disease process

drug administration—process by which a drug enters the body by ingestion, injection, application, inhalation, instillation, etc.

drug disposition—all processes that occur to the drug after absorption and that can be subdivided into distribution and elimination

drug distribution—the process of reversible transfer of a drug to and from the site of measurement, usually the blood

drug elimination—the irreversible loss of a drug from the site of measurement, usually subdivided into metabolism or excretion

drug formulary—a list of medicinal agents selected by the medical staff considered to be the most useful in patient care

drug information—information about drugs and the effects of drugs on people, the provision of which is a part of each pharmacist's practice

drug label—information placed on a drug container that includes data required by drug regulations

drug manufacturer—the company responsible for developing and producing and distributing pharmaceutical products

drug misadventures—what can go wrong in the "therapeutic adventure" of using a medication; encompass errors in prescribing judgment, system errors in the process of bringing drug products to the ultimate users, and idiosyncratic (individual and unusual sensitivity that is not dose related) responses to medication

drug order—a course of medication therapy ordered by the physician or dental practitioner in an organized health care setting

drug recalls—voluntary recall of a drug because of a health hazard potential

drug regimen review—process to provide appropriate drug therapy for patients as part of the health care team

Drug Topics Red Book—reference guide listing pharmaceuticals, medicinals, and sundries sold in drug stores, with currently available prices

drug use process—an organized, complex, and controlled system of manufacturing, purchasing, distributing, storing, prescribing, preparing, dispensing, administering, using, controlling, and monitoring of a drug's effects and outcomes to ensure that drugs are used safely and effectively

drug wholesaler—the company responsible for delivering medication, medical devices, appliances, etc. to pharmacies and retailers

druggist—historically, a person who compounds, dispenses, and sells drugs and medicine

drugs of choice—the preferred or best drug therapy that can be prescribed for a specific disease state, based upon majority medical opinion

drug-use control—the system of knowledge, understanding, judgments, procedures, skills, controls, and ethics that ensures optimal safety in the distribution and use of medication

drug-use process—the series of steps necessary to move a drug product from purchase to patient use

dumbwaiters—an inhouse elevator used to transport medications and supplies

duodenum—that area of the small intestine that is the first 25 cm after the stomach, responsible for significant drug absorption

durable medical equipment (DME)—includes health-related equipment that is used for long periods of time, is not disposable, and is rented or sold to clients for home care, such as wheelchairs, hospital beds, walkers, canes, crutches; *also see* **home medical equipment**

elastomer—an elastometric substance

elastometric—a polymer material with elastic properties

electrocardiogram—a graphic record of the heart's action by electronic measurement

electroencephalogram—a tracing or electronic recording of brain waves

electrolytes—naturally occurring ions in the body that play an essential role in cellular function, maintaining fluid balance and establishing acid-base balance; an ionizable substance in solution (e.g., sodium, potassium chloride)

electronic mail (e-mail)—a form of transmitting, storing, and distributing text in electronic form via a communications network

electrostatic copying machine—a photocopier

emboli—a blood clot; a moving or transferred blood clot

embolism—obstruction or occlusion of a blood vessel by a transported blood clot

emergency room—a hospital unit where patients are treated for conditions that require immediate attention

emesis—clinical term for vomiting

emetic—an agent that causes vomiting

emphysema—lung disease caused by constriction of airway passages

employee performance evaluations—a routine, formal process by the supervisor to provide feedback on the employee's performance versus the expected performance listed in the employee's action plan

emulsifying agent—a substance used in preparing an emulsion

emulsion—a heterogeneous system of at least one immiscible liquid intimately dispersed in another in the form of droplets, stabilized by the presence of an emulsifying agent

endogenously—originating within the organism

enforcement—the process of making sure that policies and procedures are carefully and consistently followed

enteral nutrition—liquid nutrient solution administered by mouth or through a feeding tube into stomach or intestines

enteric-coated tablet—a special tablet coating that prevents the release of a drug until it enters the intestine

enterohepatic cycling—drug taken up by the bile, secreted into the small intestine, and may be reabsorbed back to the blood

epidemic—a disease that attacks many people in the same region at the same time

epidural—infusion therapy directly into spinal cord fluid

equivalent weight—the gram molecular weight divided by the highest valent ion in the molecule

erythrocyte—a red blood cell

estrogen—a hormone that produces secondary sex characteristics in the female

ethics—the study of precepts or principles used to assist us in making the correct choice when faced with alternative possibilities in a moral situation

etiology—the study of all the factors that may be involved in the development of disease

excretion—the process whereby the undigested residue of food and the waste products of metabolism are eliminated

expectorant—a substance that promotes the ejection of mucus or an exudate from the lungs, bronchi, and trachea

expiration date—the last date of sale as determined by the manufacturer. Any sale after this date is unethical and may result in a levy of fines by pharmacy and or health inspectors.

exposure control plan—guidelines to follow in the event of an exposure to an infectious disease, including infection control training

extemporaneous—prepared at the time it is required, with materials on hand

extended-release capsules—capsules that are formulated in such a way as to gradually release the drug over a predetermined time period

facsimile equipment—fax machine; sends order over telephone lines

FDA—*see* **Food and Drug Administration**

febrile—body temperature above normal

federal and state statutes—laws enacted by a legislative body that dictate the conduct of persons or organizations subject to the law

fibrillation—rapid, ineffectual heartbeat

first-pass effect—occurs when a drug is rapidly metabolized in the liver after oral administration with minimum bioavailability

floor stock—medications provided to the nursing unit for administration to the patient by the nurse, who is responsible for preparation and administration

fluidextract—a liquid preparation of a herb containing alcohol as a solvent or preservative

Food and Drug Administration (FDA)—promulgates rules, regulations, and standards; inspects drug and food facilities to ensure public safety regarding drug products

Food, Drug, and Cosmetic Act—the federal statute through which the FDA promulgates its rules and regulations

format—standardized method of documentation for consistency

formulary—a listing of drugs of choice as determined by safety, efficacy, effectiveness and cost approved by the medical staff for use within the institution

franchise—authorization by a manufacturer to a distributor to sell a product

free flow—a dangerous condition in which all of the infusion is accidentally administered in a short period of time

galenical—a standard preparation containing one or several organic ingredients (e.g., elixir)

gargle—a substance used to rinse or medicate the mucous membrane of the throat and mouth (e.g., Listerine)

gastric—pertaining to the stomach

gastroesophageal reflux disease (GERD)—excess stomach acid causing a burning sensation in the esophagus due to eructation of small amounts of acid into the esophagus

generic drug name—the nonproprietary (nonbrand) name of a drug

generic drugs—drugs labeled by their "official" name and manufactured by a drug firm after the original patent expires

genetically engineered drugs—exact duplication of a substance already available in the human body

geriatric pharmacy practice—pharmacy practice that focuses on the medical and pharmaceutical care of the elderly

glucose tolerance test—a test for diabetes, based on the ability of the liver to store glycogen

glycoside—a compound containing a sugar molecule (e.g., digitalis)

graduate—a marked (or graduated) conical or cylindrical vessel used for measuring liquids

group purchasing—a group of hospitals or pharmacists that buy drugs directly from the manufacturer

habituation—acquired tolerance for a drug

hard copy—information on a printed sheet

hardware—equipment, software, and sets of instructions that control and coordinate the activities of the hardware and direct the processing of data; refers to the actual computer system (e.g., IBM, Digital)

health care delivery—organized programs developed to provide physical, mental, and emotional health care in institutions for home-bound and ambulatory patients

health maintenance organization (HMO)—a prepaid health insurance plan that provides comprehensive health care for subscribers, with emphasis on the prevention and early detection of disease and continuity of care. HMOs are either not-for-profit or for-profit, are designated as either an independent practice association (IPA) or a staff model, and are often owned and operated by insurance carriers. HMOs were developed as a means to control health care delivery, access, and cost.

hemodialysis—procedure by which impurities or wastes are removed from the blood

hemophilia—hereditary blood-coagulation disorder

hemorrhage—severe bleeding

hemostat—an agent used to arrest hemorrhage

HEN—home enteral therapy

hepatitis—Inflammation of the liver

hepatitis B (HBV)—a virus that causes acute infection of the liver that is transmitted through infectious bodily fluids

hepatitis C (HBC)—a virus that causes acute and chronic infection of the liver that is transmitted through infectious bodily fluids

herb—a leafy plant used as a healing remedy or a flavoring agent

herbal—a plant with therapeutic properties that can be used for nutritional or medical purposes

heroin—an illicit drug derived from morphine; also known as brown sugar, salt, horse

high efficiency particulate air (HEPA)—used in laminar flow hoods

Hippocrates—a Greek physician, called the "Father of Medicine"

HIS—*see* **hospital information system**

HIV—human immunodeficiency virus

home health care—provision of health care services to a patient in his or her place of residence

home health services—the provision of health care services by a health care professional in the patient's place of residence on a per visit basis

home infusion—intravenous drug therapy provided in patient's own home

home medical equipment (HME)—equipment used at home (e.g., hospital beds, crutches); *see* **durable medical equipment**

home pharmaceutical service—dispensing and delivery of medications to patients who have their clinical status monitored at home

homeostasis—a tendency toward stability in the internal body environment, a state of equilibrium

homogeneous—of uniform composition throughout

horizontal hospital integration—situation in which a number of hospitals share administrative, clinical, and technological functions

hormone—a chemical substance, produced by cells or an organ, that has a specific regulatory effect in the body

hospice—an institution that provides a program of palliative and supportive services to terminally ill patients and their families in the form of physical, psychological, social, and spiritual care

hospital—a network of health care services for treatment, care of the sick, study of disease, therapy, and the training of health care professionals

hospital information systems (HIS)—systems that integrate information from many parts of the hospital

human genome initiative—program of research that studies all human genes

human immunodeficiency virus (HIV)—a virus that weakens the immune system and may progress to the development of AIDS

humor—a fluid or semifluid substance in the body; originally phlegm, blood, bile (e.g., aqueous humor is a fluid produced in the eye—not tears)

hydration therapy—replaces fluid loss

hydroalcoholic—mixture of water and alcohol

hydrolysis—any reaction in which water is one of the reactants

hydrophilic—water loving

hydrophilic drug molecules—drug molecules that are polar and water loving

hydrophobic drugs—drugs whose molecules are nonpolar and lipid loving or water hating

hygroscopic—moisture absorbing

hyperalimentation—intravenous feeding; total parenteral nutrition (TPN), literally

hyperglycemia—high blood glucose level

hypersensitivity—excessive response of the immune system to a sensitizing antigen

hypersensitivity reaction—the reaction that occurs when a person is exposed to a compound previously and has generated antibodies against the compound

hypertension—disorder characterized by elevated blood pressure

hypnotic—a drug used to induce sleep

hypoglycemic—a drug that lowers the level of glucose in the blood; used primarily by diabetics

hypolipodemic—an agent to reduce lipids (fat) in the blood

hypometabolic—low basic metabolic rate

hypotension—low blood pressure

ideal drug therapy—safe, effective, timely, and cost-conscious medication use

immunity—the condition of being resistant to a particular disease (e.g., polio)

immunomodulators—agents that adjust the immune system to a desired level

incompatibility—lack of compatibility; an undesirable effect when two or more substances are mixed together

incubation—the period between exposure to an infective disease process and the symptoms of infection

independent pharmacy—a retail pharmacy owned and operated by an individual pharmacist or group of individuals as contrasted to chain drug stores

indirect contact transmission—infection through contact with a contaminated object

infection—the state or condition in which the body (or part of it) is invaded by an agent (microorganism or virus) that multiplies and produces an injurious effect (active infection)

infection control—the use of appropriate procedures and education to minimize the transfer of infections from one to another

infiltration—occurs when an intravenous solution is infused into the surrounding tissues instead of directly into the vein as intended

inflammation—the condition characterized by pain, heat, redness, and swelling

infusion—the introduction of a solution into a vein by gravity or by an infusion control device or pump

infusion pump—regulates the flow of an intravenous solution

infusion therapy—introduction of fluid into the body usually by intravenous route

in-house pharmacy—pharmacy located within the facility

injection—the introduction of a fluid substance into the body by means of a needle and syringe

inoculum—microorganism or other material introduced into a system

inpatient—a patient who requires the use of a hospital bed and is registered in the hospital to receive medical or surgical care

input devices—keyboards, light pens, optical scanners, bar code readers

institutional pharmacy—pharmacy services provided in hospitals, nursing homes, health maintenance organizations, prisons, mental retardation facilities, or other settings wherein groups of patients are provided formal, structured pharmacy programs

intensive care unit (ICU)—a unit within a hospital where the patient receives constant and vigilant attention

intermittent injection—the administration of a drug over 15 minutes to 4 hours after which there is a period of no drug administration followed again by cycles of administration and periods of no administration

intoxication—state of being poisoned by a drug or being inebriated with alcohol

intradermal—situated or applied within the skin

intramuscular—within the muscle

intraocular—within the eye

intrasynovial—into the fluid of a joint

intrasynovial (IS)—injection directly into joint fluid

intrathecal—within the subdural space of the spinal cord

intravenous (IV)—within a vein; administering drugs or fluids directly into the vein to obtain a rapid or complete effect from the drug

inventory—a complete listing of the exact amounts of all the drugs in stock at a particular time

investigational drugs—drugs that have not received approval for marketing by the Food and Drug Administration

iontophoresis—use of an electric current to cause an ionized drug to pass through the skin into the system circulation

iso-osmotic—having the same tone

isotonic—having the osmotic pressure

IV admixture—intravenous solutions to which medications are added

IV push—the administration of a drug by directly pushing the barrel of the syringe to inject its contents directly into a vein; also known as bolus

jaundice—yellow appearance of skin and mucous membranes resulting from the deposition of bile pigment

job description—a guideline written by the employer for the employee that outlines the requirements and limits of the job

Joint Commission on Accreditation of Healthcare Organization (JCAHO)—not-for-profit organization whose standards are set to ensure effective quality services (e.g., optimal standards for the operation of hospitals)

judge—the trier of law (and of fact if there is no jury)

jury—generally composed of from six to twelve persons. The jury is the trier of facts.

laboratory—a hospital department where chemical or biological testing is performed for the purpose of aiding diagnosis

lacrimal fluids—tears

leaching—effect of removing a soluble substance from a solution

legend medication—a drug that is only available to a patient with a prescription from a licensed prescriber; also known as prescription medication

leukemia—a disease characterized by an extremely high white blood cell count

levigation—mixing of particles with a base vehicle, in which they are insoluble, to produce a smooth dispersion of the drug by rubbing with a spatula on a tile

liability—that responsibility imposed upon a party who breaches a duty owed to another person

lipophilic—lipid-loving

liposome—a small membrane that entraps and later releases an active ingredient

local area networks (LAN)—permit different systems (mainframe, minicomputers, and microcomputers), as well as computers made by different manufacturers, to communicate and share data

long-term care—health care provided in an organized medical facility for patients requiring chronic or extended treatment

long-term care facility—for individuals who do not need hospital care but are in need of a wide range of medical, nursing, and related health and social services

lotions—liquid preparations intended for external application

lozenge—a small, medicated or flavored disk intended to be dissolved in the mouth

LSD—lysergic acid diethylamide, a hallucinogen; also known as beast, black sunshine, the chief

Maimonides—Rabbi Moses ben Maimon, Spanish-born teacher and physician

mainframe—the largest, most powerful type of computer system; is able to service many users at once and process several programs simultaneously; has large primary and secondary storage capacities

malaria—an infectious fever-producing disease, transmitted by infected mosquitos

malfeasance—commission of a substandard act

malignant—a type of tumor that invades healthy tissue and becomes progressively worse

malpractice—a deviation from the standard of care that arises out of a professional relationship; also called *professional negligence*

managed care—provision of health care services in the most cost-effective way

MAO inhibitors—a class of drugs that act as antidepressants by inhibiting the enzyme monoamine oxidase

marijuana—substance, from hemp, that has an effect on mood, perception, and psychomotor coordination; also known as sinse, weed, herb, grass, dope, reefer, maryjane

mastectomy—removal of the breast

materia medica—the branch of pharmacy that deals with drugs and their source, preparation, and use

materials management—the division of a hospital pharmacy responsible for the procurement, control, storage, and distribution of drugs and pharmaceutical products

matrix management—an organizational concept that emphasizes the interrelationship between departments and the common area of decision-making

Medicaid—a state health care coverage program with some federal funding assistance for persons with low income, minimal assets, and no health care coverage as mandated by Title XIX of the Social Security Act. Medicaid may go by different names in different states; often known as *medical assistance programs*.

medical records—the hospital department responsible for the maintenance and review of patients' medical charts

Medicare—a federal health care coverage program for those 65 years of age and over, certain disabled persons, and persons with end-stage renal disease as mandated by Title XVIII of the Social Security Act of 1965. Medicare includes Part A and Part B, which cover both hospital care and outpatient services.

medication administration record (MAR)—a record maintained by the nursing staff containing information about the patient's medication and its frequency of administration

medication administrator—person who administers or gives medication to patients; *see also* **medication technician**

medication related problems (MRPs)—Undesirable events a patient experiences involving drug therapy that interfere with a desired patient outcome

medication technician—an individual responsible for administering drugs to a patient; also known as the medication administrator

medium—solvent used in dissolution testing

memory—the storage of both data and instructions internally in the computer

meninges—the membrane that surrounds the brain and spinal cord

meningitis—inflammation of the meninges

meniscus—the outer surface of a liquid having a concave or crescent shape, caused by surface tension

metabolism—the process by which an organism converts food to energy needed for anabolism

metabolite—a chemical synthesized within cells as part of a metabolic pathway

metastasis—the spread of disease from one organ to another

micronized drug particles—very small drug particles that have a diameter in the smallest size range

microorganism—a microscopic plant or animal

milliequivalent (mEq)—one-thousandth of an equivalent weight

milling—reducing the particle size

Millis Study Commission—published a report in 1975 titled "Pharmacist for the Future." Its main premise stated that pharmacy is a knowledge profession.

minicomputer, microcomputer, or personal computer systems—systems used for well-defined and specialized applications

miotic—a drug that causes constriction of the pupil

mnemonic codes—short entries that are easy to remember and represent a longer instruction used to assist in the entry of data

moiety—a part of a molecule that exhibits a particular set of chemical and pharmacologic characteristics

molecular form—the drug form which elicits biological responses regardless of dosage form

monastery—the dwelling place for persons under religious vows who live in ascetic simplicity

morbidity—a disease state; the ratio of the sick to the well in a given area

morgue—a place where a corpse is kept until released for burial

mortality—occurrence of death; the ratio of deaths to the living in a given area

mucolytic—a substance that liquifies, dissolves, or digests mucus

multiple sclerosis—a degenerative disease of the central nervous system

mydriatic—an agent that dilates the pupil of the eye

myocardial infarction (MI)—injury to the heart muscle (myocardium) due to inadequate oxygen supply caused by the occlusion of a coronary artery

NAHC—National Association for Home Care

narcotic—a drug that is habit forming and addictive and produces relief from pain

narcotic antagonists—agents that oppose or overcome effects of a narcotic

nephritis—inflammation of the nephron

nephron—functional unit of the kidney

neurosonology—laboratory section of the neurology department specifically referring to EEG, EMG, carotid Doppler, brain mapping, etc.

NKA—no known allergies

noncompliance—forgetting or purposefully not taking medications as prescribed

nosocomial—an infection or illness that occurs as a result of the patient's stay in the hospital or health facility

objective—the purpose or goal toward which effort is directed

obstructive jaundice—jaundice that results from an impediment to the flow of bile from the liver to the duodenum

occlusion—blockage of a blood vessel

Occupational and Safety Act—federal law that assures every working man and woman in the nation safe and healthful working conditions; established the Occupational Safety and Health Administration (OSHA)

ointment—oil-based, semisolid, external dosage form, usually containing a medicinal substance

oleaginous—resembling or having the properties of oil

oncology—the study or knowledge of tumors; commonly refers to the study of cancer and related diseases

one-compartment model—the simplest case in pharmacokinetics in which the body is thought to behave as a single homogeneous compartment

operating room—a unit in the hospital where major surgical procedures are performed

operational manual—lists only those policies and procedures that affect the internal working of the pharmacy department

orphan drugs—drugs used for diseases and conditions considered rare in the United States, for which adequate drugs have not yet been developed and do not generate incentives for drug manufacturers to research and develop

osteoporosis—disorder characterized by abnormal porosity of bone, usually in older women

ostomy—an artificial opening into the gastrointestinal tract

outcome competency—the measurable, desired ability, knowledge, and skill achieved upon completion of program

outpatient department—an area of the hospital where various medical services are provided to patients who do not require a hospital bed (outpatients)

output devices—video display terminal (VDT), cathode ray tubes (CRT), printers, and plotters

over-the-counter (OTC) drug—a drug that can be sold without a prescription

oxytocic—an agent that causes uterine contractions

palliative—a treatment that provides relief, but no cure for a condition

pandemic—a global epidemic disease

parenteral—a sterile, injectable medication; introduction of a drug or nutrient into a vein, muscle, subcutaneous tissue, artery, or spinal column; often refers to intravenous infusions of nutritional solutions; *see also* **total parenteral nutrition**

parenteral solution—sterile solutions intended for subcutaneous, intramuscular, or intravenous injection

passive diffusion—movement of drug molecules from an area of high concentration to one of a lower concentration

pathogen—any disease-producing organism

pathology—study of the characteristics, causes, and effects of disease

patient controlled analgesia (PCA) pump—a device used to administer continuous infusion, but that also allows the patient to provide boluses of pain medication as the need arises

patient medication profile—a record kept in the pharmacy of patient data and current drug therapy. It contains such information as initiation and discontinuation of medication orders and dosage form and strength. It also indicates any allergies, diagnosis, or other information pertinent to drug therapy.

patient package insert—an informational leaflet written for the lay public describing the benefits and risks of medications

patient profile—a document that is used to incorporate patient information, allergies, sensitivities, and all medications the patient is receiving, both active and discontinued

Patient's Bill of Rights—a declaration ensuring that all patients, inpatients, outpatients, and emergency service patients are afforded their rights in a health care institution

PC—personal computer

PCA—patient controlled analgesia

PCP—phencyclidine, a hallucinogen; also known as busy bee, buzz, zombie

peptic ulcer disease (PUD)—ulceration of the stomach or duodenal lining

peptides—a compound of two or more amino acids

per diem reimbursement—payment on a preset daily rate

percutaneous—through the skin

peripheral devices—sent to a computer for processing and receive information from the CPU once the data have been processed

peripheral parenteral nutrition (PPN)—a short-term therapy used to provide nutrients directly into the peripheral veins; these solutions are lower in concentration of dextrose than TPN to prevent pain, irritation, and tissue damage

personal care and support services—the provision of nonprofessional services for patients in their place of residence

pertussis—whooping cough; an acute infectious disease of the respiratory tract

pH—a measurement of acidity or alkalinity

pharmaceutical alternates—drug products that contain the same therapeutic moiety and strength but differ in the salt, ester, or dosage form

pharmaceutical care—is the direct, responsible provision of medication-related care for the purpose of achieving definite outcomes that improve a patient's quality of life

pharmaceutical services—focus on rational drug therapy and include the essential administrative, clinical, and technical functions to meet this goal

pharmaceutics—that area of the pharmaceutical sciences that deals with the chemical, physical, and physiological properties of drugs and dosage forms and drug-delivery systems

pharmacist—a person who has (1) completed five, six, or seven years of formal education in a pharmacy school and (2) is licensed to prepare and distribute drugs and counsel on the use of medication in the state in which he/she practices

pharmacogenetics—the study of the relationship between heredity and response to drugs

pharmacognosy—the study of therapeutic agents derived from natural sources (e.g., plants)

pharmacokinetics—that branch of pharmaceutics that deals with a mathematical description of drug absorption, distribution, metabolism, and excretion and their relationship to the dosage form

pharmacology—the science that deals with the origin, nature, chemistry, effects, and uses of drugs

pharmacopeia—an authoratative treatise on drugs and their purity, preparation, and standards

pharmacotherapeutics—pertaining to the use of drugs in the prevention or treatment of disease

pharmacotherapy—the treatment of disease with medications

pharmacy—the professional practice of discovering, preparing, dispensing, monitoring, and educating about drugs

Pharmacy and Therapeutics Committee—the liaison between the department of pharmacy and the medical staff. Consisting of physicians who represent the various clinical aspects, this committee selects the drugs to be used in the hospital. The pharmacy director is the secretary and a voting member of this committee.

Pharmacy Code of Ethics—rules established for the profession by pharmacists that guide proper conduct for pharmacists

pharmacy intern—a person obtaining practical experience and training in pharmacy to meet the requirements of the state board of pharmacy for licensure as a pharmacist

pharmacy mission—to help people make the best use of medication

pharmacy resident—a graduate from an accredited pharmacy school enrolled in a program designed to develop expert skills in pharmacy practice

pharmacy service—(1) the procurement, distribution, and control of all pharmaceuticals used within the facility; (2) the evaluation and dissemination of comprehensive information about drugs and their use; and (3) the monitoring, evaluation, and assurance of the quality of drug use

pharmacy technician—a person skilled in various pharmacy service activities not requiring the professional judgment of the pharmacist; has received formal or informal skill training to participate in numerous pharmacy activities in concert with and under the supervision of a registered pharmacist

pharmacy, contemporary—a health service concerning itself with the knowledge of drugs and their effects on the body.

pharmacy, traditional—the art and science of compounding and dispensing medications.

PharmD degree—the doctor of pharmacy degree earned after a six- or seven-year course of study; emphasizes clinical (patient-oriented) professional skills

phlebitis—inflammation of the veins

phlegm—viscous mucus secreted orally

physical therapy (PT)—physical manipulation for the purpose of rehabilitation

physician—an authorized practitioner of medicine

physician assistant—an authorized practitioner of medicine who works under the responsible supervision of a licensed physician

physician order entry system—direct entry of the physician's order by the physician into the computer which can then be accessed by pharmacy

phytochemist—person who studies plant chemistry and applies these chemicals to science

PICC—peripherally inserted central catheter

piggyback—refers to a small-volume IV solution (25–250 mL) that is run into an existing IV line over a brief period of time; (e.g., 50 mL over 15 minutes)

pill—a small globular or oval medicated mass intended for oral administration

plasma—the fluid portion of the blood in which the blood cells are suspended

pleadings—the initial court papers; generally the summons, complaint, and answer

pneumatic tube system—a method of sending medication orders through the hospital by placing it in a "tube" and sending it to a dispatcher who then forwards it to the specific location

pneumonia—inflammation of lungs usually due to infection

podiatrist—a specialist in foot care

Poison Prevention Packaging Act—federal law mandating special packaging requirements that make it difficult for children under the age of five to open the package or container

policy—a defined course to guide and determine present and future decisions; established by an organization or employer who guides the employee to act in a manner consistent with management philosophy

polymer—a high-molecular-weight substance made up of identical base units

polymorphic state—a condition in which a substance occurs in more than one crystalline form

polyurethanes—substances sometimes used for linkage in elastomers

postpartum—occuring after childbirth, or delivery

PPN—peripheral parenteral nutrition

practice plan—an agreed-upon guide, written by pharmacists, on how pharmacy will be practiced in a particular setting

preferred provider organization (PPO)—an insurance plan that provides comprehensive health care through contracted providers

preferred vendor—the drug firm selected as the wholesaler

preponderance of the evidence—the burden of proof (greater than 50 percent) that a plaintiff has to meet in a civil case to obtain a favorable verdict

prescriber—a person in health care who is permitted by law to order drugs that legally require a prescription; includes physicians, physician assistants, podiatrists, dentists

prescription—permission granted orally or in writing from a physician for a patient to receive a certain medication on an outpatient basis that will help relieve or eliminate the patient's problem

prescription medication—a drug that is only available to a patient with a prescription from a licensed prescriber; also known as legend medication

preservatives—substances used to prevent the growth of microorganisms

prime vendor—drug wholesaler who contracts directly with hospital pharmacies for the purpose of their high-volume pharmaceuticals

PRN (pro res natum)—drug to be given as needed when a clinical situation arises

procedures—guidelines on the preferred way to perform a certain function; particular actions to be taken to carry out a policy

product line management—an organization concept that emphasizes the end product or category of services being delivered

prognosis—the expected outcome of the course of the disease

programs—instructions for a computer

propellant—substance used to help expel the contents of a pressurized container

prophylaxis—prevention of or protection against disease

prospective payment system (PPS)—a method of third-party reimbursement with predetermined reimbursement rates; *see also* **diagnosis-related group (DRG)**

proteins—macromolecules consisting of amino acids

protocol—a written description of how an activity, procedure, or function is to be accomplished

psychiatric—relating to the medical treatment of mental disorders

psychotropic—a drug used to treat mental and emotional disorders

pulmonary—pertaining to the lungs

purified protein derivative (PPD)—product used as a skin test for tuberculosis antibodies

quality assurance—a method of monitoring actual versus desired results in an effort to ensure a certain level of quality that meets predetermined criteria

quality assurance program—a format that elaborates special basic quality assurance steps

quality of life—a meaningful life for the patient at the optimum level of functioning for as long as possible

quality standards—the minimum results needed to achieve a desired level of quality

quasi-legal standards—recognized standards that are similar to law

radiation therapy—the use of X-rays in the treatment of a disease

radiology (X-ray) department—an area of the hospital where diagnosis and treatment are performed using X-rays, radioisotopes, and other similar methods

radiopaque—having the property of absorbing X-rays

radiopharmacy—a branch of pharmacy dealing with radioactive diagnostics

reconstitute—add a sterile solvent to a sterile active ingredient for injectable purposes

recovery room (RR)—area in the hospital where patients are monitored and treated immediately after leaving the operating room

Red Cross–Red Crescent—an international health-oriented institution that provides emergency and ongoing assistance in situations of need

refractory—resistant to treatment or a stimulus

regulation—an authoritative rule dealing with details of procedure

regulatory law—the area of law that deals with governmental agencies and how they enforce the intent of the statutes under which they operate

renal—pertaining to the kidney

residents' rights—refers to those rights that residents have within the long-term care facility, such as confidentiality and maintenance of dignity

respiration—the breathing process

retailer—the company responsible for delivering product to patients

ribonucleic acid (RNA)—a single-stranded structure that is the molecular basis for protein synthesis

robotics—technology based on a mechanical device, programmed by remote control to accomplish manual activities such as picking medications according to a patient's computerized profile

rubella—German measles

rule of three—the process of pharmacy personnel checking a medication being prepared and dispensed three times before it is administered to the patient

rules and regulations—promulgated by government agencies at the local, state, and federal levels

sanitarium—an institution for the treatment of chronic disease such as tuberculosis or nervous disorders

satellite pharmacy—where distribution occurs from a decentralized pharmacy staffed by at least a pharmacist and technician. The satellite usually handles all the needs of the units for which they are responsible.

scanners—optical recognition devices that can read preprinted characters or codes

secondary storage—data and programs maintained on tapes or discs

sedative—a drug used to allay anxiety and excitement; often used to help a patient sleep

sepsis—presence of pathogenic organisms in the blood

serum—the clear fluid of the blood separated from solid parts

side effects—known effects of a drug experienced by most people taking the drug; these are usually minor

signs—objective bodily evidence of distress found by physical examination

site survey—the visit by representatives of ASHP to review the training program to ascertain compliance with the standards

soft copy—visual display units

software—the actual programs for the computer system

solution—a homogeneous mixture of one or more substances dispersed in a dissolving solvent; clear liquid with all components completely dissolved

solution balance—single unequal arm balance used for weighing large amounts

solvation—process by which a solute is incorporated into the solvent

solvent—a substance used to dissolve another substance

stability—a condition that resists change; for example a drug maintains potency

standard—a reference to be used in evaluating institutional programs and services

standard of care—the acceptable level of professional practice that exists by which the actions of a professional are judged

standards of practice—rules that pharmacists establish for the profession that represent the preferred way to practice

staphylococcus (plural, staphylococci)—microorganism of the family *Micrococcaceae* that is the most common cause of localized suppurative infections

STAT—(*statim*) to be given immediately

state board of pharmacy—body established to ensure that the public is well served professionally by pharmacists

sterile—free from microorganisms

sterilization—the act or process of rendering sterile; the complete destruction of microorganisms by heat or bactericidal compounds

stop order—stop medication. An automatic stop order requires a physician's renewal order for the medication, and after review by the pharmacist, should be discontinued.

structure criteria—specify necessary resources (e.g., equipment)

styptic—an agent that stops or slows bleeding by contracting blood vessels when applied locally

subcutaneous—under the skin

subcutaneously—under the skin; introduced beneath the skin (e.g., subcutaneous injections)

sublingual—under the tongue

sudorific—a substance that causes sweating; also called a *diaphoretic*

supportive pharmacy personnel—another term for **pharmacy technician**

suppositories—solid dosage forms for insertion into body cavities (e.g., rectum, vagina, urethra) where they melt at body temperature

surface active agents—substances that lower the surface tension of liquids

surfactants—surface active agents, commonly known as *wetting agents*

suspending agents—chemical additive used in suspensions to "thicken" the liquid and retard settling of particles

suspension—liquid containing finely divided drug particles uniformly distributed

symptom—subjective evidence of a disease; evidence of disease as perceived by the patient

syncope—fainting; a transient loss of consciousness due to inadequate blood flow to the brain

syndrome—a group of signs and symptoms that characterize a particular abnormality

synergies—groups working together in cooperation

synergism—a joint action of agents in which the total effect of the combination is greater than the sum of their individual independent effects

synthesize—to produce by bringing elements together to form a chemical compound

syrup—a concentrated sugar solution that may have an added medicinal

system software—contains the operating system that includes master programs for coordinating the activities of the hardware and software in a computer system

systemic—relating to the body as a whole, rather than individual parts or organs

systemic action—affects the body as a whole

systemic side effect—an effect on the whole body, but secondary to the intended effect

systolic—the force exerted by the blood when the ventricles are in a state of contraction

table of contents—an index for easy referral to the appropriate policies and procedures

tablet—a solid dosage form of varying weight, size, and shape that contains a medicinal substance

tachycardia—rapid heart rate

tare—a weight used to counterbalance the container holding the substance being weighed

tax-free alcohol—ethyl alcohol obtained at cost under applicable federal regulations to be used only for diagnostic and therapeutic purposes

telephone order—an order for a drug or other form of treatment that is given over the phone to an authorized receiver by an authorized prescriber

teratogenic—substance that interferes with normal prenatal development

testosterone—a hormone that produces secondary sex characteristics in the male

Theophrastus—a Greek philosopher and botanist who classified plants by pharmaceutical actions

therapeutic—provision of treatment of a disease, infirmity, or symptom by various methods

therapeutic alternates—drug products that contain different therapeutic moieties but that are of the same pharmacologic or therapeutic class

therapeutic effect—a healing, curative, or ameliorating effect

therapeutic equivalent—a drug product that, when administered in the same amount, will provide the same therapeutic effect and pharmacokinetic characteristics as another drug to which it is compared

therapeutic substitution—the substitution of one drug product with another that differs in composition but is considered to have the same or very similar pharmacologic and therapeutic activity

therapy—treatment of disease

thrombophlebitis—inflammation of a vein with a secondary blood clot formation

thrombosis—development or presence of a blood clot

tincture—an alcoholic or hydroalcoholic solution containing a medicinal substance

title—indicates the subject that is covered

TO—abbreviation for telephone order; sometimes referred to as VO (verbal order)

tocolytic—substance that delays or prolongs birth process

topical—pertaining to the surface of a part of the body

total parenteral nutrition (TPN)—intravenous nutrition comprised of any or all of the following: amino acids, dextrose, lipids, vitamins, minerals, trace elements, electrolytes, and water in a prepared sterile solution that infuses into a large central venous blood vessel. TPN provides all of the essential nutrients needed for patients to survive if they are unable to ingest nutrients. *See also* **parenteral.**

toxic—a toxin that has been detoxified by moderate heat and chemical treatment that retains its antigenicity

toxic effect—acute or chronic poisoning through use of pharmaceuticals

toxicity—degree to which something is poisonous

toxicology—the scientific study of poisons and their actions, detection, and treatment of conditions caused by them

toxin—a poison

toxin, bacterial—a noxious or poisonous product that causes the formation of antibodies called antitoxins

TPN—total parenteral nutrition

trachea—windpipe

tracheotomy—an incision into the trachea

training program—the whole course of study (didactic, laboratory, and experiential) to prepare the student for a career

tranquilizer—a drug to relieve anxiety or agitation

transdermal—entering through the dermis or skin, as in administration of a drug applied to the skin in ointment or patch form

triturate—to reduce particle size and mix one powder with another

troche—a small tablet intended to dissolve in the mouth to deliver medication to the mouth or throat

tuberculin skin test—a test performed to identify exposure to the tuberculosis bacillus

unit dose—a single-use package of a drug. In a unit-dose distribution system, a single dose of each medication is dispensed prior to the time of administration.

universal claim form (UCF)—a pharmacy prescription claim form that is utilized to serve as the basis for reimbursement of prescriptions dispensed

Universal-Standard Precautions—a set of standards mandated by OSHA based upon CDC recommendations to reduce the risk of occupational exposure to disease

urticaria—eruption or rash associated with severe itching.

USP—*United States Pharmacopeia*

utilization review—work of committee that determines how use of resources meets criteria and standards

vaccination—introduction of a vaccine into the body to produce immunity to a particular disease (e.g., smallpox inoculation)

vaccine—a suspension of attenuated or killed bacteria, viruses, or rickettsiae administered for the prevention, amelioration, or treatment of infectious diseases (e.g., tetanus)

valence—those electrons that are associated with bonds between elements

vasconstriction—narrowing of blood vessels

vascular—related to or containing blood vessels

vasoconstrictor—a process, drug, or substance that causes constriction of blood vessels

vasodilation—relaxation of smooth muscles of the vascular system that produces dilation of the blood vessel

vasodilator—an agent or drug that causes dilitation of the blood vessels; increases the caliber of the blood vessels

vector-borne transmission—infection through contact with infection carrying insects or animals

ventricular fibrillation—rapid ineffectual action of the ventricle of the heart

verbal order—an order for a drug or other treatment that is given verbally to an authorized receiver by an authorized prescriber

verified—reviewed and approved as true and authentic

vertical health integration—a process that provides a continuum of care for the patient from hospital to ambulatory care, to home care, to long-term care

vertical hood—biological containment hood used to prepare anticancer drugs and other selective injectables

vertical laminar flow hood—an air filter process to maintain a particulate-free environment

vertigo—a sensation the patient experiences that the external world is revolving around the patient; dizziness

video display terminal (VDT)—displays computer activities; sometimes referred to as *CRT* (cathode ray tube)

virus—a submicroscopic agent of infectious disease that is capable of reproduction

viscosity—an expression of the resistance of a fluid to flow

vitamin—a general term for a number of organic substances that occur in many foods in small amounts required for normal growth and maintenance of life

VO—voice order

volatile—evaporates at low temperature

volumetric check—an accuracy check for the rate of flow for an intravenous infusion

written order—an order for a drug or other form of treatment that is written on the appropriate form by an authorized prescriber

Index

AACP (American Association of Colleges of Pharmacy), 140, 142, 143, 144, 145, 271
AAPS (American Association of Pharmaceutical Scientists), 140, 145
AAPS PharmSci, 145
AAPT (American Association of Pharmacy Technicians), 140, 141, 143, 271, 463
  Code of Ethics for Pharmacy Technicians, 130
AARP (American Association of Retired Persons), 114
  and medication noncompliance, 119
Abbokinase, 334
Abbreviations
  amount, 182
  to avoid, 441–444
  dosage, 182
  medical, 154–156
  metric, 188
  preparations, 182
  routes, 183, 326–328
  special instructions, 183
  timing, 184
Abelcet, 341
Absorbine Jr., 351
Absorbing agents, 339
ACA (American College of Apothecaries), 142, 143
Academy of Managed Care Pharmacy (AMCP), 140, 143, 145
Academy of Pharmacy Practice and Management (APPM), 142
Academy of Students of Pharmacy (ASP), 142
Acarbose, 337
ACCP (American College of Clinical Pharmacy), 141, 143, 271
Accreditation, technician training
  and ASHP (American Society of Health-System Pharmacists), 462–464
    Model Curriculum for Pharmacy Technician Training, 463
  program, 463–464
  and workforce needs, 461–462

Accreditation (defined), 481
Accupril, 336, 477
Accusource Monitoring System, 40
Accutane, 477
ACE (angiotensin converting enzyme) inhibitors, 334, 336, 477, 478, 479, 481
Acetaminophen, 154, 160, 331, 332, 350, 351
  elixir, 185
  with oxycodone, 480
Acetazolamide, 158, 161, 477
Acetohexamide, 161, 477
Acetylsalicylic acid, 12, 332. *See also* Aspirin
Achlorhydria, 481
Achromycin, 157
Acid disorder medications, 356–358
Acidity, 11
Acidosis, 481
AcipHex, 339, 477
ACPE (American Council on Pharmaceutical Education), 140, 144, 271, 481
Acquired immune deficiency syndrome. *See* AIDS
Actifed, 157
Actiq, 216, 332
Activase, 157, 334
Actonel, 331, 477
Actos, 337, 477
Actron, 351
AcuDose-Rx, HBOC/McKesson, 288
Acutrim, 176
Acyclovir, 39, 160, 341
Adalat, 157
  CC, 334, 336
Adenocard, 333
Adenosine, 333
Admission/discharge and transfer system (ADT), 427, 481
Admixture (defined), 481
Adrenalin, 442
Adriamycin, 477
ADT (admission/discharge and transfer system), 427, 481
Adverse drug reactions (ADRs), 122, 415, 481. *See also* Side effects
  information sources, 267

MedWatch FDA form, 80, 81, 140–141
  reporting, 80, 81
Advil, 157, 351
AeroBid, 344
Aerosol (defined), 481
Aerosols, 174
Afrin, 157, 353
AIDS (acquired immune deficiency syndrome), 17
  and health care worker infection control, 296–297
  home infusion therapy, 38–39, 41
  medication, 61, 478
Aim Plus ambulatory pump, 46
Alavert, 345
Albuterol, 160, 161, 344, 477
Alcohol, tax-free/taxable, 78–79
Alcott, Louisa May, 10
Aldactazide, 471
Aldactone, 336
Aldomet, 157, 161, 337, 477
Aldoril, 161, 477
Alendronate, 331
Aler-Dryl, 353
Aleve, 332, 351
Alginate, 357
Alkalinity, 11
Alkaloids, 12, 481
Alkalosis (defined), 481
Alka-Seltzer, 350, 351
Alkeran, 477
Allegra, 345
Allergies, 151, 481
  aspirin, 351
  to aspirin, 356
  and herbal preparations, 369
  to medications, 236
  medications for, 345
  nonprescription medications, 352–353
  pollen, 369
  and profiles/reviews/counseling, 90–91
  and reactions, 51, 122
Allopathy (defined), 5, 481
Allopurinol, 160, 477
Alpha-adrenergic blockers, 336, 478, 479

Alpha-1 antitrypsin, 43
Alprazolam, 160, 161, 343, 477
Altace, 336, 477
Alteplase, 157, 334
AlternaGEL, 157, 339, 357
Alternative medicine. *See also*
    Herbals
  information resources, 267
  National Center for
    Complementary and Alternative
    Medicine, 371
  statistics, USA, 117
Altrovent, 161
Alu-Cap, 357
Aluminum-containing antacids, 339
Aluminum hydroxide, 157, 170, 357
  concentrated, 157
Aluminum phosphate, 357
Alupent, 161, 344, 477
Alza Corporation
  Ocusert System, 176–177
  OROS (oralosmosis), 176
Amantadine, 341
Amaryl, 337, 477
Ambien, 343, 477
Ambulatory care, 481. See *also* Home
    infusion therapy
Ambulatory infusion centers, 37–38
Amcill, 161
AMCP (Academy of Managed Care
    Pharmacy), 140, 143, 145
Amen, 477
American Association of Colleges of
    Pharmacy (AACP), 140, 142, 143,
    144, 145, 271
American Association of
    Pharmaceutical Scientists
    (AAPS), 140, 145
American Association of Pharmacy
    Technicians (AAPT), 140, 141,
    143, 271, 463
  *Code of Ethics for Pharmacy
    Technicians*, 130
American Association of Retired
    Person (AARP), 114
  and medication noncompliance,
    119
American College of Apothecaries
    (ACA), 142, 143
American College of Clinical
    Pharmacy (ACCP), 141, 143, 271
American Council on Pharmaceutical
    Education (ACPE), 140, 144, 271,
    481
American Druggist Blue Book, 481
American Hospital Formulary Service,
    145, 266, 400
*American Journal of Health System
    Pharmacists*, 145
*American Journal of Hospital
    Pharmacy*, 266
*American Journal of Pharmaceutical
    Education*, 145

American Journal of Pharmacy, 145
American Lung Association, 271
American Medical Association, 271
American Pharmaceutical
    Association, 362, 463
  Code of Ethics for Pharmacists, 130,
    131
American Pharmacists Association
    (APhA), 140, 143, 145, 271, 466
  academies, 142
  history/overview, 141–142
  meetings, large, 142
American Society for Pharmacy Law,
    271
American Society of Association
    Executives, 141
American Society of Consultant
    Pharmacists (ASCP), 143, 145,
    271
American Society of Health-System
    Pharmacists. *See* ASHP
America's Pharmacist, 145
Amikacin, 38, 341
Amikin, 341
Amiloride, 477
Aminoglycosides, 38, 340, 341
Amiodarone, 161, 333, 477
Amitone, 357
Amitriptyline, 158, 161, 343, 477
Amlodipine, 159, 334, 336, 477
Ammonium chloride, 171
Amoxicillin, 157, 342, 480
Amoxicillin/clavulanate, 342
Amoxil, 157, 161, 342
Amphetamines, 151, 482
Amphojel, 157, 357
Amphotericin B, 38, 158, 341
Ampicillin, 38, 342
Ampicillin/sulbactam, 38, 342
Ampule handling, 234, 235
Amrinone, 161, 477
Anabolic agent, 482
Anabolism, 151, 482
Anacin, 351
Anafranil, 161, 478
Analgesics, 151, 217, 332, 471, 477,
    478, 479, 480, 482
  scheduling, 246
Anaphylaxis, 151, 482
  anaphylactic shock, 51
  home infusion therapy, 43
Anaprox, 332
Ancef, 157
Anesthetics, 151, 332, 478
Aneurysm, 151, 482
Angelica, 371, 372
Angina pectoris, 333
Angiotensin converting enzyme
    (ACE) inhibitors, 335, 336, 477,
    478, 479, 481
Angiotensin II receptor blockers
    (ARBs), 335, 336
Anhydrous bases, 175

Anhydrous (defined), 482
Anionic (defined), 482
Annals of Pharmacotherapy, 266
Antacids, 168, 170, 339, 357–358, 482
Antiacne drug, 477
Anti-Alzheimer drugs, 477, 480
Antianemia agents, 471
Antianxiety agents, 343, 477, 478, 480
Antiarrhythmic agents, 477, 479, 482
Antibacterials, 477, 480
Antibiotics, 45, 340, 341–342, 471,
    477, 479, 480, 482
  broad-spectrum, 16
  home infusion therapy, 30, 38–39
  and infection control, 296
  mycin-type, 247
  powder form, 234
  syrup form, 168
Anticholinergics, 344, 477, 482
Anticoagulants, 356, 471, 477, 482
Anticonvulsants, 342, 478, 479, 480
Antidepressants, 343, 455, 477, 478,
    479, 480
Antidiabetes agents, 477, 478
Antidotes, 8, 482
Antiemetics, 42, 217, 372, 471, 480
Antifungals, 38, 171, 341–342, 455,
    479, 480
Antigens, 151, 482
Antiglaucoma drug, 477
Antigout agents, 477
Antihistamines, 344, 345, 352, 471,
    478, 480, 482
  nonsedating, 353
Antihypertensives, 117, 455, 477, 478,
    479, 480
Anti-infectives, 217, 373, 477
Anti-inflammatory agents, 331, 350,
    351, 477
Antimalarials, 477, 479
Antimicrobials, 455
Antimotility agents, 339
Antineoplastic agents, 89, 471, 477,
    478, 479, 480, 482. *See also*
    Chemotherapy
Antiobesity agents, 480
Antiparkinson agents, 478, 480
Antiplatelet agents, 479, 480
Antipruritic (defined), 482
Antipsoriasis agents, 480
Antipsychotic agents, 477, 478, 479,
    480
Antipyretics, 151, 350, 482
Antipyrine, 157
Antiseptics, 151, 170, 373, 482
Antispasmodics, 12
Antitoxins, 12, 16, 482
Antitussives, 151, 352, 353, 482
Antiulcer drugs, 477
Antivert, 157, 345
Antivirals, 340, 341, 478, 479, 480
Antiviral therapy, 340
  home infusion therapy, 39, 42

Anxiety, 343, 352
APhA. *See* American Pharmacists Association
Apothecary symbols, 157
Apothecary system of weights
conversion, 190–192
liquid measure, 191
notation, 191
APPM (Academy of Pharmacy Practice and Management), 142
Apresazide, 161, 477
Apresoline, 157, 161, 337, 477
Arabian historical influence, 9
Aralen, 477
ARBs (angiotensin II receptor blockers), 335, 336
Area under concentration time curve (AUC), 321, 322
Aredia, 477
Argatroban, 334
Aricept, 157, 477
Aripiprazole, 477
Arixtra, 334
Arlidin, 477
Armour Thyroid, 338
Arrhythmia, 151, 332
medications, 332–333, 477, 479
Arsenic, 12
Arsphenamine, 12
Artane, 157, 477
Arteriosclerosis, 151, 482
Arthritis, 151, 372, 482
septic, 38
Arthropan, 351
Art of Healing (Galen), 6
Asacol, 477
Ascites, 151, 482
ASCP (American Society of Consultant Pharmacists), 143, 145, 271
Ascriptin, 351
Aseptic process, 42, 151, 482. *See also* Infection control
chlorhexidine gluconate, 233
handwashing, 233, 243, 301–302
IV medications, 116
laminar airflow hoods, 230–234, 294, 295, 496
parenteral admixtures, 226–227
and pharmaceutical infection control, 295
povidone-iodine, 233
principles, 296
ASHP (American Society of Health-System Pharmacists), 76, 140, 141, 143, 145, 271, 466, 481–482
alternative medicine survey, 117
Guidelines for Selecting Pharmaceutical Manufactures and Suppliers, 395
Guidelines on Managing Drug Product Shortages, 398

handling cytotoxic/hazardous drugs, 236
IV admixture recommendations, 116
labeling recommendations, 295
meetings, large, 142
Model Curriculum for Pharmacy Technician Training, 463
overview, 142
practice standards, 93
"Provision of Medication Information by Pharmacists," 260
sterile guidelines, 44, 294
Technical Assistance Bulletin on the Evaluation of Drugs for Formularies, 395
and technician training accreditation, 462–464
Web site, 260
"White Paper on Pharmacy Technicians," 128
ASP (Academy of Students of Pharmacy), 142
Asparaginase, 477
Aspercerem, 351
Aspergel, 351
Aspirin, 154, 331, 332, 350, 351, 356
allergy, 351
containers, 88
history, 12
Association Web sites, 271
Asthma, 69, 343
Atacand, 336
Atarax, 157, 161, 343, 477
ATC Profile, AutoMed Technologies, 288, 289
Atenolol, 160, 161, 336, 477
ATF (Bureau of Alcohol, Tobacco and Firearms), Department of the Treasury, and alcohol, tax-free/taxable, 78
Atherosclerosis, 151, 482
Ativan, 157, 161, 343, 477
Atorvastatin, 159, 335
Atromid-S, 335
Atropine, 12
Atrovent, 344, 477
Attapulgite, 339, 355, 356
AUC (area under concentration time curve), 321, 322
Augmentin, 342
Auralgan, 157
Automated pharmacy systems, 123, 299, 446, 482
AutoMed Technologies, ATC Profile, 288, 289
Avandia, 439, 477
Avapro, 336
Avelox, 341, 477
Axid, 157, 339, 357
Aygestin, 340

Azactam, 342
Azathioprine, 442
Azithromycin, 160, 341
Azmacort, 344
Aztreonam, 342

Bacitracin, 161, 477
Bactrim, 157
Bacteremia, 294
Bactericides, 151, 340, 341–342, 482
Bactrim, 342
Bactroban, 161, 477
Balard, Antoine, 12
Banting, Frederick, 13
Barbiturates, 471, 477
BARD Mini-infuser, 48
Basaljel, 357
Bayer aspirin, 351
Beclomethasone, 160, 344
Beclovent, 344
Beconase, 344
Bedlam (Bethlehem Hospital, London), 11
Bedsore, 485
Behring, Emil von, 12, 16
Benadryl, 158, 182, 345, 353
Benazepril, 336
Ben-Gay, 351
Bentyl, 158
Benylin, 353, 477
Benzene hexachloride, 171
Benzocaine, 157
Benzodiazepines, 343, 480
Benztropine, 158
Best, Charles, 13
Beta-2 adrenergic agonists, 344
Beta-adrenergic blockers, 333, 334, 336, 477, 478, 479
Beta-interferon, 43
Betapace, 333
AF, 333
Bethlehem Hospital, London (Bedlam), 11
Bextra, 332
Biaxin, 158, 341
XL, 341
Bile, 5, 11
Bile acid resins, 335
Bill of rights, patient, 100–101, 491
Bioavailability, 482
area under concentration time curve (AUC), 321, 322
assessment methods, 320–321
studies, 321–322
Biodegradable (defined), 482
Bioengineering, 394, 483
Bioequivalence studies, 321–322
Biohazard symbol, 302
Biopharmaceutics, 483
and administration routes, 315–316

area under concentration time curve (AUC), 321, 322
assessment, bioavailability, 319–320
bioavailability, 319
bioequivalence studies, 321–322
medication distribution, physiologic, 319–320
medication elimination, 320, 329
metabolism, 320, 329, 330
studies, bioavailability, 321–322
Biopsy, 151
Biotechnology, 17
Bisacodyl, 158, 339, 354
Bismuth subsalicylate, 355, 356
Bisoprolol, 336
Bisphosphonates, 331
Black cohosh, 372
Black Plague, 10–11, 483
Blood and history, 5, 10, 11
Bloodborne disease transmission, 243, 305–306, 483
Blood clots, 333. *See also* Thrombosis
Blood pressure
   and decongestants, 344
   diastolic, 151, 334
   hypertension, 69, 117, 152, 334–335, 352, 453
   medications, 117
   screening, 70
   systolic, 154, 494
Blood urea nitrogen (BUN), 151, 480
Blue Book, American Druggist, 481
Board of Pharmaceutical Specialties (BPS), 142
Body surface area (BSA), 196–197, 476
Bolus (defined), 483
Bone disorder medications, 331–332
Bonine, 345
Boric acid, 175
Botanicals. *See* Herbals
BPS (Board of Pharmaceutical Specialties), 142
Bradycardia, 151, 332, 483
Brandes, Rudolph, 12
Brethine, 158, 344
Bretylate, 333
Bretylium, 333
Brevibloc, 477
Brevital, 477
Bromide, 166
Bromine, 12
Brompheniramine, 158, 345, 353
Bronchitis, 38
Bronchodilators, 372
BSA (body surface area), 196–197, 476
Buchner, Johannes, 12
Bufferin, 351
Buffer systems, 167
Bumetanide, 336

Bumex, 336, 477
BUN (blood urea nitrogen), 151, 480
Bupivacaine, 332
Buprenex, 477
Bupropion, 343, 477
Bureau of Alcohol, Tobacco and Firearms (ATF), Department of the Treasury, 78–79
BuSpar, 158, 343
Buspirone, 158, 343, 477
Butorphanol, 160

CAD (coronary artery disease), 333, 334, 336–337
CADD pump, 44, 47
Cafergot, 477
Caffeine, 13
Calamine lotion, 168
Calan, 158, 333, 334, 336
Calciferol, 477
Calcitonin, 331
Calcitriol, 477
Calcium, 331
   antacids, 339
   carbonate, 166, 170, 357
   palmitate, 169
Calcium-channel blockers, 333, 334, 336, 477, 479
Calcium polycarbophil, 355, 356
Calculations
   area under concentration time curve (AUC), 321, 322
   bioavailability, 319, 321
   and error prevention, 203
   fractional doses, 192–194
   IV administration, 197–201. *See also* IV administration calculation
   measurement conversion, 187–192. *See also* Measurement conversion
   pediatric dosage, 196–197
   percentage solutions, 202–203
   pharmaceutical information resources, 269
   of proportion, 185–187
   of ratio, 185
   Roman numeral values, 184
   weight-based dosages, 194–196
Camillus de Lellis, Saint, 8
Camphor, 352
Canadian historical influences, 13
Cancer, 39, 42. *See also* Oncology
   chemotherapy, 42, 326
   pain management, 41
Candesartan, 336
Candida (defined), 483
Capoten, 158, 336
Capsaicin, 351, 352
Capsules, 166, 171
   compounding principles, 217–218
Captopril, 158, 336

Capzasin, 351
Carafate, 158, 339, 477
Carbamazepine, 160, 342
Carbonic anhydrase inhibitors, 480
Carboplatin, 477
Carcinogen (defined), 483
Carcinoma, urothelial, 369
Cardene, 477
Cardiac conditions, 43
   American Heart Association, 271
   congestive heart failure (CHF), 151, 362, 484
   high heart rate, 352, 353
   medications, 88, 117, 333, 334, 336–337, 471, 478, 479
   myocardial infarction (MI), 490
   palpitations, 352
Cardioquin, 333
Cardiotonics, 12
Cardiovascular medications, 332–335, 455
Cardizem, 158, 333, 334, 336, 477
CARDS (Computer Access to Research on Dietary Supplements), 371
Cardura, 158, 336, 478
Carminatives, 6, 483
Carvedilol, 336
Castor oil, 354
Catabolism, 151, 483
Cataflam, 161, 478
Catapres, 158, 161, 337, 478
   TTS, 337
Cataract surgery, 15
Cathartics, 5, 339, 471
Cationic (defined), 483
Causae et Curae (Hildegard of Bingen), 7
Caventou, Joseph, 13
CDC (Centers for Disease Control and Prevention)
   antiretroviral recommendations, 306
   compound admixture infection control, 294
   and droplet transmission, 299
   on hepatitis B virus (HBV), 302
   multidose vials (MDVs) recommendations, 295
   universal-standard precautions, 297, 300, 495
Ceclor, 158, 341
Cefaclor, 158, 341
Cefadroxil, 341
Cefazolin, 38, 45, 157, 159
Cefepime, 38
Cefotan, 158
Cefotaxime, 38, 161, 478
Cefotetan, 38, 158
Cefoxitin, 161, 478
Cefpodoxime, 341
Ceftazidime, 38, 158, 160
Ceftriaxone, 38, 45, 160

Cefuroxime, 38, 478
Cefzil, 341
Celebrex, 332, 439, 478
Celecoxib, 332
Celera, 478
Celexa, 343, 439
Celsus (herbalist), 11
Centers for Disease Control and Prevention. *See* CDC
Centers for Medicare and Medicaid Services (CMS). *See also* Medicare
drug distribution systems, 277
LTC oversight, 58
PPS (Prospective Payment System), 31
and reimbursement, 454–455
Central nervous system
depression, 357
stimulation, 352
and sulfanilamide elixir tragedy (1937), 363
Cephalexin, 159, 341
Cephalosporins, 38, 340, 341, 478, 480
Cerebyx, 342, 439, 478
Certification. *See also* Pharmacy Technician Certification Board (PTCB)
examinations, 142
pharmacy technicians, 141
Certified pharmacy technicians (CPhTs), 142, 465. *See also* Pharmacy Technician Certification Board (PTCB)
Cetirizine, 345
CFR (Code of Federal Regulations), Title 27 (tax-free alcohol), 78
Chain pharmacies, 67–68
Chamomile flower (matricaria), 370
Charaka, 9
Charcoal, activated, 355, 356
Chemical sterilization, 220
Chemotherapy, 12
agents, 236. *See also* Antineoplastic agents
home infusion therapy, 42
CHF (congestive heart failure), 151, 362, 484
Chicken pox/varicella, 300, 304, 351
Child-resistant containers, 87
aspirin, 88
Chinese historical influence, 8
Chloramphenicol, 16, 176
Chlorhexidine gluconate, 233
Chlorine, 12
Chlorophenothane, 171
Chlorpheniramine, 158, 345, 353
Chlorpromazine, 160, 161, 442, 446, 478
Chlorpropamide, 158, 337, 446, 478
Chlor-Trimeton, 158, 345, 353, 471
Cholesterol, 169, 334, 372

testing, 70
Cholinergics (defined), 483
Choline salicylate, 351
Chooz, 357
Christian influence (historical), 7–8
Chronic obstructive pulmonary disease (COPD), 343, 344, 478
Chronulac, 339
Ciba-Geigy
Acutrim, 176
Transderm-Nitro, 176
Transderm-Scop, 177–178
Cilastatin/imipenem, 38, 342
Cimetidine, 160, 339, 357, 358
Cipro, 158
XR, 341
Ciprofloxacin, 158, 341
Cisapride, 159
Cisplatin, 477
Citracal, 331
Citric acid, 171
Citroma, 354
Citrucel, 354
Citalopram, 343
Clarinex, 345
Clarithromycin, 158, 341
Claritin, 158, 345
Class A prescription balance, 483
Class 100 environment, 44, 220, 294, 483
Clavulanate/amoxicillin, 342
Clay tablets, Mesopotamian, 8
Clean rooms, sterile environments, 44
Clemastine fumarate, 353
Cleocin, 158
Climara, 331, 340
Clindamycin, 38
diphenhydramine, 158
Clinoril, 478
Clofibrate, 335
Clomiphene, 478
Clomipramine, 478
Clonazepam, 159, 342, 343
Clonidine, 158, 161, 478, 479
Clopidogrel, 159
Clotrimazole, 159, 341
Clozaril, 478
CMS. *See* Centers for Medicare and Medicaid Services
Coagulation (defined), 484
Cocaine, 151, 442, 484
Codeine, 13, 330, 332, 479
prescription/nonprescription status, 352
Code of Ethics for Pharmacists, 130, 131
Code of Ethics for Pharmacy Technicians, 130
Code of Federal Regulations (CFR), Title 27 (tax-free alcohol), 78
Code sets/electronic transaction standards, 92

Codes of professional behavior
Code of Ethics for Pharmacy Technicians, 130
communication issues, 133–134
and decision-making, 130, 132–133
drug distribution issues, 133
ethical principles, 132
overview, 129–130
practical application, 133–134
risk/benefit response, 134–135
Cogentin, 158
Colace, 158, 339, 354, 471
Colds, 344
nonprescription medications, 352–353
Colesevelam, 335
Colestid, 335
Colestipol, 335
Colony stimulating factor, 42, 43
Colostomy, 151, 484
Combipres, 478
Combivent, 478
Combivir, 478
Common medical terms, 150–154
Communication skills, 67
Community practice
clinical services, 69–70
reimbursement, 453–454
types, 67–68
Compazine, 158, 327–328, 442, 471
Complementary medicine. *See also* Alternative medicine; Herbals
information resources, 267
National Center for Complementary and Alternative Medicine, 371
Compliance, medication, 118–119, 328
Compounding equipment
automated, 449–450
capsule filling machines, 218
counter balance, 208
digital electronic balances, 212–213
electronic mortar and pestle (EMP), 213
graduates, 211–212
heating/magnetic stirring, 213
mini-ointment mills, 213
mortar and pestle, 210–211
packaging, 214
prescription balance, 208, 210
solution balance, 208
spatulas, 209, 211
tube heat-sealers, 214
weighing papers, 209, 210
weights, pharmaceutical, 209
Compounding information resources, 267
Compounding principles, 484
capsules, 217–218
creams, 215
enteral preparations, 218–219

flavoring, 216
gummy bears, 216
liquids, 214
lollipops, 216
lotions, 218
ointments, 215
pleuronic lecithin organogel
(PLO), 215–216
solids, 214
sterilization, 219–220
suppositories, 217
suspensions, 214–215
transdermal gels, 215–216
troches, 216
Compounding services, 68–69
and drug orders, 283–284
equilibrium verification, 210
equipment cleaning, 221–222
extemporaneous, 207–222
flavoring, 216
and history, 259
infection control, 294
levigation, 215, 489
measurement, 211–212
measurement reading, 212
mixing, 211
sterilization, 219–220
technician role, 283–284
triturating, 210–211
weighing techniques, 210–212
Comprehensive Drug Abuse and
Prevention Control Act, 84,
106–108, 484
Computer Access to Research on
Dietary Supplements (CARDS),
371
Computerization, drug distribution
systems, 280–281
Computers
admission/discharge and transfer
system (ADT), 427, 481
ancillary systems, 427–428
business systems, 428
clinical support, 430–431
in community practice, 66–67
Computer Access to Research on
Dietary Supplements (CARDS),
371
computerized physician order
entry (CPOE), 243
drug distribution systems, 280–281
drug orders, 243
electronic data interchange (EDI),
430
and formulary system, 415
future, pharmacy information
systems, 431–432
hardware, 420, 423–424
hospital information systems
(HIS), 427–428, 430
and hospital pharmacies, 429–431
information servers, 425
information technology (IT),
425–426
inventory, pharmacy, 401–402, 429
long-term care (LTC), 61
in LTC, 61
networks, 424–425
overview, 419–420
policy and procedure manuals, 389
purchasing, pharmacy, 429–430
receiving, pharmacy, 429–430
software, 424
system management, 425–426
terminology, 420, 421–423
Confidentiality, 44, 101, 243–244
Congestive heart failure (CHF), 151,
362, 484
Constipation, 338, 352, 353, 356, 357,
358
medications, 338, 339, 353–355
Constipation (defined), 484
The Consultant Pharmacist, 145, 271
Consumer Product Safety
Commission, 87
Contact lenses, 176
Container types, 403
aspirin, 88
child-resistant, 87
and disability, 88
for IV medications, 228–229
noncomplying, 87–88
OTC (over-the-counter) drugs, 88
parenteral compounding,
228–229
polyvinyl chloride (PVC), 228, 229
Containment, biological
class II, 42
laminar flow hoods, 116, 230–234,
294, 295, 496
vertical hood, 42
Contamination, pharmaceutical,
294–295
Contemporary medical practice,
14–15
Contraceptives, combined oral, 340
Controlled Substances Act (CSA),
484
controlled substances (defined),
484
and DEA (Drug Enforcement
Administration), 84, 106
drug schedules, 84–85, 106–108
inventory requirements, 87
order forms, 86, 87
records, 85–86
registration, 86–87
reports, 85–86
substance destruction, 87
symbols, 85
Conversion. *See* Measurement
conversion
COPD (chronic obstructive
pulmonary disease)
medications, 343, 344, 478
Cordarone, 161, 333
Coreg, 336
Corgard, 158, 336, 338
Coronary artery disease (CAD)
medications, 333, 334, 336–337
Correctol, 354
Corticosteroids, 478, 479, 480
Cortisone, 16
Corvert, 161
Cosmas (historical physician), 7
Cost containment, LTC (long-term
care), 61
Costs, medication, 119, 395, 396. *See
also* Reimbursement
Co-trimoxazole, 342
Cough, 352, 478
Coumadin, 158, 334, 471, 477
Counseling, pharmaceutical, 69–70
and educational level, 251–252
and patient profiles/drug review,
90–91
Counterirritants, 352, 484
Courtois, Bernard, 12
Covera, 333, 334, 336
Cowpox vaccine, 12
COX-2 inhibitors, 332, 480
Cozaar, 158, 336, 478
CPhTs (certified pharmacy
technicians), 142, 465. *See also*
Pharmacy Technician
Certification Board (PTCB)
CPOE (computerized physician
order entry), 243
and formulary system, 415
Crack cocaine, 151
Cranberry, 371
Creams, compounding principles,
215
Creatinine clearance, 151, 484
Credentialing. *See also* Pharmacy
Technician Certification Board
(PTCB)
Commission on Credentialing, 484
in hospitals, 24
Medicare certification, 31–32
Crohn's disease, 39
Cromolyn, 344
intranasal, 352, 353
Crusaders' historical influence, 9
CSA of 1970. *See* Controlled
Substances Act of 1970
Custodial care, historical
development, 14
Cyclobenzaprine, 478
Cyclophosphamide, 478
Cycloserine, 478
Cyclosporine, 478
Cyotec, 158
Cyproheptadine, 478
Cystic fibrosis, 38
Cytarabine, 442
Cytomegalovirus, 39
Cytomel, 338
Cytosar, 478

Cytotec, 339, 478
Cytotoxicity, 39, 42, 236, 485
   Guidelines for Cytotoxic (Antineoplastic) Drugs, 89
   prevention, 42
   safe handling, 236
Cytovene, 478
Cytoxan, 478

Dalmane, 343
Dalteparin, 158, 334
Damian (historical pharmacist), 7
Danazol, 478
Dantrium, 478
Darvocet-N, 332, 471, 478
Daunorubicin, 478
DEA (Drug Enforcement Administration), 76, 84, 106
   Comprehensive Drug Abuse and Prevention Control Act, 484
   disposing/destroying substances, 87
   wholesaler licenses, 109
Decadron, 158
Decision-making
   ethics, 130, 132
   process, 132–133
Declaration of Helsinki, 129
Decongestants, 151, 344, 345, 352, 353, 480, 485
Decubitus ulcer, 151, 485
Deferoxamine, 478
Deinstitutionalization, 14
Delayed-action tablets, 173, 174
Deltasone, 158, 344
Demerol, 158, 183, 332
Depakote, 158, 342
Department of Health and Human Services (HHS), 92
Department of the Treasury, Bureau of Alcohol, Tobacco and Firearms (ATF), 78–79
Depot therapy, 168
Depression, 340, 343, 364, 373
Dermatological agents, 471
Desipramine, 161, 478
Desloratadine, 345
Desogen, 340
Desogestrel/ethinyl estradiol, 340
Desoxyephedrine, 352
Desyrel, 158, 343
Dexamethasone, 158, 159
Dextromethorphan, 352, 353
   and guaifenesin, 352
Dextrose solutions, 155
DiaBeta, 158, 337, 478, 480
Diabetes, 13, 69, 352, 439, 455
   American Diabetes Association, 271
   diabetes mellitus, 151, 155, 335, 336, 485

and dosage scheduling, 245–246
glucose tolerance test, 152, 487
home infusion therapy, 38
hyperglycemia, 51, 335
hypoglycemic drug scheduling, 246
oral drug, 477, 478
testing, 70
Type I/Type II, 335
Diabinese, 158, 337
Diagnosis
   diagnosis-related groups (DRGs), 30, 287, 485
   in hospitals, 22, 23, 24
Dial-a-Flow, 45
Diamox, 158, 161, 480
Diaphoretics, 372
Diarrhea, 338, 357
   medications, 338, 339, 355–356, 479
Diarrhea (defined), 485
Diazepam, 343
Dibucaine, 332
DIC. *See* Drug information centers
Diclofenac, 332
Dictionaries, medical, 268
Dicyclomine, 158
Didanosine, 341
Dietary Supplement and Health Education Act (DSHEA), 361
   labeling, 364
   Office of Dietary Supplements, 371
Dietary supplements, 364–365. *See also* Herbals
Dietary Supplements Web sites, National Institutes of Health (NIH), 371
Dietary Supplement Verification Program (DSVP), 370, 371, 485
Diflucan, 38, 158, 341
Digitalis, 12
Digitalis lanata, 362, 369
Digitalis purpurea, 362
Digitoxin, 161, 362, 478
Digoxin, 12, 159, 161, 333, 362, 471, 478
   and apical pulse rate, 249
   and St. John's wort, 370
Dilacor, 334, 336
   XR, 333
Dilantin, 158, 342
Dilaudid, 332
Diltiazem, 158, 333, 334, 336
Diluent (defined), 151
Dimenhydrinate, 158, 161, 478
Dimetane, 353
Dimetapp, 158, 345, 353
Dioscorides, Pedanios, 5–6
Diovan, 336
Diphenhydramine, 43, 158, 161, 182, 345, 353, 478

Diphenoxylate, 339
Diphosphonate, 477
Diphtheria, 12
   vaccine, 16
Diprivan, 332
Disability and drug containers, 88
Disclosure, patient, 101
Disease state management, 69–70
Disinfectant (defined), 485
Disopyramide, 333
Dispensatories, 11
Dispensatorium Pharmacopolarum, 11
Dispensing. *See also* Drug distribution systems
   home infusion therapy, 43–44
   pharmacy technicians, 284–285
   process, 114–115
   and retail pharmacy types, 113–114
   unit-dose, 405
Disposal
   and pharmaceutical management, 394
   sharps, 303, 305
Ditropan, 158
Diupres, 478
Diuresis (defined), 485
Diuretics, 5, 336, 372, 471, 477, 478, 479, 480, 485
Divalproex sodium, 158
Dizziness, 154, 352, 356, 358
DME (durable medical equipment), 32, 486
Doan's, 351
Dobutamine, 43, 478
Documentation
   drug information centers (DIC), 265
   home infusion therapy, 50
   patient information refusal, 91
   patient medication profiles, 90, 91, 280, 282
Docusate, 339
Docusate sodium, 158, 354
Dofetilide, 333
Dolophine, 332
Domagk, Gerhard, 12
Donepezil, 157
Donnagel, 356
Dopamine, 478
Dosage forms
   aerosols, 174
   and dissolution, 166
   gastrointestinal therapeutic system (GITS), 176
   isotonic solutions, 174–175
   liquid, 166–169. *See also* Liquid dosage forms
   ocular systems, 176–177
   ointments, 5, 166, 175, 215, 491
   OTC (over-the-counter drugs), 350
   overview, 165–166

pastes, 175
solid, 170–173. *See also* Solid
  dosage forms
suppositories, 175
transdermal systems, 177–178
Doxazosin, 336
  mesylate, 158
Doxorubicin, 478
Doxycyline, 160, 342
Doxylamine, 353
Dramamine, 158
DRGs (diagnosis-related groups), 30,
  287, 485
Dristan, 353
Drixoral, 353
Dropsy, 362
Drug
  development, 16
  physiochemical properties, 166
  recalls, 79
  review, prospective, 90
  samples, 113
  therapy, pharmaceutical, 121–122
  types, 106–108
Drug compatibility
  information resources, 267
  IV/parenteral, 227
Drug-control laws, federal *vs.* state,
  76–77
Drug delivery. *See* Dosage forms
Drug distribution systems, 106,
  108–109, 133, 405–406. *See also*
  Dispensing
  advancements, 287–289
  and bar codes, 281
  centralized dispensing, 278
  computerization, 280–281
  decentralized dispensing, 278
  electromechanical systems, 279
  floor stock system, 115, 276, 277
  individual prescription system,
    276–277
  and medical information system
    (MIS), 280
  and medication administration
    record (MAR), 280, 444, 445
  robotics, 288
  unit-dose system, 115–116, 250,
    277–278, 285, 286
Drug-drug interactions, 90, 122
Drug Enforcement Administration.
  See DEA
Drug Facts and Comparisons, 266
Drug information centers (DIC)
  documentation, 265
  drug information defined, 261
  Drug Information Request
    Documentation Form, 261,
    262–263
  information synthesis, 265
  obtaining background information,
    261, 264
  overview, 259–260

"Provision of Medication
  Information by Pharmacists"
  (ASHP), 260
  question answering system,
    261–265
  requestor demographics, 261, 262
  resources, 265–270
Drug/medication administration. *See*
  Medication/drug administration;
  individual listings of drugs
Drug/medication response. *See*
  Medication/drug response
Drug orders. *See also* Prescriptions
  authorized prescribers, 242
  entry flow chart, 472
  and errors, 436–445. *See also* Error
    prevention/management
  information needed, 242–243,
    278–279
  interpretation, 181–184
  medication administration record
    (MAR), 152, 243, 280, 444, 445
  and medication
    administrator/technician,
    243–244
  pharmacist role, 282–283
  physician order entry process,
    281–282
  STAT, 242
  technician role, 283–285
  transmittal to pharmacy, 279,
    282–283
  verbal, 242
Drug Quality Reporting System
  (DQRS), FDA, 79
Drug therapy, pharmaceutical
  in hospitals, 22, 23, 24
Drug Topics Red Book, 486
Drug use process, 105–106, 107, 123
Drug utilization evaluations (DUEs),
  415
DSHEA (Dietary Supplement and
  Health Education Act), 1994, 361
  labeling, 364
  Office of Dietary Supplements, 371
DSVP (Dietary Supplement
  Verification Program), 370, 371,
  485
DUEs (drug utilization evaluations),
  415
Dulcolax, 158, 339
  contraindicated liquids, 247
Duodenum
  and medication absorption,
    317–318, 486
Durable medical equipment (DME),
  32, 486
Duragesic, 158, 332
Durham-Humphrey Amendments, 79
Duricef, 341
Dyazide, 158, 336, 471
Dynacin, 161
Dynapen, 161

E. coli, 300
Ear drug/medication administration,
  248
Eastern historical influence, 8–9
Ebers papyrus, 9, 411
Echinacea, 370, 373
Eclipse elastometric device, 46
Ecotrin, 351
Edecrin, 478
Edict of 1231 (Magna Carta of
  pharmacy), 11
EDI (electronic data interchange), 92,
  430
Education. *See also* Patient teaching
  historical, 140
  and professional associations, 142,
    461–464
E.E.S., 158, 341
Effexor, 158
  XR, 343
Efficacy, 363–364
  generic drugs, 395
Egyptian historical influence, 9
Ehrlich, Paul, 12
Elastometric device, 46
Elavil, 158, 343
Eldepryl, 478
Electrocardiogram (defined), 151,
  486
Electroencephalogram, 151, 155, 486
Electrolytes (defined), 486
Electronic data interchange (EDI),
  92, 430
Electronic transaction/code sets
  standards, 92
Elixir of sulfanilamide tragedy
  (1937), 363
EMBASE (European Medline), 266
Embolisms, 51, 151, 486
Emergicenters, 17
Emesis, 486
  hyperemesis, 42
Emetics, 5
Emphysema, 43, 486
Emulsifying agents, 169, 486
Emulsions, 168–169
  mixing, 169
  stability, 169
Enalapril, 160, 161, 336, 478
Encephalitis, West Nile, 300
Endocarditis, 38
Endocrine disorder medications,
  335, 337–338
English historical influence, 12–13
Enoxaparin, 159, 334
Enteral nutrition (EN), 40–41. *See
  also* TPN (total parenteral
  nutrition)
  enteral preparation compounding
    principles, 218–219
Enteric-coated tablets (ECT), 173,
  250, 486
Enterophepatic cycling, 486

Environmental considerations, pharmaceuticals, 400, 406–407

Ephadron Nasal, 345

Ephedra, 371

Ephedrine, 345, 352

Epidemics, 4, 487

Epilepsy medications, 340, 342

Epinephrine, 43, 344, 352

Equalactin, 356

Equivalent weight (defined), 152, 487

Error prevention/management, 122, 203

   abbreviations to avoid, 441–444

   ambiguous orders, 439–441

   and confirmation bias, 446

   filling prescriptions, 444–449

   and illegible handwriting, 436–437

   look-alike drug names, 161, 437–438, 446

   and MARs (medication administration records), 444, 445

   and medication orders, 436–443

   medication-related problems (MRPs), 121, 490

   and medication selection, 445–448

   monitoring systems, 450

   preparing medications, 444–449

   prescription-filling steps, 444–445

   sound-alike drug names, 161, 439, 477–480

   and sterile admixture preparation, 449–450

   USP/ISMP Medication Error Reporting Program, 447–448

Errors prevention/management, 122

Ery-Tab, 158, 341

Erythrocyte (defined), 152, 487

Erythromycin, 341

   base, 158, 159

   estolate, 159

   ethylsuccinate, 158

Erythropoietin, 42, 43, 456

Escitalopram, 343

Esidrix, 336

Eskalith, 338

Esomeprazole, 339

Estrace, 331, 340

Estraderm, 331, 340

Estradiol, micronized, 331, 340

Estratab, 331, 340

Estrogenic drugs, PPIs (patient package inserts), 80

Estrogens, 152, 331, 479

   conjugated, 331, 340

   esterified, 331, 340

   receptor modulators, 478

   transdermal, 331, 340

Estrone, 16

Estrostep, 340

Ethical decision-making, 130, 132

Ethinyl estradiol/desogestrel, 340

Etidronate, 478

Etomidate, 478

Eulexin, 478

European Medline (EMBASE), 266

Evista, 331, 478

Ex-Lax, 354

Expectorants, 5, 152, 477, 487

Expiration dates, 406, 487

Eyedrop/eye ointment drug/ medication administration, 247, 352

Factors VIII, IX, 43

Famciclovir, 341

Famotidine, 159, 339, 357

Famvir, 341

FDA (Food and Drug Administration), 76, 487

   and bar code labeling rule, 281, 404

   certification, 398

   creation, 363

   Drug Quality Reporting System (DQRS), 79

   field checks, 81

   Form 3490, 80, 81

   "good manufacturing standards," 79

   and herbals, 161, 365, 369, 370

   home care company requirements, 49

   IND (investigational new drug) exemption, 82

   inspection, 79

   investigational drugs, 82, 474

   and IRB (institutional review board), 84

   Medical Products Reporting Program, 140–141

   MedWatch form, 80, 81, 140–141, 271

   New Drug Application (NDA), 82, 83

   new drug marketing approval, 83

   Office of Generic Drugs, 446

   patient package inserts (PPIs), 80

   and patient package inserts (PPIs), 80

   recalls, 80–81

   "Rx only" designation, 106

   safety/efficacy studies, 322

   Safety Information and Adverse Event Reporting Program, 371

   seizure, 79

Febrile (defined), 152, 487

Federal Hazardous Substances Act, 87–88

Felodipine, 334, 336

Femara, 478

FemHRT, 478

Fenofibrate, 335

Fenoprofen, 161, 478

Fentanyl, 158, 216, 332

Feverfew, 370, 372

Fexofenadine, 345

Fiberall, 339

FiberCon, 339, 354

Fibrates, 335

Fibrillation, 152, 154, 333, 495

Filtration sterilization, 220

Fioricet, 478

Fiorinal, 478

Fire safety, 89

Flagyl, 158, 342

   ER, 342

Flavoring, compounding principles, 216

Fleet Babylax, 354

Fleming, Alexander, 12

Flexall, 351

Flomax, 478

Floor stock, in-house drug distribution, 115, 276, 277

Florey, Howard, 12

Flovent, 344

Floxin, 158

Flu. See Influenza

Fluconazole, 38, 158, 341

Flumadine, 341

Flunisolide, 344

Fluorescein, 176

Fluorine, 13

Fluoroquinolones, 340, 341, 477, 479, 480

Fluothane, 332

Fluoxetine, 160, 343

Flurazepam, 343

Flurbiprofen, 161, 478

Fluticasone, 344

Fluvoxamine, 159

FMI (Food Marketing Institute), 144

Folic acid, 478

Folinic acid, 478

Fondaparinux, 334

Food, Drug, and Cosmetic Act, 76, 79, 363, 487

Food and Drug Administration. See FDA

Food Marketing Institute (FMI), 144

Formulary system, 487

   additions to formulary, 475

   adverse drug reactions (ADRs), 415

   American Hospital Formulary Service, 145, 266, 400

   attributes, 412

   clinical evaluation drug defined, 474

   closed-formulary reimbursement, 454, 484

   and computerized physician order entry (CPOE), 415

   and consensus, 412–413

   deletions from formulary, 475

drug definitions/categories,
    474–475
drug utilization evaluations
    (DUEs), 415
and economic impact, 413–414
and effectiveness/quality, 414
formulary drug defined, 474
inclusivity, 413
investigational drug defined, 474
National Formulary (NF), 362, 400
nonformulary drug defined, 475
overview, 411–412
Pharmacy and Therapeutics
    Committee, 473
process of, 412–416
publication frequency, 415–416
restricted drug defined, 474
revision, 415
surveillance activities, 415
USP, *Good Manufacturing Practices,*
    473
USP-NF, 362, 370, 400
Fortaz, 158, 341
Fosamax, 331
Foscarnet, 39
Fosinopril, 336
Fosphenytoin, 342
Foxglove, 362, 369
Fractional dose calculation, 192–194
Fragmin, 158, 334
Franklin, Benjamin, 13, 14
Frederick II, Emperor of Germany, 11
Free flow complication, 49, 51, 487
French historical influence, 12–13
Fungal disease medications, 38, 171,
    340, 341–342, 455
Fungemia, 294
Fungizone, 158, 341
Furosemide, 159, 336, 480

Gabapentin, 159, 342
Galen, Claudius, 6
Galenical (defined), 487
Gammaglobulin, 43
Ganciclovir, 39, 42
Gantanol, 161, 478
Gantrisin, 161, 478
Garamycin, 158, 341
Gargles, 5
Garlic, 370, 372
Gastroesophageal reflux disease
    (GERD), 356, 487
    medications, 338, 339, 356, 487
Gastrointestinal disorder
    medications, 338, 339, 353–358
Gastrointestinal therapeutic system
    (GITS), 176
Gatifloxacin, 341
Gaviscon, 339, 357
Geiger, Philipp, 12
Gel dosage forms, 168
    compounding principles, 215–216

Gemfibrozil, 159, 335
Generic products, 322
    therapeutic equivalency, 395
Genetic variability, patient, 330
Geneva Convention of Medical Ethics,
    129
Gentamicin, 38, 341
George III, King, 13
GERD (gastroesophageal reflux
    disease), 338, 339, 356, 487
Geriatrics. *See also* Long-term care
    (LTC)
    American Geriatrics Society, 271
    and dosage strength, 245
    and drug containers, 88
    health care coordination, 22
    information resources, 268
    and psychotropics, 61
    and swallowing, 166
German historical influence, 11–12
Gheel, Belgium (psychiatry), 11
Ginger, 370, 372
Ginkgo, 370, 372
Ginseng, 370, 371, 372
GITS (gastrointestinal therapeutic
    system), 176
Glaucoma, 353
    antiglaucoma drug, 477
Glimeperide, 337
Glipizide, 159, 161, 337, 478
Glucophage, 337
Glucose tolerance test, 152, 487
Glucotrol, 159, 337, 478
Glyburide, 158, 159, 161, 337, 478
Glycerin, 12, 339, 354
Glycopyrrolate, 160
Glycosides, 362, 478, 479, 487
Glynase, 337
GM-CSF (granulocyte macrophage
    colony stimulating factor), 43,
    456
Goldenseal, 372
Goldenseal root, 370
GoLYTELY, 339
Gonadotropin inhibition, 478
Good Manufacturing Practices (USP),
    473
Governmental Web sites, 271
Government intervention/medical
    practice, 15
GPOs (group purchasing
    organizations), 397
Granule dosage forms, 171
Greek influence (historical), 4–6
Group purchasing organizations
    (GPOs), 397
Growth hormone, 43
Guaifenesin, 160, 352
    and dextromethorphan, 352
*Guidelines for Cytotoxic
    (Antineoplastic) Drugs,* 89
Guidelines for Selecting
    Pharmaceutical Manufactures

and Suppliers, 395
Gummy bears, 216
Gynecologic medications, 338, 340

H. pylori, 356
Halcion, 159, 343
Haldol, 159, 479
Haley's M.O., 169
Halogens, 13
Haloperidol, 159
Halothane, 332
Handbook of Nonprescription Drugs,
    145
Handwashing
    health care worker infection
        control, 301
    patients in isolation, 243
Hawthorn, 370
Hazard Communication Standard
    (HCS), 88–89
Hazardous drugs/chemicals, 88–89
HBOC/McKesson
    AcuDose-Rx, 288
    ROBOT-Rx, 289
HBV (hepatitis B virus). *See*
    Hepatitis B virus (HBV)
HCFA (Health Care Financing
    Administration). *See* Centers for
    Medicare and Medicaid Services
    (CMS)
HCS (Hazard Communication
    Standard), 88–89
HCTZ, 471
HCV. *See* Hepatitis C virus
HDMA (Healthcare Distribution
    Management Association), 109
Headaches, 358, 372
Healthcare Distribution Management
    Association (HDMA), 109
Health Care Financing
    Administration (HCFA). *See*
    Centers for Medicare and
    Medicaid Services (CMS)
Health care professional
    environment, 127–128
Health care worker infection control
    antiretroviral prophylaxis, 306
    bloodborne pathogen exposure,
        305–306
    handwashing, 301
    needle-stick prevention, 301, 303,
        305
    occupational exposures, 305–307
    overview, 296
    post-exposure prophylaxis (PEP),
        305–306
    PPE (personal protective
        equipment), 297, 300–301
    sharps injury prevention, 301, 303,
        305
    worker herpes infection, 307
Health education in hospitals, 22, 23

Health Insurance Portability and Accountability Act (HIPAA), 91–93
Health maintenance organizations (HMOs), 17, 487
  care provision management, 30
  and JCAHO accreditation, 95
Heart conditions. *See* Cardiac conditions
Heat sterilization, 219–220
Hematology, information resources, 269
Hemodialysis (defined), 488
Hemolytic streptococci, 12
Hemophilia, 43
Hemophilia (defined), 488
HEN (home enteral nutrition), 40–41. *See also* Enteral nutrition (EN)
HEPA (high-efficiency particulate air) filter, 220, 230–231, 232, 234
Heparin, 43, 334
Heparin locks, 230
Hepatitis, 152, 330
Hepatitis B vaccine, 16
Hepatitis B virus (HBV), 302, 488
  and health care worker infection control, 297
  risk from needlestick, 306
  vaccine, 16, 299
Hepatitis C virus (HCV), 488
  and health care worker infection control, 297
  risk from needlestick, 306
Hep-Lock Liquaemin, 334
Herbal Medicine: Expanded Commission E Monographs, 371
Herbals. *See also* Alternative medicine
  allergic reactions, 369
  angelica, 371, 372
  aristolochic acid adulteration, 369
  black cohosh, 372
  chamomile flower (matricaria), 370
  chemical structure, 365–368
  Computer Access to Research on Dietary Supplements (CARDS), 371
  contamination potential, 369–370
  content/concentration, 369
  cranberry, 371
  Dietary Supplement Verification Program (DSVP), 370, 371, 485
  Digitalis lanata, 362, 369
  Digitalis purpurea, 362
  drug interaction potential, 370
  echinacea, 370, 373
  efficacy, 364–365
  ephedra, 371
  feverfew, 370, 372
  foxglove, 362, 369
  garlic, 370, 372
  ginger, 370, 372

ginkgo, 370, 372
ginseng, 370, 371, 372
goldenseal, 370, 372
good manufacturing practices (GMP), 364, 369, 370
hawthorn, 370
heavy metal contamination potential, 369
hypersensitivity, 369
IBIDS (International Bibliographic Information on Dietary Supplements), 371
information sources, 370–371
kava kava, 371
licorice, 371
ma huang, 371
matricaria flower (chamomile), 370
MedWatch, 371
metabolites, 365–368
milk thistle, 371, 372
National Center for Complementary and Alternative Medicine, 371
nettle root, 371
Office of Dietary Supplements (ODS), 371
overview, 361–362
preparation, 368
purple coneflower, 373
routes, 368
safety, 368–370
saw palmetto, 370, 373
St. John's wort, 364, 370, 373
traditional uses, 372–373
valerian, 370, 373
Herbarum, De Viribus (Abbott Odo), 7
Heroin, 152
Herpes zoster/shingles, 39, 304, 307
Hexadrol, 159
H2 (histamine receptor) antagonists/blockers, 339, 356–358, 480
  and cimetidine, 358
HHS (Department of Health and Human Services), 92
High-efficiency particulate air (HEPA) filter, 220, 230–231, 232, 234
HIPAA (Health Insurance Portability and Accountability Act), 91–93
Hippocrates, 4–5, 11
Hippocratic Corpus, 4–5, 129, 130
HIS (hospital information system), 427–428, 430
Histamine receptor (H2) antagonists, 356–358, 480
  and cimetidine, 358
Histamine receptor (H2) blockers, 339
HIV (human immunodeficiency virus), 488
  confidentiality, 44

  and health care worker infection control, 297
  home infusion therapy, 38–39
  medication "overload," 61
  risk from needlestick, 306
HME (home medical equipment), 32, 488
  and home infusion therapy, 34–35
HMG-CoA reductase, 334
HMG-CoA reductase inhibitors, 335
HMOs (health maintenance organizations), 17, 487
  care provision management, 30
  and JCAHO accreditation, 95
Hohenheim, Philippus Aureolus Theophrastus Bombast von, 11
Home enteral nutrition (HEN), 40–41. *See also* Enteral nutrition (EN)
Home health care
  dietitian services, 31
  equipment management, 32
  evolution of, 29–31
  home infusion therapy. *See* main heading Home infusion therapy
  managed care, 30–31
  medical social worker services, 31
  occupational therapy, 31
  personal care/support services, 32
  pharmaceutical services, 29–30, 31, 33
  physical therapy, 31
  PPS (Prospective Payment System), 31
  private duty, 32
  services, 31–33
  speech therapy, 31
Home infusion therapy, 30, 31, 32, 68
  AIDS (acquired immune deficiency syndrome), 38–39, 41
  ambulatory infusion centers, 37–38
  anaphylaxis kits, 43
  antibiotic therapy, 30, 38–39
  antiviral therapy, 39, 42
  billing clerk role, 52
  and biological containment, 42
  CADD pump, 44, 47
  and cancer, 41, 42
  case manager role, 52
  chemotherapy, 42
  complications, 50–51
  device types, 44–49
  dispensing of medication, 43–44
  disposable devices, 35, 46
  documentation need, 50
  driver/delivery representative role, 52
  drugs administered, 42–43
  EN (enteral nutrition), 40–41
  equipment management, 49–50
  equipment management services, 34–35
  FDA requirements, 49

HIV (human immunodeficiency virus), 38–39
HME-based providers, 37
and home health agencies, 37
hydration, 42
infusion devices. *See* main heading Infusion devices
infusion therapy specialty providers, 37
IV medications, 33–34, 41
legalities, 34, 43–44
and LTC, 35, 36
nursing services, 34, 43
pain management, 30, 41–42
patient service representative role, 52
and pharmacies, 33–34, 36–37
PICC (peripherally inserted central catheters), 34
Port-a-Cath, 38
preparing medications, 43–44
provider types, 35–38
purchasing manager role, 52
record-keeping, 34
technican roles, 51–52
TPN (total parenteral nutrition), 30, 38
warehouse supervisor/technician role, 52
Home medical equipment (HME), 32, 488
Homeopathy, 5
Homeostasis, historic concept, 4, 5
Homepump, 46
Hoods
class 100 clean environment, 220, 294, 483
laminar flow hoods, 116, 230–234, 294, 295, 496
vertical hood, 42, 496
Hormones, 217
discoveries, 16
Hospice care, 61
Hospitalers, Order of St. John of God, 9
Hospitals
administration, 24–25
committees, 26
departments, 23–24
drug purchasing, group, 108
functions, 21–23
governing body, 23
historical development, 13–14, 16
hospital information systems (HIS), 427–428, 430
in-house drug distribution, 115–116
medical staff, 23–24
organization, 23–26
patient processing, 22
satellite pharmacies, 116, 278
Hospital Sketches (Louisa May Alcott), 10

Humalog, 337
Human immunodeficiency virus (HIV). *See* HIV (human immunodeficiency virus)
Humulin, 16, 337
Hycodan, 161, 478
Hycomine, 161, 478
Hydralazine, 157, 161, 337, 446, 478
Hydration, home infusion therapy, 42
Hydrea, 471
Hydrochloride, 167
salt, 442
Hydrochlorothiazide, 158, 159, 336, 442
Hydrocodone, 332, 478
Hydrocortisone, 215, 442, 471, 478
HydroDIURIL, 159, 336
Hydrogel contact lenses, 176
Hydrogesic, 478
Hydromorphone, 332, 478
Hydrophilics, 167, 488
Hydropres, 478
Hydroxide, 354
Hydroxyzine, 157, 160, 161, 343, 446, 478
Hygroscopic substances, 170, 173
Hygroton, 479
Hyperalimentation, 152. *See also* TPN (total parenteral nutrition)
Hyperemesis, 42
Hyperglycemia, 51, 335, 488
Hyperlipidemia, 69, 334
medications, 334, 335, 455, 478, 479, 480
Hypersensitivity, 488
Hypertension, 69, 117, 152, 334–335, 352, 453
medications, 117, 455, 477
Hyperthyroidism, 337, 342
Hypnotic agents, 343, 477, 480
Hypoglycemic agents, 337, 477, 478, 479, 480
Hypothyroidism, 337
Hytone, 478
Hytrin, 159, 336

IBIDS (International Bibliographic Information on Dietary Supplements), 371
Ibuprofen, 157, 159, 160, 332, 350, 351
ICHP (Illinois Council of Health-Systems Pharmacists), 466
ICU (intensive care unit), 489
Icy Hot, 351
IDIS (Iowa Drug Information Service), 266
Ileum and medication absorption, 318
Illinois Council of Health-Systems Pharmacists (ICHP), 466
Ilosone, 159
Ilotycin, 159

Imdur, 159, 334
Imipenem/cilastatin, 38, 342
Imipramine, 160, 161, 343, 478
Immunology, information resources, 268
Immunomodulators, 16, 488
Immunostimulants, 16, 372, 373
Immunosuppression, 16, 39, 43, 478
Imodium, 339, 356
Incubation, 152
Independent pharmacies, 67
Independent practice association (IPA), 487
Inderal, 159, 161, 336, 479
LA, 336
Inderide, 479
India's historical influence, 9
Indinivar and St. John's wort, 370
Indocin, 159, 161, 332, 479
Indomethacin, 159, 332
Infantile paralysis, 14
Infection control, 12, 488. *See also* Aseptic process; Health care worker infection control; Sterile preparation
airborne precautions, 304
American Society of Health-System Pharmacists (ASHP), 294
and antibiotics, 296
biohazard symbol, 302
CDC (Centers for Disease Control and Prevention) recommendation, 294
cleaning, 302
compound admixture infection control, 294
contact precautions, 305
decontamination, 302
droplet precautions, 304
engineering controls, 302–303
goals, 296
hospital isolation, 303–305
Intravenous Nursing Society Standards of Practice, 294
needlestick prevention devices, 303, 305
pharmaceutical contamination, 294–295
quality control, 295
regulated medical waste) handling, 302–303
and respirators, 304
sharps disposal, 303, 305
universal-standard precautions, 297
work place, 302–303
Infections
airborne transmission, 300, 481
colonization, 299
common vehicle transmission, 300
contact transmission, 299
direct-contact transmission, 299
droplet transmission, 299–300, 485

Infections (*Cont.*):
  gram-positive, 12
  and home infusion therapy, 51
  hosts, 299
  indirect-contact transmission, 299
  infectious agent sources, 298
  routes, 299–300
  vector-borne transmission, 300
Infectious disease
  information resource, 268
  medications, 340, 341–342
Infiltration, IV, 50, 488
Influenza, 351
Influenza vaccine, 16
Information technology (IT), 425–426
Infusion (defined), 152
Infusion devices. *See also* Home
    infusion therapy
  CADD pump, 44, 47
  checks of, 50
  elastometric external pump, 45
  equipment management, 49–50
  external pump, nonmechanical,
    45–46
  FDA (Food and Drug
    Administration) requirements,
    49
  free flow potential, 49, 51, 487
  implantable pump, 48, 49
  microinfusion pump, 47
  PCA pump, 41–42, 47, 491
  peristaltic pump, mechanical,
    46–47
  piston pump, mechanical, 47–48
  programming of, 47, 48
  rate controller, nonmechanical, 45
  selection factors, 49
  spring-controlled pump, 46–47
  syringe pump, mechanical, 48
INH, 306, 342
Inhalation therapy, 174
Injectable drug/medication
    administration, 166, 249
Inoculum (defined), 489
Inotropic agents, 477
Insecticides, 171
Insomnia, 352, 373
Institute for Safe Medication
    Practices (ISMP), 271, 446
  drug distribution systems, 277
  high-risk drug identification, 245
Institutional review board (IRB),
    84
Insulin, 13, 16, 335, 337
  glargine, 479
  neutral protamine Hagedorn, 156
  protamine zinc, 156
  zinc suspension, 479
Insurance
  EDI (Electronic Data Interchange),
    92
  and HIPAA implementation, 92
  reimbursement, 453–454

Insurance Reform. *See* HIPAA (Health
    Insurance Portability and
    Accountability Act)
Intal, 344
Intensive care unit (ICU), 489
Intern, pharmacy, 153
Internal medicine, information
    resources, 268
International Bibliographic
    Information on Dietary
    Supplements (IBIDS), 371
*International Pharmaceutical
    Abstracts,* 145
International Pharmaceutical
    Abstracts (IPA), 266
International Pharmacopoeia (WHO),
    13
Internet as resource, 270
Internet pharmacies, 114
Interpersonal skills, 67
Intraconazole, 341
Intravenous (IV). *See* IV topics
Intravenous medications. *See* IV
    medications
Intravenous Nursing Society
    Standards of Practice, 294
Inventory, 489
  computerized control, 401–402
  controlled substances, 87, 401
  CSA (Controlled substances Act)
    of 1970, 87
  and JCAHO (Joint Commission on
    Accreditation of Healthcare
    Organizations), 401
  just-in-time (JIT) strategy, 398
  pharmaceutical management, 394,
    398, 401–402
  restocking, 445
  rotation, 401
  safety, 401
  security, 400–402
  tax-free alcohol, 78, 401
  turnover rate, 402
Investigational drugs, 79
  and FDA, 82, 474
  and formulary system, 474
  handling, 83
  investigational new drug (IND)
    exemption, 82
  labeling, 108
  studies, 82–83
Iodine, 12
Iontophoresis, 152, 489
Iowa Drug Information Service (IDIS),
    266
IPA (independent practice
    association), 487
IPA (International Pharmaceutical
    Abstracts), 266
Ipratropium, 344
Irbesartan, 336
IRB (institutional review board), 84
Iron dextran, 42, 43

ISMP. *See* Institute for Safe
    Medication Practices
Isolation, hospital, 303–305
Isoniazid, 155, 342
Iso-osmotic (defined), 489
Isoptin, 333, 334, 336
Isorbide mononitrate, 334
Isordil, 161, 334, 479
  chewable, packaging, 88
Isosorbide dinitrate, 160, 334
  chewable, packaging, 88
Isosorbide mononitrate, 159
Isotonic (defined), 489
Isotonic/iso-osmotic solutions,
    174–175
IT (information technology), 425–426
IV administration calculation
  flow rate, 198–200
  piggyback infusion, 200–201
IV medications
  administration set, 228, 229
  admixture in-house drug
    distribution, 116
  aseptic process, 116
  and concentration, 227
  containers, 228–229
  and DEHP plasticizer, 228
  drug compatibility, 227
  and drug response, 326
  drug stability, 227
  home infusion therapy, 33–34, 41,
    45
  and infiltration, 50, 488
  intermittent injection, 489
  laminar airflow hoods, 230–234,
    294, 295, 496
  large-volume parenterals (LVPs),
    228
  and liver metabolism, 318
  and parenteral admixtures,
    227–228
  piggyback infusion, 155, 156,
    200–201, 229–230, 234, 492
  and polyvinyl chloride (PVC)
    containers, 228, 229
  and PVC (polyvinyl chloride)
    containers, 228, 229
  and sepsis, 50
  small-volume parenterals (SVPs),
    228
  solution types, 228–229
Jaundice, 489
Jaundice (defined), 152
JCAHO (Joint Commission on
    Accreditation of Healthcare
    Organizations), 76, 271, 489
  accreditation, 94–95, 99–100
  Comprehensive Accreditation
    Manuals, 95, 99
  drug distribution systems, 277
  inventory, 401
  IV admixture recommendations,
    116

and medical equipment/supplies, 32
overview, 94
prescription requirements, 279
and reimbursement, 458
and samples, 113
standards, 95–96
survey process, 96–99
survey results, 99–100
unit-dose dispensing, 405
Web site, 100
Jejunum and medication absorption, 318
Jenner, Edward, 12, 16
Jewish influence (historical), 6–7
JIT (just-in-time) inventory strategy, 398
Joint Commission on Accreditation of Healthcare Organizations. *See* JCAHO
Joint disorder medications, 331–332
Journal of American Pharmacists Association, 145, 271
Journal of Managed Care Pharmacy, 145
Journal of the American Medical Association, 266
Journal of the Philadelphia College of Pharmacy, 145, 271
Just-in-time (JIT) inventory strategy, 398

Kaolin, 355
and pectin, 356
Kaopectate, 339, 356
Kardex, nursing, 116
Kava kava, 371
K-Dur, 337
Keflex, 159, 341, 471
Kefzol, 159
Kenalog, 159
Ketoconazole, 159, 341
Ketoprofen, 332, 350, 351
Key, Nitro-Dur, 177
Kidney function and dosage strength, 245
Kilogram, 155
Klonopin, 159, 161, 342, 343, 478
Klor-Con, 337
Koch, Robert, 16
Konsyl, 354
K-Phos Neutral, 479
Kwell, 159

Labeling. *See also* Packaging; PPIs (patient package inserts)
admixtures, 33–34
ASHP (American Society of Health-System Pharmacists) recommendations, 295
bar codes, 281, 404–405

Dietary Supplement and Health Education Act (DSHEA), 1994, 364
herbals, 364
investigational drugs, 108
legislation, 79
pharmaceutical management, 394, 402–405
by pharmacy technicians, 284–285
and record-keeping, 220–221
requirements, 403–404
Labetalol, 336, 477
Laboratory data interpretation, information resources, 268
Lactobacillus, 355, 356
Lactulose, 339
Lamictal, 342, 479
Laminar airflow hoods, 116
cleaning, 232
contamination risks, 233
parenteral admixture services, 230–231
types, 231
Lamisil, 479
Lamotrigine, 342
Lanoxin, 159, 479
Lansoprazole, 339, 477
Lantus, 337, 479
Lao-tsu, 8
Large intestine and medication absorption, 318
Lasix, 159, 336, 471, 479
Latin. *See* Abbreviations
Law. *See* Legalities
Laxatives, 217, 339, 353–355
contraindicated liquids, 247
Laxative salts, 171
Legalities
American Society for Pharmacy Law, 271
drug-control laws, 76–77
home infusion therapy, 34, 43–44
information resource, 269
legal responsibilities, 254–255
The NABP Survey of Pharmacy Law (2001), 129
outpatient *vs.* hospital pharmacy law, 43–44
quasi-legal standards, 76
Safe Medical Devices Act (SMDA) of 1990, 35
Legend medication. *See* Prescriptions
Lente, 337, 479
Lerukeran, 477
Leucovorin calcium, 478
Leukemia, 152, 489
Levalbuterol, 344
Levaquin, 159
Levigation, 215, 489
Levofloxacin, 159
Levothroid, 159, 338
Levothyroxine, 159, 160, 338

Levoxyl, 338
Lexapro, 343
Licorice, 371
Lidex, 471
Lidocaine, 332, 333
Lidoderm patch, 327
Lifecare Omniflow, 48
Lindane, 159
Lioresal, 161, 479
Liothyroxine, 338
Liotrix, 338
Lipitor, 159, 335
Lipophilic membranes, 176
Liposome (defined), 489
Liquid dosage forms, 166–169
advantages, 166
bromide, 166
buffer systems, 167
compounding principles, 214
disadvantages, 166–167
emulsions, 168–169
gels, 168
hydroalcoholic solvent system, 167
with insoluble matter, 167–169
jellies, 168
o/w & w/o emulsifying agents, 169
pH change, 167
potassium iodide, 166
with soluble matter, 167
suspensions, 167–168
Lisinopril, 159, 160, 161, 336, 479
Lithium, 16, 338
carbonate, 479
Lithobid, 338, 479
Lithostat, 479
Lithotabs, 338, 479
"Lititz Pharmacopoeia" (USA Revolutionary War), 10
Liver
alcoholic disease, 330
impairment and dosage strength, 245
metabolism, 318–319, 329, 330
Lodine, 479
Lollipops, 216
Lomotil, 339, 479
Long-term care facility (LTCF), regulation, 58, 77–78
Long-term care (LTC), 68. *See also* Medicaid; Medicare assisted living, move to, 61
computer use, 61
and consultant pharmacists, 60, 61
facility types, 57–58
and 5 medication "rights," 59, 244–246
hospice provision, 61
income sources, 58–59
nursing, 60, 61
overview, 57
pharmaceutical challenges/future, 60–61

Long-term care (LTC) (*Cont.*):
  and pharmaceutical personnel, 60
  pharmacy providers, 36
  population of, 59–60
  and prescription overload, 60–61
  private payment, 58
  regulation of, 58
  reimbursement, 455–456
  third-party payers, 58–59
Loniten, 337
Look-alike drug names, 161, 437–438,
    446. *See also* Sound-alike drug
    names
Lo/Ovral, 340
Loperamide, 339, 355, 356
Lopid, 159, 335, 439, 479
Lopressor, 159, 336
Lorabid, 479
Loratadine, 158, 345
Lorazepam, 157, 161, 343, 477
Lorcet, 332
Lortab, 332
Losartan, 158, 336
Lotensin, 336, 479
Lotions, 168
    compounding principles, 218
Lotrimin, 159, 341
Lovastatin, 335, 479
Lovenox, 159, 161, 334
Low-Ogestrel-28, 340
Loxitane, 480
Lozenges, 152, 173
LTCF (long-term care facility),
    regulation, 58, 77–78
Ludiomil, 479
Luminal, 342
Luvox, 159, 161
Lyme disease, 38, 300

Maalox, 339, 357
Macrobid, 342
Macrodantin, 342
Macrolides, 340, 341, 480
Magna Carta of pharmacy, 11
Magnesium, 171, 354
    carbonate, 170
    citrate, 354
    hydroxide, 357
    oxide, 357
    salicylate, 351
    sulfate, 442
    trisilicate, 170
Magnesium/aluminum antacids, 339
Mag-Ox, 357
Ma huang, 371
Mail-order pharmacies, 91, 114
Maimon, Moses ben (Maimonides),
    7, 489
Malaria, 13, 300, 490
    antimalarials, 477, 479
Malt soup extract, 354
Maltsupex, 354

Managed care
  and drug therapy, 61
  and HMOs (health maintenance
    organizations), 30
  and home health care, 30–31
  managed care organizations
    (MCOs), 411
  reimbursement, 453–454
Management. *See* Pharmaceutical
    management Al-Mansur
    Hospital, Cairo, 9
Manuals. *See* Policy and procedure
    manuals
MAO (monoamine oxidase)
    inhibitors, 152, 490
Marcaine, 332
Marijuana, 490
MAR (medication administration
    record), 152, 243, 280, 444, 445,
    490
M*A*S*H, 10
Mast cell stabilizing agents, 344
Material safety data sheets (MSDS),
    88–89
Materia Medica (Dioscorides), 5, 10
Matricaria flower (chamomile), 370
Matrix management, 25
Maxair, 344
Maxzide, 336
MCOs (managed care organizations),
    411
MDR (multi-drug resistant) TB, 307
Measles
    rubeola, 300, 304
    vaccine, 16
Measurement conversion
    apothecary system of weights,
      190–192
    metric system, 187–190
Meclizine, 157, 345
MedFlo, 46
Medicaid, 32, 57, 58, 490. *See also*
    Centers for Medicare and
    Medicaid Services (CMS)
    DRGs (diagnosis-related groups),
      485
    federal Conditions of
      Participation, 77
    Medicaid allowable cost (MAC),
      454
    Pharmaceutical Services, 77
    reimbursement, 453–454
    Title XIX, 77
Medical information system (MIS),
    280
Medical practice, contemporary,
    14–15
Medical Products Reporting
    Program, FDA, 140–141
Medical records. *See also* Record-
    keeping
    HIPAA-defined health information,
      93

in hospitals, 22, 23, 24
patient access, 92
PHI (protected health
    information), 93
protection, 92
rights, 101
Medical terms, common, 150–154
Medicare, 29–30, 32, 57, 58, 490. *See
    also* Centers for Medicare and
    Medicaid Services (CMS)
    certification, 31–32
    DRGs (diagnosis-related groups),
      30, 287, 485
    federal Conditions of
      Participation, 77, 95
    and home health services, 31–32
    and JCAHO accreditation, 95
    Pharmaceutical Services, 77
    and reimbursement, 453, 454–455
    Title XVII, 77
Medication administration record
    (MAR), 152, 243, 280, 444, 445,
    490
Medication delivery systems. *See*
    Drug distribution systems
    ATC Profile, AutoMed
      Technologies, 288, 289
    dumbwaiters, 286
    medication dispensing units, 287
    pneumatic tube system, 285–286
    robotics, 286
    ROBOT-Rx, HBOC/McKesson, 289
    transportation courier, 285
    unit-dose picking area, 286
Medication/drug administration,
    117–118. *See also* Prescriptions;
    separate listings of drugs
    absorption factors, 166, 316–318
    administrator and drug orders,
      243–244
    anatomic absorption factors,
      317–318
    collaborative drug therapy
      agreement, 70
    costs, 119. *See also*
      Reimbursement
    and crushing, 250
    diffusion/absorption, 317
    discontinuance, 249–250
    dissolution/absorption, 316–317
    dosage form/absorption, 316
    dosage form verification, 245
    dose verification, 245
    drug identification information
      resources, 267
    drug interaction information
      resources, 267
    drug standards, 19th century, 15
    drug verification, 244–245
    and Durham-Humphrey
      Amendments, 79
    ear preparations, 248
    effervescent tablets, 350

and empty stomach, 317
errors, 122. *See also* Error
    prevention/management
eyedrop/eye ointment, 247
and fatty foods, 317, 328
foreign information resources, 267
general information resources, 268
genetically engineered drugs, 42
herbal interaction potential, 370
high-risk drug identification, 245
history, 51
and immunosuppression, 39
information/literature evaluation,
    267
information resources, 265–270
injectable, 249
internal vs. external, 250–251
and liver metabolism, 318–319,
    329, 330
medication-related problems
    (MRPs), 121, 490
nonapproved use, physician,
    83–84
non-USA information resources,
    267
nose preparations, 248
oral, 246–247
orders. *See* Drug orders
and patient teaching, 251–253
patient verification, 244
physiologic absorption factors,
    317–318
prescription "overload," 61, 66
and prescription processing, 66–67
preservatives, 166
professional responsibilities,
    253–254
profiles, patient, 90, 91, 116, 280,
    282
"5 rights," 59, 244–246
route, 481
route verification, 245
rule of three, 494
safety, 122. *See also* Error
    prevention/management
schedule verification, 245–246
and solubility, 316–317
statistics, USA, 117
stop-order policy example, 471
suppository, 248–249
suspensions, 167–168
technician double-checking, 244
technicians and drug orders,
    243–244
therapeutic drug monitoring
    (TDM), 249–250
topical, 247
transdermal, 248
Medication/drug response. *See also*
    Side effects
additive interactions, 330
and administration route, 325–328
antagonistic interactions, 330

and compliance, patient, 118–119,
    328
drug-disease interaction, 330
and drug distribution, physiologic,
    329
drug-drug interaction, 329
drug-food interaction, 317, 328
enzyme induction/inhibition, 329
and genetics, 330
and IV administration, 326
and medication absorption, 329
and medication elimination, 329
and metabolism, 329, 330
and patient age, 330
and patient variability, 328–330
synergistic interactions, 330
weight, patient, 330
Medication Error Reporting Program,
    447–448
Medication orders. *See* Drug orders
MEDLINE, 266, 270
Medrol, 479
Medroxyprogesterone, 340
    /conjugated estrogens, 340
MedStation Rx System, Pyxis, 288
MedWatch, 80, 81, 140–141, 271, 371
Mefoxin, 159
Mellaril, 159
Menest, 331, 340
Meningitis, 490
Meniscus (defined), 490
Menopause, 372
Menstruation, 372
Menthol, 351, 352
Meperidine, 332
Mercurochrome, 9
Mercury, 9, 11
Meropenen, 342
Merperidine, 158
Merrem IV, 342
Merthiolate, 9
Mesopotamian clay tablets, 8
Metabolism, 152, 320, 329, 330
    liver, 318–319, 329, 330
Metabolite (defined), 490
Metamucil, 339, 354
Metaproterenol, 344
Metformin, 337
Methadone, 332
Methimazole, 338
Methotrexate, 441, 442, 479
Methylcellulose, 354
Methyldopa, 157
Methylprednisolone, 43
Metoclopramide, 42, 160, 339, 479
    hydrochloride, 479
Metolazone, 479
Metoprolol, 159, 336
    extended release, 160
    tartrate, 479
Metric system conversion, 187–192
Metronidazole, 158, 342
Mevacor, 335

Mexiletine, 333
Mexitil, 333
Miacalcin, 331
Micardis, 336
Michigan Pharmacists Association
    (MPA), 466
Miconazole, 341
Microgram, 155
Micro-K, 337
Micronase, 159, 337
Micronor, 340
Midazolam, 343
Military historical influence, 9–10
Milk thistle, 371, 372
Milliequivalent, 490
MI (myocardial infarction), 490
Mineral oil, 339, 354
*Minhaj (Handbook for the Apothecary
    Shop)*, 9
Minipress, 159, 336
Minitran, 334
Minocin, 161, 342, 479
Minocycline, 342
Minoxidil, 337, 479
Miotic, 152
Miotic (defined), 490
MiraLax, 339
Mircette, 340
Mirtazapine, 343
MIS (medical information system),
    280
Misoprostol, 158, 339, 479
Mithradates VI, 8
Mitoxantrone, 442
Mitrolan, 354, 356
Model State Pharmacy Practice Act
    and Model Rules, 468
Moiety (defined), 490
Moissan, Henri, 13
Momentum, 351
Monistat, 341
Monitoring, pharmaceutical, 34
    patient self-monitoring, 91
    therapeutic drug monitoring
        (TDM), 249–250
Monoamine oxidase (MAO)
    inhibitors, 152, 490
Monopril, 336, 479
Morbidity (defined), 490
Morphine, 11, 13, 330, 332, 478
    sulfate, 155, 442
Motrin, 159, 332, 351
Moxifloxacin, 341
MPA (Michigan Pharmacists
    Association), 466
MRPs (medication-related
    problems), 121, 490
MS Contin, 332
MSDS (material safety data sheets),
    88–89
Mucolytic, 152, 490
Mulin, 337
Multidose vials (MDVs), 295

Multiple compressed tablets (MCT), 173
Multiple sclerosis, 43, 490
Mumps vaccine, 16
Muscle relaxants, 478, 479, 480
Mycelex, 159, 341
Mycifradin, 341
Mycin-type antibiotics, contraindicated liquids, 247
Mycostatin, 159, 341
Mydriatic, 152
Mydriatic (defined), 490
Mylanta, 339, 357
Myleran, 477
Mylicon, 159
Myocardial infarction (MI), 490

NABPLEX (North American Pharmacist Licensure Exam), 144
NABP. *See* National Association of Boards of Pharmacy
NACDS (National Association of Chain Drug Stores), 140, 143–144, 271
Nadolol, 158, 336, 338
Nafcillin, 38
NAHC (National Association for Home Care), 29
Nambumetone, 332
Naphazoline, 352
Naprosyn, 159, 332
Naproxen, 332, 350, 351
  sodium, 159
Narcotics, 42
NARD (National Association of Retail Druggists). *See also* National Community Pharmacists Association (NCPA)
Nasalcrom, 344
Nateginide, 337
National Academy of Sciences
  drug efficacy, 363–364
  and medical errors, 404
National Association for Home Care (NAHC), 29
National Association of Boards of Pharmacy (NABP), 140, 271, 466
  and automated pharmacy systems, 299
  Model State Pharmacy Practice Act and Model Rules, 468
  The NABP Survey of Pharmacy Law (2001), 129
  overview, 144
National Association of Chain Drug Stores (NACDS), 140, 143–144, 271
National Association of Retail Druggists (NARD). *See also* National Community Pharmacists Association (NCPA)

National Center for Complementary and Alternative Medicine, 371
National Community Pharmacists Association (NCPA), 140, 141–142, 145
  overview, 142–143
  and reimbursement, 458
National Coordinating Council for Medication Error Reporting and Prevention, 271
National Council on Patient Information and Education (NCPIE) and medication noncompliance, 119
National Drug Code (NDC), 92
National Formulary (NF), 362, 400
National institute for Pharmacist Care Outcomes (NIPCO), 142–143, 458
National Institute of Occupational Safety and Health (NIOSH) and respirators, 304
National Institutes of Health (NIH), 371
National Pharmacy Technician Association (NPTA), 140, 145
Natural products. *See* Herbals
Nausea, 358. *See also* Vertigo
Navane, 479
NCPA. *See* National Community Pharmacists Association
NCPIE (National Council on Patient Information and Education) and medication noncompliance, 119
NDC (National Drug Code), 92
Nebcin, 159, 341
Nedocromil, 344
Needle sticks, 236–237, 301, 303, 305
Nelfinavir, 479
Neoloid, 354
Neomycin, 341
Neosynephrine, 345, 353
Nephritis, 152, 491
Nephrology information resource, 268
Nephron, 491
Nephrotoxicity, 369
Nettle root, 371
Neurologic disorder medications, 340, 342, 343
Neurontin, 159, 342, 479
Neurosonology, 491
Neutra-Phos-K, 479
Nevirapine, 479
Nexium, 339
Niacin, 11, 335
Niaspan, 335
Nicardipine, 446, 479
Nicotine, 11
Nicotine transdermal patches, 178
Nicotinic acid, 11
Nifedipine, 157, 159, 334, 336, 446, 479

NIH (National Institutes of Health), 371
NIOSH (National Institute of Occupational Safety and Health) and respirators, 304
NIPCO (National Institute for Pharmacist Care Outcomes), 142–143, 458
Nitrates, 334
Nitro-Bid, 334
Nitrodisc, 177
Nitro-Dur, 177
Nitrofurantoin, 342
Nitroglycerin, 334, 442
  dosage forms, 177, 326
  packaging, 88
  and polyvinyl chloride (PVC) containers, 228, 229
  systemic effect, 236
Nitropress, 337
Nitrostat, 334
Nizatidine, 157, 339, 357
Nizoral, 159, 341
Nolvadex, 471
Nomogram, 476
Noncompliance, medication, 118–119, 328
Nonprescription medications. *See also* OTC (over-the-counter drugs)
  acid disorder, 356–358
  allergies, 352–353
  analgesics, 350–352
  antacids, 357–358
  colds, 352–353
  constipation, 353–355
  decongestants, 352, 353
  for diarrhea, 35–356
  dosage forms, 350
  information resources, 268
  overview, 349–350
  peptic disorder, 356–358
Nonsteroidal anti-inflammatory drugs (NSAIDs), 331, 350, 351, 478, 479
Norethindrone, 340
  /ethinyl estradiol, 340
Norflex, 442
Norfloxacin, 442
Norgestimate
  /ethinyl estradiol, 340
Norgestrel, 340
  /ethinyl estradiol, 340
Norlutate, 479
Norlutin, 479
Normodyne, 336
Noroxin, 479
Norpace, 333
Norpramin, 478
Nor-QD, 340
North American Pharmacist Licensure Exam (NABPLEX), 144
Nortriptyline, 161, 477

Nortryptiline, 343
Norvasc, 159, 334, 336, 479
Norvir, 479
Nose preparation drug/medication administration, 248
Nosocomial (defined), 491
Nosocomial infection, 243
NovaLog, 337
Novocain, 332
Novolin (7/30, L, N, R), 337
NPH-regular combinations, 337
NPTA (National Pharmacy Technician Association), 140, 145
NSAIDs (nonsteroidal anti-inflammatory drugs), 331, 350, 351, 478, 479
NuLYTELY, 339
Nupercaine, 332
Nuprin, 351
Nuremberg Code, 129
Nursing
    5 medication "rights," 59, 244–246
    home health care, 31, 32
    and home infusion therapy, 34, 43
    and LTC, 60, 61
Nystatin, 159, 341

OBRA 90 (Omnibus Budget Reconciliation Act) of 1990, 90–91
Obstetric medications, 338, 340
Occupational and Safety Act, 88–89, 491
Occupational Safety and Health Administration. *See* OSHA
Ocufen, 479
Ocuflox, 479
Ocular dosage systems, 176–177
Ocusert System, Alza Corporation, 176–177
ODS (Office of Dietary Supplements), 371
Office of Dietary Supplements (ODS), 371
Off-patent products, 322
Ofloxacin, 158
Ointments, 5, 166, 175, 491
    compounding principles, 215
OKT-3, 43
Oleaginous bases, 175
Oleaginous (defined), 491
Omeprazole, 159, 339
Omnibus Budget Reconciliation Act (OBRA) 1990, 90–91
Omnicell Sure-Med, 288
Oncology
    American Cancer Society, 271
    drug safety, 401
    information resources, 269
Oral contraceptives, combined, 340

Oral drug/medication administration, 246–247
Oralosmosis (OROS), 176
Orasone, 344
Oretic, 159, 336
Organizational theory, 25
Organization Web sites, 271
Orinase, 161, 479
Ornade, 161, 479
OROS (oralosmosis), 176
Orphan drugs, 84, 491
Orthoclone, 43
Ortho-Cyclen, 340
Ortho-Novum, 340
Ortho Tri-Cyclen, 340
Orudis KT, 332, 351
OSCAL, 331
OSHA (Occupational Safety and Health Administration), 491
    and air contaminants, 89
    and combustibility, 89
    cytotoxics safe handling, 236
    and flammability, 89
    Guidelines for Cytotoxic (Antineoplastic) Drugs, 89
    HCS (Hazard Communication Standard), 88–89
    MSDS (material safety data sheets), 88–89
    Occupational and Safety Act, 88–89, 491
    PEL (permissible exposure limit), 89
    and reimbursement, 458
    and safety devices, 303
    universal-standard precautions, 297, 300, 495
Osmolality, 227–228
Osteoarthritis medications, 332
Osteomyelitis, 38
Osteoporosis, 491
    medications, 331–332
Ostomy (defined), 491
OTC (over-the-counter) drugs, 108, 491
    acid disorder, 356–358
    allergies, 352–353
    analgesics, 350–352
    antacids, 357–358
    colds, 352–353
    constipation, 353–355
    containers, 88
    and cost containment, 61
    decongestants, 352, 353
    for diarrhea, 35–356
    dosage forms, 350
    efficacy studies, 364
    information resources, 268
    overview, 109–110, 349–350
    and patient medication profiles, 90
    peptic disorder, 356–358
    statistics, USA, 117
Otrivin, 353

Outpatient hospital pharmacies, 114
Ovcon, 340
Over-the-counter drugs. *See* OTC
Overview, 65–66
Ovral, 340
Ovrette, 340
Oxazepam, 343
Oxybutynin, 158
Oxycodone, 332, 480
    with acetaminophen, 480
OxyContin, 332
OxyIR, 332
Oxymetazoline, 157, 352, 353
Oxytocic, 153
Oxytocic (defined), 491

Pacerone, 333
Packaging. *See also* Labeling
    blister packages, 483
    child-resistant containers, 87, 88
    container types, 403
    noncomplying containers, 87–88
    Poison Prevention Packaging Act, 87–88, 493
    prescription-only (legend) drugs, 88
    repackaging, 402–405
Paclitaxel, 479
PACs (political action committees), 142, 143
Pain management, 11, 13, 42, 331–332, 455
    home infusion therapy, 30, 41–42
    PCA (patient-controlled analgesia) pump, 41–42
Palliative, 153
Palliative (defined), 491
Pamelor, 343
Pancreatic enzymes, 480
Pandemic, 12, 491
Pantoprazole, 339
Paracelsus, 11
Paraplatin, 479
Parenteral compounding, 491. *See also* IV topics
    additive, 481
    ampule handling, 234, 235
    compatibility, drug, 227
    containers, 228–229
    and DEHP plasticizer, 228
    handwashing, 233
    heparin locks, 230
    high-efficiency particulate air (HEPA) filter, 230–231, 232, 234
    hypertonicity, 227–228
    hypotonicity, 227–228
    isotonicity, 227
    IV administration set, 228, 229
    IV products, 227–228
    laminar airflow hoods, 230–234, 294, 295, 496

Parenteral compounding services
(*Cont.*):
large-volume parenterals (LVPs),
228
and needles, 234–235, 236–237
osmolality, 227–228
parenteral solution, defined, 153
and particulate matter, 227
and pH, 228
and phlebitis, 227
piggyback infusion, 155, 156,
229–230, 234, 492
and polyvinyl chloride (PVC)
containers, 228, 229
preparation steps, 233–234
product preparation, 230–235
and PVC (polyvinyl chloride)
containers, 228, 229
pyrogens, 227
routes, 226
safety, 235–237
small-volume parenterals (SVPs),
228
solution types, 228–229
and stability, 227, 295
sterility, 226–227, 449–450
and syringes, 234–235
technician role, 237
vial handling, 234
Parlodel, 479
Paroxetine, 159, 343, 479
Pastes, 175
Pathology, 153
humoral pathology theory, 4–5, 6
Patient-controlled analgesia (PCA)
pump, 41–42, 45, 47, 491
Patient medication profiles, 90, 116,
153, 280, 282, 491
and drug distribution systems,
280, 282
medication, 90, 91
Patient package inserts (PPIs), 80,
491
Patient's bill of rights, 100–101, 491
Patient teaching
and age, 251–252
and educational level, 251–252
and learning method, 252
patient profiling/counseling, 91
plan for, 252
process of, 252–253
readiness, 251
Patient variability
additive interactions, 330
age, 330
antagonistic interactions, 330
compliance, 118–119, 328
drug-disease interaction, 330
and drug distribution, 329
drug-drug interaction, 329
drug-food interaction, 317, 328
enzyme induction/inhibition, 329
genetics, 330

and medication absorption, 329
and medication elimination, 329
and metabolism, 329, 330
synergistic interactions, 330
weight, 330
Paxil, 159, 343, 479
CR, 343
PBM (pharmacy benefits
management), 114, 411
PCA (patient-controlled analgesia)
pump, 41–42, 45, 47, 491
PCP (phencyclidine), 491
Pectin, 355
and kaolin, 356
PediaCare, 353
Pediatrics, 168
American Academy of Pediatrics,
271
body surface area (BSA), 196–197
and diarrhea medication, 356
dosage calculation, 196–197
and dosage strength, 245
information resources, 269
Reye's syndrome, 350–351
salicylate side effects, 350–351, 356
scarlet fever, 304
and swallowing, 166
transdermal gels, 215
viral infection, 304
Pegaspargase, 477
Pellet dosage forms, 173
Pelletier, Pierre, 13
PEL (permissible exposure limit),
OSHA, 89
Pelvic inflammatory disease, 38
Penicillamine, 479
Penicillin, 10, 12, 16, 340, 342, 479,
480
contraindicated liquids, 246–247
G, 38, 342
Procaine Penicillin G, 168
Pennsylvania Hospital, 13, 14
Pentazocine, 332
Pentothal, 332
Pentoxifylline, 160
Pen T'sao, 8
Pepcid, 159, 339, 357
PEP (post-exposure prophylaxis),
305–306
Peptic disorder medications,
356–358
Peptic ulcer disease (PUD), 356, 491
Pepto-Bismol, 356
Percocet, 332, 479
Percodan, 479
Perdiem, 354
Pericolace, 471
Peripherally inserted central
catheters (PICC), 34
Peripheral parenteral nutrition
(PPN), 40, 491
Peripheral vascular disease (PVD),
334

Permissible exposure limit (PEL),
OSHA, 89
Perphenazine, 160
Persian historical influence, 9
Personal protective devices, 243
Personal protective equipment
(PPE), 297, 300–301
Pertussis, 153, 492
PESH (Public Employee Safety &
Health Administration),
universal-standard precautions,
297
pH, 153
and compound flavoring, 216
and drug-food interaction, 328
and liquid dosage forms, 167
and medication absorption, 329
and medication solubility, 316–317
Pharmaceutical care, 119–121,
128–129
Pharmaceutical contamination,
294–295
Pharmaceutical management
bar codes, 281, 404–405
computerized inventory control,
401–402
cost analysis, 395, 396
disposal, 394, 406–407
distribution systems, 405–406. *See
also* Drug distribution systems
drug receiving control, 399
drug selection, 395
and drug shortages, 397–398
drug storage, 399–400
and emergency drugs, 406
environmental considerations,
400, 406–407
expiration dates, 406, 487
GPOs (group purchasing
organizations), 397
group purchasing, 396
Guidelines on Managing Drug
Product Shortages, 398
inventory, 394, 398, 401–402
just-in-time (JIT) inventory
strategy, 398
labeling, 394, 402–405
procurement, 394, 395–399
purchase orders, 398–399, 430
purchasing, 396–397
recapture, 394, 406–407
record-keeping, 398–399
repackaging, 394, 402–405
returned medications, 406
safety, 401
security, 400–402
source selection, 395
turnover rate, inventory, 402
vendor relationships, 396
Pharmaceutical manufacturer
distribution, 108
Pharmaceutical Research, 145
Pharmacist scarcity, 123

Pharmacogenetics, 492
Pharmacognosy, 5, 492
Pharmacokinetics, 269, 483, 492
Pharmacopoeias
    and drug standards (19th
        century), 15
    historical, 11–12
    *International Pharmacopoeia
        (1951)*, 13
Pharmacotherapy, 6
Pharmacy automation, 123
Pharmacy benefits management
    (PBM), 114, 411
Pharmacy organization, history. *See
    also* main headings of groups
Pharmacy Technician Certification
    Board (PTCB), 140, 142, 143. *See
    also* CPhTs (certified pharmacy
    technicians)
    communication vehicles, 468
    examination practices, 466–467
    involvement opportunities, 467
    item writers, 467
    overview, 465–466
    and regulation, 468
    Stakeholder Policy Council, 467
    structure, 466
    Web sites, 467
Pharmacy Technician Certification
    Examination (PTCE), 467
Pharmacy Technician Educators
    Council (PTEC), 140, 143
Pharmacy technicians
    and ASHP, 128
    certification, 141
    *Code of Ethics for Pharmacy
        Technicians,* 130
    compounding procedures,
        283–284
    CPhTs (certified pharmacy
        technicians), 142
    dispensing medication, 284–285
    and drug information, 270, 272
    and error prevention/
        management. *See* Error
        prevention/management
    evaluation form sample, 381–382
    future, 468–469
    and medication labeling, 284–285
    *The NABP Survey of Pharmacy Law
        (2001)*, 129
    regulation, 468
    and reimbursement enhancement,
        458
    role, 128–129
    training program accreditation,
        461–464
    training/recognition, 141
Pharmacy Today, 145
Pharyngitis, streptococcal, 304
Phencyclidine (PCP), 491
Phenergan, 159, 345
    expectorant, 471

Phenobarbital, 16, 342, 471
Phenylephrine, 176, 345, 352, 353
Phenylpropanolamine, 158
Phenytoin, 158, 342
Philadelphia College of Pharmacy,
    140
Phillips Milk of Magnesia, 354, 357
PHI (protected health information),
    93
Phlebitis, 50
    and particulate matter, 227
Phlegm, 5, 11
Physiochemical properties, drug, 166
Phytochemistry, 13
PICC (peripherally inserted central
    catheters), 34
Pills, 5
Pilocarpine, 176–177
Pindolol, 479
Pioglitazone, 337
Piperacillin/tazobactam, 342
Pipracil, 342
Pirbuterol, 344
Plasma, 10
Platinol, 479
Plavix, 159, 479
Plendil, 334, 336
Pletal, 479
Pleuronic lecithin organogel (PLO),
    215
Pneumonia, 38, 304
Poisoning, information resource,
    269
Poison Prevention Packaging Act,
    87–88, 493
Policy and procedure manuals
    administrative section, 387
    approval process, 385–386
    clinical section, 388
    composition of, 382–384
    contents, 386–388
    date, 382–383
    distributional section, 387–388
    distribution of, 388–389
    evaluation form sample, 381–382
    example, 384
    format, 382–384
    need for, 379–380
    operational manuals, 386
    and PCs (personal computers),
        389
    problems, 389–390
    signatures, 383
    title, 382
Poliomyelitis, 14
Polio vaccine, 14, 16
Political action committees (PACs),
    142, 143
Polycarbophil, 339, 354, 355
Polyethylene glycol, 339
Polymorphic state (defined), 493
Pontocaine, 332
Port-a-Cath, 38

Post-exposure prophylaxis (PEP),
    305–306
Potassium chloride, 171, 219, 442
Potassium iodide, 166
Povidone-iodine, 233
Powder dosage forms, 170–171
    absorbent, 171
    dispersible, 170
    divided, 170–171
    dusting, 171
    storage, 170–171
PPD (purified protein derivative),
    493
PPE (personal protective
    equipment), 297, 300–301
PPIs (patient package inserts), FDA
    regulations, 80
PPN (peripheral parenteral
    nutrition), 40, 491
PPO (preferred provider
    organization), 493
PPS (Prospective Payment System),
    31, 493
Practice standards, ASHP, 93
Prandin, 337, 477
Pravachol, 335, 479
Pravastatin, 335
Prayer of Maimonides, 7
Prazosin, 159, 336
Precose, 337
Prednisolone, 479
    methylprednisolone, 43
Prednisone, 158, 344, 479
Preferred provider organization
    (PPO), 493
Pregnancy/breastfeeding
    information resource, 269
    vomiting, 42
Premarin, 331, 340, 479
Premphase, 340
Prempro, 340
Preparation types, 182
Prescription interpretation,
    181–184
Prescriptions, 106. *See also* Drug
    orders; Medication/drug
    administration; separate drug
    listings
    and drug orders, 112–113
    information on, 110–111, 161
    "overload," 61, 66
    overview, 110
    processing, 66–67
    security, 401
    types, 112
Prevacid, 339, 479
Prilosec, 159, 161, 339, 479
Primatene Mist, 344
Primaxin, 38, 342
Principen, 342
Principles, pharmaceutical care,
    120–121
Prinivil, 159, 336, 479

Privacy
  health information, 92
  professional pharmaceutical
    requirements, 93
Procainamide, 159, 333
Procainamide sustained release, 159
Procaine, 332
Procaine Penicillin G, 168
Procanbid, 333, 479
Procan SR, 159, 479
Procardia, 159
  XL, 334, 336
Procedures. *See* Policy and
  procedure manuals
Prochlorperazine, 158, 327–328, 478
Product line management, 25
Professional drug administration
  responsibilities, 253–254
Professional organizations. *See also*
  main headings for individual
  groups
  and drug quality, 140–141
  and education, 140
  history, 139–141
  publications, 145
Progestational drugs, PPIs (patient
  package inserts), 80
Progesterone, 340
Progestins, 340, 477, 479
Promethazine, 159, 161, 345, 478
Prometrium, 340
Pronestyl, 159, 333
  SR, 250
Prontonix, 339
Prontosil, 12, 16
Propafenone, 333
Propofol, 332
Proportion calculation, 185–187
Propoxyphene, 332
Propranolol, 159, 336, 479
Propulsid, 159, 479
Propylhexedrine, 352
Propylthiouracil, 338
Propyl-Thyracil, 338
Proscar, 479
Prospective drug review, 90
Prospective Payment System (PPS),
  31, 493
Prostaglandins, 478, 479
Prostatic hypertrophy, benign, 352,
  353, 373
Protected health information (PHI),
  93
Proton pump inhibitors, 339, 477
Proventil, 160, 344, 479
Provera, 340, 479
Provider 6000 multichannel pump,
  47
Providone-iodine, 43
"Provision of Medication Information
  by Pharmacists" (ASHP), 260
Prozac, 160, 161, 343, 479
Pseudoephedrine, 157, 345, 352, 353

oral form, 352
Psychiatry, 9, 11
  medications, 340, 343
  psychiatric care, historical
    development, 13–14
Psychotropics, 61, 455
Psyllium, 339, 354
PTCB. *See* Pharmacy Technician
  Certification Board
PTCE (Pharmacy Technician
  Certification Examination), 467
PTEC (Pharmacy Technician
  Educators Council), 140, 143
Public Employee Safety & Health
  Administration (PESH),
  universal-standard precautions,
  297
PUD (peptic ulcer disease), 356, 491
Pure Food Act, 1906, 361, 362–363
Purge, 354
Purified protein derivative (PPD),
  493
Purple coneflower, 373
PVD (peripheral vascular disease),
  334
Pyrogens
  and compounding, 219
  and parenteral admixtures, 227
Pyro-Test, 219
Pyxis MedStation Rx System, 288

Q-Test, 219
Quakers, 13
Quality control, 295
Quasi-legal standards, 76
Quinaglute, 333
Quinamm, 479
Quinapril, 336
Quinidex, 333
Quinidine, 161, 333, 471, 479
Quinine, 13, 161, 479

Rabeprazole, 339
Radiation therapy, 243
Radiopaque suspensions/ emulsions,
  168, 169
Rafamate, 480
Raloxifene, 331
Ramipril, 336
Ranitidine, 160, 339, 357
Ratio calculation, 185
Raudixin, 16
Read-alike drug names, 161
ReadyMED, 46
Recalls, drug, 80–81
Record-keeping. *See also* Medical
  records
  drug repackaging, 81
  extemporaneous compounding,
    220–221
  home infusion therapy, 34

labeling, products, 220–221
master formula record, 221
pharmaceutical management,
  398–399
Red Book, Drug Topics, 486
Reglan, 160, 339
Regroton, 479
Regulated medical waste handling,
  302–303
Regulation. *See also* OBRA 90
  (Omnibus Budget Reconciliation
  Act) of 1990; OSHA
  (Occupational Safety and Health
  Administration)
  and alcohol, tax-free/taxable,
    78–79
  botanicals, 364–365
  Bureau of Alcohol, Tobacco and
    Firearms (ATF), Department of
    the Treasury, 78–79
  Bureau of Chemistry, 363
  and CFR, Title 27 (tax-free
    alcohol), 78
  and counseling, patient, 90–91
  DEA, 76
  Department of Agriculture
    Chemistry Division, 363
  Dietary Supplement and Health
    Education Act (DSHEA), 1994,
    361
  dietary supplements, 364–365
  Drug Amendments of 1962, 363
  drugs, 362–364
  and effectiveness, 363–364
  FDA (Food and Drug
    Administration), 76
  FDA (Food and Drug
    Administration) creation, 363,
    397
  federal, 78–80
  Food, Drug, and Insecticide
    Administration, 363
  Food, Drug and Cosmetic Act, 363,
    487
  herbals, 364–365
  HIPAA (Health Insurance
    Portability and Accountability
    Act), 91–93
  history, 362–364
  Kefauver-Harris Amendments,
    363
  mail-order pharmacies, 91
  OTC/prescription distinction, 363
  and patient medication profiles,
    90, 91
  prescription/OTC distinction, 363
  and prospective drug review, 90
  Pure Food Act, 1906, 361, 362–363
  quasi-legal standards, 76
  state board of pharmacy, 77
  sulfanilamide elixir tragedy (1937),
    363
  thalidomide, 363

Reimbursement
  acute care, 456–457
  average wholesale price (AWP), 454, 482
  closed-formulary contracts, 454
  cognitive services, 457–458
  for community pharmacy services, 453–454
  long-term care (LTC), 455–456
  Medicaid allowable cost (MAC), 454
  Medicare, 453, 454–455
  parenteral ambulatory pharmacy services, 454–455
  and pharmacy technicians, 458
  prescription insurance coverage, 454
  retrospective-payer system, 458
  wholesaler acquisition cost, 454
Relafen, 332
Remeron, 343
Reminyl, 477, 480
Renaissance influence (historical), 8, 11
Renal impairment, 357, 363
Repackaging, 81
  pharmaceutical management, 394, 402–405
Repackaging, drugs, record-keeping, 81
Repaglinide, 337
Resident, pharmacy, 153
Respiratory disorder medications, 343, 344, 345
Restoril, 343
Retail pharmacy types, 113–114
Retrovir, 160, 341, 479, 480
Reye's syndrome, 350–351
Rhythmol, 333
Ribavirin, 341
Rice, Charles, 15
Ridaura, 478
Rifadin, 342
Rifampin, 342, 480
Right to refuse treatment, 101
Rimantadine, 480
Ringer's solution, 42
Riopan, 357
Risendronate, 331
Ritonavir, 480
RMW (regulated medical waste) handling, 302–303
Roberts, Jonathan (first US hospital pharmacist), 13
Robinul, 160, 480
Robiquet, Pierre, 13
Robitussin, 160, 353, 471
Robotics, 494
  drug distribution systems, 288
  medication delivery systems, 286
Rocephin, 38, 160, 341
Rofecoxib, 332

Rolaids, 339
Roman influence (historical), 6
Roman numeral values, 184
Roosevelt, President Franklin, 14
Rosiglitazone, 337
Routes, 183. *See also* main IV topics
  abbreviations, 183, 326–328
  of administration, 481
  biopharmaceutics, 315–316
  buccal, 173, 326, 483
  determination of, 316
  epidural, 41, 45, 487
  extravascular barriers, 316
  of herbals, 368
  infections, 299–300
  inhalation, 174, 327
  injection, 41
  intra-arterial (IA), 226, 326
  intracardiac (IC) route, 226
  intradermal (ID), 152, 226, 489
  intramuscular (IM), 41, 45, 152, 168, 226, 327
  intrasynovial, 45, 489
  intrathecal (IT), 41, 45, 152, 226, 489
  nasal, 248, 328
  ophthalmic/otic, 247, 328
  oral, 246–247, 326
  patches, 41, 61, 247
  percutaneous, 491
  rectal, 327–328. *See also* Suppositories
  subcutaneous (SC), 41, 45, 226, 327
  sublingual, 173, 318, 326
  topical, 247, 327, 351–352
  transdermal, 41, 61, 177–178, 248, 318, 327
  translingual, 326
  vaginal, 217, 328
Rubella vaccine, 16
Rubeola/measles, 300, 304
Rufen, 160
Rules and regulations. *See* Regulation
Rush, Benjamin, 13–14

Sabin, Albert, 14
Safe Medical Devices Act (SMDA) of 1990, 35
Safety
  bloodborne disease transmission, 243
  medication, 122
  and medications, 235–236
  needle sticks, 236–237, 301, 303, 305
  and nosocomial infection, 243
  parenteral admixture services, 235–237
Salicin, 12. *See also* Aspirin
Salicylates, 350–351, 356

Salicylic acid, 171, 215
Saline, 339
Salk, Jonas, 14
Salmeterol, 344
Salmonellosis, 300
Salt, 11
  salt-restricted diets, 350
Salvarsan, 16
Samples, drug, 113
Sarafem, 439, 480
Saw palmetto, 373
Saw palmetto fruit, 370
Schedules, drug, 84–85, 106–108
Scheele, Karl, 12
Scopolamine, 177–178
Screening, community, 70
Searle, Nitrodisc, 177
Secretin, 215
Security, 400–402
Sedatives, 477, 480
Seldane, 471
Self-care, patient, 109
  medication, 118
Senior citizens. *See* Geriatrics
Senna, 339, 354
  leaves, 364
Senokot, 339, 354, 471
Sepsis, 38, 50, 494. *See also* Infection
Septic shock, 294
Septra, 160, 342
Serax, 343
Serevent, 344
Serophene, 439, 480
Seroquel, 480
Serotonin reuptake inhibitors, 343
Sertraline, 160, 343
Serturner, Frederick, 11
Serum therapy, 12, 16. *See also* Vaccines
Serzone, 480
Shingles/*Herpes zoster*, 39, 304, 307
Shortages, drug, 397–398
Side effects, 122. *See also* Adverse drug reactions (ADRs)
  antacids, 357
  defined, 494
  H2 (histamine receptor) antagonists, 358
  nonprescription medications, 351, 352
  NSAIDs (nonsteroidal anti-inflammatory drugs), 351
  OTC antihistamines, 353
  salicylates, 350–351, 356
Sidekick, 47
Simethicone, 159
Simvastatin, 160, 335
Sina, Ibn (Avicenna), 9
Slo-bid, 439
Slow-K, 337
Small intestine and medication absorption, 317–318
Smallpox vaccine, 12, 16

SMDA (Safe Medical Devices ACT) of 1990, 35
Smoking cessation, 69, 178
Soaps, 169
Social Security Act, 490
Sodium bicarbonate, 170, 171, 339, 357
  and alginic acid, 357
Sodium biphosphate, 171
Sodium chloride, 219
Sodium lauryl sulfate, 169
Sodium nitroprusside, 337, 442
Sodium oleate, 169
Sodium phosphate, 354
Sodium salt form, 167
Sodium sulfate, 171
Solid dosage forms
  capsules, 171
  compounding principles, 214
  granules, 171
  powders, 170–171
  tablets, 171–173, 174. See also Tablets
Solu-Medrol, 43
Solution, 166
Solvation (defined), 494
Sonata, 343
Sorbitan esters, synthetic nonionic, 169
Sorbitrate, 160
Soriatane, 480
Sotalol, 333
Sound-alike drug names, 161, 439, 477–480
Special instructions, 183
Spiranolactone, 336
Sporanox, 341
St. John's wort, 370, 373
  and digoxin, 370
  and indinivar, 370
  and warfarin, 370
Stability
  information resources, 267
  IV/parenteral, 227, 295
Stadol, 160
Staphylococcus, 494
Starlix, 337
STAT drug orders, 242
Statutes
  Comprehensive Drug Abuse and Prevention Control Act, 84, 106–108, 484
  Controlled Substances Act (CSA), 84–85, 87, 106–108, 484
  Dietary Supplement and Health Education Act (DSHEA), 361, 364, 371
  Durham-Humphrey Amendments, 79
  Federal Hazardous Substances Act, 87–88
  Food, Drug, and Cosmetic Act, 76, 79, 363, 487

Health Insurance Portability and Accountability Act (HIPAA), 91–93
  OBRA 90 (Omnibus Budget Reconciliation Act) of 1990, 90–91
  Occupational and Safety Act, 88–89, 491
  Orphan Drug Act, 84
  and OSHA, 88–89
  Poison Prevention Packaging Act, 87–88, 493
  Pure Food Act, 1906, 361, 362–363
  Safe Medical Devices Act (SMDA) of 1990, 35
  Social Security Act, 490
Stavudine, 341
Sterile preparation, 494. See also Aseptic process; Infection control
  and AIDS, 39
  and blood, 39
  compounding principles, 219–220
  heat sterilization, 219–220
  and home infusion therapy, 33
  parenteral compounding, 226–227, 449–450
Steroids, 43, 344
  corticosteroids, 478, 479, 480
Stomach and medication absorption, 317
Stop-order policy example, 471
Storage. See also Inventory
  and pharmaceutical management, 399–400
  powdered forms, 170–171
Streptase, 334
Streptococcal pharyngitis, 304
Streptococci, hemolytic, 12
Streptokinase, 334
Streptomycin, 14–15, 16, 341
Styptic, 153, 494
Sucralfate, 158, 339
Sucrets, 353
Sudafed, 345, 353, 471
Sudorifics, 5, 494
Sulfadiazine, 480
Sulfa drugs, 12
Sulfamethoxazole, 157, 160
Sulfanilamide elixir tragedy (1937), 363
Sulfasalazine, 480
Sulfonamides, 10, 478, 480
Sulfur, 11
  precipitated, 215
Sumycin, 342
Suppositories, 175
  compounding principles, 217
Suppository drug/medication administration, 248–249
Sure-Med, Omnicell, 288
Surfactants, 494
Surgery, 243, 249

supply services, 68
surgical care, historical development, 14, 15
Suspending agents, 494
Suspensions, 167–168, 214–215
Sustained-action tablets, 173, 174, 250
Swedish historical influence, 12
Symbols, apothecary, 157
Symmetrel, 341
Sympathomimetic agents, 477, 478, 479
Synalar, 471
Syncope, 154, 494
Synthetics, 16
Synthroid, 160, 338
Syphilis, 12

Tablets, 166
  buccal tablets, 173
  compression methods, 172
  delayed-action, 173, 174
  disintegration in gastrointestinal (GI) fluid, 316
  dispensing tablets (DT), 172
  effervescent, 350
  enteric-coated tablets (ECT), 173, 250, 486
  film-coated tablets (FCT), 173
  hypodermic tablets (HT), 172
  lozenges, 152, 173
  multiple compressed tablets (MCT), 173
  pellets, 173
  standard compressed tablets (CT), 172
  sublingual or buccal tablets (ST), 173
  sugar-coated tablets (SCT), 173
  sustained-action, 173, 174, 250
  tablet triturates (TT), 172
Tachycardia, 154, 333, 495
Tagamet, 160, 339, 357
Talwin, 332
Tambocor, 333
"Tao te Ching" (The Way), 8
Tapazole, 338
Tare (weighing), 218
Tartaric acid, 171
Task Force for Compliance, 119
Taxol, 479
Tazicef, 160
Tazidime, 160
Tazobactam/piperacillin, 342
TDM (therapeutic drug monitoring), 249–250
Teaching. See Patient teaching
Technical Assistance Bulletin on the Evaluation of Drugs for Formularies, 395
Technician program accreditation, 461–464

Technicians. *See* Pharmacy technicians
Tegretol, 160, 342, 480
Telmisartan, 336
Temazepam, 343, 480
Tempra, 351
Tenormin, 160, 336
Tequin, 341, 480
Terazosin, 336
   hydrochloride, 480
Terbinafine, 480
Terbutaline, 161, 344
   sulfate, 158
Terfenadine, 480
Terminology
   abbreviations, 154–156, 182–184, 188
   apothecary symbols, 157
   medical terms, common, 150–154
   pharmacy, 154–156
   prefixes/suffixes, 150, 188
Testing
   community, 70
   Pyro-Test, 219
   Q-Test, 219
Testosterone, 16
Tetanus, 12
   vaccine, 16
Tetracaine, 332, 442
Tetracycline, 157, 176, 340, 342, 471
Tetrahydrozoline, 352
Thalidomide, 363
Theo-Dur, 160
Theophrastus, 5, 495
Theophylline sustained release, 160
Therapeutic advances, recent centuries, 15–16
Therapeutic drug monitoring (TDM), 249–250
Therapeutic Mineral Ice, 351
Therapeutics/pharmacology, pharmaceutical information resources, 269
Thiopental, 332
Thioridazine, 159
Thorazine, 16, 160
Thrombosis, 43
   thrombi, 333
   thrombolytic agents, 334
   thrombophlebitis, 50, 495
Thyroid
   Armour Thyroid, 338
   hyperthyroidism, 337, 342
   hypothyroidism, 337
   medications, 117, 335, 337–338
   thyroid USP, 338
Thyrolar, 338
Thyroxine, 16
Tiazac, 333, 334, 336
Ticar, 342
Ticarcillin, 342
Ticlid, 480
Tigan, 471

Tikosyn, 333
Tilade, 344
Time keeping, 184
Timolol, 161, 477
Tinctures, 6, 495
Tobramycin, 38, 159, 160, 341
Tobrex, 160
Tocainide, 333
Tocolytic therapy, 43
Today's Technician, 145
Tofranil, 160, 343
Tolazamide, 161, 480
Tolbutamide, 161, 480
Topical drug/medication administration, 247, 327, 351–352
Toprol XL, 160, 336
Torsemide, 480
Total parenteral nutrition (TPN). *See also* Enteral nutrition (EN); TPN (total parenteral nutrition)
Toxicity, 495
   cytotoxicity, 39, 42, 236, 485
   cytotoxics safe handling, 236
   Guidelines for Cytotoxic (Antineoplastic) Drugs, 89
   nephrotoxicity, 369
Toxicology information resource, 269
t-PA, 157
TPN (total parenteral nutrition), 30, 38, 494. *See also* Enteral nutrition (EN)
   and free flow, 49, 51, 487
   overview, 39
   parenteral solution, 153
   PPN (peripheral parenteral nutrition), 40, 491
Tracheotomy (defined), 495
Tramadol, 160, 332
Trandate, 336
Tranquilizers, 154, 456
Transdermal drug/medication administration, 177–178, 248, 331
Transderm-Nitro, 176
Transderm-Scop, 177–178
Transplant patients, 43
Trazodone, 158, 343
Treatment, in hospitals, 22, 23
Tremors, 352
Trental, 160
Triamcinolone, 159, 344, 442
Triaminic, 353
Triamterene, 158, 336
Triazolam, 159, 343
Tricor, 335
Triethanolamine stearate, 169
Trifluoperazine, 480
Triglycerides, 334
Trihexyphenidyl, 157, 480
Trilafon, 160
Trimethoprim /sulfamethoxazole, 342

sulfate, 157, 160
Trimox, 161, 342, 480
Triprolidine, 157
Troches, 5, 216
Trolamine salicylate, 351, 352
Trovafloxacin, 160
Trovan, 160
TST (tuberculin skin test), 306
Tubercle bacillus, 15
Tuberculosis (TB), 14–15, 38, 39
   and contagion, 306
   infection *vs.* disease, 306
   INH prophylactic treatment, 306
   medications, 480
   multi-drug resistant (MDR) TB, 307
   Mycobacterium tuberculosis, 300, 306
   purified protein derivative (PPD), 493
   tuberculin skin test (TST), 306
Tums, 331, 339
Tylenol, 160, 332, 351
   elixir, 185
   w/codeine, 332
Tylox, 332
Typhus vaccine, 16

Ultram, 160, 332, 480
Ultrase, 480
Unasyn, 38, 342
Unit-dose in-house drug distribution, 115–116, 250, 277–278, 285, 286
Universal-standard precautions, 297, 300, 495
Urinary tract infection, 38
Urination decrease, 353
Urokinase, 43, 334
Uro-Mag, 357
Urticaria, 154
U.S. Pharmacopoeia (USP), 271, 362
   first, 15
   herbal monographs, 370–371
   sterile preparation guidelines, 44
   storage considerations, 400
U.S. Sanitary Commission (Civil War), 10
USP-ISMP (Institute for Safe Medication Practices), 446
   Medication Error Reporting Program, 447–448
USP-NF, 362, 370, 400
USP (U.S. Pharmacopoeia), 271, 362
   first, 15
   sterile preparation guidelines, 44
   storage considerations, 400

Vaccination (defined), 495
Vaccines, 12, 14, 16, 154, 299, 303
Vaginal anti-infectives, 217
Valacyclovir, 341
Valdecoxib, 332

Valerian, 370, 373
Valium, 16, 343
Valproic acid, 158, 342
Valsartan, 336
Valtrex, 341
Vancenase, 344, 480
Vanceril, 160, 344, 480
Vancomycin, 38
Vantin, 341
Variability. *See* Patient variability
Varicella/chicken pox, 300, 304, 351
Vasoconstriction, 154
Vasodilator agents, 16, 154, 333, 337, 477, 479, 495
Vasosulf, 161, 480
Vasotec, 160, 336, 471
Vatronol, 345
Velafaxine, 343
Velosef, 161, 480
Velosulin, 337
Venlafaxine, 158
Ventolin, 160, 344, 477
VePesid, 480
Verapamil, 158, 159, 333, 334, 336
Verelan, 333, 334, 336
Verifuse ambulatory pump, 47
Versed, 343, 480
Vertigo, 154, 352, 356, 358
Veterans Affairs system, 412
Veterinary medicine
    compounding, 215, 216
    information resource, 269
Vfend, 341
VIACTIV, 331
Vial handling, 234, 295
    multidose vials (MDVs)
    contamination, 295
Vibramycin, 160, 342
Vicks Sinex, 353
Vicodin, 161, 332
Vidarabine, 442
Videx, 341

Vinblastine, 446
Vincristine, 446
Viral disease medications, 340, 341–342
Virazole, 341
Viscosity, 154
Vision blurred, 353
Vistaril, 160, 343, 480
Vitamins, 169
    vitamin B complex, 11, 478
    vitamin D, 331, 477
Vivelle, 331, 340
Volatile drugs, 170
Volmax, 478
Voltaren, 332
Volumetric check, 495
Vomiting, 42, 352, 358
Voriconazole, 341
Vytone, 478

Waksman, Selman, 14–15
WalkMed pump, 47
Warfarin, 158, 334, 356
    and St. Johns wort, 370
Web site, information resources, 271–272
Weight-based dosage calculation, 194–196
Welchol, 335
Wellbutrin, 343
Wellness promotion, as hospital
    function, 22, 23
Western historical influences, 10–13
West Nile encephalitis, 300
Wholesaler distribution, 108–109
Whooping cough vaccine, 16
WHO (World Health Organization), 13, 271
Wiley, Harvey W. (Bureau of Chemistry), 363
Withering, William, 12, 362

Wool fat, 169
World Health Organization (WHO), 13, 271
World Medical Association, 129

Xanax, 160, 161, 343, 480
Xeloda, 480
Xenical, 480
Xopenex, 344
Xydis technology, 480
Xylocaine, 332, 333
Xylometazoline, 352, 353

Zaleplon, 343
Zantac, 160, 161, 339, 357, 480
Zebeta, 478, 480
Zerit, 341
Zestril, 160, 336
Ziac, 336
Zidovudine, 160, 341, 442
Zinacef, 480
Zinc
    sulfate, 442
    undecylenate, 171
Zithromax, 160, 341, 480
Zocor, 160, 335, 478, 480
Zofran, 480
Zoloft, 160, 343, 480
Zolpidem, 343
Zonegran, 342
Zonisamide, 342
Zostrix, 351
Zosyn, 342, 480
Zovirax, 160, 341, 480
Z-Pack, 341
Zyban, 343
Zyloprim, 160
Zyprexa, 439, 480
Zyrtec, 345, 480
Zyvox, 480